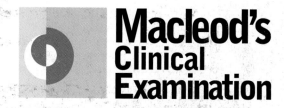

Macleod's
Clinical
Examination

John Macleod
(1915–2006)

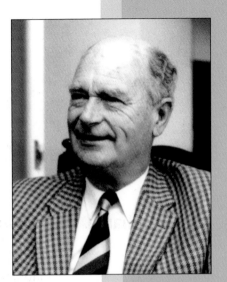

John Macleod was appointed consultant physician at the Western General Hospital, Edinburgh, in 1950. He had major interests in rheumatology and medical education. Medical students who attended his clinical teaching sessions remember him as an inspirational teacher with the ability to present complex problems with great clarity. He was invariably courteous to his patients and students alike. He had an uncanny knack of involving all students equally in clinical discussions and used praise rather than criticism. He paid great attention to the value of history taking and, from this, expected students to identify what particular aspects of the physical examination should help to narrow the diagnostic options.

His consultant colleagues at the Western welcomed the opportunity of contributing when he suggested writing a textbook on clinical examination. The book was first published in 1964 and John Macleod edited seven editions. With characteristic modesty he was very embarrassed when the 8th edition was renamed *Macleod's Clinical Examination*. This, however, was a small way of recognizing his enormous contribution to medical education.

He possessed the essential quality of a successful editor — the skill of changing disparate contributions from individual contributors into a uniform style and format without causing offence; everybody accepted his authority. He avoided being dogmatic or condescending. He was generous in teaching others his editorial skills and these attributes were recognized when he was invited to edit *Davidson's Principles and Practice of Medicine*.

For Elsevier:

Commissioning Editor: Laurence Hunter

Development Editor: Helen Leng

Project Manager: Kerrie-Anne McKinlay

Designer: Stewart Larking

Illustration Manager: Gillian Richards

Illustrators: Robert Britton; Oxford Illustrators

Macleod's

Clinical Examination

Edited by

Graham Douglas BSc(Hons) MBChB FRCPE
Consultant Physician
Aberdeen Royal Infirmary
Honorary Reader in Medicine
University of Aberdeen

Fiona Nicol BSc(Hons) MBBS FRCGP FRCPE
GP Principal and Trainer
Stockbridge Health Centre, Edinburgh
Honorary Clinical Senior Lecturer
University of Edinburgh

Colin Robertson BA(Hons) MBChB FRCPE FRCS Ed
Consultant and Honorary Professor in Emergency Medicine
Royal Infirmary of Edinburgh
University of Edinburgh

Illustrated by
Robert Britton
Oxford Illustrators

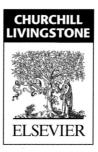

CHURCHILL LIVINGSTONE

ELSEVIER

Edinburgh London New York Oxford Philadelphia St Louis Sydney Toronto 2009

12th Edition

CHURCHILL LIVINGSTONE
ELSEVIER

First edition 1964
Second edition 1967
Third edition 1973
Fourth edition 1976
Fifth edition 1979
Sixth edition 1983
Seventh edition 1986
Eighth edition 1990
Ninth edition 1995
Tenth edition 2000
Eleventh edition 2005
Twelfth edition 2009

ISBN 9780443068485
 Reprinted 2010, 2011
International ISBN 9780443068454
 Reprinted 2009, 2010

British Library Cataloguing in Publication Data
A catalogue record for this book is available from the British Library

Library of Congress Cataloging in Publication Data
A catalog record for this book is available from the Library of Congress

Notice
Knowledge and best practice in this field are constantly changing. As new research and experience broaden our knowledge, changes in practice, treatment and drug therapy may become necessary or appropriate. Readers are advised to check the most current information provided (i) on procedures featured or (ii) by the manufacturer of each product to be administered, to verify the recommended dose or formula, the method and duration of administration, and contraindications. It is the responsibility of the practitioner, relying on their own experience and knowledge of the patient, to make diagnoses, to determine dosages and the best treatment for each individual patient, and to take all appropriate safety precautions. To the fullest extent of the law, neither the publisher nor the editors assumes any liability for any injury and/or damage to persons or property arising out of or related to any use of the material contained in this book.

The Publisher

Printed in China

Preface

The skills of history taking and physical examination are central to the practice of clinical medicine. This book describes these and is intended primarily for medical undergraduates who often have patient contact from their first days of study. It should also be of value to primary care and postgraduate hospital doctors, particularly those studying for higher clinical examinations or returning to a clinical environment after a period of research or specialized study. Nurse practitioners and other paramedical staff are involved increasingly in medical assessment and we hope that the book will provide a reference for them.

Much clinical teaching occurs in primary care as well as in hospital. This is reflected in the editorial team and contributors. Because English has no epicene third person pronoun, we have used the male pronoun in the book to aid clarity. Please be assured that this does not reflect any prejudice on our part.

This edition has three sections: Section 1 details the principles of history taking and general examination; Section 2 covers symptoms and signs in individual systems; and Section 3 reviews specific situations. The text has been extensively edited to improve consistency and there are several new chapters, including The skin, hair and nails, The endocrine system, The visual system, Assessment for sedation and anaesthesia, and Confirming death. The number of Objective Structured Clinical Examination (OSCE) boxes has been increased to 52 to assist with revision, and the key points at the end of each chapter distil clinical experience.

In response to feedback from readers, this edition contains more figures and diagrams, while the number of photographs has increased to 336. Many students find reading text laborious and pictorial information is often assimilated more easily. Clinical acumen is also, at least in part, based on pattern recognition. Line drawings illustrate surface anatomy and techniques of examination, and photographs show normal and abnormal clinical appearances.

The evidence base for much of clinical examination is scanty. We have tried to exclude techniques of little clinical value and excessively rare features. While recognizing the merits of anecdote and individual clinical experience, rigorous evaluation of many clinical symptoms and signs is lacking. This offers challenges and opportunities. It is possible to open this book at almost any page and find a topic which is crying out for evidence-based analysis. We hope that one function of the book will be to stimulate this enquiry and would encourage these responses and incorporate them in future editions.

This 12th edition of *Macleod's Clinical Examination* — full text and illustrations — is available in an online version, as part of Elsevier's 'Student Consult' electronic library. It continues to be closely integrated with *Davidson's Principles and Practice of Medicine,* and is best read in conjunction with that text.

The Editors

Acknowledgements

The editors are very grateful to all of the contributors and editors of previous editions; in particular, we owe an immeasurable debt to Dr John Munro for his teaching and wisdom.

We greatly appreciate the constructive suggestions and help that we have received from past and present students, colleagues and focus groups in the design and content of the book. We wish to thank the many individuals who have provided advice and support, particularly Jackie Fiddes for designing the manikins and for her computer skills, and Drs Tom Ford, Anni Dougherty and Laura Robertson for their helpful suggestions.

We particularly wish to thank Steven Hill of the Department of Medical Illustration, University of Aberdeen, and Dr Alan Denison of the Department of Radiology and Dr Graeme Currie of the Chest Clinic, both at Aberdeen Royal Infirmary, for providing clinical photographs.

Finally we wish to thank Helen Leng, development editor, Wendy Lee, copy editor, and Laurence Hunter, commissioning editor, at Elsevier for their tolerance, support and encouragement.

J.G.D.
F.N.
C.E.R.

Picture and table credits

We are grateful to the following individuals and organizations for permission to reproduce the figures and tables listed below:

Chapter 3

Figs 3.27A–D Forbes CD, Jackson WF. Color Atlas of Clinical Medicine. 3rd edn. Edinburgh: Mosby; 2003.

Chapter 6

Figs 6.7 and 6.11 Haslett C, Chilvers ER, Boon NA, Colledge NR, eds. Davidson's Principles and Practice of Medicine. 19th edn. Edinburgh: Churchill Livingstone; 2002. Figs 6.10, 6.20A–D and 6.44A Forbes CD, Jackson WF. Color Atlas of Clinical Medicine. 3rd edn. Edinburgh: Mosby; 2003.

Chapter 9

Fig. 9.12 Pitkin J, Peattie AB, Magowan BA. Obstetrics and Gynaecology: An Illustrated Colour Text. Edinburgh: Churchill Livingstone; 2003. Figs 9.13A&B Haslett C, Chilvers ER, Boon NA, Colledge NR, eds. Davidson's Principles and Practice of Medicine. 19th edn. Edinburgh: Churchill Livingstone; 2002.

Chapter 11

Fig. 11.17 Epstein O, Perkin GD, de Bono DP, Cookson J. Clinical Examination. 2nd edn. London: Mosby; 1997.

Chapter 12

Figs 12.14B&C Forbes CD, Jackson WF. Color Atlas of Clinical Medicine. 3rd edn. Edinburgh: Mosby; 2003. Fig. 12.15 Nicholl D, ed. Clinical Neurology. Edinburgh: Churchill Livingstone; 2003. Figs 12.29A–D Epstein O, Perkin GD, de Bono DP, Cookson J. Clinical Examination. 2nd edn. London: Mosby; 1997.

Chapter 13

Figs 13.27A&B and 13.31C Bull TR. Color Atlas of ENT Diagnosis. 3rd edn. London: Mosby-Wolfe; 1995.

Chapter 14

Fig. 14.2 Haslett C, Chilvers ER, Boon NA, Colledge NR, eds. Davidson's Principles and Practice of Medicine. 19th edn. Edinburgh: Churchill Livingstone; 2002. Fig. 14.11A Forbes CD, Jackson WF. Color Atlas of Clinical Medicine. 3rd edn. Edinburgh: Mosby; 2003.

Chapter 15

Figs 15.8, 15.10, 15.12A&B, 15.13 and 15.29 Lissauer T, Clayden G. Illustrated Textbook of Paediatrics. 2nd edn. Edinburgh: Mosby; 2001. Fig. 15.19 Child Growth Foundation. Fig. 15.21 Dr Jack Beattie, Royal Hospital for Sick Children, Glasgow.

Chapter 17

Fig. 17.9 European Resuscitation Council. Box 17.1 Adapted from Hillman K, Parr M, Flabouris A et al 2001 Redefining in-hospital resuscitation: the concept of the medical emergency team. Resuscitation 48(2): 105–110.

How to get the most out of this book

The purpose of this book is to document and explain how to:

- talk with a patient
- take the history from a patient
- examine a patient
- formulate your findings into differential diagnoses
- rank these in order of probability
- use investigations to support or refute your differential diagnosis.

Initially, when you approach a section, we suggest that you glance through it quickly, looking at the headings and how it is laid out. This will help you to see in your mind's eye the framework you will be using.

Learn to speed-read. It is invaluable in medicine and in life generally. Most probably, the last lesson you had on reading was at primary school. Most people can dramatically improve their speed of reading *and* increase their comprehension by using and practising simple techniques.

Try making mind maps of the details to help you recall and retain the information as you progress through the chapter. Each of the systems chapters is laid out in the same order:

- Introduction and anatomy
- Symptoms and definition
- The history: what questions to ask and how to follow them up
- The physical examination: what and how to examine

- Investigations: those done at the patient's side (near-patient tests); laboratory investigations; and invasive investigations, including X-rays
- Key points, including some clinical points that will help you see how an experienced clinician thinks about problems.

Your purchase of this book entitles you to access the complete text online and to search using key words or using the index. You can view all the illustrations and use the hypertext-linked page cross-references to navigate quickly through the book. There are integrated links which provide bonus content from other textbooks, including *Davidson's Principles and Practice of Medicine*.

Return to this book to refresh your technique if you have been away from a particular field for some time. It is surprising how quickly your technique will deteriorate if you do not use it regularly. Practise at every available opportunity so that you become proficient at examination techniques and gain a full understanding of the range of normality.

Ask a senior colleague to review your examination technique regularly; there is no substitute for this and for regular practice. Listen also to what patients say — not only about themselves but also about other health professionals — and learn from these comments. You will pick up good and bad points that you will want to emulate or avoid.

Finally, enjoy your skills. After all, you are learning to be able to understand, diagnose and help people. For most of us, this is the reason we became doctors.

Objective Structured Clinical Examination boxes
OSCEs

Most undergraduate and postgraduate clinical examinations, including PACES for MRCP(UK), have an Objective Structured Clinical Examination (OSCE) format. This edition contains 52 OSCE revision panels, listed below, summarizing common clinical examples which may arise in examinations.

Examine this patient with ...

Clinical skills video

Included with your copy of this book is a DVD of clinical examination videos, custom made for the Twelfth Edition. Filmed using qualified doctors, with hands-on guidance from the Macleod's authorship team, these videos offer you the chance to watch trained professionals performing many of the examination routines described in the book. By helping you to memorize the essential examination steps required for each major system and by demonstrating the proper clinical technique, these videos should act as an important bridge between textbook learning and bedside teaching. The videos will be available to you to view again and again as your clinical skills develop and will prove invaluable as you prepare for your clinical OSCE examinations.

Each examination routine is accompanied by a detailed explanatory voiceover but for maximum benefit the videos should be viewed in conjunction with the book. To facilitate this, sections of the videos are also linked to the online text thus allowing you to view the relevant examination sequences as you progress through each chapter.

Contents of the DVD-Rom

- Examination of the cardiovascular system
- Examination of the respiratory system
- Examination of the gastrointestinal system
- Examination of the neurological system
- Examination of the ear
- Examination of the muscoloskeletal system
- Examination of the thyroid gland

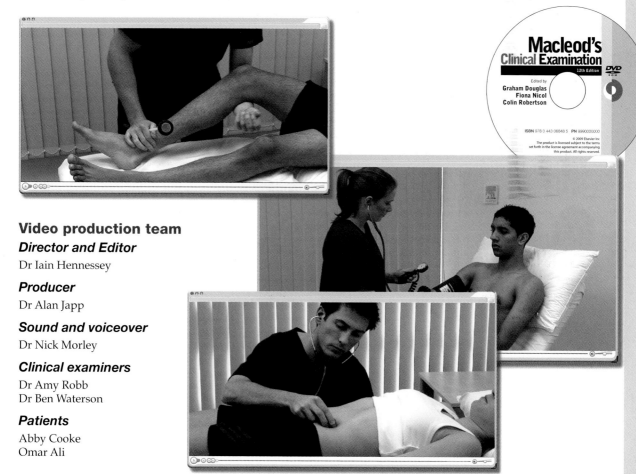

Video production team

Director and Editor
Dr Iain Hennessey

Producer
Dr Alan Japp

Sound and voiceover
Dr Nick Morley

Clinical examiners
Dr Amy Robb
Dr Ben Waterson

Patients
Abby Cooke
Omar Ali

Contributors

Elaine D C Anderson MD FRCS(Edin)
Consultant Breast Surgeon, Western General
Hospital; Clinical Director, South-East Scotland Breast
Screening Programme, Edinburgh

John S Bevan BSc(Hons) MBChB(Hons) MD FRCPE
Consultant Endocrinologist, Aberdeen Royal
Infirmary; Honorary Reader in Endocrinology,
University of Aberdeen

Andrew W Bradbury BSc MD MBA FRCS(Edin)
Sampson Gamgee Professor of Vascular Surgery,
and Head of Quality Assurance and Enhancements,
College of Medical and Dental Sciences, University of
Birmingham; Consultant Vascular and Endovascular
Surgeon, Heart of England NHS Foundation Trust,
Birmingham

Sineaid Bradshaw MBChB BSc DRCOG MRCGP
Paediatric GP Fellow; General Practitioner,
Wester Hailes Medical Practice, Lothian NHS Trust,
Edinburgh

Nicki R Colledge BSc(Hons) FRCPE
Consultant Geriatrician, Liberton Hospital and Royal
Infirmary of Edinburgh; Honorary Senior Lecturer,
University of Edinburgh

Richard A Cowie BSc MBChB FRCS(Edin) FRCS(SN)
Consultant Neurosurgeon, Hope Hospital, Salford

Allan Cumming MBChB FRCPE FRCP(Lond)
Professor of Medical Education and Director of
Undergraduate Learning and Teaching, University
of Edinburgh; Honorary Consultant Physician, Renal
Medicine, Lothian University Hospitals Division

Richard J Davenport DM FRCP(Edin)
Consultant Neurologist, Western General Hospital
and Royal Infirmary of Edinburgh; Honorary Senior
Lecturer, University of Edinburgh

Graham Devereux MA MD PhD FRCPE
Professor of Respiratory Medicine, University of
Aberdeen; Honorary Consultant, Aberdeen Royal
Infirmary

Graham Douglas BSc(Hons) MBChB FRCPE
Consultant Physician, Aberdeen Royal Infirmary;
Honorary Reader in Medicine, University of
Aberdeen

Jamie Douglas BSc MedSci MBChB
General Practice Specialist Registrar, Manchester

Michael J Ford MBChB(Hons) MD FRCPE
Consultant Physician, Western General
Hospital, Edinburgh; Honorary Professor
of Student Learning, University of
Edinburgh

David J Gawkrodger MD FRCP FRCPE
Consultant Dermatologist, Royal Hallamshire
Hospital, Sheffield; Honorary Professor of
Dermatology, University of Sheffield

Ailsa E Gebbie FRCOG MFFP
Consultant Gynaecologist, Family Planning Services,
NHS Lothian, Edinburgh; Honorary Senior Lecturer,
University of Edinburgh

Jane H Gibson MD FRCP(Edin) FRCP(Lond)
Consultant Rheumatologist, Fife Rheumatic
Diseases Unit, Cameron Hospital, Fife

Alasdair J Gray MBChB MD FRCS(Edin) FCEM
Consultant in Emergency Medicine,
Royal Infirmary of Edinburgh;
Honorary Reader,
University of Edinburgh

Neil R Grubb BSc(Hons) MBChB MRCP MD
Consultant Cardiologist and Honorary Senior
Lecturer, Royal Infirmary of Edinburgh

Iain A M Hennessey MBChB(Hons) BSc(Hons) MRCS
Specialty Registrar in Paediatric Surgery, Royal
Manchester Children's Hospital, Manchester

James S Huntley MA DPhil(Oxon) FRCS(Edin)(Orth&Tr)
Consultant Orthopaedic Surgeon, Royal
Hospital for Sick Children, Yorkhill, Glasgow

Alan G Japp MBChB(Hons) BSc(Hons) MRCP
Specialty Registrar in Cardiology, Royal Infirmary
of Edinburgh

Ian Laing MA MD FRCPE FRCPCH
Consultant Neonatologist, Royal Infirmary of
Edinburgh

Robert B S Laing MD FRCPE
Consultant Physician in Infectious Diseases,
Aberdeen Royal Infirmary

Alastair MacGilchrist MD FRCPE
Consultant Gastroenterologist/Hepatologist, Royal
Infirmary of Edinburgh

George Masterton BSc MD FRCPsych FRCPE
Consultant Psychiatrist, Royal Infirmary of Edinburgh

Robert P Mills MS MPhil FRCS
Consultant Otolaryngologist, Royal Infirmary of Edinburgh; Honorary Reader in Otolaryngology, University of Edinburgh

Nicholas C D Morley MA(Cantab) MBChB MRCS
Specialist Registrar in Radiology, South-East Scotland Rotation

Fiona Nicol BSc(Hons) MBBS FRCGP FRCPE
GP Principal and Trainer, Stockbridge Health Centre, Edinburgh; Honorary Clinical Senior Lecturer, University of Edinburgh

John Olson MD FRCP(Edin), FRCOphth
Consultant Ophthalmic Physician, Aberdeen Royal Infirmary; Honorary Clinical Senior Lecturer, University of Aberdeen

Rowan W Parks MD FRCSI FRCS(Edin)
Senior Lecturer in Surgery and Honorary Consultant Surgeon, Royal Infirmary of Edinburgh

James Y Paton MD FRCPCH
Reader in Paediatric Respiratory Medicine, University of Glasgow; Honorary Consultant in Paediatric Respiratory Medicine, Royal Hospital for Sick Children, Glasgow

Stephen R Payne MS FRCS FEBUrol
Consultant Urological Surgeon, Central Manchester and Manchester Children's Healthcare Trust

Brian Pentland FRCPE
Consultant Neurologist, Astley Ainslie Hospital, Edinburgh; Honorary Professor, Queen Margaret University; Senior Lecturer, University of Edinburgh

Colin Robertson BA(Hons) MBChB FRCPE FRCS(Ed)
Consultant and Honorary Professor in Emergency Medicine, Royal Infirmary of Edinburgh, University of Edinburgh

Hamish Simpson DM(Oxon) FRCS(Edin&England)
Professor of Orthopaedics and Trauma, University of Edinburgh

Norman C Smith MD FRCOG
Consultant Obstetrician and Honorary Clinical Senior Lecturer, Aberdeen Maternity Hospital

David Snadden MCISc MD FRCGP FRCP
Vice Provost Medicine and Professor, Northern Medical Program, University of Northern British Columbia; Regional Associate Dean, Northern British Columbia and Affiliate Professor, Department of Family Practice, University of British Columbia, Canada

James C S Spratt BSc MBChB MD FRCP FESC FACC
Consultant Interventional Cardiologist, Forth Valley Acute Hospitals

Timothy Walsh BSc(Hons) MBChB(Hons) FRCP FRCA MD MSc
Consultant in Critical Care, Royal Infirmary of Edinburgh; Honorary Professor, Clinical and Surgical Sciences, University of Edinburgh

Contents

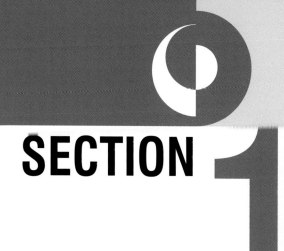

SECTION 1

History taking and general examination

Graham Douglas
Fiona Nicol
Colin Robertson

Approach to the patient

1

1

PROFESSIONAL OBLIGATIONS

Your professional obligations, the expectations placed upon you by the public, the law and your colleagues, start on your first day as a student and continue throughout your working life. You have demonstrated considerable intellect and application to get into and through Medical School, but there is more to being a good clinician than intellectual and technical proficiency. While some individuals have greater 'natural' technical ability, particularly where spatial awareness and manipulation are required, to an extent these things can be taught. Fundamentally, however, a good clinician is someone who is interested in people. The qualities that patients look for in a doctor (Box 1.1) may appear obvious, but should underpin all your clinical contacts.

One way to reconcile these expectations with your inexperience and incomplete knowledge or skills is to put yourself in the situation of the patient and/or their relatives. Consider how you would wish to be cared for in their situation, acknowledging that you are different and your preferences may not be theirs. Most doctors have their approach to, and care of, patients radically altered by their own experiences as a patient or a relative. Some of this process is empathy — where you respond in a way that demonstrates that you have made the connection between the patient's emotion and its cause. Doctors, nurses and everyone involved in healthcare have a profound influence on how patients experience illness and their sense of dignity. When you are dealing with patients, always preserve their dignity by observing the following:

- **A**ttitude — 'How would I be feeling in this patient's situation?'
- **B**ehaviour — Always treat patients with kindness and respect
- **C**ompassion — Recognize the human story that accompanies each illness
- **D**ialogue — Acknowledge and understand the individual.

1.1 The qualities that patients look for in a doctor

- Humaneness
- Competence
- Accuracy
- Honesty
- Openness
- Responsiveness
- Involving the patient in the decision-making process
- Trustworthiness
- Time to listen

1.2 The duties of a registered doctor*

- The care of your patient is your first concern
- Protect and promote the health of patients and the public
- Provide a good standard of practice and care
    - Keep your professional knowledge and skills up to date
    - Recognize and work within the limits of your competence
    - Work with colleagues to serve your patients' interests best
- Treat patients as individuals and respect their dignity
    - Treat patients politely and considerately
    - Respect patient confidentiality
- Work in partnership with the patient
    - Listen to your patients and respond to their concerns and preferences
    - Give information in a way they can understand
    - Respect their right to reach decisions with you about their care
    - Support patients in caring for themselves to improve and maintain their health
- Be honest and open, and act with integrity
    - Act without delay if you have a good reason to believe that you or a colleague may be putting patients at risk
    - Never discriminate unfairly against patients or colleagues
    - Never abuse your patient's or the public's trust in you or the profession

*Adapted from the General Medical Council (UK).

CONFIDENTIALITY AND CONSENT

As a student and as a doctor you will be given private and intimate information about patients and their families. This information is confidential, even after a patient's death. This is a general rule and its legal application varies between countries. In the UK, the guidelines issued by the General Medical Council (GMC) (Box 1.2) should be followed. There are exceptions to the general rules governing patient confidentiality, where failure to disclose information would put the patient or someone else at risk of death or serious harm, or where disclosure might assist in the prevention, detection or prosecution of a serious crime. If you find yourself in this situation as a student, contact the senior doctor in charge of the patient's care immediately and inform them of the situation.

Take all reasonable steps to ensure that your meeting with and examination of a patient is private. Never discuss patients where you can be overheard or leave patients' records, either on paper or on screen, where they can be seen by other patients, unauthorized staff or the public. Make sure you have obtained consent or other valid authority before undertaking any examination or investigation, providing treatment, or involving patients in teaching or research. Even where you have signed consent to disclose information about the patient, ensure you only disclose what is being asked for; if in doubt, discuss your report with the patient so that he is clear about what information is going to a third party.

Always make a clear record of your findings in the patient's case notes after the consultation. These case notes are confidential and should be stored securely. They also constitute a legal document that could be used in a court of law. Keeping accurate and up-to-date case notes is an essential part of good patient care (p. 35).

PERSONAL RESPONSIBILITIES

Always look after yourself and maintain your own health. Register with a general practitioner (GP) and consult him, rather than indulging in self-diagnosis and treatment. If you know that you have, or think that you might have, a serious condition you could pass on to patients, or if your judgement or performance could be affected by a condition or its treatment, you must consult your GP and be guided as to the need for secondary referral. Heed your doctor's advice regarding investigations, treatment and changes to your working practice. Protect yourself, your patients and your colleagues by being immunized against common but serious communicable diseases where vaccines are available: for example, hepatitis B.

Your professional position is a privileged one and must not be used to establish or pursue a sexual or improper emotional relationship with a patient or someone close to them. Do not give medical care to anyone with whom you have a close personal relationship. Do not express your personal beliefs, including political, religious or moral ones, to your patients in ways that exploit their vulnerability or are likely to cause them distress.

DRESS AND DEMEANOUR

The way you dress is important in establishing a successful patient–doctor relationship. Your dress style and demeanour should never make your patient or your colleagues uncomfortable or distract them. Expressing your personality is of secondary importance. Smart, sensitive and modest dress sense is appropriate. Exposing the chest, midriff and legs may create offence and impede communication. Sleeves should be either short, three-quarter length or rolled up away from the wrists prior to examination of patients or when carrying out procedures. This will enable effective hand decontamination to be carried out and reduce risk of cross-infection. Tie back long hair and keep jewellery simple and limited so as not to impede hand washing or examination. Some medical schools or hospitals require students and medical staff to wear white coats for reasons of professionalism and identification. In the past, white coats were perceived to be a barrier to cross-infection, although more recent evidence contradicts this. If you wear a white coat, it should be clean and smart.

Whenever you see a patient or relative, introduce yourself fully and clearly. A friendly smile helps to put your patient at ease. Always wear a name badge which is easily visible to the patient (not pinned on at waist level). The way you speak to and address a patient depends upon their age, background and cultural environment. In general, older patients prefer not to be called by their first name, and it is best to ask adult patients how they would prefer to be addressed.

COMMUNICATION SKILLS

Much of the art of medicine lies in communication. Doctors who communicate well are able to identify a patient's problem more rapidly and accurately, while their patients benefit from a better understanding of their condition and its management. Good communication skills are the most important part of being a good doctor. These should always include:

- maintaining good eye contact
- checking the patient's prior knowledge or understanding
- active listening
- encouraging verbal and non-verbal communication
- avoiding jargon
- eliciting and addressing the patient's agenda
- ability to discuss difficult issues
- going at a pace that is comfortable for the patient.

Conversely, poor communication skills are associated with increased medico-legal vulnerability and burnout. Reviewing your patient interview and examination by video with a senior clinician is a chastening and enlightening process, and is helpful for clinicians at all levels. Never be complacent about your communication skills; they will develop with experience but can always be improved.

EXPECTATIONS AND RESPECT

Stereotypes and literary and media depictions of doctors frequently involve miraculous intuition, the confirmation of rare and brilliant diagnoses, and the performance of dramatic life-saving interventions. Reality is different. Much of medicine involves seeing and treating patients with common conditions and chronic diseases for which conventional medicine may only be able to provide palliation.

The best doctors are invariably the most humble. Much of this stems from their recognition that humans are infinitely more complex, demanding and fascinating than one can imagine. Additionally, they understand that much so-called medical 'wisdom' is at best incomplete, and often simply wrong.

HAND WASHING AND CLEANLINESS

Transmission of microorganisms from the hands of healthcare workers is the main source of cross-infection

1.3 Infections that can be transmitted on the hands of healthcare workers..

Healthcare-acquired infections (HAIs)

- Meticillin-resistant Staphylococcus aureus (MRSA)
- *Clostridium difficile*

Diarrhoeal infections

- *Salmonella*
- *E. coli* 0157:H7
- *Shigella*
- Norovirus

Respiratory infections

- Influenza
- Respiratory syncytial virus (RSV)
- Common cold

Other infections

- Hepatitis A

in hospitals, primary care surgeries and nursing homes. Healthcare-acquired infections (HAIs) now complicate up to 10% of hospital admissions and in the UK 5000 people die from them each year (Box 1.3).

Hand washing is the single most effective way to prevent the spread of infection. However, doctors and nurses often fail to wash their hands after examining patients because of lack of hand hygiene agents or facilities for hand washing, and perceived lack of time. It is your responsibility as a clinician to prevent the spread of infection and you must routinely wash your hands after every clinical examination.

- If your hands are visibly soiled, wash thoroughly with soap and water
- If your hands are not obviously dirty, wash with soap and water or use an alcohol-based rub or gel
- Always wear surgical gloves when contact with blood, mucous membranes or non-intact skin could occur.

David Snadden
Robert Laing
George Masterton
Fiona Nicol
Nicki Colledge

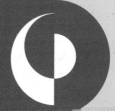

History taking

TALKING WITH PATIENTS

People visit doctors because something unexpected has happened to them, usually an ongoing problem, a relatively minor complaint or something that 'isn't right' (Box 2.1). The decision to consult may have been made after speaking to family, friends or other health professionals, trying various remedies, or looking for information on the Internet to explain or heal their illness or problem. Most patients have formed some idea of what might be wrong with them and have worries or concerns they wish to discuss.

The general practitioner (GP) is usually the first point of contact. Even a straightforward visit can be a big event for patients. They have to decide to attend the surgery, make an appointment, work out what they are going to say and possibly arrange time off work or for child care. They then have to sit in a waiting room. Think about how this affected you the last time you had to do it (Box 2.2). A visit to hospital, where 'serious' things happen, may further increase people's anxiety and apprehension. All patients seek explanation and meaning for their symptoms. Whatever the setting, you must work out why patients have come to see you, what they are most concerned about, and then agree with them the best course of action.

The first and major part of the consultation is talking with the patient. Communication is integral to the clinical examination and is most important both at the start of the interview, to gather information, and at the end, to find common ground and engage your patients in their management. These are the principles of patient-centred medicine.

Patient-centred medicine

Patient-centred medicine emphasizes the communication skills that will help you understand the patient as a whole person, and which should be part of any clinical

encounter. Good communication supports the building of trust between doctor and patient and helps you provide clear and simple information (Boxes 2.3 and 2.4). It allows you and the patient to understand each other and to agree goals together. Communication means much more than 'taking a history'; it is the only way to effectively involve patients in their healthcare. Poor communication leads to misunderstanding, conflicting messages and patient dissatisfaction, and is the root cause of complaints and litigation.

A number of consultation models provide frameworks to help you develop your own consulting style (Box 2.4).

2.3 Effective communication skills

Improve patient satisfaction

- Patients understand what is wrong
- They understand what they can do to help

Improve doctor satisfaction

- Patients are more likely to follow advice when they agree mutual goals with their doctor

Improve health by positive support and empathy

- Improving health outcomes
- Enhancing the relationship between doctor and patient

Use time more effectively

- Active listening helps the doctor recognize what is wrong
- Active listening leads to fewer patient complaints

2.1 Reasons why people visit doctors

- They have reached their limits of tolerance
- They have reached their limits of anxiety
- They have problems of living presenting as symptoms
- For prevention
- For administrative reasons

2.2 Attending a GP's surgery

Think about the last time you sat in a doctor's waiting room.
- How did you feel?
- What were your ideas and expectations?
- What happened?

2.4 Consulting with patients (BASICS)

Beginning

- Setting up
- Preparation
- Introduction

Active listening

- The patient's experience of his illness

Systematic enquiry

- Disease-oriented systematic enquiry

Information-gathering

- Clinical examination

Context

- Understanding your patient as a person

Sharing

- Information
- Agreeing action and goals

Beginning

Setting up

Where will you see your patient?

Ideally, choose a quiet, private space. This is often difficult in hospital, where privacy may be afforded only by curtains — which means no privacy at all. Be sensitive to your patients' privacy and dignity in all circumstances. If you have other staff or students with you, introduce them and ask the patient's permission for them to be there. If your patient is in a hospital bed but is mobile, use a side room or interview room. If there is no alternative to speaking to patients at their bedside, let them know that you understand your conversation may be overheard and give them permission not to answer sensitive questions if they feel uncomfortable about it.

How long will you have?

Consultation length varies. In UK general practice the average length is 13 minutes. This is usually adequate, as the doctor may have seen the patient on several occasions and is already familiar with the family and social background. In hospital 5–10 minutes may be adequate for returning outpatients, but for new and complex problems 30 minutes or more may be needed. If you are a student learning to talk with and examine patients, allow 30 minutes at least.

How will you sit?

Arrange the seating in a non-confrontational way. If you use a desk, arrange the seats at the corner of the desk. This is less formal and helps communication (Fig. 2.1A). If you use a computer, make sure the screen and keyboard do not get in the way. Turn away from the screen to talk to your patient. At a bedside, pull up a chair and sit level with your patient to see them easily and gain eye contact.

Non-verbal communication

First impressions are important. Your demeanour, attitude and dress influence your patient from the outset. At all times be professional in dress and behaviour (p. 5) and show concern for your patient's situation. Avoid interruptions such as the telephone (Fig. 2.1B).

Pick up non-verbal cues from your patients. Are they distressed? What is their mood, and how do their demeanour and body language change during the consultation? These are clues to difficulties patients are having that they cannot express verbally. If people feel uncomfortable during a line of questioning, their body language may become 'closed': that is, they may cross their arms and legs and break off eye contact (Fig. 2.1B).

Starting your consultation

Make sure you are talking to the correct patient. Introduce yourself, so your patient knows who you are and what you do. It may be appropriate to shake

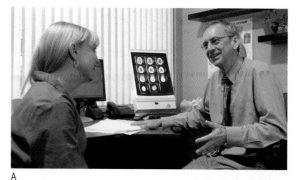

A

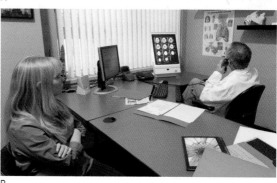

B

Fig. 2.1 Seating arrangements.

hands and to use the patient's and your own names to confirm identity. Tell patients if you are in training; they are usually eager to help. Look at the patient records and at any transfer or admission letters before you start the conversation. Note facts that are easily forgotten, e.g. blood pressure readings or family tree, but writing notes should not interfere with the consultation.

The principles of communication are important. Put these into practice, even though the words you use may change depending on the situation. Here are some ideas on how to get an interview going.

Good morning, Mrs Jones. I have got the right person, haven't I? I'm Mr Brown. I'm a fourth-year medical student. I've been asked to come and talk to you and examine you.

It might take me 20–30 minutes, if that's alright with you.

I see that you can't really get out of bed so we'll need to talk here. I'll pull the screens round. I'm sorry it's not very private. If I ask you a question that you don't want to answer in case other people overhear, then just say so.

I'll need to make a few notes so I don't forget anything important. Now, if I'm writing things down, it doesn't mean I'm not listening to you. I still will be.

Are you happy with all that?

Active listening

Hearing the patient's own story about his or her illness experience and what has actually happened is vital. Ask patients to tell you what has brought them into hospital. In the community, try 'How can I help you today?' or 'What has brought you along to see me today?'. Patients know doctors are busy and most will tell you their problem within 1–2 minutes, so do not interrupt.

Active listening means encouraging patients to talk by looking interested, making encouraging comments or noises, e.g. 'Tell me a bit more' or 'Uhuh', and giving them the impression that you have time for them. Active listening helps gather information and allows patients to tell their story in their own words. Clarify anything you do not understand. Tell them what you think they have said and ask if your interpretation is correct (reflection).

The way you ask a question is important:

- Open questions encourage the patient to talk. They start with a word like 'where' or 'what', or a phrase like 'tell me more about …', and are most useful initially when you are finding out what is going on and encouraging the patient to talk
- Closed questions, e.g. 'Have you had a cough today?', seek specific information as part of a systematic enquiry. They invite 'yes' or 'no' answers.

Both types of question have their place.

Can we start with you telling me what has happened to bring you into hospital? (*Opening*)

Well, I've been getting this funny feeling in my chest over the last few months. It's been getting worse and worse but it was really awful this morning. I got really breathless and felt someone was crushing me.

Tell me a bit more about the crushing feeling. (*Open questioning*)

Well, it was here, across my chest. It was sort of tight.

And did it go anywhere else? (*Clarifying*)

No. Well, maybe up here in my neck.

So what you are saying is that you had this tight pain in your chest this morning that went on a long time and you felt it in your neck? (*Summarizing*)

You said you've had the pain for the last few months. Can you tell me more? (*Reflecting and open questioning*)

Well, it was the same but not that bad, though it's been getting worse recently.

OK. Can you remember when it first started? (*Clarifying*)

Oh, 3 or 4 months ago.

Does anything make it worse? (*Open questioning*)

Well, if I go up steps or up hills that can bring it on.

What do you do?

Stop and sometimes take my puffer.

Your what? (*Clarifying*)

This spray the doctor gave me to put in my mouth.

Can you show me it, please?

OK.

And what does it do? (*Clarifying*)

Well, it takes the pain away, but I get an awful headache with it.

So, for a few months you've had this tightness in your chest, which gets worse going up hills and upstairs and which goes away if you use your spray. But today it came on and lasted longer but felt the same. Have I got that right? (*Summarizing*)

No, it was much worse this morning.

Once you have established what has happened, find out about your patient's FIFE:

F   Feelings related to the illness
I   Ideas on what is happening to him
F   Functioning in terms of the impact on daily life
E   Expectations of the illness and you the doctor.

Patients will have feelings and ideas about what has happened to them, and these may or may not be accurate. A patient with chest pain might think they have indigestion while you are considering angina. Ask 'Do you have any thoughts about what might be happening to you?'. A simple question like 'What were you thinking I might do today?' can avoid unnecessary prescriptions or investigations. Modern medicine may be unable to 'cure' a problem, and the important issue is what you can do to help a patient to function.

Dealing with feelings

Illness can cause anger and frustration and you will encounter angry or distressed patients. Getting angry yourself or ignoring their emotion does not help. If you feel angry with your patients, it is likely that they feel angry themselves. Exploring the reasons for the emotion often defuses the situation. Recognize that your patient is angry and ask him to explain why. If an apology is needed, give it; it may defuse the situation. Use phrases such as, 'You seem angry about something' or 'Is there something that is upsetting you?'. This technique of reflecting what you see back to the patient works with other emotions too. Recognize the emotion, show empathy and understanding, encourage your patient to talk and offer what explanations you can.

You will also meet talkative or over-familiar patients. With talkative patients or those who want to deal with a lot of things at once, try: 'I only have a short time left with you, so what's the most important thing we need to deal with now?'. If they have a long list of complaints, suggest: 'Of the six things you've raised today, I can only deal with two, so tell me which are the most important to you and we'll deal with the rest next time.'

Set professional boundaries if your patient becomes over-familiar: 'Well, it would be inappropriate for me to discuss personal issues with you. I'm here to help you so let's focus on your problem.'

Empathy

Being empathic helps your relationship with patients and improves their health outcomes. What is empathy and how do you express it? Empathy is not sympathy, the expression of sorrow; it is much more. It is helping your patients feel that you understand what they are going through. Try to see the problem from their point of view and relate that to them. Consider a young teacher who has recently had disfiguring facial surgery to remove a benign tumour from her upper jaw. Her wound has healed, but she has a drooping lower eyelid and significant facial swelling. She returns to work. Think how you would feel and imagine yourself in this situation. Express empathy through questions which show you can relate to your patient's experience.

… So, are you all healed up from your operation now?

Yes, but I still have to put drops in my eye.

And what about the swelling under your eye?

That gets worse during the day, and sometimes by afternoon I can't see that well.

And how does that feel at work?

Well, it's really difficult. You know, with the kids and everything. It's all a bit awkward.

I can understand that that must make you feel pretty uncomfortable and awkward. That must be very difficult. How do you cope? Thinking about it makes me wonder if there are any other areas that are awkward for you, maybe in other aspects of your life, like the social side …

Understanding your patient's context

The context of our lives has a major influence on how we deal with illness. Finding out about your patient's context is a crucial part of gathering information. It is far more than just a 'social history'. You must understand your patients' personal constraints and supports, including where they live, who they live with, where they work, who they work with, what they actually do, their cultural and religious beliefs, and their relationships and past experience. It is about them as a person. It may not be appropriate to explore these sensitive areas with everyone, but they are important in any long-term doctor–patient relationship. Understanding the whole person modifies the information you give and the way you give it, the treatment you advise and the drugs you use.

Establish your patient's job and explore in some depth what this job entails, as this may have a bearing on the illness. A single job description can cover many tasks, so find out what your patient actually does, whether there are any stresses involved, and whether there are any relationships at work that might affect the patient: for example, a bullying boss or a harassing colleague.

In the following dialogue, Patient A is under stress and Patient B may be suffering the consequences of exposure to fungal spores which can cause farmer's lung. However, their initial answer to the first question is the same.

Doctor: So, tell me what your job is.

Patients A and B: I work on a farm.

Doctor: Yes, but what do you actually do?

Patient A: Well, I own the farm and mostly do the bookwork and buying and selling of animals.

Patient B: I'm a labourer on the farm.

Doctor: So, what are you doing at the moment?

Patient A: It's been a terrible year with the drought. The yields are down and I'm trying to get another loan from the bank manager.

Patient B: Well, just now we work in the barn first thing in the mornings, cleaning up and then laying feed for the cattle. It's very mouldy this year. After that, we're in the fields doing the early ploughing.

Find out about your patient's home circumstances. Try asking, 'Is there anyone at home with you?' or 'Is there anyone that can help?', and be equally tactful enquiring about relationships and the home environment. If a 15-year-old newly diagnosed diabetic is about to go home, find out about the home circumstances: who is at home and are the relationships supportive? Different arrangements should be made for a patient whose mother is a health worker in a stable home, compared to one from a deprived background, who has a lone parent and poor relationships.

Patients' beliefs influence healthcare. Religious beliefs affect how they cope with a disability or a dying relative, and whether they will accept certain treatments. Be sensitive to, and tolerant of, these issues.

Sharing information and agreeing goals

We have seen how excellent communication is vital in order to reach agreement with your patient about what is wrong and what is the best course of action; now your patient needs to understand your use of words. Clarify and summarize what you say. Use words that your patient understands and tailor your explanation to your patient; you would use very different terms when dealing with a lawyer, as opposed to a farm labourer.

Explain what you have found and what you think this means. Give important information first and check what has been understood. Provide the information in small chunks and warn the patient how many important things are coming: for example, 'There are two important things I want to discuss with you. The first is …'.

Use simple language and ensure your patient understands the treatment options and likely prognosis. What you say should be accurate and unambiguous, and the information should be given sensitively. There is no place for being abrupt or for brutal honesty.

2

Engaging your patient

Make sure patients are involved in any decisions. Share your ideas with them, make suggestions and encourage them to contribute their thoughts. Be sensitive to your patients' body language. If they seem unclear about something or disagree with you, reflect this back to them. Use phrases like 'Are you comfortable with what I'm saying?' or 'Is there anything that I've said that isn't clear to you or has maybe confused you?'. Help patients' decision-making by giving them written information to take home or by suggesting other sources of information: for example, self-help groups or the Internet. Check they have understood you and discuss any investigations or treatment you think might be needed, including risks or side-effects.

In this way, you will be able to negotiate a mutually agreed plan. For example, a patient with cancer may have the choice of surgery or radiotherapy. By involving them and discussing the pros and cons of treatments, you will enable them to reach a decision that you both understand and agree with. Patients will have to live with the consequences of the treatment, which will be much easier to accept if they have chosen the treatment themselves.

Try to agree realistic goals. These might be areas that your patient needs to work on. For example, if patients are trying to stop smoking, then you may set goals together that involve when they are going to stop, what help they will need, e.g. support groups, nicotine replacement therapy or both, how they will identify risky situations, e.g. socializing, and handle these to avoid being tempted to have a cigarette.

Finally, arrange for follow-up if necessary or give patients some idea about when to return. This depends on how they are feeling and on any treatment you have suggested. End a complex discussion by briefly summarizing what you have agreed, or ask your patient to summarize for you (Box 2.5).

Situations which influence communication

Transference/countertransference

Transference occurs when your patient unconsciously projects on to you thoughts, behaviours and emotional reactions that originate from other significant relationships in their past. People who are very ill or who have just been given some news about a specific diagnosis, the implications of which are overwhelming, may behave in uncharacteristic ways. They might return to a position of dependency and seek care and comfort that was absent in their past. If you do not provide this, patients may get very angry. These are difficult concepts, but they play a major part in any doctor–patient relationship. You cannot avoid transference because it is an unconscious process, but be aware that

2.5 Talking with patients
• Speak clearly and audibly
• Do not use jargon
• Do not use unnecessarily emotive words
• Listen to their story
• Find out about them as people
• Clarify
• Negotiate mutual goals
• Summarize

it is happening. This helps you understand unexpected behaviour. Transference can be used positively, to enhance communication with your patient.

Countertransference is when a doctor's response to patients is related to significant past relationships in the doctor's own life. Repeated failure to listen to a patient's stories of failed relationships may echo a doctor's own experiences. Signs of countertransference are not listening, misjudging your patient's feelings, repeatedly going over the same story and always running late with the same patient. Being self-aware is the most important way to deal with this and talking to someone about troubling relationships helps us to gain personal insight.

Sensitive situations

Doctors sometimes need to ask personal or sensitive questions and examine intimate parts. This needs time and care. If you are talking to a patient who may have a sexually transmitted disease, broach the subject sensitively. Indicate that you are going to ask questions in this area, and make sure the conversation is entirely private. Here are some examples of questions that might work.

Because of what you're telling me, I need to ask you some rather personal questions. Is that OK?

Can you tell me if you've had any casual relationships recently?

Are you worried that you might have picked anything up — I mean, in a sexual way?

You've told me that you think you're at risk. Can I ask if you have a regular sexual partner?

Follow this up with: 'Is your partner male or female?' If there is no regular partner, ask how many sexual partners there have been in the past year and how many have been male and how many female.

Ask permission sensitively if you need to examine intimate areas. First warn your patient; then seek permission to carry out an examination, explaining what you need to do. Offer a chaperone, and record that person's name and position. If patients decline the offer, respect their wishes and record this in the notes.

So, I need to examine you down below since that seems to be where the problem is. I'll need to examine you with my hands. I'll have gloves on. I'll also need to look at you down below through a small instrument. It would be helpful if we had a chaperone who can help us. Would that be OK?

Give clear instructions about what clothes need to be removed. Sometimes it is appropriate to delay an intimate examination until sufficient time, appropriate facilities or a chaperone can be made available.

Breaking bad news

Breaking bad news is one of the most difficult communication tasks you will face. Speak to the patient in a quiet, private environment; ideally, if the patient agrees, conduct the interview in the presence of a relative or partner, and if possible with a nurse or counsellor. Be honest. Your patients may only wish to be given a few facts, and may appear not to hear or retain what you say. This is called denial or 'ambivalence about knowing', and is a normal defence mechanism. Go at your patients' pace; find out how much more they want to know and continually check their understanding. They will need time to reflect on what you have said and may need to return at another time. 'How long do I have?' is a common question. Be careful not to give a specific time — you will usually be wrong. Even in the most difficult circumstances, do not take away hope. There is always something that can be done for a patient.

Patients who are too ill to talk or who are confused

If your patient is very ill, confused or mentally ill, obtain what information you can from third parties.

Communication difficulties

Try to establish some form of communication with patients who do not speak the same language as you, those who are deaf or those who have expressive problems, e.g. dysphasia, dysarthria or stammering:
- Use an interpreter
- Write things down
- Employ lip-reading or sign language
- Involve someone who is used to communicating with your patient.

Transcultural issues

Patients from a culture that is not your own may have different social rules (Box 2.6). Ideas around eye contact, touch and personal space may be different. In Western cultures, maintaining eye contact for long periods is normal; in most of the rest of the world, this is seen as confrontational or rude. Shaking hands with the opposite sex is strictly forbidden in certain cultures. Death may be dealt with differently in terms of what family expectations of physicians may be, who will

2.6 Transcultural awareness

- Appropriateness of eye contact
- Appropriateness of hand gestures
- Personal space
- Physical contact between sexes, e.g. shaking hands
- Cultures and beliefs surrounding illness
- What should happen as death approaches?
- What should happen after death?

expect to have information shared with them and what rites will be followed. Be aware of differences in your patients' cultures and beliefs, and accept them. When in doubt, ask the patient. This lets them know that you are aware of and sensitive to these issues.

Third party information

In all circumstances, confidentiality is your first priority. You may need to obtain information about your patient from someone else: usually a relative and sometimes a friend or carer. Obtain your patient's permission and have the patient present to maintain confidentiality. Third parties may approach you without your patient's knowledge. Find out who they are, what their relationship to your patient is, and whether your patient knows the third party is talking to you. Tell third parties that you can listen to them but cannot divulge any clinical information without the patient's express permission. They may tell you about sensitive matters, such as mental illness, sexual abuse, or drug or alcohol addiction. This information needs to be sensitively explored with your patient to confirm the truth.

2.7 Key points: talking with patients

- Patient-centred medicine
  Requires good communication
  Supports the building of trust between doctor and patient
  Improves health.
- Actively listen to encourage patients.
- Identify your patient's feelings, ideas, functioning and expectations (FIFE) and address these.
- Clarify any medical or other terms the patient uses.
- Ask questions in an objective and non-judgemental way.
- Share information and engage the patient in agreeing a plan.

GATHERING INFORMATION
The presenting complaint

Diagnosis

The next step is to establish your patient's presenting complaint. To make a diagnosis, experienced clinicians

2

2.8 Terms used by patients that should be clarified

- Allergy
- Angina
- Arthritis
- Diarrhoea
- Dizziness
- Eczema
- Fits
- Heart attack
- Migraine
- Pleurisy
- Vertigo

recognize patterns of symptoms. By seeing as many patients as possible and observing colleagues, you will, with experience, refine your questions according to the presenting complaint. After obtaining details of the nature and circumstances of the presenting complaint, you should be able to produce a differential diagnosis before you examine the patient.

Ensure that patients tell you about the principal problem in their own words and record this. Use your knowledge to direct your questioning. Clarify what they mean by any term they use. How patients use some terms should be explored (Box 2.8).

Each answer makes the probability of a particular diagnosis more or less likely, while helping to exclude other possibilities. In the dialogue that follows, the patient is a 65-year-old male smoker. His age and the fact that he is a long-term smoker increase the probability of certain diagnoses related to smoking. A persistent cough for 2 months increases the likelihood of lung cancer and chronic obstructive pulmonary disease (COPD). The chest pain does not exclude COPD since the man could have pulled a muscle by coughing, but the pain is less likely to be due to this than to be pleuritic pain from infection. In turn, an infection could be caused by obstruction of an airway by lung cancer. Haemoptysis lasting 2 months dramatically increases the chance of lung cancer. When the patient confirms his weight loss, the positive predictive value of all these answers is very high for lung cancer, so you should examine him and plan investigations accordingly.

What would you say is the main problem? (*Open question*)

I've had a cough that I just can't seem to get rid of. I think it started after I'd been ill with the flu about 2 months ago. I thought it would get better but it hasn't and it's driving me mad.

Can you tell me a bit more about the cough? (*Open question*)

Well, it's bad all the time. I cough and cough, and bring up some phlegm. I can't sleep at night sometimes and I wake up feeling rough because I've slept so poorly. Sometimes I get pains in my chest because I've been coughing so much.

Follow up by asking key questions to clarify the cough — page 156. **Tell me about the pains.** (*Open question*)

Well, they're here on my side when I cough.

Does anything else bring on the pains? (*Open and prompting question*)

No.

Follow this up by asking key questions about the pain — Box 2.10. **What colour is the phlegm?** (*Closed question, focusing on the symptom offered*)

Clear.

Have you ever coughed up any blood? (*Closed question*)

Yes, sometimes.

How often? (*Closed question*)

Oh, most days.

How much? (*Closed question, clarifying the symptom*)

Just streaks, but sometimes a bit more.

Do you ever get wheezy or feel short of breath with your cough?

A bit.

How has your weight been? (*Open question, seeking additional confirmation of serious pathology*)

I've lost about 6 kilos.

What sort of pathology does the patient have?

Think about which pathological process may account for the symptoms. Diseases are either congenital or acquired, and there are only certain pathological processes that cause acquired disease (Box 2.9). The onset, progression, timescale and associated symptoms elicited in the presenting complaint should guide you to the likely pathology. Box 2.9 is only a guide to get you started because presenting complaints do not always fit into the textbook table.

What about physical signs?

Some illnesses have no physical signs, e.g. migraine or angina. Other conditions almost always cause physical signs, e.g. fractured neck of femur or stroke. Other diseases are more likely in the presence of physical signs but cannot be excluded in their absence. Experience helps you to rank the reliability of signs in supporting your diagnosis. For example, the patient with a history suggestive of transient ischaemic attacks may have a carotid bruit but its absence would not exclude this diagnosis. On the other hand, the breathless patient in whom you suspect an asthmatic attack would be expected to have audible wheeze on chest auscultation. The absence of wheeze and presence of inspiratory crackles would suggest pulmonary oedema. Always reconsider your diagnosis if you do not find an expected physical sign.

Pain

Pain is common. Its characteristics suggest the likely cause (Box 2.10). Clarify the patient's symptoms to make a differential diagnosis. These principles apply to any presenting symptom — such as bleeding, headache, shortness of breath — but with appropriate modification, e.g. you cannot have a site of shortness of breath.

2.9 Deciding on the type of pathology

Type of pathology	Onset of symptoms	Progression of symptoms	Associated symptoms/pattern of symptoms
Infection	Usually hours	Usually fairly rapid over hours or days	Fevers, localizing symptoms, e.g. pleuritic pain and cough
Inflammation	Often quite sudden	Weeks or months	Localizing symptoms of variable severity, often coming and going
Metabolic	Very variable	Hours to months	Steadily progressive in severity with no remission
Neoplastic	Gradual	Weeks to months	Weight loss, fatigue
Toxic	Abrupt	Rapid	Dramatic onset of symptoms; vomiting often a feature
Trauma	Abrupt	Little change from onset	Diagnosis usually clear from history
Vascular	Sudden	Hours	Rapid development of associated physical signs
Degenerative	Gradual	Months to years	Gradual worsening interspersed with periods of more acute deterioration

2.10 Characteristics of pain (SOCRATES)

Site

- Somatic pain often well localized, e.g. sprained ankle
- Visceral pain more diffuse, e.g. angina pectoris

Onset

- Speed of onset and any associated circumstances

Character

- Described by adjectives, e.g. sharp/dull, burning/tingling, boring/stabbing, crushing/tugging, preferably using the patient's own description rather than offering suggestions

Radiation

- Through local extension
- Referred by a shared neuronal pathway to a distant unaffected site, e.g. diaphragmatic pain at the shoulder tip via the phrenic nerve (C_3, C_4)

Associated symptoms

- Visual aura accompanying migraine with aura
- Numbness in the leg with back pain suggesting nerve root irritation

Timing (duration, course, pattern)

- Since onset
- Episodic or continuous
  If episodic, duration and frequency of attacks
  If continuous, any changes in severity

Exacerbating and relieving factors

- Circumstances in which pain is provoked or exacerbated, e.g. food
- Specific activities or postures, and any avoidance measures that have been taken to prevent onset
- Effects of specific activities or postures, including effects of medication and alternative medical approaches

Severity

- Difficult to assess, as so subjective
- Sometimes helpful to compare with other common pains, e.g. toothache
- Variation by day or night, during the week or month, e.g. relating to the menstrual cycle

Associated symptoms

Any severe pain can be associated with nausea, sweating and faintness as part of the vagal and sympathetic response but some associated symptoms suggest a particular underlying cause. For example, visual disturbance may precede migraine; palpitation (suggesting an arrhythmia) might occur in association with angina. Pain disturbing sleep suggests a physical cause while exhaustion changes the patient's perception of pain and ability to cope with it.

Effects on lifestyle

Ask 'How do you cope with the pain?' This helps you to gain insight into the patient's coping strategies (FIFE, p. 10). Areas to think about in relation to chronic pain are illustrated in Figure 2.2.

Attitudes to illness

Many symptoms, such as pain and fatigue, are subjective and patients with identical conditions can present dramatically different histories.

- Pain threshold and tolerance. These vary considerably, not only between patients but also in the same person in different circumstances. Patients vary in their willingness to speak about their discomfort (Box 2.11)
- Past experience. Personal and family experience influences the response to symptoms. A family history of sudden death from heart disease may well affect how a person interprets and reacts to chest pain
- Gains. Most illness brings some gains to the patient. These vary from attention from family and friends to financial allowances and avoiding work or stress. Patients may not be conscious of these as demotivating factors in their illness but sometimes deliberately exaggerate symptoms.

Examples of questions that can be used to ask about common symptoms are shown in Box 2.12.

2.11 Pain threshold

Increased

- Exercise
- Analgesia
- Positive mental attitude
- Personality

Decreased

- Sleep deprivation
- Depression
- Financial and personal worries
- Anxiety and fear about the cause
- Past experience

2.12 Questions that can be used to ask about common symptoms

System	Question
Cardiovascular	Do you ever have chest pain or tightness? Do you ever wake up during the night feeling short of breath? Have you ever noticed your heart racing or thumping?
Respiratory	Are you ever short of breath? Have you had a cough? Do you ever cough anything up? Have you ever coughed up blood?
Gastrointestinal	Are you troubled by indigestion or heartburn? Have you noticed any change in your bowel habit recently? Have you ever seen any blood or slime in your stools?
Genitourinary	Do you ever have pain or difficulty passing urine? Do you have to get up at night to pass urine? If so, how often? Have you noticed any dribbling at the end of passing urine? Have your periods been quite regular?
Musculoskeletal	Do you have any pain, stiffness or swelling in your joints?
Endocrine	Do you tend to feel the heat or cold more than you used to? Have you been feeling thirstier or drinking more than usual?
Neurological	Have you ever had any fits, faints or blackouts? Have you noticed any numbness, weakness or clumsiness in your arms or legs?

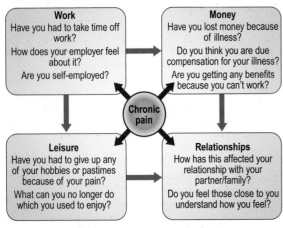

Fig. 2.2 The effects of chronic pain: questions you might ask.
Note that pain affects several areas of a patient's life but that these are interlinked.

Past history

Past medical history may be relevant to the presenting complaint: e.g. previous angina in a patient with chest pain, or haematemesis and a past history of multiple minor injuries, which raise the possibility of alcohol abuse.

Strike a balance between asking open questions about the past history and obtaining relevant, meaningful information (Box 2.13).

Drug history

Ask about prescribed drugs and any other medications. Include over-the-counter remedies and alternative medicine treatments, particularly herbal or homeopathic remedies, laxatives, analgesics and vitamin/mineral supplements. Note the name of each drug, dose, dosage regimen and duration of treatment, along with any significant side-effects. If hospitalized patients claim to be taking unlikely combinations or amounts of drugs, verify this with their GP. For those being dispensed drugs to treat an addiction, e.g. methadone, inform the dispensing pharmacy and ask for the prescription to be halted for the duration of the hospital admission (Box 2.14).

Compliance, concordance and adherence

Patients who take their medication as prescribed by the doctor are said to be compliant but the term suggests

paternalism on the part of the prescriber. Adherence is a less paternalistic word. Concordance implies that the patient and doctor negotiate and reach agreement on management.

Half of all patients do not take medicines as directed. Ask patients to describe how and when they take their medication. Check to see if they know the names of the drugs and what they are for. Give them permission to admit that they do not take all their medicines by saying 'That must be difficult to remember'.

Drug allergies/reactions

Ask if your patient has ever had an allergic reaction to medication. Clarify exactly what patients mean by allergy. Enquire particularly before prescribing an antibiotic, especially penicillin. Ask about other allergies, such as foodstuffs, animal hair, pollen or metal. Record true allergies prominently in the patient's case records, drug chart and computer notes.

Family history

Use open questions such as 'Are there any illnesses that run in your family?'. The presenting complaint may direct you to a particular line of enquiry: for example, 'Is there any history of heart disease in your family?'. Many illnesses, such as thyroid disease and coronary artery disease, are associated with a positive family history but are not due to a single gene disorder (Box 2.15).

Document illness in first-degree relatives: that is, parents, siblings and children. If there is a suspicion of an inherited disorder, e.g. Huntington's disease or haemophilia, go back three generations for details of racial origins and consanguinity (Fig. 2.3). Note whether your patient or any close relative has been adopted. Record the health of other household members, since this may suggest environmental risks to the patient's health.

Social history

The social history helps you to understand the context of the patient's life and possible relevant

2.13 Past history

- Have you had any serious illness that brought you to see your doctor?
- Have you had to take time off work because of ill health?
- Have you had any operations?
- Have you attended any hospital clinics?
- Have you ever been in hospital? If so, why was that?

2.14 Example of a drug history

Drug	Dose	Duration	Indication	Side-effects, patient concerns
Aspirin	75 mg daily	5 years	Started after myocardial infarction	
Amitriptyline	25 mg at night	6 months	Poor sleep	Feels drowsy in morning
Atenolol	50 mg daily	5 years	Started after myocardial infarction	Causes cold hands (? compliance)
Codydramol (paracetamol + dihydrocodeine)	Up to 8 tabs daily	4 weeks	Back pain	Causes constipation

2

factors (Box 2.16). Focus on the relevant issues; for example, ask an elderly woman with a hip fracture if she lives alone, whether she has any friends or relatives nearby, what support services she receives and how well suited her house is for someone with poor mobility.

The patient's illness may affect others. There may be an infirm relative at home for whom the patient cares; alternatively, there may be no one at home to look after the patient because, although she is married, her husband works abroad for three weeks out of four. Problems must be addressed for successful discharge from hospital to the community.

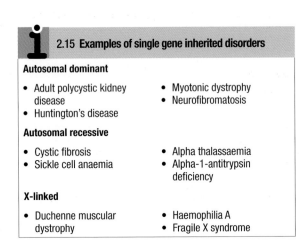

2.15 Examples of single gene inherited disorders

Autosomal dominant

- Adult polycystic kidney disease
- Huntington's disease
- Myotonic dystrophy
- Neurofibromatosis

Autosomal recessive

- Cystic fibrosis
- Sickle cell anaemia
- Alpha thalassaemia
- Alpha-1-antitrypsin deficiency

X-linked

- Duchenne muscular dystrophy
- Haemophilia A
- Fragile X syndrome

Lifestyle

Exercise

Do your patients take part in any sports or take any other regular exercise? If so, find out how often they do so and how strenuous it is. Do they usually use the stairs or the lift at work? Have they had to reduce their exercise because of illness?

Diet

Do your patients have any dietary restrictions and how have they decided on these? Some patients believe that they have a food intolerance and may stick to rigid exclusion diets backed up by no medical evidence. Ask about the frequency and times of meals and the variety and types of foods eaten, as well as snacking habits.

Occupational history

Work profoundly influences health, while unemployment is associated with increased morbidity and mortality. Some occupations are associated with particular illnesses (Box 2.17).

Take a full occupational history from all patients. Try asking, 'Please tell me about all the jobs you have done in your working life'. Clarify exactly what the patient does when at work: in particular, any chemical or dust exposure (p. 162), any sick colleagues and use of protective devices. Symptoms that improve over the weekend or during holidays suggest an occupational disorder. Hobbies may also be associated with certain

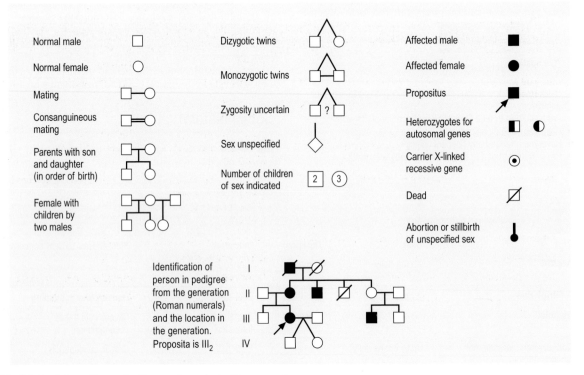

Fig. 2.3 Symbols used in constructing a pedigree chart, with an example.

2.16 The social history

Upbringing

- Birth injury or complications
- Early parental attachments and disruptions
- Schooling, academic achievements or difficulties
- Further or higher education and training
- Behaviour problems

Home life

- Emotional, physical or sexual abuse*
- Experiences of death and illness
- Interest and attitude of parents

Occupation

- Current and previous (clarify exactly what a job entails)
- Exposure to hazards, e.g. chemicals, asbestos, foreign travel, accidents and compensation claims
- Unemployment: reason and duration
- Attitude to job

Finance

- Circumstances, including debts
- Benefits from social security

Relationships and domestic circumstances

- Married or long-term partner
- Quality of relationship

- Problems
- Partner's health, occupation and attitude to patient's illness
- Who else is at home? Any problems, e.g. health, violence, bereavement?
- Any trouble with the police?

House

- Type of home, size, owned or rented
- Details of home, including stairs, toilets, heating, cooking facilities, neighbours

Community support

- Social services involvement, e.g. home help, meals on wheels
- Attitude to needing help

Sexual history*

Leisure activities

- Hobbies and pastimes
- Pets

Exercise

- What, where and when?

Substance misuse*

*Only ask if it is relevant to the history.

2.17 Examples of occupational disorders

Occupation	Factor	Disorder	Presents
Shipyard workers, boilermen	Asbestos	Pleural plaques Asbestosis Mesothelioma	Over 20 years later
Dairy farmers	*Leptospira hadjo* Fungus spores on mouldy hay	Lymphocytic meningitis Farmer's lung (extrinsic allergic alveolitis)	Within 1 week Within 4–18 hours
Divers	Surfacing from depth too quickly	Decompression sickness Central nervous system, skin, bone and joint symptoms	Immediately and up to 1 week
Industrial workers	Chemical exposure, e.g. chromium	Dermatitis on hands	Variable
Bakery workers	Flour dust	Occupational asthma	Variable
Healthcare workers	Cuts, needlestick injuries	Hepatitis B and C	Incubation period >3 months
Work involving noisy machinery	Excessive noise	Sensorineural hearing loss	Develops over months

2.18 Incubation periods of travel-related infections

Disease	Incubation period	Travel to presentation	Usual symptoms
Falciparum malaria	8–25 days	Up to 6 weeks	Fever
Vivax malaria	8–27 days	Up to 1 year	Fever
Typhoid fever	10–14 days	Up to 3 weeks	Fever, headache
Dengue fever	3–15 days	Up to 3 weeks	Fever, headache
Schistosomiasis	2–63 days	Up to 10 weeks	Itch, fever, haematuria, abdominal discomfort
Hepatitis A	28–42 days	Up to 6 weeks	Jaundice
HIV infection	12–26 weeks	Up to ?12 years	Weight loss, pneumonia

illnesses: e.g. psittacosis pneumonia and extrinsic allergic alveolitis in those who keep birds.

Travel history

One in eight people travelling outside Europe or North America attends a GP on returning with possible travel-related illness. Travellers risk unusual or tropical infections, and air travel itself increases certain conditions, such as middle ear problems or deep vein thrombosis. The incubation period is useful in deciding on the likelihood of an illness (Box 2.18).

List the countries your patients visited and the dates they were there. Enquire about the type of accommodation and the activities undertaken: for example, water sports and sexual contacts. Note any travel vaccination or malarial prophylaxis taken.

Sexual history

Only take a full sexual history if this is appropriate (p. 247). Ask questions sensitively and objectively (Box 2.19). Signal your intentions with a statement: for example, 'As part of your medical history, I need to ask you some questions about your relationships. Is this all right?'.

2.19 Sexual history questions

- Do you have a regular sexual partner at the moment?
- Is your partner male or female?
- Have you had any (other) sexual partners in the last 12 months?
- How many were male? How many female?
- Do you use barrier contraception — sometimes, always or never?
- Have you ever had a sexually transmitted infection?

Tobacco

Ask if your patient has ever smoked; if so, enquire as to how long, what (cigarettes, cigars or pipe) and how much. Use 'pack years' (Box 2.20) to estimate the risk of tobacco-related health problems (Fig. 2.4) (p. 162). Ask non-smokers about exposure to passive smoking at work or home.

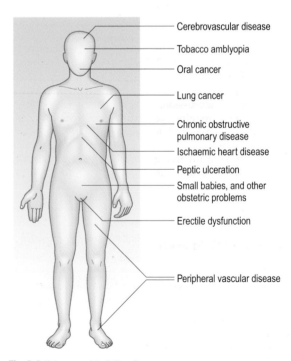

- Cerebrovascular disease
- Tobacco amblyopia
- Oral cancer
- Lung cancer
- Chronic obstructive pulmonary disease
- Ischaemic heart disease
- Peptic ulceration
- Small babies, and other obstetric problems
- Erectile dysfunction
- Peripheral vascular disease

Fig. 2.4 Tobacco-related disorders.

Alcohol

Asking bluntly 'How much alcohol do you drink?' may upset patients. Try 'Do you ever drink any alcohol?'. Work out with them how much and when. Use open questions, giving permission for them to tell you, and do not judge them. Follow up with closed questions covering:

- what?
- when?
- how much? (Box 2.21).

Other useful questions are:

- When did you last have a drink?
- What's the most you ever drink?

The number of units of alcohol consumed each week can be calculated in one of two ways (Box 2.22).

Alcohol problems

- Hazardous drinking: This is 'at-risk' drinking and is the regular consumption of more than:
  24 g of pure ethanol (3 units) per day for men
  14 g of pure ethanol (2 units) per day for women.

It increases depression, obesity, liver disease and hypertension, impairs cognitive function and is associated with risk of violent death in men and breast cancer in women.

Binge drinking involving a large amount of alcohol causes acute intoxication and is more likely to result in trauma, e.g. a head injury, than if the same amount is consumed over 4 or 5 days. Everyone should have at least 2 days per week when they drink no alcohol.

- Harmful drinking: This is drinking that has caused physical or mental health damage or disruption to social circumstances
- Alcohol dependence: The use of alcohol takes a higher priority than other behaviours that previously had greater value (Box 2.23)

Early identification of alcohol problems is important because of the health risks to patients and their families (Fig. 2.5). Screening tests help detect problem drinking. The CAGE questionnaire is easy to remember but is not sensitive (Box 2.24). The FAST questionnaire is more sensitive but has a more complex scoring system (Box 2.25).

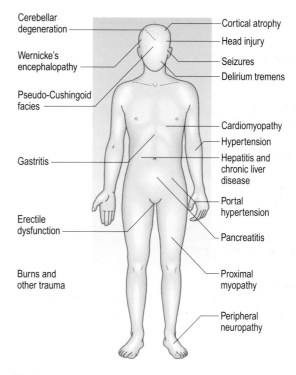

Fig. 2.5 Alcohol-related disorders.

Labels: Cerebellar degeneration; Cortical atrophy; Head injury; Wernicke's encephalopathy; Seizures; Delirium tremens; Pseudo-Cushingoid facies; Cardiomyopathy; Hypertension; Gastritis; Hepatitis and chronic liver disease; Portal hypertension; Erectile dysfunction; Pancreatitis; Burns and other trauma; Proximal myopathy; Peripheral neuropathy

Non-prescribed drug use

Ask any patient with symptoms possibly associated with drug misuse about their use of non-prescribed drugs, remembering that about 30% of the adult population in Britain has used drugs (mainly cannabis) at some time (Boxes 2.26 and 2.27).

2.22 Calculating units of alcohol

Method 1

Standard measure (1 unit) = 1 small glass of wine

1 half-pint of beer

1 short of spirits

Method 2

Standard measure (1 unit) = 25 ml of 40% alcohol

= 10 ml ethanol

x% proof = x units of alcohol per litre

Examples

1 litre of 40% proof spirits contains 400 ml ethanol or 40 units

750 ml (standard bottle) contains 30 units alcohol

1 litre of 4% beer contains 40 ml ethanol or 4 units

500 ml can contains 2 units of alcohol

Alternatively, use an online calculator, e.g. http://www.drinkaware.co.uk/how-many-units.html

2.23 Features of alcohol dependence

- A strong, often overpowering, desire to take alcohol
- Inability to control starting or stopping drinking and the amount that is drunk
- Tolerance, where increased doses are needed to achieve the effects originally produced by lower doses
- Withdrawal state when drinking is stopped or reduced — including tremor, sweating, rapid heart rate, anxiety, insomnia, and occasionally seizures, disorientation or hallucinations (delirium tremens). It is relieved by more alcohol
- Neglect of other pleasures and interests
- Continuing to drink in spite of being aware of the harmful consequences

2.24 The CAGE questionnaire

- Have you ever felt you should **C**ut down on your drinking?
- Have people **A**nnoyed you by criticizing your drinking?
- Have you ever felt bad or **G**uilty about your drinking?
- Do you ever have a drink first thing in the morning to steady you or help a hangover (an **E**ye opener)?

Positive answers to two or more questions suggest problem drinking; confirm this by asking about the maximum taken

2.25 The FAST questionnaire

For the following questions please circle the answer that best applies

1 drink = ½ pint of beer or 1 glass of wine or 1 single measure of spirits

1. MEN: How often do you have EIGHT or more drinks on one occasion?

    WOMEN: How often do you have SIX or more drinks on one occasion?
    - Never (0)
    - Less than monthly (1)
    - Monthly (2)
    - Weekly (3)
    - Daily or almost daily (4)

2. How often during the last year have you been unable to remember what happened the night before because you had been drinking?
    - Never (0)
    - Less than monthly (1)
    - Monthly (2)
    - Weekly (3)
    - Daily or almost daily (4)

3. How often during the last year have you failed to do what was normally expected of you because of drinking?
    - Never (0)
    - Less than monthly (1)
    - Monthly (2)
    - Weekly (3)
    - Daily or almost daily (4)

4. In the last year has a relative or friend, or a doctor or other health worker been concerned about your drinking or suggested you cut down?
    - Never (0)
    - Yes, on one occasion (2)
    - Yes, on more than one occasion (4)

Scoring FAST

First stage

If the answer to question 1 is *Never*, then the patient is probably not misusing alcohol

If the answer is Weekly or Daily or Almost daily, then the patient is a hazardous, harmful or dependent drinker

50% of people are classified using this one question

Second stage

Only use these questions if the answer is *Less than monthly* or *Monthly*

Score questions 1–3: 0, 1, 2, 3, 4

Score question 4: 0, 2, 4

Minimum score is 0

Maximum score is 16

Score for hazardous drinking is 3 or more

2.26 Non-prescribed drug history

- What drugs are you taking?
- How often and how much?
- How long have you been taking drugs?
- Any periods of abstinence? If so, when and why did you start using drugs again?
- What symptoms do you have if you cannot get drugs?
- Do you ever inject? If so, where do you get the needles and syringes?
- Do you ever share needles, syringes or other drug paraphernalia?
- Do you see your drug use as a problem?
- Do you want to make changes in your life or change the way you use drugs?

2.27 Complications of drug misuse

Infections

- Hepatitis B and C
- HIV
- Abscesses, cellulitis and necrotizing fasciitis
- Septic pulmonary thromboembolism or lung abscesses
- Aspiration pneumonia
- Endocarditis
- Tetanus
- Wound botulism
- Sexually transmitted disease: many work in the sex industry to finance their habit

Injury

- Thrombophlebitis and deep vein thrombosis
- Arterial injury and occlusion
- Skin ulceration

Overdose

- Respiratory failure
- Rhabdomyolysis and renal failure

Chaotic life style leading to

- Poor nutrition
- Poor dental hygiene
- Failure to care for dependants
- Debt
- Prison

Systematic enquiry

Systematic enquiry uncovers symptoms that may have been forgotten. Ask 'Is there anything else you would like to tell me about?'. Then run through the symptoms in Box 2.29 with every patient until you are experienced enough to hone these down. Follow up any positive response by asking questions to increase or decrease the probability of certain diseases.

Some examples of targeted systematic enquiry are as follows:

- The smoker with weight loss: Are there any respiratory symptoms, e.g. unresolving chest infection or haemoptysis to suggest lung cancer? Are there any symptoms that suggest another cause for the weight loss, e.g. altered bowel habit due to colon cancer?
- The patient with recurrent mouth ulcers: Do any alimentary symptoms suggest Crohn's disease or coeliac disease? Are there any locomotor symptoms to suggest Behçet's disease?
- The patient with palpitation: Are there any endocrine symptoms to suggest thyrotoxicosis or is there a family history of thyroid disease?
- The patient who arouses your suspicions, e.g. smelling of alcohol: Ask questions about symptoms that might be related, such as numbness in the feet due to alcoholic neuropathy.

Completing the history taking

With all the relevant information assembled, you should have a list of differential diagnoses.

Before you examine the patient:

- Briefly summarize what the patient has told you
- Reflect this back to the patient. This allows the patient to:
    - Correct anything you have misunderstood
    - Add anything that may have been forgotten
- Tell the patient what you are going to examine and gain his permission to do so.

2.28 Key points: gathering information

- Summarize your understanding of the problems and reflect it back to the patient.
- Quantify the patient's use of tobacco, alcohol and non-prescribed drugs.
- Patients' previous experience and attitude influence their symptoms and presentation.
- Check drug history and other facts with the patient's GP.
- You should have a good idea of the differential diagnosis after obtaining the history.

THE PSYCHIATRIC HISTORY

Taking a psychiatric history is an essential skill for all clinicians because mental disorders are very common (40% of primary care consultations), often co-exist with physical disorders and are common causes of mortality, disability and working years lost.

Psychiatric assessment consists of four elements:

- the history
- mental state examination
- selective physical examination
- collateral information.

2.29 Systematic enquiry: cardinal symptoms

General health

- Well-being
- Appetite
- Weight change
- Energy
- Sleep
- Mood

Cardiovascular system

- Chest pain on exertion (angina)
- Breathlessness:
    Lying flat (orthopnoea)
    At night (paroxysmal nocturnal dyspnoea)
    On minimal exertion — record how much
    Palpitation
    Pain in legs on walking (claudication)
    Ankle swelling

Respiratory system

- Shortness of breath (exercise tolerance)
- Cough
- Wheeze
- Sputum production (colour, amount)
- Blood in sputum (haemoptysis)
- Chest pain (due to inspiration or coughing)

Gastrointestinal system

- Mouth (oral ulcers, dental problems)
- Difficulty swallowing (dysphagia — distinguish from pain on swallowing, odynophagia)
- Nausea and vomiting
- Vomiting blood (haematemesis)
- Indigestion
- Heartburn
- Abdominal pain
- Change in bowel habit
- Change in colour of stools (pale, dark, tarry black, fresh blood)

Genitourinary system

- Pain passing urine (dysuria)
- Frequency passing urine (at night, nocturia)
- Blood in the urine (haematuria)
- Libido

- Incontinence (stress and urge)
- Sexual partners — unprotected intercourse

Men

- If appropriate:
    Prostatic symptoms including difficulty starting — hesitancy
    Poor stream or flow
    Terminal dribbling
    Urethral discharge
    Erectile difficulties

Women

- Last menstrual period (consider pregnancy)
- Timing and regularity of periods
- Length of periods
- Abnormal bleeding
- Vaginal discharge
- Contraception
- If appropriate:
    Pain during intercourse (dyspareunia)

Nervous system

- Headaches
- Dizziness (vertigo or light-headed)
- Faints
- Fits
- Altered sensation
- Weakness
- Visual disturbance
- Hearing problems (deafness, tinnitus)
- Memory and concentration changes

Musculoskeletal system

- Joint pain, stiffness or swelling
- Mobility
- Falls

Endocrine system

- Heat or cold intolerance
- Change in sweating
- Excessive thirst (polydipsia)

Other

- Bleeding or bruising
- Skin rash

History

Psychiatric interviewing has three purposes:

- to obtain a history
- to assess the present mental state

- to establish rapport that will facilitate further management (Boxes 2.30 and 2.31).

Practise taking a complete history to become familiar with the components and to gain the skills and insight to guide you as to when to be comprehensive. Collecting information that initially seems unconnected

2.30 Content of a psychiatric history

- Referral source
- Reason for referral
- History of presenting complaint(s)
- Systematic enquiry into other relevant problems and symptoms
- Past medical/psychiatric history
- Prescribed and non-prescribed medication
- Substance use: illegal drugs, alcohol, tobacco, caffeine
- Family history (including psychiatric disorders)
- Personal history

2.31 Personal history

- Childhood development
- Losses and experiences
- Education
- Occupation(s)
- Financial circumstances
- Relationships
- Partner(s) and children
- Housing
- Leisure activities
- Hobbies and interests
- Forensic history

2.32 What to ask: sensitive topics

- You said a few minutes ago that sometimes you wish you had died in your sleep. I need to ask you a bit more about that thought. Have you ever considered doing something that would make that happen?
- You've just told me that you feel your life isn't worth living. Do you ever think in the same way about your children's lives?
- You indicated that something terrible happened to you when you were a child. Do you want to tell me more about that now?

to the presenting complaint may increase your understanding of how and why the illness evolved. It is useful to consider these factors under the headings:

- predisposing
- precipitating
- perpetuating.

For example, a patient presenting with depression may have had a mother who suffered from depression and died when the patient was a child (predisposing factors). The partner may have left recently when investigations for a breast lump were being carried out (precipitating factors). The patient is abusing alcohol and not taking the antidepressant medication the GP has prescribed (perpetuating factors).

Sensitive topics

In certain circumstances, such as when the patient is in police custody or at a sexual dysfunction clinic, make it obvious that sensitive questions are required and tactful questioning will usually then be straightforward. However, if the topic seems irrelevant to the patient, or too embarrassing or stressful, this can damage rapport and so impair management. This applies particularly to:

- sexual issues, e.g. sexual dysfunction, gender identity
- major traumatic experiences, e.g. rape, childhood sexual abuse, witnessing a death
- illicit drug misuse
- crime
- suicidal or homicidal ideas
- delusions or hallucinations.

It is important to develop good rapport at the first interview. Consolidate this before raising a sensitive topic; a subject's relevance and context then become clearer to the patient and there is time to deal with it properly. Sometimes it is imperative to cover such material without delay: for instance, when you need to establish the drug-taking habits of a teenager who presents with acute psychotic illness, or the risk to mother and baby in a woman with postnatal depression. In these cases, tell the patient about the nature of and reason for your sensitive enquiries, reflecting the patient's own comments (Box 2.32).

Mental state examination

The mental state examination (MSE) is a systematic evaluation of the patient's mental condition at the time of interview. The aim is to establish signs of disorder that, taken with the history, enable you to make, suggest or exclude a diagnosis. While making your specific enquiries, you need to observe, evaluate subjectively, draw inferences from and incorporate aspects of the history. This is daunting, but with good teaching, practice and experience you will learn the skills.

Mental state examination involves:
- observation of the patient
- incorporation of relevant elements of the history
- specific questions exploring various mental phenomena
- short tests of cognitive function.

Content is channelled by the history and potential diagnoses so that, for example, detailed cognitive assessment in an elderly patient presenting with confusion is crucial; similarly, mood and suicide risk are closely evaluated when the presenting problem is depression (Box 2.33).

Appearance

Appearance is assessed by observing:
- general elements, e.g. attire, signs of self-neglect
- facial expression

2.33 Elements of the Mental State Examination (MSE)

- Appearance
- Behaviour
- Speech
- Mood
- Thought form
- Thought content
- Perceptions
- Cognition
- Insight
- Risk assessment

2.35 Speech: definitions

Term	Definition
Clang associations	Thoughts connected by having a similar sound rather than by meaning
Mutism	Absence of speech without impaired consciousness
Neologism	An invented word, or a new meaning for an established word
Pressure of speech	Rapid, excessive, continuous speech (due to pressure of thought)

2.34 Behaviour: definitions

Term	Definition
Agitation	A combination of psychic anxiety and excessive, purposeless motor activity
Compulsion	An unnecessary, purposeless action that the patient is unable to resist performing repeatedly
Disinhibition	Loss of control over normal social behaviour
Motor retardation	Decreased motor activity, usually a combination of fewer and slower movements
Posturing	The maintenance of bizarre gait or limb positions for no valid reason

---

2.36 Mood: definitions

Term	Definition
Blunting	Loss of normal emotional sensitivity to experiences
Catastrophic reaction	An extreme emotional and behavioural over-reaction to a trivial stimulus
Flattening	Loss of the range of normal emotional responses
Incongruity	A mismatch between the emotional expression and the associated thought
Lability	Superficial, rapidly changing and poorly controlled emotions

---

- scars, tattoos
- signs of physical disease, e.g. spider naevi, exophthalmos.

Behaviour

Behaviour is largely assessed by observing:
- cooperation, rapport, eye contact
- social behaviour, e.g. aggression, disinhibition
- overactivity, e.g. agitation, compulsions
- underactivity, e.g. stupor, motor retardation
- abnormal activity, e.g. posturing, involuntary movements (Box 2.34).

Speech

Speech is largely assessed by observing:
- articulation, e.g. stammering, dysarthria
- quantity, e.g. mutism, garrulousness
- rate, e.g. pressured, slowed
- volume, e.g. whispering, shouting
- tone and quality, e.g. accent, emotionality
- abnormal language, e.g. neologisms, dysphasia, clanging (Box 2.35).

Mood

Mood is assessed by observing (objective), and by taking elements from the history and making specific enquiries (subjective) (Boxes 2.36 and 2.37).

Pervasive disturbance of mood is the most important feature of depression, mania, and anxiety and associated disorders, but mood changes commonly occur in other mental disorders such as schizophrenia and dementia.

Incidentally, the terms mood and affect are often used interchangeably, but they are subtly different. Mood refers to the pervasive emotional state, whereas affect is the observable expression of emotions, which is variable over time. A usefully analogy is to think of a patient's mood as a climate, in which case the patient's affect is the current weather.

Abnormalities of mood consist of:
- pervasive or predominant abnormal affect/mood, e.g. depressed, elated, anxious, fearful, angry, suspicious, irritable, perplexed
- range, e.g. flattened, expanded
- reactivity, e.g. blunted, labile, catastrophic
- appropriateness, e.g. incongruous.

2.37 Mood: what to ask

- How has your mood been lately?
- Have you noticed any change in your emotions recently?
- Has your family commented recently on your mood?
- Do you still enjoy things that normally give you pleasure?

2.38 Thought form: definitions

Term	Definition
Circumstantiality	Trivia and digressions impairing the flow but not direction of thought
Concrete thinking	Inability to think abstractly
Flights of ideas	Rapid shifts from one idea to another, retaining sequencing
Loosening of associations	Logical sequence of ideas impaired. Subtypes include knight's move thinking, derailment, thought blocking and, in its extreme form, word salad
Perseveration	Inability to shift from one idea to the next
Pressure of thought	Increased rate and quantity of thoughts
Word salad	Meaningless string of words, often with loss of grammatical construction

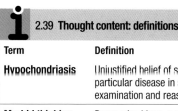

2.39 Thought content: definitions

Term	Definition
Hypochondriasis	Unjustified belief of suffering from a particular disease in spite of appropriate examination and reassurance
Morbid thinking	Depressive ideas, e.g. themes of guilt, burden, unworthiness, failure, blame, death, suicide
Obsessional thinking	Repetitive, intrusive, senseless thoughts or preoccupations the person cannot stop
Phobia	A senseless avoidance of a situation, object or activity stemming from a belief that has caused an irrational fear
Preoccupations	Beliefs that are not inherently abnormal but which have come to dominate the patient's thinking
Ruminations	Repetitive, unproductive thoughts

2.40 Thought content: what to ask

- What thoughts have been particularly on your mind lately?
- Do you have any thoughts that are of special significance or concern for you?
- What have your main worries been recently?

Thought form

Thought form is largely assessed by observation (Box 2.38).

Loosening of associations in its various guises is sometimes termed formal thought disorder, and is a core feature of schizophrenia. Subjectively, this may be reported as having difficulty thinking clearly. Manic expression is characterised by pressure of thoughts and flights of ideas, whereas with depression these processes are slowed and impoverished; this is also characteristic of dementia.

Elements are:

- rate, e.g. pressure of thought, retardation
- flow, e.g. flights of ideas, circumstantiality, perseveration
- sequencing, e.g. loosening of associations
- abstract thinking, e.g. concrete thought.

Record examples of speech from the history to show how a person thinks.

Thought content

Thought content is assessed from the history and specific enquiries (Box 2.39). Note thought content from what the patient has discussed during history taking and then explore it by further questioning.

Thought content may be divided into:

- preoccupations
- abnormal beliefs.

Preoccupations

Preoccupations commonly occur in abnormal mood states: for example, the worries and fears of anxious people or the morbid thoughts found in depression. Hypochondriasis, and obsessional and phobic disorders are other conditions in which ruminations are frequently found (Box 2.40).

Abnormal beliefs

Abnormal beliefs fall into two categories:

- those that are not diagnostic of mental illness, e.g. overvalued ideas, superstitions, magical thinking
- those that invariably signify mental illness, i.e. delusions.

The main difference is that delusions either lack a cultural basis for understanding the belief or have been derived from abnormal processes.

Overvalued ideas are beliefs of great personal significance that are abnormal because of their effects on a person's behaviour or well-being. For example, in anorexia nervosa people may still believe they are

2.41 Abnormal beliefs: definitions

Term	Definition
Delusion	An abnormal belief, held with total conviction, which is maintained in spite of proof or logical argument to the contrary and is not shared by others from the same culture
Delusional perception	A delusion which arises from the false interpretation of a real perception, e.g. a diner who asks a waiter for a glass of water is believed to be a Russian spy making contact with an assassin
Magical thinking	An irrational belief that certain actions and outcomes are linked, often culturally determined by folklore or custom, e.g. fingers crossed for good luck
Overvalued ideas	Beliefs that are held, valued, expressed and acted on beyond the norm for the culture to which the person belongs
Thought broadcasting	The belief that the patient's thoughts are heard by others
Thought insertion	The belief that thoughts are being placed in the patient's head from outside
Thought withdrawal	The belief that thoughts are being removed from the patient's head

2.42 Abnormal beliefs: what to ask

- Have there been times when you've thought something strange is going on?
- Do you ever think you're being followed or watched?
- Do you ever feel other people can interfere with your thoughts or actions?

fat when they are seriously underweight — and they respond to their belief rather than their weight (Box 2.41).

Delusional beliefs matter greatly to the person, resulting in powerful emotional and important behavioural consequences. This means they are always of clinical significance. They are classified by their content, such as:

- paranoid
- religious
- grandiose
- hypochondriacal
- of guilt
- of love
- of jealousy
- of infestation
- of thought interference
- of control.

Bizarre delusions are easy to recognize, but not all delusions are weird ideas. For example, a person who is convinced that his partner is unfaithful may or may not be deluded. What matters is how the belief arose. Even if a partner were unfaithful, it would still amount to a delusional jealousy if the belief were held for some unaccountable reason, such as finding a dead bird in the garden.

Delusions are subdivided into primary and secondary. Primary delusions arise without a trigger and are characteristic of schizophrenia. Secondary delusions are products of other abnormal mental processes such as:

- abnormal mood
- hallucinations
- clouded consciousness
- another delusion.

Delusions can sometimes be understood as the patient's way of trying to make sense of his experience, while their content often gives a clue that may help type the underlying illness; e.g. delusions of guilt suggest severe depression whereas grandiose delusions typify mania. There are some delusions which are characteristic, but not diagnostic, of schizophrenia, most notably a primary delusional perception (Box 2.42). These include 'passivity phenomena': namely, the belief that thoughts, feelings or acts are no longer controlled by a person's free will:

- delusions of thought interference (thought insertion, withdrawal or broadcasting)
- delusions of external control
- this is not a passivity phenomenon (but is said to be diagnostic of schizophrenia).

Perceptions

Perceptions are assessed from the history and specific enquiries, sometimes backed up by observation (Box 2.43).

We take for granted the ease with which people distinguish between their inner and outer worlds. We know what is real and what it feels like to be real. However, this can be disrupted in mental illnesses so that normal perceptions become strange and unfamiliar while abnormal perceptions seem real. These anomalies fall into several categories:

- depersonalization, derealization
- altered perceptions: sensory distortions, illusions
- false perceptions: hallucinations, pseudohallucinations.

Depersonalization and derealization are common; they are usually normal and are associated with tiredness or stress. They can also occur in most types of mental illness. With altered perceptions there is a real external object but its internal perception has been distorted. Sensory distortions, such as unpleasant amplification of light (photophobia) or sound (hyperacusis), can occur in physical diseases, but are also common in anxiety states and drug intoxication or

2.43 Perceptions: definitions

Term	Definition
Depersonalization	A subjective experience of feeling unreal
Derealization	A subjective experience that the surrounding environment is unreal
Hallucination	A false perception arising without a valid stimulus from the external world
Illusion	A false perception that is an understandable misinterpretation of a real stimulus in the external world
Pseudohallucination	A false perception which is perceived as part of one's internal experience

2.44 Perceptions: what to ask

- Do you ever hear voices when nobody is talking?
- What do they say?
- Where do they come from?
- Have you had any visions?
- Have you ever felt that you were not real or that the world around you wasn't real?

2.45 Cognition: definitions

Term	Definition
Clouding of consciousness	A reduced level of consciousness observed as drowsiness (coma in extreme cases)
Confabulation	Plausible but false memories that cover memory gaps

withdrawal. Diminution of perceptions, including pain, can occur in depression and schizophrenia.

Illusions commonly occur among people with established impairment of vision or hearing. They are also found in predisposed patients who are subjected to sensory deprivation, notably after dark in a patient with clouding of consciousness.

True hallucinations arise from no external stimuli. Their presence usually indicates severe mental illness, although they can occur naturally when going to sleep (hypnagogic) or waking up (hypnopompic). Hallucinations are categorized according to mode of sensory presentation, notably:

- auditory
- visual
- olfactory
- gustatory
- tactile.

Virtually any form of hallucination can occur in any severe mental disorder. By far the most common, however, are auditory and visual hallucinations, the former being associated with schizophrenia and the latter with delirium. Some auditory hallucinations are characteristic of schizophrenia, such as voices discussing the patient in the third person, or giving a running commentary on the person's activities.

Pseudohallucinations are common. They may occur in mental illness, but not infrequently they are experienced by an anxious or dramatic patient, sometimes as an inner voice. The key distinction from a true hallucination is that these phenomena occur within the patient rather than arising externally. Characteristically they have an 'as if' quality, so that they often lack the vividness and reality of true hallucinations. Consequently, the affected person is not upset or distressed by them; nor does the person feel the need to respond, as happens with true hallucinations (Box 2.44).

Cognition

Cognition is largely evaluated by standard tests but is also assessed from the history and observation.

Cognitive functions are brain processes that include:
- level of consciousness
- orientation
- memory
- attention and concentration
- intelligence.

Mental disorders are rarely associated with a reduced level of consciousness. The exception is delirium, in which this is common; it is then termed clouding of consciousness and is assessed by observation (Box 2.45).

Orientation is a key aspect of cognitive function, being particularly sensitive to impairment. Disorientation is the hallmark of the 'organic mental state' found in delirium and dementia. Abnormalities may be evident during the interview. Check the patient's knowledge of the current time and date, recognition of where he is (place) and identification of familiar people (person).

Memory function is divided into:
- Working memory: concerned with registering new information. Test by asking the patient to repeat the names of three objects (such as apple, table, penny); any mistake is significant. Alternatively, ask the patient to repeat a sequence of random numbers (digit span), where a person with normal function can produce at least five digits accurately
- Short-term memory: assessed by checking the patient's recollections of what has been discussed; tests then confirm and quantify any deficits. Give the patient some new information; once this has registered, check retention after 5 minutes. Do the same with the names of three objects; any error is significant. Alternatively, use a six-item name and address, where more than one error indicates impairment. Ask patients to remember the information and tell them that their recollection will be checked in a few minutes

• Long-term memory: assessed mainly from the personal history that the patient provides. Gaps and mistakes are often obvious, but some patients may confabulate so check the account with a family member if possible. Failing long-term memory is characteristic of dementia, although this store of knowledge can be remarkably intact in the presence of severe impairment of other cognitive functions. Confabulation, unconscious filling in of gaps in memory with fabricated facts, is associated with Korsakoff's psychosis, a complication of chronic alcoholism.

Impairment of attention and concentration occurs in many mental disorders and is not diagnostic. Impaired attention is observed as increased distractibility, with the patient responding inappropriately to extraneous stimuli, which may be either real, e.g. a noise outside the room, or unreal, e.g. auditory hallucinations. Concentration is the patient's ability to stick with a mental task. It is tested by using simple, repetitive sequences, such as asking the patient to repeat the months of the year in reverse or to do the 'serial 7s' test, in which 7 is subtracted from 100, then from 93, then 86 etc. Note the finishing point, the number of errors and the time taken.

Intelligence is estimated clinically from a combination of the history of educational attainment and occupations, and the evidence provided at interview of vocabulary, general knowledge, abstract thought, foresight and understanding. If in doubt as to whether the patient has a learning disability, or if there is a discrepancy between the history and presentation, a psychologist should formally test IQ.

Insight

Insight is assessed from the history and specific enquiries (Box 2.46).

Whether your patient is aware of the nature of his disorder has a crucial bearing on management, because lack of insight may lead to lack of cooperation with treatment. Occasionally, patients have no insight, but more often insight is partial (Box 2.47).

Risk assessment

A crucial part of every psychiatric history is the assessment of risk. Consider risk in terms of:

• Who is at risk. This is usually the patient and/or his family. Sometimes the threat may be directed at other specified individuals, such as neighbours, celebrities or health service staff, or more widely at people selected by age, ethnic group or some other factor such as sexual orientation or pregnancy. It can occasionally be random

• Nature of the risk:
   violence, including suicide or self-harm, homicide and attacks on others
   health, through refusal to accept, or non-compliance with, necessary care and treatment for a significant physical or mental illness

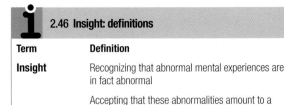

2.46 Insight: definitions

Term	Definition
Insight	Recognizing that abnormal mental experiences are in fact abnormal
	Accepting that these abnormalities amount to a mental illness
	Accepting the need for treatment

2.47 Insight: what to ask

• Do you think anything is wrong with you?
• What do you think is the matter with you?
• If you are ill, what do you think needs to happen to make you better?

welfare, through patients' inability to care appropriately for themselves or for people who are dependent on them, resulting in problems such as inadequate nutrition, heat, shelter or hygiene.

Evaluate risk in all psychiatric assessments, but in depth when:

• the presentation includes threats of self-harm or reports of command hallucinations
• the past history includes self-harm or violent behaviour
• the social circumstances show a recent, significant loss
• the mental disorder is strongly associated with risk, e.g. depression or a paranoid state (Box 2.48).

Screening questions for mental illnesses

There is no single question you can ask that clinches the diagnosis for any specific type of mental disorder.

Some features are closely associated with particular mental illnesses:

• passivity phenomena and schizophrenia
• re-experiencing an ordeal and post-traumatic stress disorder
• phobia of normal weight and anorexia nervosa.

However, these features may occur in other mental disorders.

Some symptoms are non-specific but important. They include:

• sleep disturbance
• impaired concentration
• anxiety.

A psychiatric diagnosis is made by identifying particular clusters of symptoms and mental state

2.48 Risk assessment: what to ask

Suicide/self-harm

- How do you feel about the future?
- Have you thought about ending your life?
- Have you made plans to end your life?
- Have you attempted to end your life?

Homicide/harm to others

- Are there people you know who don't deserve to live?
- Are there people you know who would be better off dead?
- Have you thought about harming somebody else?
- Have you been told to harm somebody else?

2.49 Screening questions for mental illnesses

When you suspect an anxiety disorder

- What physical symptoms have you been experiencing?
- How calm have you been feeling recently?
- Have there been any particular concerns or worries on your mind recently? If so, can you please tell me about them?

When you suspect a depressive disorder

- How has your mood been recently?
- Are you still enjoying things the way you used to?
- How do you view the future just now?

When you suspect schizophrenia

- Have you any beliefs that you think other people might find odd?
- Have you had any unusual experiences recently?
- Have you had any difficulty controlling your thinking?
- Have you heard people's voices when there's no one around? If so, where do you think the voices are coming from and what are they saying?

changes in the patient. Cover certain areas routinely when you suspect a particular mental illness (Box 2.49).

The physical examination

Physical and mental disorders are associated, so always consider the physical dimension in any patient presenting with a psychiatric complaint. The scale and content will depend on the age and health of patients, the nature of their mental disorder and their cooperation at the time. Usually, general observation, coupled with basic cardiovascular and neurological examination, will suffice.

Collateral history

The role and recording of third party information has already been described (p. 13). Collateral history is particularly important in psychiatric assessment, and sometimes is the key element, such as when the patient:

- has a severe learning disability or confusional state
- has a mental disorder that prevents effective communication
- is too disturbed
- refuses to be assessed.

Psychiatric rating scales

The use of psychiatric rating scales as clinical tools in psychiatric assessment is increasing. Most scales were developed as validated and reliable instruments that could be used in research studies to make a confident diagnosis or to be sensitive to severity or change in severity of illness. Some scales require special training; all must be used sensibly.

In routine practice, scales are employed to assess cognitive function when an organic brain disorder is suspected. Commonly used scales include:

- AMT (Abbreviated Mental Test): takes less than 5 minutes and is scored out of 10 (Box 2.50)
- MMSE (Mini Mental State Examination): takes about 5–10 minutes and is scored out of 30 (Box 2.51).

In general, scales are too inflexible and limited in scope to replace a well-conducted standard psychiatric interview, but they can be useful adjuncts for either screening or measuring response to treatment. Other well-known instruments include:

- general morbidity:
  GHQ (General Health Questionnaire)
- mood disorder:
  HADS (Hospital Anxiety and Depression Scale)
  BDI (Beck Depression Inventory)
- alcohol:
  CAGE questionnaire (Box 2.24)
  FAST questionnaire (Box 2.25).

2.50 The Abbreviated Mental Test

(Each question scores 1 mark; a score of 8 or less indicates confusion)

- Age
- Date of birth
- Time (to the nearest hour)
- Year
- Hospital name
- Recognition of two people, e.g. doctor, nurse
- Recall address
- Dates of First World War
- Name of the monarch
- Count backwards 20–1

2

2.51 Mini Mental State Examination (MMSE)

Orientation

- What is the year, season, date, day and month? (1 point for each; maximum total 5 points)
- Where are we: town, county, country, which hospital, surgery or house, and which floor? (1 point for each; maximum total 5 points)

Registration

- Name 3 objects, e.g. apple, table, penny, taking 1 second to say each one. Then ask the individual to repeat the names of all 3 objects. Give 1 point for each correct answer. Repeat the objects' names until all 3 are learned (up to 6 trials). Record the number of trials needed (maximum total 3 points)

Attention and calculation

- Spell 'world' backwards. Give 1 point for each letter that is in the right place, e.g. DLROW = 5 points, DLORW = 3 points
- Alternatively, do serial 7s: ask the person to count backwards from 100 in blocks of 7, i.e. 93, 86, 79, 72, 65. Stop after 5 subtractions. Give one point for each correct answer. If one answer is incorrect, e.g. 92, but the following answer is 7 less than the previous answer, i.e. 85, count the second answer as being correct. 1 point for each subtraction (maximum total 5 points)

Recall

- Ask for the 3 objects repeated above, e.g. apple, table, penny. Give 1 point for each correct object (maximum total 3 points)

Language

- Point to a pencil and ask the person to name this object (1 point). Do the same thing with a wrist-watch (1 point). (Maximum total 2 points)
- Ask the person to repeat the following: 'No ifs, ands or buts' (1 point). Allow only one trial (1 point)
- Give the person a piece of blank white paper and ask him/her to follow a 3-stage command: 'Take a paper in your right hand, fold it in half and put it on the floor' (1 point for each part that is correctly followed). (Maximum total 3 points)
- Write 'CLOSE YOUR EYES' in large letters and show it to the patient. Ask him or her to read the message and do what it says (give 1 point if the person actually closes his/her eyes)
- Ask the individual to write a sentence of his/her choice on a blank piece of paper. The sentence must contain a subject and a verb, and must make sense. Spelling, punctuation and grammar are not important (1 point)
- Show the person a drawing of 2 pentagons which intersect to form a quadrangle. Each side should be about 1.5 cm. Ask them to copy the design exactly as it is (1 point). All 10 angles need to be present and the two shapes must intersect to score 1 point. Tremor and rotation are ignored.

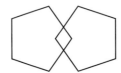

MEDICALLY UNEXPLAINED SYMPTOMS

Patients often present with symptoms that do not fit the characteristic patterns of specific diseases. Fewer than 30% of primary care patients have symptoms which can be explained by physical disease (Fig. 2.6). Sixty to eighty per cent of the 'healthy' population experience physical symptoms in any one week, while 10–20% of the healthy population are worried about the possibility of physical illness. When these persist they are called medically unexplained symptoms.

Symptoms may not fit a simple model of cause and effect and you must understand the context in which symptoms arise in patients' lives. This will help you to avoid adopting a cynical or judgemental approach, and maximize your understanding of patients. In turn, you will be better equipped to enable patients to deal with their symptoms more effectively.

This does not mean that symptoms are 'all in the mind' or are fabricated, only that we are unable to give a physical explanation for them. Doctors must understand patients as individuals and help them to cope with the distress that symptoms provoke. Thinking of the mind and body as separate and of disorders as organic or functional is unhelpful. Symptoms result from complex interactions between biological, social and psychological factors, each component being unique to the individual.

Only 5% of patients presenting with new symptoms to their GP have symptoms attributable to recognized physical disease. Symptoms resolve in 2 weeks without medical intervention in 75%. The remaining 25% may have medically unexplained symptoms and require a management approach focusing on their feelings, ideas, functioning and expectations (FIFE; p. 10). Most people with symptoms never consult a doctor. So what makes those seeking help different? (Fig. 2.7).

2.52 Key points: the psychiatric history

- Get as much background information and history from other sources as you can (with the patient's permission, if this is indicated).
- Concentrate initially on establishing rapport by helping your patients feel at ease and enabling them to tell their story as they wish.
- Be willing to modify the extent, order and content of the assessment to take account of your patient's background and presentation.
- Observe your patients closely to gain objective evidence of their mental state, especially non-verbal information.
- Your patients' speech gives you access to their thought form and content, mood and cognitive functioning.
- Consider your own response to your patients; you can often sense their mood. Do you feel sad, angry, irritated or confused, for example?
- Use brief formal tests to assess cognitive function.
- Consider standardized rating scales as a screening tool (and sometimes to monitor progress).
- Do not forget the importance of selective physical examination.
- Remember to assess these key issues: potential risks to self or others, degree of distress and disability, capacity to take decisions, insight into illness.

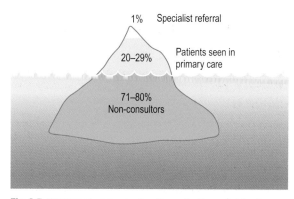

Fig. 2.7 What happens to people with medically unexplained symptoms.

2.53 Common functional syndromes[1]

Syndrome	Symptoms
Chronic fatigue syndrome	Persistent fatigue[2]
Irritable bowel syndrome	Abdominal pain, altered bowel habit (diarrhoea or constipation) and abdominal bloating
Chronic pain syndrome	Persistent pain in one or more parts of the body, sometimes following injury but which outlast the original trauma[2]
Fibromyalgia	Pain in the axial skeleton with trigger points (tender areas in the muscles)[2]
Chronic back pain	Pain, muscle tension or stiffness localized below the costal margin and above the inferior gluteal folds, with or without leg pain[2]

[1]In all cases, physical examination and investigation fail to reveal an underlying physical cause.
[2]Symptoms must have lasted more than 3 months.

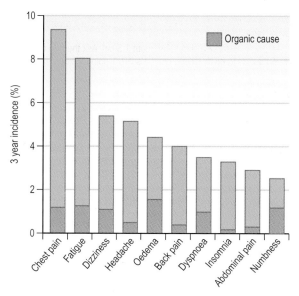

Fig. 2.6 Common symptoms presenting in primary care: showing the percentage with an organic cause.

How to recognize medically unexplained symptoms

Many symptoms are non-specific. When symptoms cluster in recognizable patterns, they are termed syndromes. When syndromes arise in the absence of identifiable physical abnormalities despite appropriate investigation, they are labelled functional syndromes. Some symptoms may indicate physical disease, but others are less likely to be associated with physical disease and should alert you to the possibility of a functional 'dis-ease' (Boxes 2.53 and 2.54).

Multiple symptoms

Patients with chronic physical disease are more likely to suffer emotional distress or psychiatric disorders such as depression. Having multiple unexplained symptoms affecting different body systems also raises the likelihood of depression. One in 6 patients have multiple symptoms, and the more symptoms patients have, the more likely they are to be suffering from psychiatric rather than physical disease. Having nine or more symptoms confers an 80% likelihood of having depression. What is cause and what is effect is not

33

2.54 Symptoms and their relationship to physical disease

More commonly	Less commonly
• Chest pain	• Fatigue
• Breathlessness	• Back pain
• Syncope	• Headache
• Abdominal pain	• Dizziness

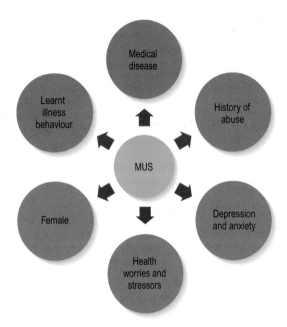

Fig. 2.8 Risk factors for symptoms with no physical cause.

known, and treating the underlying depression may not resolve the symptoms.

Risk factors

Certain risk factors increase the likelihood of multiple unexplained symptoms. Explore these where symptoms suggest the possibility of a functional problem (Fig. 2.8).

Management

Avoiding excessive investigation and treatment may improve outcome. In primary care, if there is no abnormality on physical examination, it is better to review the patient than to investigate initially because 75% of patients have self-limiting symptoms. This reduces both potential harm to patients and cost. 'Standard' investigations and management seeking to exclude all physical illness are costly and unhelpful, risk side-effects and do not give patients lasting reassurance. Explain what is not causing their symptoms, e.g. sharp left-sided intermittent chest pain lasting a few seconds in an otherwise fit 26-year-old

2.55 Examples of possible patient's concerns about common non-organic conditions

Symptoms	Patient's concern	Common diagnosis
Abdominal pain, relieved by defecation Bloating Low back pain Rabbit pellet stools Tired all the time	Bowel cancer	Irritable bowel syndrome
Band-like headache Onset during the day Not relieved by analgesics	Brain tumour	Tension headache
Sharp intermittent left-sided chest pain	Heart attack	Musculoskeletal chest pain

man is not angina, and reassure them about the good prognosis (Box 2.55).

Even complex and definitive investigations, such as coronary angiography, do not reassure patients for very long. Drug therapy is often ineffective, and even strong analgesics may have little effect on pain. Symptoms cause distress and patients want help in dealing with the effect of these on their lives. Avoid labelling patients in a way that prejudices your approach to them.

Try asking the patient two key questions:
• 'What do you think may have caused your symptoms and are you worried about it?'
• 'Have you thought of anything that might help your symptoms?'

Aim to address these concerns and ideas. Whether you see patients in primary or secondary care is important. There is a huge difference between primary and secondary care in the prevalence of disease in patients (Box 2.56).

Many patients with severe physical disability manage to function well and work in full-time jobs. Others with apparently modest symptoms are unable to function

 2.56 Differences in approach between primary and secondary care

The usual approach of the hospital specialist

• To reduce uncertainty
• To explore possibility
• To marginalize error

The usual approach of the GP

• To accept uncertainty
• To explore probability
• To marginalize danger

Adapted from Marshall Marinker

effectively or cope with the demands of full-time work. The lack of correlation between symptoms, disease and social functioning occurs in patients' response to treatment, so that even when they have a physical disease, treatment may not improve their symptoms. For example, triple therapy for *Helicobacter pylori*-associated gastritis in a patient with a peptic ulcer may cure the peptic ulcer but not relieve the dyspeptic symptoms (Box 2.57).

2.57 Key points: medically unexplained symptoms

- Some symptoms are less likely to be due to underlying pathology than others.
- The more symptoms a patient has:
  the more likely they are to have depression
  the less likely they are to have physical disease.
- Treating the depression does not always improve the symptoms.
- Treating the underlying disease does not always cure the symptoms.
- Focus on helping the symptom if there is no underlying organic disease.
- 75% of symptoms in primary care are self-limiting.
- Only 5% of patients presenting to their GP have symptoms attributable to serious physical disease.

DOCUMENTING THE FINDINGS: THE CASE NOTES

The case notes, or records, are the written record of a patient's medical condition. They include your initial findings, proposed investigations and plan of management, together with information about the patient's progress. Information is recorded for each episode of illness over time and shared by all the healthcare staff caring for a patient. Notes must therefore be accurate, legible, dated and signed. Primary care records contain the whole story of a patient's health rather than discrete episodes of hospital care, and follow the patient between practices (Box 2.58).

You may write notes while talking with a patient, but do not let this interrupt the discussion and maintain as much eye contact as possible. Active listening is difficult if you are writing, so make brief notes to remind yourself of the important points, and write up the full history afterwards. Write up the physical findings after you have completed the examination. Only record objective findings and never make judgemental or flippant comments.

Although structured proformas for recording history and examination findings are used in many hospitals, it is not necessary to record every detail in every patient. Only record negative findings if they are relevant.

2.58 Information in the case record

- History and examination findings
- Investigations and results
- Management plan
- Assessments by other health professionals, e.g. dietitians, health visitors
- Information and education provided to patients and their relatives
- Correspondence about the patient
- Patient's progress
- Advance directives or 'living will'
- Contact details for next of kin

2.59 Describing wounds

Position

- Where on the body, including which aspect of a limb

Size and orientation

- e.g. 5 cm × 3 mm vertical scratch

Appearance

- e.g. Colour, shape

Type of lesion

- Abrasion: loss of the outer skin due to impact with a rough surface
- Scratch: linear abrasion due to drawing of a sharp point over the skin
- Bruise: bleeding within the tissues beneath the skin
- Laceration: tearing of the skin due to blunt trauma; ragged edges
- Incised wound: cut or gash; sharp edges
- Penetrating wound: depth is greater than length; breaches full skin thickness

For example, in a patient with breathlessness, the negative details of the respiratory enquiry are important but negative responses to the gastrointestinal enquiry can be condensed to a single entry of 'none'. You may use abbreviations but they should not be obscure or ambiguous (Fig. 2.9). The prefix '°' is often used to signify 'no': for example, '°tenderness'. Use diagrams to show the site and size of superficial injuries or wounds, and for the abdomen to illustrate the position of tenderness, masses or scars (Fig. 8.14, p. 199). Describe injuries accurately; you may be asked to give legal evidence from the notes many months later (Box 2.59).

Unitary or 'multidisciplinary' notes allow the whole team to record their findings in one document rather than each keeping separate case records. Unitary records can be cumbersome but encourage shared care, avoid duplication and make it easy to access information.

Date : 03.08.09
Time : 14.00

MARY BROWN aged 86
32 Tartan Cresc.
Edinburgh
DOB 12.09.33

Emergency admission to CCU via GP: Dr Wells, High St., Edinburgh

History from patient

PC	Chest pain	2 hours
	Breathlessness	1 hour
	Dizziness	30 mins

HPC

Severe pain 'like a band around chest' while watching TV which has now lasted 2 hours despite using GTN.
Radiates to jaw and inner aspect of L arm.
Has gradually become breathless over the last hour and dizzy in last 30 minutes.

First began 6 months ago: episode of lower retrosternal chest pain after walking about 1/2 mile uphill:
        • no associated palpitation or SOB.
Two further episodes over the next 3 months.

3 months ago: increasing frequency of pain
                • now brought on by walking 200 yards on the flat or climbing 1 flight of stairs
                • worse after heavy meals
                • other features of pain as before.

2 months ago: visited GP who diagnosed angina. Prescribed GTN which gave effective relief.

1 week ago: three episodes of chest pain at rest, all immediately relieved by GTN.

Smokes 20/day since aged 19.
°Blackouts °pain in calves on exertion.

PH	Tonsillectomy	1952	Hospital X
	Perforated peptic ulcer	1977	Hospital Y
	COPD	Since 1990	General practitioner

°MI, °DM, ° J, °HBP, °Stroke, °RF, °TB

DH

		DOSE	FREQUENCY	DURATION
	Salbutamol inhaler	2 puffs	As necessary	3 years
	Zopiclone	7.5mg	At night	6 months
	Senokot (self medication)	2 tabs	2–3 times per week	10 years
	GTN spray	1 puff	As required	2 months
	Allergies			

FH

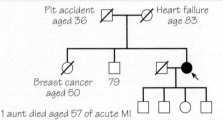

Pit accident aged 36 — Heart failure age 83

Breast cancer aged 50   79

1 aunt died aged 57 of acute MI

1

Fig. 2.9 Case notes: example

Demographic Details

Always record
- The patient's name and address, date of birth and age
- Any national health identification number such as CHI in the UK
- Source of referral e.g. from Accident and Emergency or General Practitioner
- GP's name and address
- Source of history e.g. patient, relative, carer
- Date and time of examination

Presenting Complaint (PC)

State the major problem in one or two of the patient's own words (or give a brief list), followed by the duration of each. Do not use medical terminology.

History of Presenting Complaint (HPC)

Describe the onset, nature and course of each symptom.
Paraphrase the patient's account and condense it if necessary.
Omit irrelevant details.
Put particularly telling comments in inverted commas.
Include other parts of the history if relevant, such as the smoking history in patients with cardiac or respiratory presentations, or family history in disorders with a possible genetic trait such as hypercholesterolaemia or diabetes.
Correct grammar is not necessary.
GTN – glyceryl trinitrate
SOB – short of breath

Past History (PH)

Tabulate in chronological order.
Include important negatives, e.g. in a patient with chest pain ask about previous myocardial infarction, angina, hypertension or diabetes mellitus and record whether these are present or absent. Jaundice is important because it may pose a risk to health care workers if due to hepatitis B or C.

COPD – Chronic obstructive pulmonary disease
MI – Myocardial infarction
DM – Diabetes mellitus
J – Jaundice
HBP – Hypertension
RF – Rheumatic fever

Drug History (DH)

Tabulate these and include any allergies particularly to drugs.
Record any previous adverse drug reactions prominently on the front of the notes as well as inside.

Family History (FH)

Record the age and current health or the causes of or the ages at death of the patient's parents, siblings and children.
Use the symbols shown in Fig. 2.3 to construct a pedigree chart.

2

SH

Retired cleaner.
Widow for 3 years. Lives alone in sheltered housing.
Smoked 20/day from age 19.
Teetotal.
HH once a week for cleaning and shopping. Daughter nearby visits regularly.

SE

CVS: See above.

RS: Long-standing cough most days with white sputum on rising in morning only. °Haemoptysis.
Wheezy in cold weather.

GI: Weight steady.
Nil else of note.

GUS: PARA 1 + 0. °PMB, °urinary symptoms

CNS: Nil of note.

MSS: Occasional pain and stiffness in right knee on exertion for 5 years.

ES: Nil of note.

O/E

Anxious, frail, cachectic lady.
Weight 45 kg. Height 1.25 m
2 cm craggy mass in upper, outer quadrant L breast. Fixed to underlying tissues.
<u>Patient unaware of this</u>
1 cm node in apex of left axilla.
°Pallor, °cyanosis, °jaundice, °clubbing.

CVS

P90 reg, small volume, normal character.
BP 140/80 JVP + 3 cms normal character, °oedema, AB 5ICS MCL, °thrills.
HS I + II + 2/6 ESM at LLSE °radiation.
°Bruits.
PP:

	Radial	Brachial	Carotid	Femoral	Popliteal	Post. Tibial	Dorsalis pedis
R	+	+	+	+	+/-	+/-	+/-
L	+	+	+	+	+	+	+

(Normal +, Reduced +/-, Absent -)

RS

Trachea central. Reduced cricosternal distance and intercostal indrawing on inspiration.
Expansion reduced but symmetrical.
PN resonant.
BS vesicular and quiet.
VR normal and symmetrical.

Fig. 2.9 (Continued)

Social History (SH)
Occupation
Marital status
Living circumstances; type of housing and with whom
Smoking
Alcohol
Illicit drug use (if appropriate)
Social support in the frail or disabled

HH – home help

Systematic Enquiry (SE)
Document positive responses that do not feature in the HPC.

CVS – Cardiovascular system
  RS – Respiratory system
  GI – Gastrointestinal system
GUS – Genito-urinary system
PMB – Postmenopausal bleeding
CNS – Central nervous system
MSS – Musculoskeletal system
  ES – Endocrine system

General / On examination (OE)
Physical appearance e.g. frail, drowsy, breathless
Mental state e.g. anxious, distressed, confused
Undernourished, cachectic, obese
Abnormal smells e.g. ketones, alcohol, uraemia, foetor hepaticus
Record height, weight and waist circumference
Skin e.g. cyanosis, pallor, jaundice, any specific lesions or rashes
Breasts, normal or describe any mass
Hands; finger clubbing, or abnormalities of skin and nails
Lymph nodes; characteristics and site

Cardiovascular System (CVS)
Pulse (P) rate, rhythm, character and volume
Blood pressure (BP)
Jugular venous pressure (JVP) height and character
Presence or absence of ankle oedema
Apex beat (AB) position, character, presence of thrills
Heart sounds (HS) any added sounds, murmurs and grade
Peripheral pulses (PP) and bruits

5ICS – 5th intercostal space
 MCL – Mid clavicular line
 ESM – Ejection systolic murmur
LLSE – Lower left sternal edge

Respiratory System (RS)
Any chest wall deformity
Trachea central or deviated
Signs of hyperinflation
Expansion and its symmetry
Percussion note (PN) and site of any abnormality
Breath sounds (BS), any added sounds and site of abnormality
Vocal resonance (VR) and site of abnormality

Abdo.
Normal oral mucosa
Upper midline scar
Hernial orifices intact
°Tenderness or guarding
°Masses
°LKKS or ascites
BS normal
PR not done
FOB negative
PV not performed

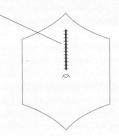
Scar

CNS
AMT 9/10
Cranial nerves II–XII: PERLA, NAD
Speech normal

	RIGHT		LEFT	
	UL	LL	UL	LL
Power	5	5	5	5
Tone	normal (n)	n	n	n
Light touch	n	n	n	n
Position	n	n	n	n
Coordination	n	n	n	n

Reflexes	K	A	B	T	S	Pl
R	++	+	++	+	+	flexor
L	++	+	++	+	+	flexor

(increased +++, normal ++, diminished +, absent -)

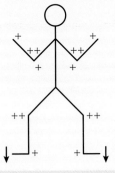

MSS
Heberden's nodes on index and middle fingers bilaterally.
Full ROM in all joints.
Crepitus in right knee. No other bony abnormality.

IMPRESSION △

Active problems
1 Chest pain suggestive of acute coronary syndrome
2 Left breast lump and axillary node suspicious of cancer
3 Smoker

Inactive problems
1 Stable COPD
2 Perforated duodenal ulcer 1977
3 Possible osteoarthritis of right knee

3

Fig. 2.9 (Continued)

Abdominal System (AS)

Mouth
  Any abnormality – own teeth or dentures
Abdomen
  Scars and site
  Shape, distended or scaphoid
  Hernial orifices
  Tenderness and guarding and site of this
  Masses and description of these
  Enlargement of liver, kidneys or spleen (shorten to LKKS)
  Ascites if present
  Bowel sounds (BS); presence and character
  Rectal examination (PR) record whether or not it was
  performed and your findings. It should not be done in patients
  with possible cardiac chest pain, as arrhythmias may be provoked
  in acute MI.
  In women; vaginal examination (VE) is only carried
  out if relevant
  In men; external genitalia

FOB – Faecal occult blood testing

Central Nervous System (CNS)

In older patients record the abbreviated mental test (AMT) score
In impaired consciousness, head injury or possible raised
intracranial pressure record the Glasgow Coma Scale (GCS)

Abnormal speech
Cranial nerves; record abnormalities only
Fundoscopy
Tabulate the remaining examination
If it is relevant record the presence or absence of tremor, gait,
abnormality, fasciculation, dyspraxia, two point discrimination,
stereognosis or sensory neglect.

PERLA – Pupils equal and react to light and accommodation
  NAD – No abnormality detected
    UL – Upper limb
    LL – Lower limb
    K – Knee
    A – Ankle
    B – Biceps
    T – Triceps
    S – Supinator
    Pl – Plantar

Musculoskeletal System (MSS)

Gait if abnormal
Muscle or soft tissue changes
Swelling, colour, heat, tenderness
Deformities in the bones of joints
Limitations of ranges of movements (ROM) in any affected joint

Clinical Diagnosis or Impression

Record your conclusions and the most likely diagnoses in order
of probability.
In patients with multiple pathology make a problem list so the key
issues are seen immediately.

△ Diagnosis

Plan

ECG performed on admission shows sinus rhythm and deep ST depression in leads II, III and aVF

Troponin at 12 hours
Repeat ECG in 1 hour
Chest X-ray
Full blood count
Urea and electrolytes, glucose

Oxygen and cardiac monitor
IV morphine and metacloprmide
Aspirin and clopidogrel
Low molecular weight heparin
Diltiazem as beta-blocker contraindicated due to COPD
Advice to stop smoking

When stable
1 Review anti-anginal management
2 Referral for mammography and fine needle aspiration of breast lump
3 Spirometry and assessment of inhaler technique

Information given

Diagnosis and treatment explained to patient and daughter
N.B. Breast lump not mentioned at this stage until discussed with senior staff

A. Doctor (signed)

A. DOCTOR   (Date and Time) capitals

Progress notes

3.8.09
1800 Ward Round – Dr Consultant

No further chest pain

O/E
P70 BP 100/70
JVP not elevated, °oedema
HS I + II and ESM as above
Chest clear
Breast lump noted

ECG at 4 hours – resolution of inferior ST changes

Impression

Acute coronary syndrome

Plan

Await troponin
Continue LMW heparin
Check liquid profile
For echocardiography in view of murmur then consider ACE inhibitor
Spirometry and assessment of inhaler technique

Consultant to discuss finding of breast lump
with patient and daughter

A. Doctor (signed)

A. DOCTOR   (Date and Time) capitals

4

42   **Fig. 2.9** (Continued)

Plan
- List the investigations required. When a result is already available, for example of an electrocardiograph, record it.
- Record any immediate management instigated
- If uncertain about an investigation or treatment, precede with a '?' and discuss with a more senior member of staff

Information given
Document what you have told the patient and any other family member. It is also important to document any diagnosis that you have not discussed.
If the patient voices any concerns or fears, document these too.

Progress Notes
Follow the same structure with these additions
- Changes in the patient's symptoms
- Examination findings
- Results of new investigations
- Clinical impression of the patient's progress
- Plans for further management, particularly drug changes.
Make progress notes regularly depending on the speed of change in the patient's condition; in an intensive therapy setting, this may be several times a day but, in a stable situation, daily or alternate days.
Date, time and sign all entries.
Record any unexpected change in the patient's condition as well as routine progress notes.

Computer records

Records may be held on paper or computer. Computers allow easy access to medical and prescribing information during the consultation. All electronic data must be stored securely; they should be accessible only to relevant staff and must be password-protected. Paperless general practices hold all patient information on computer and this can be downloaded on to portable palmtops for domiciliary use. Smart cards carried by patients holding their entire medical record are being developed.

Confidentiality

The case record is confidential and constitutes a legal document that may be used in a court of law. Details cannot be shared with anyone who is not involved in a patient's care, unless the patient gives fully informed written consent. This includes insurance companies, lawyers, the police and research workers. You may only break confidence if a patient is posing a risk to themself or other members of the public.

Patients increasingly have the right to receive a copy of their paper case record; in the UK, for example, the Health Records Act of 1990 governs this. Some patients already hold their own records, usually when antenatal or diabetic care is shared between hospital and community. Patients may have the right to see any personal information held on computer, including their medical records (in the UK this is granted by the Data Protection Act 1998). You can stop patients seeing a part of their record if you think it would seriously harm their physical or mental health or that of any other individual. Remember this when you record information about third parties, particularly in cases of sexual abuse.

Letter-writing

Letters must be written when referring a patient to a specialist, and to the GP following an outpatient consultation or hospital admission. The hospital discharge letter (or summary) is structured in a standard format, which can be adapted for referral and outpatient letters. The text of the letter should be brief; concentrate on the main issues but include any unexpected findings or complications and relevant investigation results. Include the reason for referral rather than the diagnosis, along with full details of the

2.60 Discharge letter headings

- Diagnosis
    Primary or active
    Inactive: list comorbidities or previous illnesses
- Procedures or operations
- History (include important social factors)
- Examination
- Investigations: only give detailed results if abnormal
- Clinical progress: brief description of course during hospital stay
- Social arrangements where relevant
- Drugs on discharge, including doses and duration of course
- Follow-up arrangements
- Information given to patients (and relatives)

patient's past history and current medication. Ensure copies of letters are sent to the patient's GP and any other specialist involved in their care.

Most letters are dictated and typed, although structured computerized letters may also be used. When using a dictation machine, remember to:

- State your name and the date of dictation
- State the patient's name and date of birth
- State other important dates: e.g. the patient's attendance at an outpatient appointment, or hospital admission
- Speak slowly and clearly. Spell out unusual medical terms
- Say 'stop' at the end of a sentence, and 'new para' as required; detailed punctuation is not needed. Use paragraph headings as in Box 2.60.

Letters are easier to dictate when you have just seen the patient rather than several days later.

2.61 Key points: documenting the findings

- Always record, date and sign your findings, investigations and management plan for the patient.
- Record objective findings only.
- Record all abnormal findings, but only record the negative findings if they are relevant.
- The notes are confidential and details must be shared only with professionals directly involved in the patient's care.
- Patients have the right to see their case notes.

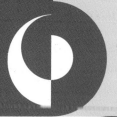

Graham Douglas
John S. Bevan

The general examination

3

3

THE SETTING FOR A PHYSICAL EXAMINATION

Regardless of the setting, privacy is essential when you examine a patient. Pulling the curtains around the bed in a ward obscures vision but not sound. Talk quietly but ensure good communication, which may be difficult with deaf or elderly patients (p. 9). The room should be warm and well lit. Subtle abnormalities of complexion such as mild jaundice are easier to detect in natural light. The height of the examination couch or bed should be adjustable, with a step to enable patients to get on to it easily. An adjustable backrest is essential, particularly for breathless patients who cannot lie flat.

Seek permission and sensitively, but adequately, expose the areas of the body to be examined; cover the rest of the patient with a blanket or sheet to ensure that he or she does not become cold. Avoid unnecessary exposure and embarrassment. A female patient will appreciate the opportunity to replace her bra after her chest examination and before you examine her abdomen. Tactfully ask relatives to leave the room before the physical examination. Sometimes it is appropriate for a relative to remain if the patient is very apprehensive, if you need a translator or if the patient requests it. Parents should always be present when you examine children (p. 411). For any intimate examination you should always offer a chaperone to prevent misunderstandings and to provide support and encouragement for the patient (p. 12). Record the chaperone's name and presence. If patients decline the offer, respect their wishes and record this in the notes.

Collect together all the equipment you need before starting the examination (Box 3.1).

SEQUENCE FOR PERFORMING A PHYSICAL EXAMINATION

After taking a history, you should have a differential diagnosis in mind. Examine the patient, trying to elicit the signs that will confirm or refute your diagnoses.

3.1 Equipment required for a full examination

- Stethoscope
- Pen-torch
- Measuring tape
- Ophthalmoscope
- Sphygmomanometer
- Tendon hammer
- Tuning fork
- Cotton wool
- Disposable Neurotips
- Wooden spatula
- Thermometer

- Magnifying glass
- Accurate weighing scales and a height-measuring device (preferably a Harpenden stadiometer)
- Disposable gloves, lubricant gel and a proctoscope may also be required
- Facilities for obtaining blood samples, urinalysis and faecal occult blood testing should be available

With experience, you will develop your own style and sequence of physical examination. A regular routine reduces errors of omission.

The sequence of examination is:

- **Inspection**
- **Palpation**
- **Percussion**
- **Auscultation** (Fig. 3.1).

Learn to integrate these smoothly into each component of the physical examination. There is no single correct way of performing a physical examination; Box 3.2 provides a suggested sequence.

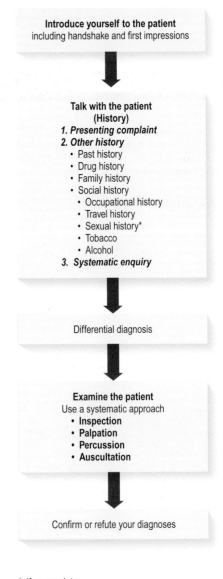

Introduce yourself to the patient
including handshake and first impressions

Talk with the patient
(History)
1. Presenting complaint
2. Other history
- Past history
- Drug history
- Family history
- Social history
  - Occupational history
  - Travel history
  - Sexual history*
  - Tobacco
  - Alcohol
3. Systematic enquiry

Differential diagnosis

Examine the patient
Use a systematic approach
- Inspection
- Palpation
- Percussion
- Auscultation

Confirm or refute your diagnoses

* if appropriate

Fig. 3.1 Overall plan of clinical assessment.

3.2 A personal system for performing a physical examination

- Handshake and introduction
- Note general appearances while talking
  Does the patient look well?
  Any immediate and obvious clues, e.g. obesity, plethora, breathlessness
  Complexion
- Hands and radial pulse
- Face
- Mouth
- Neck
- Thorax
  Breasts
  Heart
  Lungs
- Abdomen
- Lower limbs
  Oedema
  Circulation
  Locomotor function and neurology
- Upper limbs
  Movement and neurology
- Cranial nerves, including fundoscopy
- Blood pressure
- Temperature
- Height and weight
- Urinalysis

FIRST IMPRESSIONS

The physical examination starts as soon as you see the patient. Assess patients' general demeanour and external appearance, and watch how they rise from their chair and walk into the room. Often your general observations point to a specific diagnosis or to the system causing problems.

The handshake

Observe your patient, even before you introduce yourself and shake hands. This may provide diagnostic clues (Box 3.3). Greet your patient in a friendly but professional manner. Note if his right hand works; in patients with a right hemiparesis you may need to shake their left hand. Avoid too firm a grip, particularly in patients with arthritis.

3.3 Information from a handshake

Features	Diagnosis
Cold, sweaty hands	Anxiety
Cold, dry hands	Raynaud's phenomenon
Hot, sweaty hands	Hyperthyroidism
Large, fleshy, sweaty hands	Acromegaly
Dry, coarse skin	Regular water exposure Manual occupation Hypothyroidism
Delayed relaxation of grip	Myotonic dystrophy
Deformed hands/fingers	Trauma Rheumatoid arthritis Dupuytren's contracture

Facial expression and general demeanour

Ask yourself:
- 'Does this patient look well?'
- 'How does this patient make me feel?' If you are aware of feeling tense, your patient may be anxious or thyrotoxic.

Facial expression and eye-to-eye contact are indicators of physical and psychological well-being (Box 3.4), but in some cultures direct eye-to-eye contact is impolite. Patients who are deliberately self-harming may cover their face with the bedclothes and be reluctant to communicate. Actively recognize the features of anxiety, fear, anger or grief, and explore the reasons for these. Some patients conceal anxieties and depression with inappropriate cheerfulness.

Clothing

Clothing gives clues about patients' personality, state of mind and social circumstances. Young people wearing dirty clothes may have problems with alcohol or drug addiction, or be making a personal statement. Unkempt elderly patients with faecal or urinary soiling may be unable to look after themselves because of physical disease, immobility, dementia or other mental illness. Anorectic patients wear baggy clothing to cover weight loss. Consider blood-borne viral infections, e.g. hepatitis B or C in patients with tattoos. A MedicAlert bracelet (Fig. 3.2) or necklace highlights important medical conditions and treatments.

Complexion

Facial colour depends on oxyhaemoglobin, reduced haemoglobin, melanin and carotene. Unusual skin colours are due to abnormal pigments: for example, the sallow

3.4 Abnormal facial expressions

Features	Diagnosis
Poverty of expression	Parkinsonism
Startled expression	Hyperthyroidism
Apathy, with poverty of expression and poor eye contact	Depression
Apathy, with pale and puffy skin	Hypothyroidism
Lugubrious expression with bilateral ptosis	Myotonic dystrophy
Agitated expression	Anxiety Hyperthyroidism Hypomania

yellow-brownish tinge seen in chronic renal failure. A bluish tinge is produced by abnormal haemoglobins, such as sulphaemoglobin or methaemoglobin, or by drugs, such as dapsone. Some drug metabolites cause striking abnormal coloration of the skin, particularly in areas exposed to light: for example, mepacrine (yellow), clofazimine (brownish-black), amiodarone (bluish-grey) and phenothiazines (slate-grey) (Fig. 3.3).

Haemoglobin

Untanned Caucasian skin is pink due to the red pigment oxyhaemoglobin in the superficial capillary–venous plexuses. A pale complexion suggests anaemia (Box 3.5). The pallor of anaemia is best seen in the mucous membranes of the conjunctivae, lips and tongue and in the nail beds (Fig. 3.4).

Pallor from vasoconstriction occurs during a faint or from fear. Vasodilatation may produce a pink complexion, even in anaemia. Perimenopausal women and patients with carcinoid syndrome may have transient pink

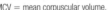

3.5 Types of anaemia

Microcytic (MCV < 80 fl)

- Chronic blood loss
- Iron deficiency
- Thalassaemia
- Sideroblastic anaemia

Macrocytic (MCV > 96 fl)

- Megaloblastic marrow
- Vitamin B12 deficiency
- Folic acid deficiency
- Excess alcohol
- Haemolytic disorders
- Liver disease
- Hypothyroidism

Normocytic (MCV 80–96 fl)

- Acute blood loss
- Anaemia of chronic disease
- Chronic renal failure
- Connective tissue disorders
- Marrow infiltration

MCV = mean corpuscular volume.

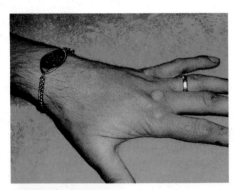

Fig. 3.2 MedicAlert bracelet.

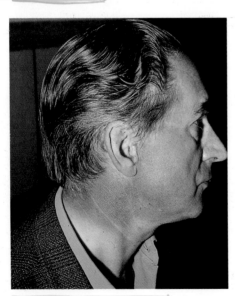

Fig. 3.3 Phenothiazine-induced pigmentation.

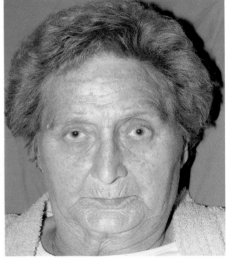

A

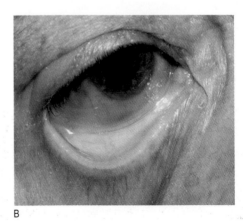

B

Fig. 3.4 Anaemia. (A) Facial pallor. **(B)** Conjunctival pallor.

flushing, particularly of the face, due to vasodilatation caused by circulating oestrogens. Facial plethora is caused by raised haemoglobin concentration with elevated haematocrit (polycythaemia; Box 3.6).

Cyanosis

Cyanosis is a blue discoloration of the skin and mucous membranes that occurs when the absolute concentration of deoxygenated haemoglobin is >50 g/l. This corresponds to an arterial oxygen saturation of <90% and usually indicates underlying cardiac or pulmonary disease. It can be difficult to detect, particularly in black and Asian patients.

Central cyanosis

This is seen at the lips and tongue (Fig. 3.5). Anaemic or hypovolaemic patients rarely have central cyanosis because severe hypoxia is required to produce the necessary concentration of deoxygenated haemoglobin. Patients with polycythaemia can become cyanosed at normal arterial oxygen saturation.

Peripheral cyanosis

This occurs in the hands, feet or ears, usually when they are cold. It is also found with central cyanosis, but is most often seen with poor peripheral circulation due to shock, heart failure, peripheral vascular disease, Raynaud's phenomenon and venous obstruction, e.g. deep vein thrombosis.

Melanin

Skin colour is greatly influenced by the deposition of melanin (Box 3.7).

3.6 Types of polycythaemia

Primary

- Polycythaemia rubra vera

Secondary

- Hypoxia
  Chronic lung disease
  Cyanotic congenital
  heart disease
  Altitude
- Excess erythropoietin
  Adult polycystic kidney
  disease
  Renal cancer
  Ovarian cancer

Vitiligo

This is a chronic condition with bilateral symmetrical depigmentation, commonly of the face, neck and extensor aspects of the limbs, resulting in irregular pale patches of skin. It is associated with autoimmune diseases, such as diabetes mellitus, thyroid and adrenal disorders, and pernicious anaemia (Fig. 3.6).

Albinism

This is an inherited disorder in which patients have little or no melanin in their skin or hair. The amount

3.7 Causes of abnormal melanin production

Condition	Mechanism
Underproduction	
Vitiligo (patchy depigmentation)	Autoimmune destruction of melanocytes
Albinism	Genetic deficiency of tyrosinase
Hypopituitarism	Reduced pituitary secretion of melanotrophic peptides, growth hormone and sex steroids
Overproduction	
Adrenal insufficiency (Addison's disease)	Increased pituitary secretion of melanotrophic peptides
Nelson's syndrome (may occur after bilateral adrenalectomy for Cushing's disease)	Increased pituitary secretion of melanotrophic peptides
Cushing's syndrome due to ectopic ACTH secretion by tumours, e.g. small cell lung cancer	Ectopic release of melanotrophic peptides by dysregulated tumour cells
Pregnancy and oral contraceptives	Increased levels of sex hormones
Haemochromatosis	Iron deposition and stimulation of melanocytes

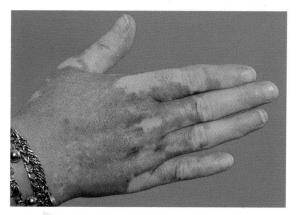

Fig. 3.6 Vitiligo.

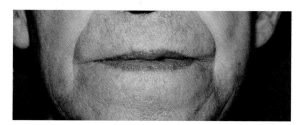

Fig. 3.5 Central cyanosis of the lips.

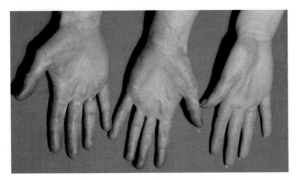

Fig. 3.7 Hypercarotenaemia.

of pigment in the iris varies; some individuals have reddish eyes, but most have blue.

Overproduction of melanin

This can be due to excess of the pituitary hormone, adrenocorticotrophic hormone (ACTH), as in adrenal insufficiency. It produces brown pigmentation of the skin, particularly in skin creases, recent scars, sites overlying bony prominences, areas exposed to pressure, e.g. belts and bra straps, and the mucous membranes of the lips and mouth, where it results in muddy brown patches (Figs 5.12A, B and C, p. 100).

Pregnancy and oral contraceptives

These may produce blotchy pigmentation of the face (chloasma). Pregnancy also causes increased pigmentation of the areolae, axillae, genital skin and a dark line in the midline of the lower abdomen (linea nigra).

Carotene

Hypercarotenaemia occurs in people who eat large amounts of raw carrots and tomatoes, and in hypothyroidism. A yellowish discoloration is seen on the face, palms and soles, but not the sclerae, which distinguishes it from jaundice (Fig. 3.7).

Bilirubin

Jaundice is detectable when serum bilirubin concentration is $>50\,\mu mol/l$ and the sclerae, mucous membranes and skin become yellow (Fig. 8.10, p. 195). In longstanding jaundice a green colour develops in the sclerae and skin due to biliverdin. Patients with pernicious anaemia have a characteristic lemon-yellow complexion due to a combination of mild jaundice and anaemia.

Iron

Haemochromatosis increases skin pigmentation due to iron deposition and increased melanin production (Fig. 3.8). Iron deposition in the pancreas causes diabetes mellitus and the combination with skin pigmentation is known as 'bronzed diabetes'.

Haemosiderin, a haemoglobin breakdown product, is deposited in the skin of the lower legs following extravasation of blood into subcutaneous tissues from

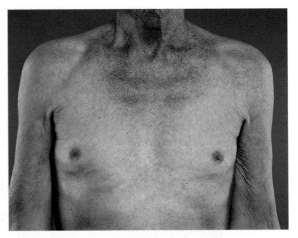

Fig. 3.8 Haemochromatosis with increased skin pigmentation.

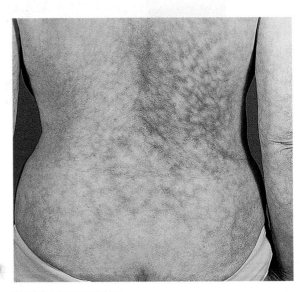

Fig. 3.9 Erythema ab igne.

venous insufficiency. Local deposition of haemosiderin (erythema ab igne or 'granny's tartan') occurs with heat damage to the skin from sitting too close to a fire or from applying local heat, such as a hot water bottle, to the site of pain (Fig. 3.9).

Odours

Everybody has a natural smell, produced by apocrine sweat acted on by bacteria; this may be altered by antiperspirants, deodorants and perfume. Excessive sweating and poor personal hygiene increase body odour and may be compounded by dirty or soiled clothing and stale urine. Excessive body odour occurs in:

- extreme old age or infirmity
- major mental illness

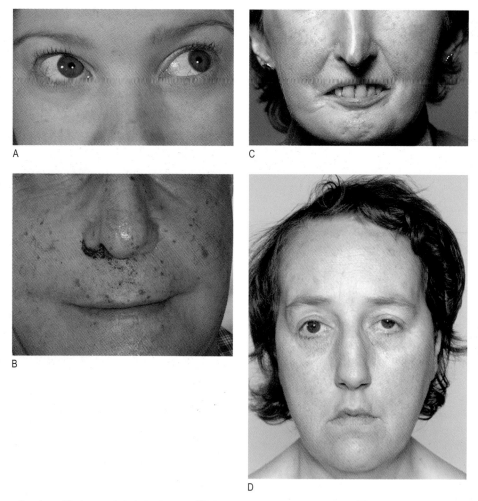

Fig. 3.10 Some disorders with characteristic facial features. **(A)** Blue sclera of osteogenesis imperfecta. **(B)** Telangiectasia around the mouth typical of hereditary haemorrhagic telangiectasia. **(C)** Systemic sclerosis with 'beaking' of the nose and taut skin around the mouth. **(D)** Dystrophia myotonica with frontal balding and bilateral ptosis.

- alcohol or drug misuse
- physical disability preventing normal hygiene
- severe learning difficulties.

Tobacco's characteristic lingering smell pervades skin, hair and clothing. Marijuana (cannabis) can also be identified by smell. The smell of alcohol on a patient's breath, particularly in the morning, suggests an alcohol problem.

Bad breath (halitosis) is caused by decomposing food wedged between the teeth, gingivitis, stomatitis, atrophic rhinitis and tumours of the nasal passages. Other characteristic odours include:

- stale 'mousy' smell of the volatile amine, methyl mercaptan, in patients with liver failure (fetor hepaticus)
- sweetness of the breath (like nail varnish remover) in diabetic ketoacidosis or starvation due to acetone
- fishy or ammoniacal smell on the breath in uraemia
- putrid or fetid smell of chronic suppuration due to bronchiectasis or lung abscess
- foul-smelling belching in patients with gastric outlet obstruction
- offensive faecal smell in patients with gastrocolic fistula.

'Spot diagnoses'

Many disorders have characteristic facial features (Fig. 3.10). For example, osteogenesis imperfecta is an

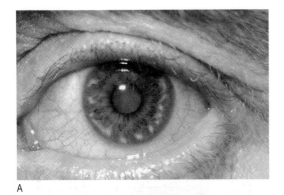

A

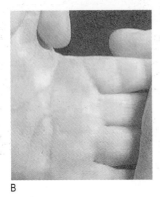

B

Fig. 3.11 Down's syndrome. (A) Brushfield's spots: grey-white areas of depigmentation in the iris. **(B)** Single palmar crease.

autosomal dominant condition causing fragile and brittle bones in which the sclerae are blue due to abnormal collagen formation. In systemic sclerosis the skin is thickened and tight, causing loss of the normal wrinkles and skin folds, 'beaking of the nose', and narrowing and puckering of the mouth. Hereditary haemorrhagic telangiectasia is also an autosomal dominant condition associated with small dilated capillaries or terminal arteries (telangiectasia) on the lips and tongue. Dystrophia myotonica is another autosomal dominant condition with characteristic features of frontal balding, bilateral ptosis and delayed relaxation of grip after a handshake.

Major chromosomal abnormalities

There are several genetic or chromosomal syndromes that should be easily recognized on first contact with the patient.

Down's syndrome (trisomy 21—47, XX/XY+21)

Down's syndrome is characterized by typical physical features, including short stature, a small head with flat occiput, upslanting palpebral fissures, epicanthic folds, a small nose with a poorly developed bridge and small ears. Grey-white areas of depigmentation are seen in the iris (Brushfield's spots; Fig. 3.11A). The hands are broad with a single palmar crease (Fig. 3.11B),

the fingers are short and the little finger is curved. The incidence of Down's syndrome increases with maternal age from 1:15 000 live births at age 20 to 1:50 at age 43. It accounts for nearly one-third of children with severe learning difficulties and patients have an increased risk of congenital heart disease, leukaemia and hypothyroidism.

Turner's syndrome (45XO)

Turner's syndrome is due to loss of a sex chromosome. It occurs in 1:2500 live female births and is the most common cause of delayed puberty in girls. Typical features include short stature, webbing of the neck, small chin, low-set ears, low hairline, short fourth finger, increased carrying angle at the elbows and widely spaced nipples ('shield-like chest').

Achondroplasia (dwarfism)

This is an autosomal dominant disease of cartilage caused by mutation of the fibroblast growth factor gene. Although the trunk is of normal length, the limbs are very short and broad. The vault of the skull is enlarged, the face is small and the bridge of the nose is flat.

THE HANDS

▶ Examination sequence

The hands
▶ Inspect the dorsal and then palmar aspects of both hands.
▶ Note changes in the:
  - Skin
  - Nails
  - Soft tissues (evidence of muscle-wasting)
  - Tendons
  - Joints.
▶ Assess temperature.

Abnormal findings

Deformity

Deformity may be diagnostic: for example, the flexed hand and arm of hemiplegia or radial nerve palsy, and ulnar deviation at the metacarpophalangeal joints in longstanding rheumatoid arthritis (Fig. 14.14, p. 367). Dupuytren's contracture is a thickening of the palmar fascia causing fixed flexion deformity and usually affecting the little and ring fingers (Fig. 3.12). Long thin fingers (arachnodactyly) are typical of Marfan's syndrome (Fig. 3.27). Trauma is the most common cause of deformity of the hand.

Colour

Look for cyanosis in the nail bed and tobacco staining of the fingers (Fig. 7.12, p. 166). Examine the skin creases for pigmentation, but note that pigmentation occurs and is normal in many non-Caucasian races (Fig. 3.13).

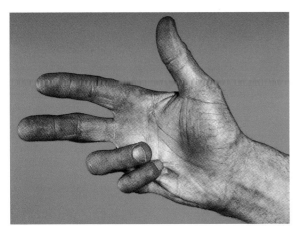

Fig. 3.12 Dupuytren's contracture.

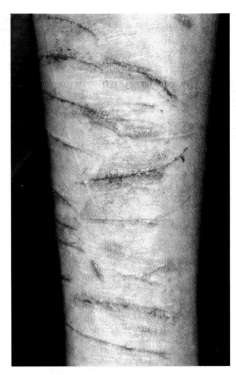

Fig. 3.14 Self-cutting.

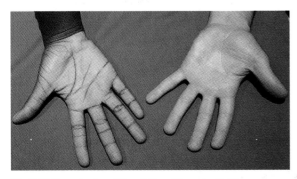

Fig. 3.13 **Normal palms.** African (left) and Caucasian (right).

Temperature

In a cool climate the temperature of the patient's hand is a good guide to peripheral perfusion. In chronic obstructive pulmonary disease (COPD), the hands may be cyanosed due to reduced arterial oxygen saturation but warm due to vasodilatation from elevated arterial carbon dioxide levels. In heart failure the hands are often cold and cyanosed because of vasoconstriction in response to a low cardiac output. If they are warm, heart failure may be due to a high-output state, such as hyperthyroidism.

Skin

The dorsum of the hand is smooth and hairless in children and in adult hypogonadism. Manual work may produce specific callosities due to pressure at characteristic sites. Disuse results in soft, smooth skin, as seen in the soles of the feet in bed-bound patients.

Look at the flexor surfaces of the wrists and forearms. Note any venepuncture marks of intravenous drug use and linear (usually transverse), multiple wounds or scars from deliberate self-harm (Figs 3.14 and 3.15).

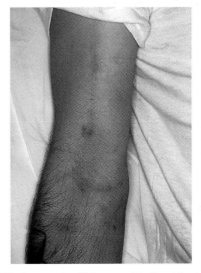

Fig. 3.15 The linear marks of intravenous injection at the right elbow.

Some patients who cut themselves have a history of physical or sexual abuse.

Nails

In chronic iron deficiency the nails become brittle, flat and eventually spoon-shaped (koilonychia). White

53

nails (leukonychia) are a sign of hypoalbuminaemia (Box 3.8). Beau's lines, due to temporary arrest of nail growth, are transverse white grooves that appear on all nails shortly after a severe illness and which move out to the free margins as the nails grow. Although one or two splinter haemorrhages are commonly seen under the nails of manual workers, multiple lesions raise the possibility of infective endocarditis. Distal nail separation (onycholysis) is a common feature of psoriasis. Dilated capillaries in the proximal nail fold are found in vasculitic conditions, such as systemic lupus erythematosus (Fig. 3.16).

Finger clubbing

Finger clubbing is an important sign and may indicate intrathoracic malignancy, e.g. lung cancer, or chronic sepsis, e.g. bronchiectasis (Figs 7.9A and B, p. 165). Autoimmune hyperthyroidism may be associated with a specific type of finger clubbing (thyroid acropachy), more pronounced in the digits on the radial side of the hand (Fig. 5.5C, p. 93).

Joints

Arthritis frequently involves the small joints of the hands. Common conditions include rheumatoid arthritis (metacarpophalangeal and proximal interphalangeal joints; Fig. 14.14, p. 367), and osteoarthritis and psoriatic arthropathy (distal interphalangeal joints; Fig. 14.15, p. 367).

Muscles

Small muscle wasting of the hands is common in rheumatoid arthritis, producing 'dorsal guttering' of the hands. In carpal tunnel syndrome, median nerve compression leads to wasting of the thenar muscles (Figs 14.32A and B, p. 379), and cervical spondylosis with nerve root entrapment causes small muscle wasting.

3.8 Causes of hypoalbuminaemia and leukonychia

Reduced albumin synthesis

- Chronic liver disease

Urinary protein loss

- Nephrotic syndrome

Protein-losing enteropathy

- Crohn's disease
- Ulcerative colitis
- Ménétrier's disease of the stomach
- Coeliac disease
- Intestinal lymphoma
- Bacterial overgrowth
- Radiation damage

Protein malnutrition

- Kwashiorkor

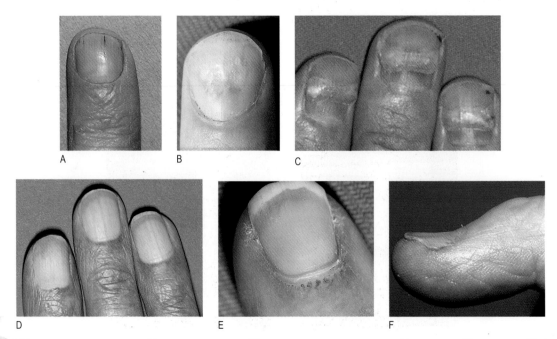

Fig. 3.16 The nail as a diagnostic aid. (A) Splinter haemorrhages. **(B)** Onycholysis with pitting in psoriasis. **(C)** Beau's lines. **(D)** Leukonychia. **(E)** Dilated capillaries in the proximal nail fold in systemic lupus erythematosus. **(F)** Koilonychia.

THE TONGUE

Ask the patient to put out his tongue (Fig. 3.17).

- Tremor can be due to anxiety, thyrotoxicosis, delirium tremens or Parkinsonism
- Fasciculation (irregular ripples or twitching of the tongue) occurs in lower motor neurone disorders, e.g. motor neurone disease
- Enlargement of the tongue (macroglossia) may occur in acromegaly, amyloidosis or tumour infiltration, e.g. with lymphangioma
- Tongue furring is normal and common in heavy smokers
- Geographic tongue is the name used to describe red rings and lines which change over days/weeks on the surface of the tongue. It is usually not significant but can be due to riboflavin (vitamin B2) deficiency
- White patches that may be scraped off the tongue are due to the fungal yeast, candida (oral thrush). Common causes include inhaled steroids, immune deficiency, e.g. HIV, and terminal illness
- Glossitis is a smooth reddened tongue due to atrophy of the papillae. It is common in alcoholics, in nutritional deficiencies of iron, folate and vitamin B12, and in 30% of patients with coeliac disease. Glossitis may cause a burning sensation over the tongue but usually a painful tongue is a symptom of anxiety or depression.

THE LYMPH NODES

Lymph nodes may be palpable in normal people, especially in the submandibular, axilla and groin regions (Fig. 3.18). Distinguish between normal and pathological nodes. Pathological lymphadenopathy may be local or generalized, and is of diagnostic and prognostic significance in the staging of lymphoproliferative and other malignancies.

Size

Normal nodes in adults are seldom >0.5 cm in diameter.

Consistency

Normal nodes feel soft. In Hodgkin's disease they are characteristically 'rubbery', in tuberculosis they may be 'matted', and in metastatic cancer they feel hard.

Tenderness

Acute viral or bacterial infection, including infectious mononucleosis, dental sepsis and tonsillitis, causes tender, variably enlarged lymph nodes.

Fixation

Lymph nodes fixed to deep structures or skin suggest malignancy.

Examination sequence

The lymph nodes

General principles

Inspect for visible lymphadenopathy.
Palpate one side at a time using the fingers of each hand in turn.
Compare with the nodes on the contralateral side.
Assess:
- Site
- Size
- Consistency
- Tenderness.

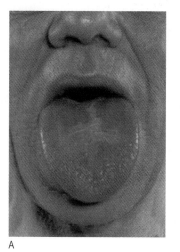
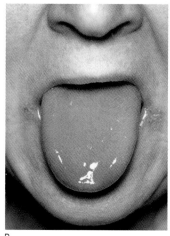

A   B

Fig. 3.17 The tongue as a diagnostic aid. (A) Large tongue (macroglossia) of acromegaly. **(B)** Smooth red tongue and angular stomatitis of iron deficiency.

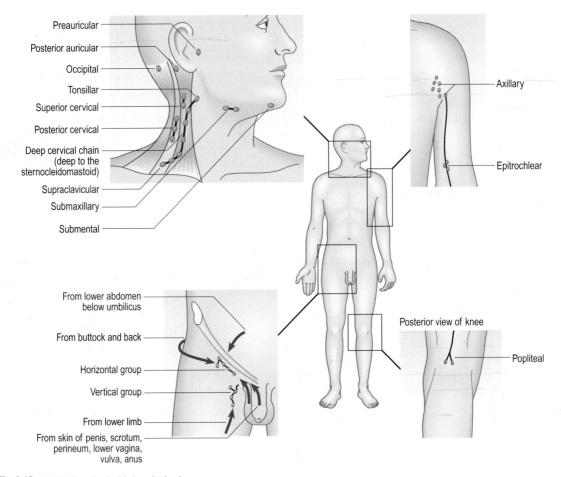

Fig. 3.18 Distribution of palpable lymph glands.

▶ Determine whether the node is fixed to:
 • Surrounding and deep structures
 • Skin.
▶ Measure the main nodes.

Cervical nodes

▶ Examine the cervical and axillary nodes with the patient sitting.
▶ From behind, examine the submental, submandibular, preauricular, tonsillar, supraclavicular and deep cervical nodes in the anterior triangle of the neck (Fig. 3.19A).
▶ Palpate for the scalene nodes by placing your index finger between the sternocleidomastoid muscle and clavicle. Ask the patient to tilt his head to the same side and press firmly down towards the first rib (Fig. 3.19B).
▶ From the front of the patient, palpate the posterior triangles, up the back of the neck and the posterior auricular and occipital nodes (Fig. 3.19C).

Axillary nodes

▶ From the patient's front or side, palpate the right axilla with your left hand and vice versa (Fig. 3.20A). Gently place your finger tips into

the apex of the axilla and then draw them downwards, feeling the medial, anterior and posterior axillary walls in turn. Keep your nails short to avoid causing discomfort.

Epitrochlear nodes

▶ Support the patient's right wrist with your left hand, grasp his partially flexed elbow with your right hand, and use your thumb to feel for the epitrochlear node. Examine the left epitrochlear node with your left thumb (Fig. 3.20B).

Inguinal nodes

▶ Examine for the inguinal and popliteal nodes with the patient lying down.
▶ Palpate over the horizontal chain, which lies just below the inguinal ligament, and then over the vertical chain along the line of the saphenous vein (Fig. 3.20C).

Abnormal findings

If you find localized lymphadenopathy, examine the areas which drain to that site. Infection commonly causes localized tender lymphadenopathy (lymphadenitis); for

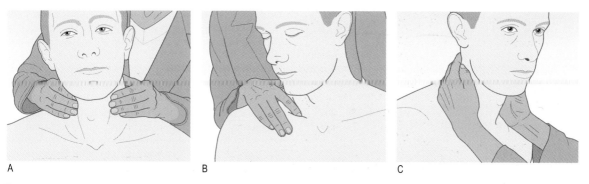

Fig. 3.19 Palpation of the cervical glands. (A) Examine the glands of the anterior triangle from behind, using both hands. **(B)** Examine for the scalene nodes from behind with your index finger in the angle between the sternocleidomastoid muscle and the clavicle. **(C)** Examine glands in the posterior triangle from the front.

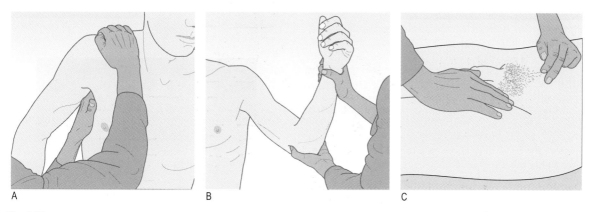

Fig. 3.20 Palpation of the axillary, epitrochlear and inguinal glands. (A) Examination for right axillary lymphadenopathy. **(B)** Examination of the left epitrochlear glands. **(C)** Examination of the left inguinal glands.

 3.9 Important common causes of lymphadenopathy

Generalized

- Viral: Epstein–Barr virus (glandular fever or Burkitt's lymphoma), cytomegalovirus, HIV
- Bacterial: brucellosis, syphilis
- Protozoal: toxoplasmosis
- Malignancy: lymphoma, acute or chronic lymphocytic leukaemia
- Inflammatory: rheumatoid arthritis, SLE, sarcoidosis

Localized

- Infective: acute or chronic, bacterial or viral
- Malignancy: secondary metastases, lymphoma (Hodgkin's or non-Hodgkin's lymphoma)

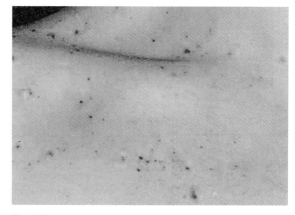

Fig. 3.21 Petechiae.

example, in acute tonsillitis the submandibular nodes are involved. If the lymphadenopathy is non-tender, look for a malignant cause, tuberculosis or features of HIV infection. Generalized lymphadenopathy occurs in a number of conditions (Box 3.9). Examine for enlargement of the liver and spleen, and for other haematological features, such as bruising under the skin (purpura) which can be large (ecchymoses) or pinpoint (petechiae; Fig. 3.21).

3

LUMPS OR SWELLINGS

Patients often present with a lump they have just found. This does not necessarily mean that it has only recently developed. Ask about any changes since they noticed it and whether there are any associated features, such as pain, tenderness or colour change. You may find a lump the patient was unaware of during examination (Box 3.10).

Size

Accurately measure the size of any lump, so that with time you can detect significant change.

Position

The origin of some lumps may be obvious, e.g. in the breast, thyroid or parotid gland; in other sites, e.g. the abdomen, this is less clear. Multiple lumps may occur in neurofibromatosis (Fig. 3.22A), skin metastases, lipomatosis and lymphomas.

Attachments

Lymphatic obstruction causes fixation of the skin with fine dimpling at the opening of hair follicles that resembles orange peel (peau d'orange) (Fig. 10.5, p. 237). This is common in malignant disease. Fixation to deeper structures may occur in a breast cancer fixed to underlying muscle.

Consistency

The consistency of a lump may vary from soft to 'stony' hard. Very hard swellings are usually malignant or calcified, or consist of dense fibrous tissue. Fluctuation indicates the presence of fluid, e.g. abscess, cyst, or soft encapsulated tumours, e.g. lipoma (Fig. 3.22B).

Edge

The edge or margin may be well delineated or ill defined, regular or irregular, sharp or rounded. The margins of enlarged organs, e.g. thyroid gland, liver, spleen or kidney, can usually be defined more clearly

than those of inflammatory or malignant masses. An indefinite margin suggests infiltrating malignancy in contrast to the clearly defined edge of a benign tumour.

Surface and shape

The surface and shape of a lump may be characteristic. Examples in the abdomen include an enlarged spleen or liver, a distended bladder or the fundus of the uterus in pregnancy. The surface may be smooth or irregular and provide a clue to the pathological process. For example, the surface of the liver is smooth in acute hepatitis but is often nodular in metastatic disease.

Pulsations, thrills and bruits

Arterial swellings (aneurysms) and highly vascular tumours are pulsatile (move in time with the arterial pulse). Other swellings may be pulsatile if they lie over a major blood vessel. If the blood flow through a lump is

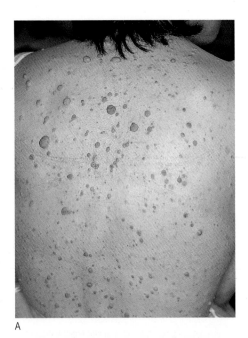

A

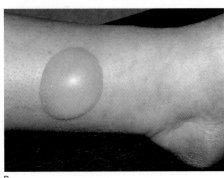

B

Fig. 3.22 Lumps and swellings. (A) Neurofibromatosis. **(B)** Blister on leg.

3.10 Features to note in any lump or swelling (SPACESPIT)

- Size
- Position
- Attachments
- Consistency
- Edge
- Surface and shape
- Pulsation, thrills and bruits
- Inflammation
    - Redness
    - Tenderness
    - Warmth
- Transillumination

increased, a systolic murmur (bruit) may be auscultated and, if loud enough, a thrill may be palpable. Bruits are also heard over arterial aneurysms and arteriovenous malformations.

Inflammation

Redness, tenderness and warmth suggest inflammation.

- Redness (erythema). The skin over acute inflammatory lesions is usually red due to vasodilatation. In haematomas the pigment from extravasated blood may produce the range of colours familiar in a bruise (ecchymosis)
- Tenderness. Inflammatory lumps, e.g. boil or abscess, are usually tender or painful, while swellings not associated with inflammation, e.g. lipomas, skin metastases and neurofibromas, are characteristically painless
- Warmth. Inflammatory lumps and some tumours, especially if rapidly growing, may feel warm due to increased blood flow.

Transillumination

In a darkened room, press the lighted end of a pen-torch on to one side of the swelling. A cystic swelling, e.g. testicular hydrocoele, will light up if the fluid is translucent, provided that the covering tissues are not too thick (Fig. 15.9, p. 407).

Examination sequence

Lumps or swellings (Box 3.10)

- Inspect the lump, noting any change in colour or texture of the overlying skin.
- Gently palpate for tenderness or change in skin temperature.
- Define the site and shape of the lump.
- Measure its size and record the findings diagrammatically.
- Feel the lump for a few moments to determine if it is pulsatile.
- Assess the consistency, surface texture and margins of the lump.
- Try to pick up an overlying fold of skin to assess whether the lump is fixed to the skin.
- Try to move the lump in different planes relative to the surrounding tissues to see if it is fixed to deeper structures.
- Compress the lump on one side; see and feel if a bulge occurs on the opposite side (fluctuation). Confirm the fluctuation in two planes.
- Auscultate for vascular bruits.
- Transilluminate.

MEASUREMENT OF WEIGHT AND HEIGHT

Weight is an important indicator of general health and nutrition. Serial weight measurements are useful in monitoring acutely ill patients and those with chronic disease. Serial height is helpful in monitoring growth in children and osteoporotic vertebral collapse in the elderly.

Measure the body mass index (BMI), rather than weight alone, as it is independent of the patient's height. BMI is calculated from the formula Weight/Height^2 (using metric units, kg/m^2). It can also be derived from a nomogram (Fig. 3.23). Obesity is defined by BMI (Box 3.11).

BMI, however, does not describe body fat distribution and excess intra-abdominal fat is an independent predictor of hypertension, insulin resistance, type 2 diabetes mellitus and coronary artery disease. Waist circumference correlates better with visceral fat and indirectly measures central adiposity. Health risk is increased when waist circumference exceeds 94 cm (37 inches) for men and 80 cm (32 inches) for women. Waist: hip ratio is strongly related to risk of coronary artery

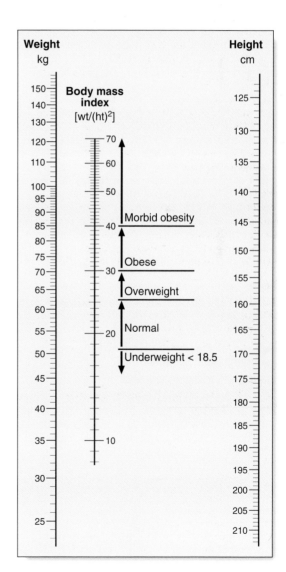

Fig. 3.23 Desirable weights of adults according to BMI.

	3.11 The relationship between BMI, nutritional status and ethnic group	
	BMI Non-Asian	**BMI Asian**
Underweight	<18.5	<18.5
Normal	18.5–24.9	18.5–22.9
Overweight	25–29.9	23–24.9
Obese	30–39.9	25–29.9
Morbidly obese	≥40	≥30

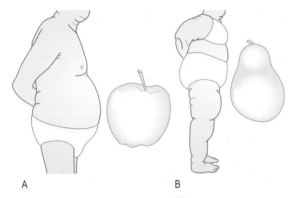

Fig. 3.24 Abdominal obesity and generalized obesity. (A) Abdominal obesity (apple shape). **(B)** Generalized obesity, where fat deposition is mainly on the hips and thighs (pear shape).

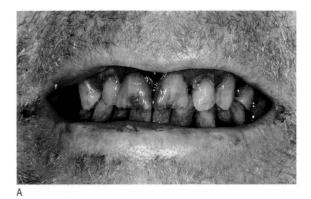

A

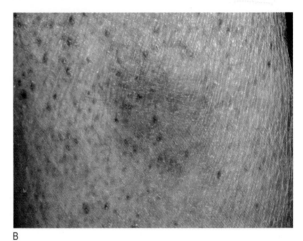

B

Fig. 3.25 Scurvy. (A) Bleeding gums. **(B)** Bruising and perifollicular haemorrhages.

disease. 'Pear shape' and a waist:hip ratio of ≤0.8 in females or <0.9 in males have a good prognosis, whereas 'apple-shaped' subjects with a greater waist:hip ratio have an increased risk of coronary artery disease and the 'metabolic syndrome' (Fig. 3.24).

Examination sequence

Measurement of height and weight

- Note any abnormalities in stature or body proportions.
- Measure height using a vertical scale and a rigid, adjustable arm-piece. In the serial assessment of growth in children and teenagers, measure height to the nearest millimetre using a calibrated stadiometer (Fig. 15.23, p. 417).
- The patient should stand erect and be weighed in his indoor clothing without shoes. Inpatients should wear their nightclothes.
- Calculate and record BMI.
- Look for abnormal fat distribution.
- Measure the waist with the patient standing. This is the girth at the level equidistant between the costal margin and iliac crest. The measurement should record the maximum diameter, so measure over any abdominal fat and not under it.
- Look for any evidence of malnutrition or specific vitamin deficiencies.

Nutritional status

Illness may produce profound changes in an individual's nutritional requirements, appetite and ability to eat. Malnutrition delays recovery from illness and surgery, and delays wound healing. Record BMI initially and repeat this at least weekly in an acute setting, and monthly in outpatients or in the community, to monitor nutritional status.

Vitamin deficiencies

Vitamins are organic substances that have key roles in certain metabolic pathways. They are fat-soluble (vitamins A, D, E and K) or water-soluble (vitamins of the B complex group and vitamin C).

Vitamin deficiencies occur in older people and alcoholic patients, and are common in children in developing countries. Consider vitamin C deficiency (scurvy) in patients with extensive bruising, particularly the elderly living alone without access to fresh fruit and vegetables (Fig. 3.25). Those with alcohol dependency may eat poorly and also become deficient in vitamin B1

3.12 Vitamins and deficiencies

Vitamin	Source	Deficiency
Fat-soluble		
Vitamin A (retinol)	Liver, milk, butter, cheese, fish oils	Xerophthalmia — night blindness Keratomalacia
Vitamin D (cholecalciferol)	Manufactured in skin under influence of sunlight	Rickets in children Osteomalacia
Vitamin E (α-tocopherol)	Vegetables, seed oils	Haemolytic anaemia Ataxia
Vitamin K	Green vegetables, dairy products	Bleeding disorder
Water-soluble		
Vitamin B1 (thiamine)	Cereals, grains, beans, pork	Beri-beri — neuropathy (dry) or heart failure (wet) Wernicke–Korsakoff syndrome
Vitamin B2 (riboflavin)	Milk	Glossitis, stomatitis
Vitamin B3 (nicotinic acid)	Meat, cereals	Pellagra — dermatitis, diarrhoea and dementia
Vitamin B6 (pyridoxine)	Meat, fish, potatoes, bananas	Polyneuropathy
Biotin	Liver, egg yolk, cereals, yeast	Dermatitis, alopecia, paraesthesiae
Folate	Liver	Megaloblastic anaemia
Vitamin B12 (cobalamin)	Animal products	Megaloblastic anaemia Neurological disorders
Vitamin C (ascorbic acid)	Fresh fruit and vegetables	Scurvy — extensive bleeding, bruising and perifollicular haemorrhages

3.13 Drugs associated with weight gain

Class	Examples
Anticonvulsants	Sodium valproate, phenytoin, gabapentin
Antidepressants	Citalopram, mirtazapine
Antipsychotics	Chlorpromazine, risperidone, olanzapine, lithium
β-blockers	Atenolol
Oral corticosteroids	Prednisolone, dexamethasone
Migraine prophylaxis	Pizotifen
Sulphonylureas/hypoglycaemic agents	Glibenclamide, gliclazide, rosiglitazone, pioglitazone
Insulin	All formulations
Protease inhibitors for HIV infection	Indinavir, ritonavir, lopinavir

(thiamine). Vitamin B12 deficiency occurs in vegans, in small bowel overgrowth, in those with ileal disease or resection, and in the autoimmune disorder, pernicious anaemia. Small bowel malabsorption and liver and biliary tract disease can lead to deficiency of fat-soluble vitamins (Box 3.12).

Common abnormalities of height and weight

Obesity

Obesity is a major worldwide health problem, largely a result of changes in lifestyle. It is caused by excess calorie intake associated with inadequate exercise. Rarely, it is secondary to hypothyroidism, Cushing's syndrome, Prader–Willi syndrome or drugs (Box 3.13). It is associated with hypertension, hyperlipidaemia, type 2 diabetes mellitus, gallbladder disease, sleep apnoea and cancer of the oesophagus, pancreas and uterus (Fig. 3.26). Obesity reduces life expectancy by about 7 years.

Weight loss

Weight loss is important clinically. It may be due to:
- reduced food intake from a poor appetite (anorexia)
- malabsorption or loss of nutrients, e.g. in prolonged diarrhoea

3

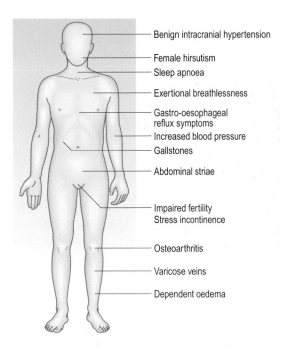

Benign intracranial hypertension
Female hirsutism
Sleep apnoea
Exertional breathlessness
Gastro-oesophageal reflux symptoms
Increased blood pressure
Gallstones
Abdominal striae
Impaired fertility
Stress incontinence
Osteoarthritis
Varicose veins
Dependent oedema

Fig. 3.26 Complications of obesity.

- metastatic cancer, e.g. of the lung, breast or gastrointestinal tract
- serious and prolonged infection, e.g. tuberculosis
- untreated advanced HIV infection
- chronic inflammation, e.g. inflammatory bowel disease.

In most of these systemic disorders, weight loss is associated with anorexia. Occasionally, weight loss can be associated with a normal or increased appetite (thyrotoxicosis, coeliac disease or type 1 diabetes mellitus). The degree to which a patient complains about weight loss does not always correlate with true weight loss. Temporary weight loss is most commonly associated with anxiety, depression or dieting (a deliberate attempt to lose weight).

Malnutrition and starvation are major problems. Malnutrition has been estimated to affect 15–40% of UK hospital admissions, and is usually due to poverty or illness. Weight loss due to malnutrition also occurs in anorexia nervosa, alcohol abuse and drug addiction.

Short stature

Short stature is usually familial, so ask about the height of the patient's parents and siblings (p. 413). Any significant childhood illness will reduce the rate of growth and may limit final height. Identify causes of short stature from associated features (Box 15.16, p. 418). Other disorders, such as renal tubular acidosis, intestinal malabsorption and hypothyroidism, may be less obvious in young people and delay the diagnosis. Loss of height is part of normal ageing but is accentuated by compression fractures of the spine due to osteoporosis, particularly in women. In post-menopausal women loss of >5cm height is an indication to investigate for osteoporosis.

Tall stature

Tall stature is less common than short stature and is usually familial. Most individuals with heights above the 95th centile are not abnormal and you should ask about the height of close relatives. Abnormal causes of increased height include:

- Marfan's syndrome
- hypogonadism
- pituitary gigantism.

In Marfan's syndrome, the limbs are long in relation to the length of the trunk, and the arm-span exceeds height (Fig. 3.27A). Additional features include long slender fingers (arachnodactyly) (Fig. 3.27B), narrow feet, a high-arched palate (Fig. 3.27C), upward dislocation of the lenses of the eyes (Fig. 3.27D), and cardiovascular abnormalities such as mitral valve prolapse, and dilatation of the aortic root with aortic regurgitation.

During puberty, the epiphyses close in response to stimulation from the sex hormones, so in some patients with hypogonadism the limbs continue to grow for longer than usual. Sitting height is less than half their total standing height. The arm-span may exceed the standing height or, more significantly, be twice the sitting height.

Pituitary gigantism is a very rare cause of tall stature due to excessive growth hormone secretion before epiphyseal fusion has occurred. In contrast, acromegaly, in which excessive growth hormone secretion occurs after growth plates have fused, only affects soft tissue and flat bones.

ASSESSMENT OF HYDRATION

Between 60 and 65% of body mass in adults is water. A male weighing 70kg has 42 litres of water, of which two-thirds is intracellular (28 litres), 12% interstitial fluid (9.4 litres) and the remainder circulating blood volume or plasma (4.6 litres). Women have a smaller percentage of total body water than men, although they sometimes have cyclical fluctuations in weight due to perimenstrual fluid retention.

Dehydration

It is easy to overlook or underestimate the severity of dehydration unless you think of it. Assess hydration in all patients, especially those with excess fluid loss, e.g. vomiting, diarrhoea, sweating, burns and polyuria, and when ambient temperature is raised. Take a detailed history of the nature and the quantity of fluid loss. If the usual weight is known, useful information is obtained by weighing the patient. Loss of skin turgor occurs in severe dehydration but adults can lose 4–6 litres before the skin becomes dry and loose. Blood pressure may be low and postural hypotension may indicate intravascular volume depletion. A dry tongue is not a reliable indicator of dehydration since it is often due to mouth breathing.

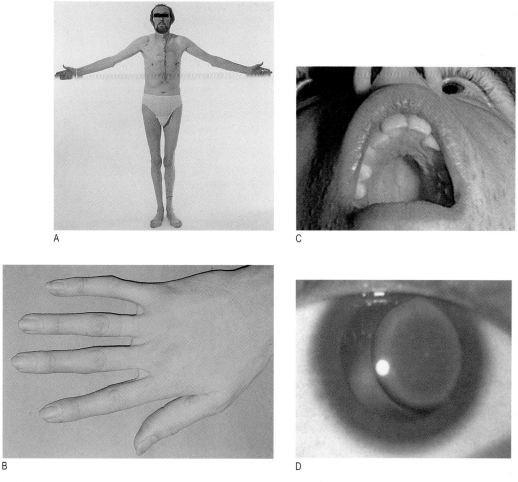

Fig. 3.27 Marfan's syndrome, an autosomal dominant condition. (A) Tall stature and reduced upper segment to lower segment ratio (note surgery for aortic dissection). **(B)** Long fingers. **(C)** High-arched palate. **(D)** Dislocation of the lens in the eye.

Oedema

Oedema is tissue swelling due to an increase in interstitial fluid. Interstitial fluid and plasma are separated by the capillary wall. The distribution of water between the vascular and interstitial spaces is determined by the balance between hydrostatic pressure, which forces water out of the capillary, and colloid osmotic (oncotic) pressure, which sucks fluid into the vascular space (Starling's forces). Oncotic pressure is largely dependent on circulating protein concentration, particularly serum albumin (Fig. 3.28).

Clinical manifestations of oedema

Oedema can be generalized, localized or postural.

The cardinal sign of subcutaneous oedema is pitting of superficial tissues. Pitting on pressure may not be demonstrable until body weight has increased by 10–15%. Day-to-day alterations in body weight are usually the most reliable index of changes in body water. Hypothyroidism is characterized by mucinous infiltration of tissues (myxoedema). In contrast to oedema, myxoedema and chronic lymphoedema do not pit on pressure.

Generalized oedema

There are two principal causes of generalized oedema (Box 3.14):

- fluid overload
- hypoproteinaemia.

Distinguish them by assessing the jugular venous pulse (JVP; p. 124). The JVP is usually elevated in fluid overload but not in hypoproteinaemia.

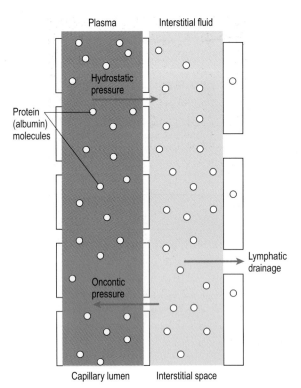

Fig. 3.28 Starling's forces.

3.14 Causes of oedema

Low plasma oncotic pressure

Low serum albumin due to:

- Increased loss — nephrotic syndrome
- Decreased synthesis — chronic liver disease
- Malabsorption — protein-losing enteropathy, e.g. Crohn's disease and coeliac disease
- Malnutrition — kwashiorkor

Increased hydrostatic pressure

High venous pressure/obstruction due to:

- Deep vein thrombosis
- Venous insufficiency
- Pregnancy
- Pelvic tumour
- Congestive heart failure
- Intravascular volume expansion, e.g. excess IV fluid, renal failure

Increased capillary permeability

- Local — soft tissue infection/inflammation
- Systemic — severe septicaemia
- Drugs, e.g. calcium channel-blockers
- Acute allergy

Lymphatic obstruction (lymphoedema) — non-pitting

- Malignant infiltration
- Congenital abnormality — Milroy's disease
- Radiation injury
- Elephantiasis — tropical (filarial) worm infestation

Fluid overload

Fluid overload may be due to heart failure or renal disease, or stem from iatrogenic causes.

- Heart failure causes oedema in the following ways:
  Renal underperfusion activates the renin-angiotensin-aldosterone system (secondary hyperaldosteronism) and releases vasopressin, leading to salt and water retention
  Renal blood flow is reduced, causing increased reabsorption of salt and water
  When the patient lies flat, blood is redistributed from the legs into the torso, increasing venous return to the heart. In the failing heart this results in increased end diastolic pressure within the left ventricle, leading to pulmonary oedema. The patient therefore experiences breathlessness on lying flat (orthopnoea)
  In very severe prolonged heart failure, chronic congestion of the liver leads to reduced albumin synthesis and reduced oncotic pressure
- Renal disease, e.g. acute glomerulonephritis, may reduce urine volume, with increased circulating and extracellular fluid volume and increased tubular reabsorption of sodium
- Iatrogenic causes result from the actions of the medical profession. These include excessive fluid replacement, especially intravenously, which

produces fluid overload. Infants, young children and patients with diminished (oliguria) or absent (anuria) urine production due to renal failure are at particular risk of fluid overload.

Hypoproteinaemia

Hypoproteinaemia, particularly hypoalbuminaemia, reduces oncotic pressure and encourages fluid to move to the interstitial space, thus causing oedema. Nephrotic syndrome causes heavy proteinuria and most patients with a hepatic cause will have features of chronic liver disease (Fig. 8.12, p. 198).

When oedema is generalized (Fig. 3.29), its distribution is determined by gravity. It is usually found in the ankles, backs of the thighs and the lumbosacral area in the semi-recumbent patient. If the patient lies flat, it may involve the face and hands, as in children with nephrotic syndrome.

Localized oedema

This may be caused by venous, lymphatic, inflammatory or allergic disorders.

Venous causes

Any increased venous pressure will increase hydrostatic pressure within capillaries, producing oedema in the

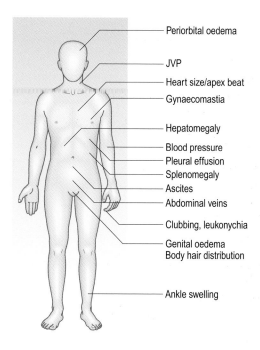

Periorbital oedema

JVP

Heart size/apex beat

Gynaecomastia

Hepatomegaly

Blood pressure

Pleural effusion

Splenomegaly

Ascites

Abdominal veins

Clubbing, leukonychia

Genital oedema
Body hair distribution

Ankle swelling

Fig. 3.29 Features to look for in oedema.

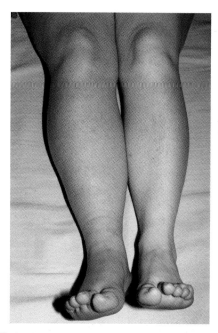

Fig. 3.30 Swollen right leg: suggesting deep vein thrombosis or inflammation, e.g. soft tissue infection or ruptured Baker's cyst.

area drained by that vein. Venous causes include deep vein thrombosis, external pressure from a tumour or pregnancy, or valvular incompetence from previous thrombosis or surgery. Conditions which impair the normal pumping action of muscles, e.g. hemiparesis and forced immobility, increase venous pressure by impairing venous return. Oedema may occur in immobile, bedridden patients, in a paralysed limb, or even in a healthy person sitting for long periods, e.g. during air travel (Fig. 3.30).

Lymphatic causes

Normally, interstitial fluid returns to the central circulation via the lymphatic system. Any cause of impaired lymphatic flow, e.g. intraluminal or extraluminal obstruction, may produce localized oedema (lymphoedema) (Fig. 3.31). If the condition persists, fibrous tissues proliferate in the interstitial space and the affected area becomes hard and no longer pits on pressure. In the UK, lymphoedema is usually due to congenital hypoplasia of lymphatics in the legs (Milroy's disease) or recurrent lymphangitis (resulting in lymphatic fibrosis), or may affect an arm after radical mastectomy and/or irradiation for breast cancer. Lymphoedema is common in some tropical countries because of lymphatic obstruction by filarial worms.

Inflammatory causes

Any cause of tissue inflammation, including infection, injury or ischaemia, liberates mediators, e.g. histamine, bradykinin and cytokines, which cause vasodilatation and increase capillary permeability. Inflammatory

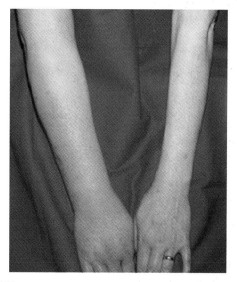

Fig. 3.31 Lymphoedema of the right arm. In this case, lymphoedema followed mastectomy and radiotherapy on the right side.

oedema is accompanied by the other features of inflammation — redness, tenderness and warmth — and is therefore painful.

Allergic causes

Increased capillary permeability occurs in acute allergic conditions. The affected area may be red and

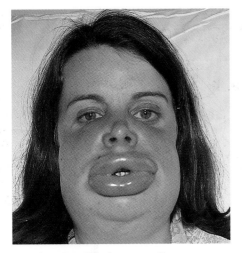

Fig. 3.32 Angio-oedema following a wasp sting.

itchy (pruritic) because of local release of histamine and other inflammatory mediators but, in contrast to inflammation, is not painful.

Angio-oedema is a specific form of allergic oedema affecting the face, lips and mouth (Fig. 3.32). Swelling may develop rapidly and may be life-threatening if the upper airway is involved.

Postural oedema

This is due to failure of muscle movement and is common in the lower limbs of inactive patients.

▶ Examination sequence

Oedema

▶ Apply firm pressure with your fingers or thumb for at least 15 seconds (Fig. 3.33). Pitting may persist for several minutes until it is obliterated by the slow return of the displaced fluid.

▶ Assess the state of hydration by looking for sunken orbits and dry mucous membranes. If severe dehydration seems likely, test skin turgor. Gently pinch a fold of skin on the neck or anterior chest wall, hold it for a few seconds and then release. Well-hydrated skin springs back into position immediately, whereas dehydrated skin subsides abnormally slowly.

▶ Record weight and urine output.

▶ Record the pulse rate and supine/erect blood pressures. Look for tachycardia >100/min and postural hypotension (a fall >15 mmHg in systolic pressure on standing).

▶ Check for oedema in the ankles and legs. In bed-bound patients, check for sacral oedema.

▶ Examine the JVP (p. 124).

TEMPERATURE

The 'normal' oral or ear temperature is 37°C but may range between 35.8°C and 37.2°C (98–99°F). There is a circadian variation, with the lowest readings occurring

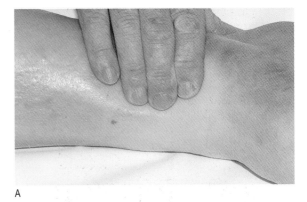

A

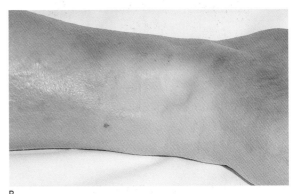

B

Fig. 3.33 Demonstration of pitting oedema.

in the early morning. Rectal temperature is about 0.5°C higher than in the mouth. The axilla is not a reliable site for measuring temperature. Use a digital thermometer under the tongue, or in the rectum or the external auditory meatus. Mercury thermometers have been replaced by electronic devices, which are safer and more accurate (Fig. 3.34).

Fever and rigors

Fever is an increase in body temperature caused by a cellular response to infection, immunological disturbance or malignancy. Rarely, it may be a response to raised ambient temperature (often in humid environments) — heat illness. Fever may make the patient's skin feel abnormally warm but a patient with a normal temperature may feel cold, so an apparently normal skin temperature does not exclude hypothermia or fever. Pyrexia (fever) of uncertain origin (PUO) is a common presenting problem and is defined as a consistently elevated temperature of >37.5° persisting for >2 weeks with no diagnosis. A rigor is uncontrollable shivering or shaking related to a rapid increase in body temperature, and may be followed by sweating. The pattern of fever is not a reliable indicator of the nature or severity of disease, although patients

3

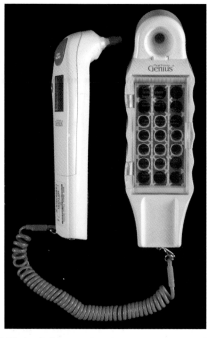

Fig. 3.34 Electronic thermometer.

with collections of pus, e.g. an abscess, commonly have a high swinging fever with rigors. In tropical countries fever and rigors are often due to malaria.

Hypothermia

Hypothermia is a core temperature <35°C and is easily missed unless rectal temperature is measured. As body temperature falls, conscious level is progressively impaired, and coma is common with core temperatures <28°C (Box 3.15), mimicking death (Box 18.1, p. 453). If hypothermia is suspected, measure temperature at more than one site e.g. external auditory meatus and rectum.

Hypothermia occurs in:

- elderly immobile patients living alone, particularly during the winter
- water immersion and near-drowning
- prolonged unconsciousness in low ambient temperatures, especially combined with alcohol intoxication (which causes peripheral vasodilatation), drug overdosage, stroke or head injury
- severe hypothyroidism.

3.15 Clinical features of hypothermia

Core temperature	Clinical features
36°C	Increased metabolic rate, vasoconstriction
35°C (hypothermia)	Shivering maximal, impaired judgement
34°C	Uncooperative
33°C	Depressed conscious level
28–32°C (severe hypothermia)	Progressive depression of conscious level, muscle stiffness
	Failure of vasoconstrictor response and shivering
	Bradycardia, hypotension, J waves present on ECG, risk of arrhythmias
28°C	Coma, patient may appear dead, absent pupillary and tendon reflexes
	Spontaneous ventricular fibrillation
20°C	Asystole/profound bradyarrhythmias

3.16 Key points: the general examination

The physical examination starts as soon as you see the patient:

- Ask yourself: 'Does this patient look well?'
- Examine patients in a warm, well-lit environment.
- Look out for features of a 'spot diagnosis'.
- Develop a systematic routine for your examination to avoid missing anything.
- Abnormalities in the hands and tongue can often indicate a diagnosis.
- Localized lymphadenopathy suggests local infection or metastatic malignancy.
- Use a systematic approach to examine a lump or swelling.
- BMI and waist:hip ratio are important prognostic risk factors for cardiovascular disease.
- Unplanned weight loss is often important and requires investigation.
- Lymphoedema and myxoedema do not pit on pressure.
- Oedema due to inflammation is tender; oedema due to acute allergy is non-painful.
- Always measure body temperature to avoid missing hypothermia or hyperthermia.
- The axilla is an unreliable site for measuring temperature.
- Increasingly, temperature is measured electronically.

SECTION 2

System examination

David J. Gawkrodger

The skin, hair and nails

4

4 EXAMINATION OF THE SKIN, HAIR AND NAILS

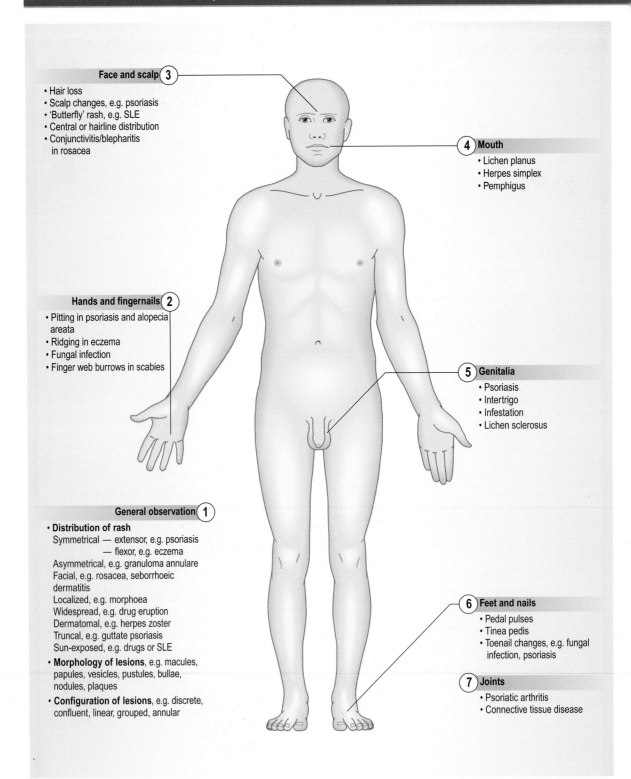

Face and scalp ③
- Hair loss
- Scalp changes, e.g. psoriasis
- 'Butterfly' rash, e.g. SLE
- Central or hairline distribution
- Conjunctivitis/blepharitis in rosacea

④ **Mouth**
- Lichen planus
- Herpes simplex
- Pemphigus

Hands and fingernails ②
- Pitting in psoriasis and alopecia areata
- Ridging in eczema
- Fungal infection
- Finger web burrows in scabies

⑤ **Genitalia**
- Psoriasis
- Intertrigo
- Infestation
- Lichen sclerosus

General observation ①
- **Distribution of rash**
  Symmetrical — extensor, e.g. psoriasis
  — flexor, e.g. eczema
  Asymmetrical, e.g. granuloma annulare
  Facial, e.g. rosacea, seborrhoeic dermatitis
  Localized, e.g. morphoea
  Widespread, e.g. drug eruption
  Dermatomal, e.g. herpes zoster
  Truncal, e.g. guttate psoriasis
  Sun-exposed, e.g. drugs or SLE
- **Morphology of lesions**, e.g. macules, papules, vesicles, pustules, bullae, nodules, plaques
- **Configuration of lesions**, e.g. discrete, confluent, linear, grouped, annular

⑥ **Feet and nails**
- Pedal pulses
- Tinea pedis
- Toenail changes, e.g. fungal infection, psoriasis

⑦ **Joints**
- Psoriatic arthritis
- Connective tissue disease

ANATOMY

Anatomy and function of the skin

The skin is the largest organ in the body, making up 16% of body weight. It protects the body from external factors and keeps the internal organs intact (Fig. 4.1 and Box 4.1).

Skin has three layers:

- the epidermis
- the dermis
- the subcutis.

Epidermis

The epidermis is a stratified squamous epithelium. It has four layers (basal, prickle, granular and horny), representing the stages of maturation of keratin. The main cell, the keratinocyte, produces keratin. Melanocytes (5–10% of the cell population) synthesize melanin and are most numerous on the face and other exposed sites, originating from the neural crest. Cells lose their nuclei in the granular layer and, as flat plates, form the horny layer. Langerhans cells are dendritic and immunologically

4.1 Functions of skin

Barrier

- Against chemicals, particles, microbes, UV radiation
- Against loss of body fluids
- Against mechanical injury

Homeostasis

- Regulation of body temperature

Sensation

- Touch
- Pressure
- Temperature
- Pain

Mobility

- Provides a surface for grip

Metabolism

- Role in vitamin D production

Immunity

- Outpost for immune surveillance

Psychology

- Sexual attraction
- Self-image

4

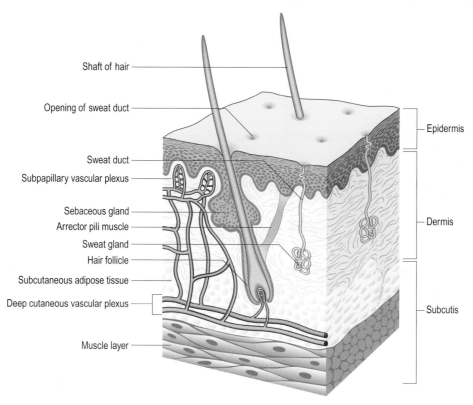

Shaft of hair
Opening of sweat duct
Sweat duct
Subpapillary vascular plexus
Sebaceous gland
Arrector pili muscle
Sweat gland
Hair follicle
Subcutaneous adipose tissue
Deep cutaneous vascular plexus
Muscle layer

Epidermis
Dermis
Subcutis

Fig. 4.1 Structure of the skin.

4

active antigen-presenting cells that form a network throughout the epidermis.

Dermis

The dermis is a supportive connective tissue matrix containing specialized structures. It is thin (0.6mm) on the eyelids and thicker (3mm or more) on the back, palms and soles. It contains fibroblasts, dendritic cells, mast cells, macrophages and lymphocytes. Collagen fibres make up 70% of the dermis and give strength and toughness. Elastin fibres provide the skin with elasticity. Glycosaminoglycans form a semisolid matrix that allows some movement of dermal structures, such as hair follicles, sweat glands, blood and lymphatic vessels, and nerves.

Subcutis

This is a loose layer of connective tissue and fat; it is of variable thickness and may be up to 3cm thick on the abdomen.

Anatomy and function of hair and nails

Hair and nails are specialized epidermal structures.

Hair

Hair has a protective and sexual function and hairs cover the surface of the skin, except for the glabrous skin of the palms and soles, the glans penis and the vulval introitus. The follicle density is greatest on the face. The hair shaft has an outer cuticle enclosing a cortex of packed keratinocytes.

There are three types of hair:

- Lanugo: fine and long; found in the fetus
- Vellus hairs: short, fine and light in colour; cover most body surfaces
- Terminal hairs: long, thick and dark; found on the scalp, eyebrows, eyelashes, and pubic, axillary and beard areas.

Amount and type of hair vary and are influenced by racial and genetic factors. Typically, Europeans have straight hair, black Africans curly hair, and Orientals sparse facial and body hair, while people from the Mediterranean area have more body hair than northern Europeans.

Hair cycle

Regular cycles of growth (anagen), resting (telogen) and shedding (catagen) occur. The cycle lasts up to 5 years for scalp hair, but less for eyebrow, axillary and pubic hair. Adjacent hairs are not in the same phase but illnesses or childbirth can synchronize the hair cycle and cause an alarming loss of large amounts of hair (telogen effluvium).

Puberty

Body hair develops with sexual maturity, with wide normal variation in its pattern. At puberty, androgens induce vellus hairs of the pubic region to develop into terminal hairs. Gonadotrophins are not involved in this process, so patients with gonadotrophin deficiency have pubic hair but no other pubertal development. Axillary hair appears 2 years after pubic hair and coincides with onset of facial hair in boys (p. 425).

Nails

The nail is a plate of hardened, densely packed keratin protecting the finger tip and facilitating grasp and tactile sensitivity in the finger pulp (Fig. 4.2). The nail matrix contains dividing cells that mature, keratinize and move forward to form the nail plate, which in the finger is 0.3–0.5 mm thick and grows at 0.1 mm/24 hours (Fig. 4.2). Toenails grow more slowly. Adjacent dermal capillaries produce the pink colour of the nail; the white lunula is the visible distal part of the matrix.

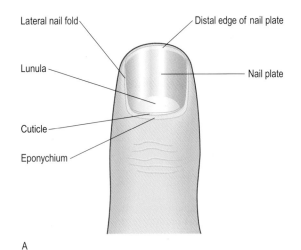

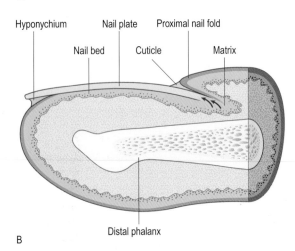

Fig. 4.2 Structure of the nail.

SYMPTOMS AND DEFINITIONS

Symptoms include:

- a rash
- itch (pruritus) and sleep disturbance
- a growth or lump
- discharge, crusting and smell
- scales falling from the skin or scalp
- disfigurement and psychological distress
- inability to work or pursue leisure activities, e.g. swimming.

Skin eruptions and lesions

The shape (morphology) of individual lesions, and their grouping (configuration) and distribution on the body help make the diagnosis.

Distribution patterns

- Symmetrical or universal eruptions suggest systemic or constitutional causes
- Asymmetrical rashes that spread from one focus are more likely to be due to fungal, bacterial or viral infection (Box 4.2)

The time and evolution of the spread and change in morphology help diagnosis.

- Flexural, in the antecubital and popliteal fossae, indicates atopic eczema, typically involving the flexures of the popliteal fossa, antecubital fossa, neck and face (Fig. 4.3)
- Extensor plaques on elbows and knees suggest psoriasis, which characteristically affects the extensor surfaces of the knees and elbows, the scalp and the sacrum (Fig. 4.4)
- Facial, on the forehead, nasolabial folds and scalp, suggests seborrhoeic dermatitis, an inflammatory reaction to yeasts. Comedones, pustules and cysts on the face suggest acne vulgaris, which also affects the chest and back, or rosacea, if there is telangiectasia with pustules. The face is commonly affected by sun damage and malignant tumours, such as basal cell cancer (Fig. 4.5)

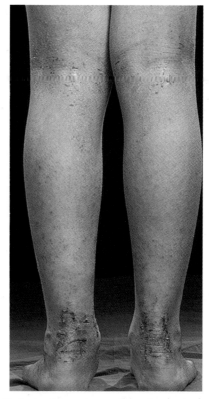

Fig. 4.3 **Distribution: flexural.** Atopic eczema in the popliteal fossae and ankles.

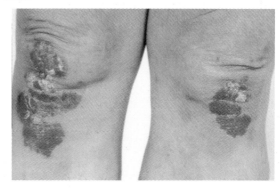

Fig. 4.4 **Distribution: extensor.** Psoriasis on the knees.

4.2 Some examples of skin lesions and systemic disease

Skin lesions	Associations	Ask about
Erythema nodosum	Sarcoidosis, tuberculosis, post-streptococcal infection, connective tissue diseases, drugs	Cough and sputum, breathlessness, sore throat, drugs
Pyoderma gangrenosum	Ulcerative colitis, rheumatoid arthritis, leukaemia	Rectal bleeding, joint symptoms
Dermatitis herpetiformis	Gluten enteropathy	Family history, change in bowel habit
Generalized purpura	Idiopathic thrombocytopenic purpura and other haematological disorders	Family history, haematuria, fever and weight loss
Dermatitis artefacta	Personality disorders	Stresses or anxieties

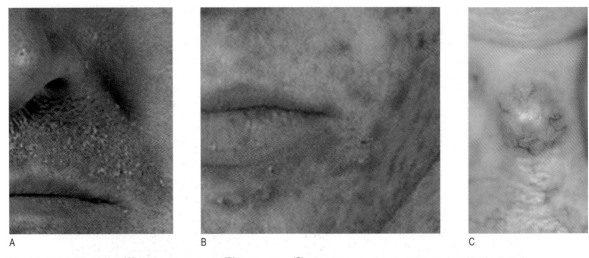

A

B

C

Fig. 4.5 Distribution: facial. (A) Seborrhoeic dermatitis. **(B)** Acne vulgaris. **(C)** Basal cell cancer showing pearly papules with telangiectasia.

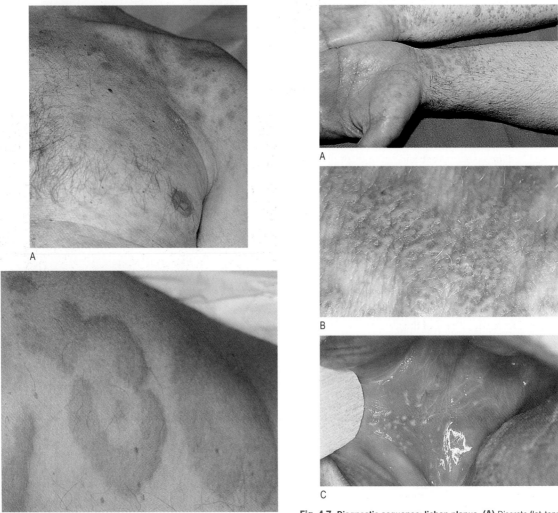

A

B

A

B

C

Fig. 4.6 Distribution: truncal. (A) Pityriasis rosea. **(B)** Urticaria.

Fig. 4.7 Diagnostic sequence: lichen planus. (A) Discrete flat-topped papules on the wrist. **(B)** Wickham's striae visible on close inspection. **(C)** White lacy network of striae on buccal mucosa.

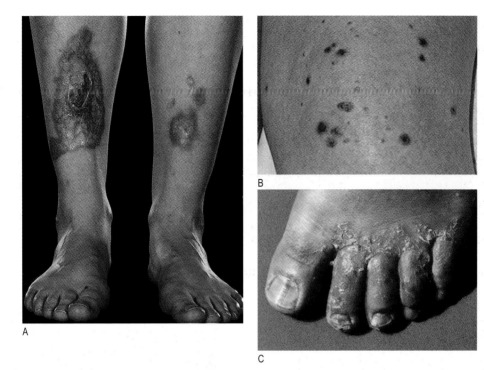

Fig. 4.8 Distribution: peripheral. (A) Necrobiosis lipoidica. **(B)** Vasculitis. **(C)** Fungal infection.

- Truncal, e.g. guttate psoriasis, following a streptococcal throat infection; pityriasis rosea, which usually starts with one lesion, the 'herald patch'; tinea versicolor, caused by *Pityrosporum* yeast; and urticaria, producing itchy wheals that clear within 24 hours (Fig. 4.6)
- Peripheral, e.g. wrist lesions, suggesting lichen planus (Fig. 4.7). Look at the buccal mucosa for the white lacy lesions of Wickham's striae to confirm this. Eruptions on the lower leg include necrobiosis lipoidica (Fig. 4.8A), erythema nodosum (due to sarcoidosis or streptococcal infection) and vasculitis caused by circulating immune complexes damaging dermal blood vessels (Fig. 4.8B). The hands or feet can be affected by fungal infection, typically 'athlete's foot' (Fig. 4.8C)
- Sun-exposed, on the face (sparing areas beneath the eyes and lower lip), the V of the neck or the posterior neck, and exposed areas of the arms and legs. Causes include connective tissue diseases, e.g. systemic lupus erythematosus (SLE), photosensitizing drugs, e.g. thiazide diuretics or non-steroidal anti-inflammatory drugs (NSAIDs) or a primary sun sensitivity condition, e.g. polymorphic light eruption or a photosensitive eczema
- Dermatomal, e.g. herpes zoster (shingles) (Fig. 4.9).

Morphology

Morphology is the shape and pattern of the skin lesions (Box 4.3 and Figs 4.10–4.13). Lesions may be:
- monomorphic (all the same appearance), as in guttate psoriasis
- pleomorphic (of differing appearance), as in chickenpox.

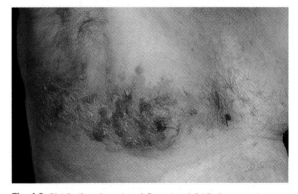

Fig. 4.9 Distribution: dermatomal. Dermatomal distribution suggests shingles.

Configuration

Configuration is the pattern in which lesions are arranged. Patterns include linear, grouped and annular (in a ring), or the Koebner phenomenon (an eruption in an area of local trauma) (Fig. 4.14). Secondary changes of crusting, erosion and excoriation complicate primary lesions.

Common patterns of hair disease

Hair loss

Hair loss (alopecia; Fig. 4.15) can be total or partial:
- Diffuse alopecia. In common male-pattern hair loss terminal scalp hairs undergo miniaturization to

> **i** 4.3 Terms used to describe skin lesions

Term	Definition	Term	Definition
Abscess	A localized collection of pus	Milium	A small white cyst that contains keratin
Atrophy	Loss of epidermis, dermis or both, thin, translucent and wrinkled skin, visible blood vessels	Nodule	A solid elevation of skin >5 mm in diameter
Bulla	A fluid-filled blister >5 mm in diameter	Papilloma	A nipple-like projection from the surface of the skin
Burrow	A tunnel in epidermis caused by a parasite, e.g. *Acarus* in scabies	Papule	A solid elevation of skin <5 mm in diameter
Callus	Local hyperplasia of horny layer on palm or sole, due to pressure	Petechia	A haemorrhagic punctate spot 1–2 mm in diameter
Comedo	A plug of sebum and keratin wedged in a dilated pilosebaceous orifice on the face	Plaque	A palpable elevation of skin >2 cm diameter and <5 mm in height
Crust	Dried exudate, e.g. serum, blood or pus, on the skin surface	Purpura	Extravasation of blood resulting in redness of skin or mucous membranes
Cyst	A nodule consisting of an epithelial-lined cavity filled with fluid or semisolid material	Pustule	A visible collection of pus in a blister
Ecchymosis	A macular red or purple haemorrhage, >2 mm in diameter, in skin or mucous membrane	Scale	Accumulation of easily detached fragments of thickened keratin
Erosion	A superficial break in the epidermis, not extending into dermis, heals without scarring	Scar	Replacement of normal tissue by fibrous connective tissue at the site of an injury
Erythema	Redness of the skin due to vascular dilatation	Stria	Atrophic linear band in skin, white, pink or purple, from connective tissue changes
Excoriation	A superficial abrasion, often linear, due to scratching	Telangiectasia	Dilated dermal blood vessels resulting in a visible lesion
Fissure	A linear split in epidermis, often just extending into dermis	Ulcer	A circumscribed area of skin loss extending into the dermis
Freckle	A macular area showing increased pigment formation by melanocytes	Vesicle	A clear, fluid-filled blister <5 mm in diameter
Lichenification	Chronic thickening of skin with increased skin markings, from rubbing or scratching	Wheal	A transitory, compressible papule or plaque of dermal oedema, red or white, indicating urticaria
Macule	A localized area of colour or textural change in the skin		

vellus hairs. This ageing phenomenon is strongly inherited and depends on androgens. Age-related hair loss in women is more diffuse. Non-scarring diffuse hair loss occurs in hypothyroidism, hypopituitarism and iron deficiency, or may be drug-induced, e.g. cytotoxic agents

- Localized non-scarring alopecia. In alopecia areata there is circumscribed loss of scalp, beard or eyebrow hair. Alopecia areata may involve the whole scalp (alopecia totalis) or all body hair (alopecia universalis). Localized hair loss can be caused by fungal infection, hair pulling, traction from braiding and secondary syphilis
- Scarring alopecia. Burns, severe infections, e.g. herpes zoster, lichen planus and SLE, may permanently scar the scalp and hair loss is permanent

- Loss of secondary sexual hair. In old age, cirrhosis and hypopituitarism, axillary and pubic hair is lost.

Excess hair

Excess hair growth takes two forms:

- Hirsutism: occurs in females. There is male-pattern growth of terminal hair, including facial and pubic hair extending towards the umbilicus (male escutcheon). It is a racial trait but may be idiopathic, and is rarely caused by an androgen-secreting tumour (Box 4.4). In these cases there are other features of virilization, e.g. male-pattern hair loss, clitoromegaly or a deep voice
- Hypertrichosis: occurs in males or females. There is excess terminal hair growth in a non-androgenic

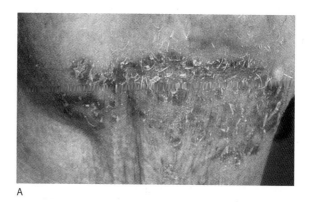

A

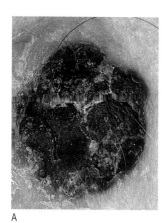

A

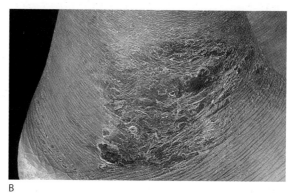

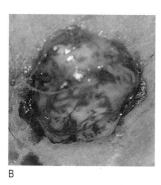

B

B

Fig. 4.10 **Nodule. (A)** Seborrhoeic wart. **(B)** Squamous cell cancer.

Fig. 4.12 **Plaque. (A)** Lupus vulgaris (tuberculosis of the skin).
(B) Tuberculoid leprosy.

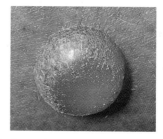

Fig. 4.13 **Bulla.** From an insect bite.

Nail abnormalities

Nail changes are useful in diagnosing internal conditions and skin diseases (Box 4.5; Fig. 3.16, p. 54).

Abnormal findings in mucous membranes and other sites

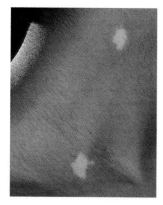

Fig. 4.11 **Macule.** Macules can be pigmented, as in a freckle, erythematous as in a haemangioma, or hypopigmented, as shown here in vitiligo, an autoimmune condition in which there is often symmetrical loss of pigment through destruction of melanocytes.

distribution. Hypertrichosis is uncommon and usually due to a systemic disorder, e.g. porphyria cutanea tarda, malignancy, anorexia nervosa, malnutrition or drugs, e.g. ciclosporin, minoxidil and phenytoin.

Changes in the mucous membranes of the mouth and genitalia accompany and may be characteristic of certain skin conditions: e.g. oral Wickham's striae in lichen planus, oral lesions in Kaposi's sarcoma

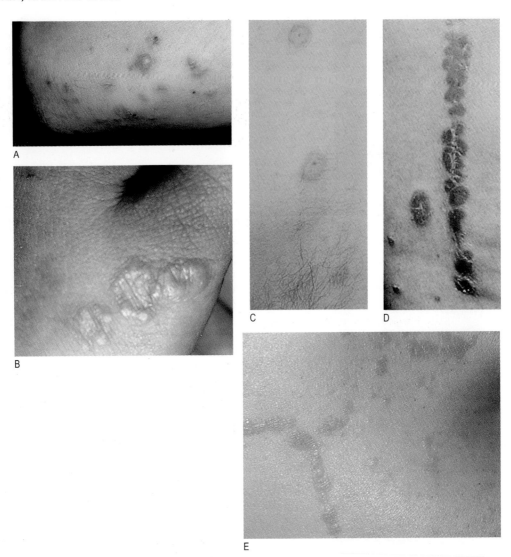

Fig. 4.14 Configuration. (A) Dermatitis herpetiformis: grouped. **(B)** Granuloma annulare: annular. **(C)** Insect bites: linear. **(D)** Psoriasis: showing the Koebner phenomenon — lesions in an area of trauma. **(E)** Viral warts: Koebner phenomenon.

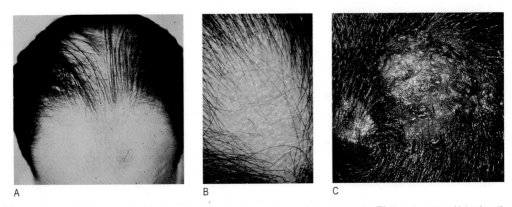

Fig. 4.15 Hair disorders. (A) Male-pattern baldness with hair loss from the temples and vertex of the scalp. **(B)** Alopecia areata with 'exclamation mark' hairs, which taper as they approach the skin. **(C)** Scalp ringworm with secondary bacterial infection and localized hair loss.

4

4.4 Causes of hirsutism

Type	Example
Pituitary	Acromegaly
Adrenal	Cushing's syndrome, virilizing tumours, congenital adrenal hyperplasia
Ovarian	Polycystic ovary syndrome, virilizing tumours
Drugs	Androgens, progestogens
Idiopathic	End-organ hypersensitivity to androgens

(Fig. 4.16A) or vulval involvement with lichen sclerosus. Fully examine patients with skin lymphoma for lymphadenopathy and hepatosplenomegaly. In patients with leg ulcers, feel the leg and foot pulses to assess the arterial supply (Fig 6 46 p 146)

THE HISTORY

Presenting complaint

Ask about when, where and how the eruption or lesions began, the initial appearance and what changes

4.5 Nail changes in systemic disease and skin disorders

Change	Description of nail	Differential diagnosis
Beau's lines	Transverse grooves	Any severe systemic illness which affects growth of the nail matrix (Fig. 3.16C, p. 54)
Brittle nails	Nails break easily, usually at distal margin	Effect of water and detergent, iron deficiency, hypothyroidism, digital ischaemia
Clubbing	Loss of angle between nail fold and nail plate. Finger tip bulbous. Nail matrix feels spongy	Familial or may signify serious cardiac or respiratory disease (Fig. 7.9, p. 165)
Colour changes	Blue	Cyanosis, antimalarials, haematoma
	Blue-green	*Pseudomonas* infection
	Brown	Fungal infection, staining from cigarettes, chlorpromazine, gold, Addison's disease
	Brown longitudinal streak	Melanocytic naevus, malignant melanoma, Addison's disease, racial variant
	Red streaks (splinter haemorrhages)	Infective endocarditis, trauma
	White spots	Trauma to nail matrix (not calcium deficiency)
	White/brown 'half and half' nails	Chronic renal failure
	White (leukonychia)	Hypoalbuminaemia, e.g. associated with cirrhosis
	Yellow	Psoriasis, fungal infection, jaundice, tetracycline
	Yellow nail syndrome	Defective lymphatic drainage — pleural effusions may occur
Combination changes	Longitudinal ridges and triangular nicks at the distal nail	Darier's disease
Koilonychia	Spoon-shaped depression of nail plate	Iron deficiency anaemia, lichen planus, repeated exposure to detergents (Fig. 3.16F, p. 54)
Nail fold erythema and telangiectasia	Dilated capillaries and erythema at nail fold	Connective tissue disorders, including systemic sclerosis, systemic lupus erythematosus, dermatomyositis (Fig. 3.16E, p. 54)
Onycholysis	Nail separates from nail bed	Psoriasis, fungal infection, trauma, thyrotoxicosis, tetracyclines (photo-onycholysis) (Fig. 3.16B, p. 54)
Onychomycosis	Thickening of the nail plate with colour change, usually whitening or brown discoloration	Fungal infection
Pitting	Fine or coarse pits in the nail	Psoriasis, eczema, alopecia areata, lichen planus
Thimble pitting	A particular type of fine regular pitting, as seen on a thimble	Alopecia areata
Coarse pitting	Larger irregular pits in the nail plate	Eczema
Ridging	Transverse (across nail)	Beau's lines (see above), eczema, psoriasis, tic-dystrophy, chronic paronychia
	Longitudinal (up/down)	Lichen planus, Darier's disease
Splinter haemorrhages	Small red streaks that lie longitudinally in the nail plate	Trauma but can signify infective endocarditis (Fig. 3.16A, p. 54)

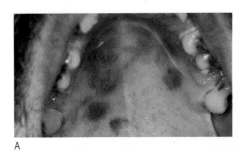

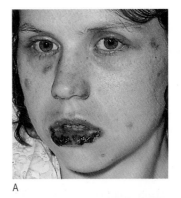

A

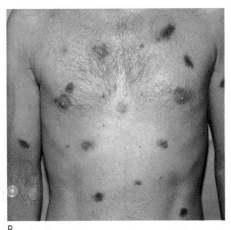

B

Fig. 4.16 Kaposi's sarcoma. **(A)** In the mouth. **(B)** On the skin.

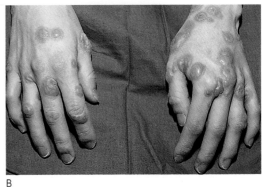

B

Fig. 4.17 Stevens–Johnson syndrome. **(A)** Facial and oral lesions. **(B)** 'Target lesions' of erythema multiforme on hands.

have occurred with time. Note associated features, such as itch and systemic upset, together with aggravating and relieving factors.

Past and drug histories

Ask about previous skin disease, atopic symptoms (hayfever, asthma, childhood eczema), medical disorders that may involve the skin, e.g. Stevens–Johnson syndrome caused by drugs (Fig. 4.17) or have cutaneous features, and prescribed or self-medicated drugs, including creams and cosmetics.

Social, family and genetic histories

Foreign travel gives exposure to tropical infections or sunlight that could cause a photosensitive eruption. Psoriasis and atopic eczema have strongly inherited traits.

Occupational and environmental histories

Chemicals encountered at work or during leisure activities may cause contact dermatitis. Suspect industrial

dermatitis if the eruption improves when the patient is away from work.

THE PHYSICAL EXAMINATION

General examination

Examining the skin is part of the general examination. When you examine the hands or face, note any abnormalities of the skin.

Specific examination

Ensure a warm, well-lit, private place is available. Offer a chaperone; record the chaperone's name or the fact that the patient has declined the offer. For widespread lesions ask patients to undress to their underclothes. Use a hand lens to examine individual lesions. A dermoscope, using a ×10 magnification illuminated lens system, is helpful for pigmented lesions (Fig. 4.18).

4

OSCEs 4.6 Examine this patient with a rash on the elbows

1. Look at whether there is involvement on the extensor areas of the elbows and knees, over the sacral area or on the trunk. (In atopic eczema, involvement is more commonly on the flexures of the elbows, behind the knees and on the face. Facial involvement is less common in psoriasis.)
2. Look at whether the nails are affected by onycholysis, subungual hyperkeratosis or brown 'oil-stain' patches — the changes of psoriasis. (In eczema, coarse pitting may be found.)
3. Look at the scalp (commonly involved in psoriasis by thick white plaques which shed large white scales).
4. Look at the hands and feet. (In palmo-pustular psoriasis, a variant not always associated with chronic plaque psoriasis, sterile pustules are found on the palms and soles.)
5. Examine for joint involvement. (Arthritis of various types is found in up to 30% of patients with psoriasis. It is not a feature of eczema.)
6. Examine the genitalia. (Psoriasis can involve the vulva and penis. These sites are less often involved in eczema.)

OSCEs 4.7 Examine this patient with a hand eruption

1. Look at the distribution:
   a. Finger tips involved, e.g. garlic allergy in a chef
   b. Small papules at the wrists extending up the forearm (lichen planus)
   c. Nails involved, e.g. pitting in psoriasis.
2. Are there skin lesions elsewhere on the body, e.g. atopic eczema affecting the antecubital or popliteal fossae, or psoriasis on the elbows, knees or scalp?
3. Look for burrows on the hands or genitalia (scabies).
4. Are there small blisters (vesicles) with redness, fissuring and scaling (eczema) or are the changes those of plaques with nail pitting (psoriasis)?
5. Consider further investigations: for example, patch testing for cell-mediated allergy, e.g. to fragrances in cosmetics, or prick testing for immediate allergy, e.g. to latex.

Look for:

- distribution
- variation in the types of lesion and in their individual shape, size and colour
- composition in terms of the nature of individual lesions
- configuration.

Examination sequence

The skin, hair and nails

Stand back and look at the skin: is it abnormal?

Note the distribution of lesions.

Observe the individual lesion for:

- Size
- Shape
- Colour
- Consistency
- Border changes
- Spatial interrelationships.

Palpate the lesions with your finger tips to establish their consistency. (Put on gloves if the skin is broken.)

Look at:

- Nails on hands and feet
- Different areas of the scalp (part the hair to see and ask the patient to point to the site of the problem to help localize it)
- Mucous membranes.

Examine local lymph nodes in any patient with a potential squamous cell cancer, malignant melanoma or cutaneous T-cell lymphoma (pp. 55–57).

Take a skin scraping for microscopy and culture if you suspect fungal infection.

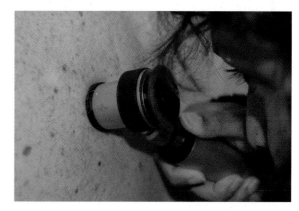

Fig. 4.18 A dermoscope. The dermoscope is helpful when looking at suspicious pigmented lesions.

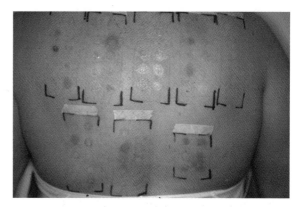

Fig. 4.19 Patch testing. Known allergens are applied to the patient's back and read at 2 and 4 days.

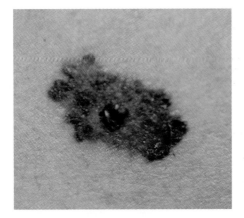

Fig. 4.20 Malignant melanoma. A darkly pigmented nodule, with irregular margins and variability of pigmentation.

PUTTING IT ALL TOGETHER

In order to diagnose skin disease you need to be familiar with the patterns of skin conditions and then mentally test multiple hypotheses for the best fit against the facts of the history and examination. Not all historic or physical findings match the classic descriptions. The diagnosis is usually suggested by the history and confirmed by the physical findings. Investigations, such as a skin biopsy, are required in a few cases, to support or refute the clinical possibilities.

OSCEs 4.8 Examine this patient with a pigmented skin lesion on the back

1. Has the mole appeared recently or has it changed? (Malignant melanoma can occur in an existing melanocytic naevus or as a new lesion.)
2. Has the mole has become bigger, has it been itchy or has it bled (malignant melanoma).
3. Is there a family history of malignant melanoma or other skin cancer? (A family history is found in 10% of patients with malignant melanoma.)
4. Does the patient have a fair skin type, i.e. does he burn easily and tan poorly or not at all? (Skin cancers are more common with a pale skin.)
5. Look at the edge of the mole, the distribution of pigment within it and whether it is inflamed or ulcerated. (Malignant melanoma commonly shows variation in pigmentation or outline and has an irregular or diffuse edge.) Remember the mnemonic **'ABCD'** — **A**symmetry, **B**order irregular, **C**olour irregular and **D**iameter >6 mm.
6. Examine the entire skin for other suspicious moles or skin cancers. (Abnormal moles are more common in patients who have a malignant melanoma.)
7. Request urgent surgical excision biopsy for histological examination.

INVESTIGATIONS

Box 4.9.

4.9 Investigations in skin disease

Investigation	Indication/Comment
Wood's light	Vitiligo, fungal infection Hand-held ultraviolet lamp shows vitiligo not apparent in ordinary light, or fluorescence in fungal infection
Blood tests, including haematology and biochemistry	Systemic disease Anaemia, kidney, liver and thyroid function may confirm systemic disease. Monitor blood parameters in patients on systemic drugs
Serology	Autoimmune disease and eczema SLE and rheumatic disease. Serum IgE or allergen-specific IgE in some patients with atopic eczema
Microscopy and fungal culture	Rashes Use a disposable scalpel to scrape the active margin of the rash, dislodging scales on to a piece of black paper
Surgical biopsy	Rashes or nodules Histology or direct immunofluorescence (vasculitis)
Doppler studies	Leg ulcers An index of the dorsalis pedis BP over brachial BP of <0.8 helps suggests arterial disease
Photography	Pigmented lesions Compare the development of the lesion over time
Patch tests	Delayed-type contact allergy, e.g. to fragrances Prepared allergens on small aluminium discs are applied to the upper back and the skin reviewed 2 and 4 days later
Prick tests	Immediate allergy, e.g. to latex Prepared allergen solutions are pricked into the dermis and reviewed 15 minutes later. Histamine and saline solutions are used as positive and negative controls

4.10 Key points: the skin, hair and nails

- Be particularly sensitive to your patient's feelings. Skin conditions are especially difficult for many people to bear.
- The timing of the start and evolution of the eruption often suggests the diagnosis.
- Look at the entire skin surface; it is easy to miss a typical patch of psoriasis on the elbow in someone whose hand eruption is not typical for psoriasis.
- Use a hand lens or dermoscope with good lighting.
- Gently feel the skin to assess texture, wearing gloves if the skin is broken.
- Always take a scraping for fungal examination in unilateral hand dermatitis.
- In scabies, treat all members of the household, not just the index case.
- A patient whose eczema is not responding to treatment may have developed allergic contact dermatitis to a topical treatment or a fungal infection.
- Ask patients what over-the-counter creams they have used; they might be reacting adversely to them.
- Always understand what your patient's occupation is; it often has a bearing on the skin problem, even if it is not causing it directly.

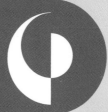

John S. Bevan

The endocrine system

5

ENDOCRINE EXAMINATION

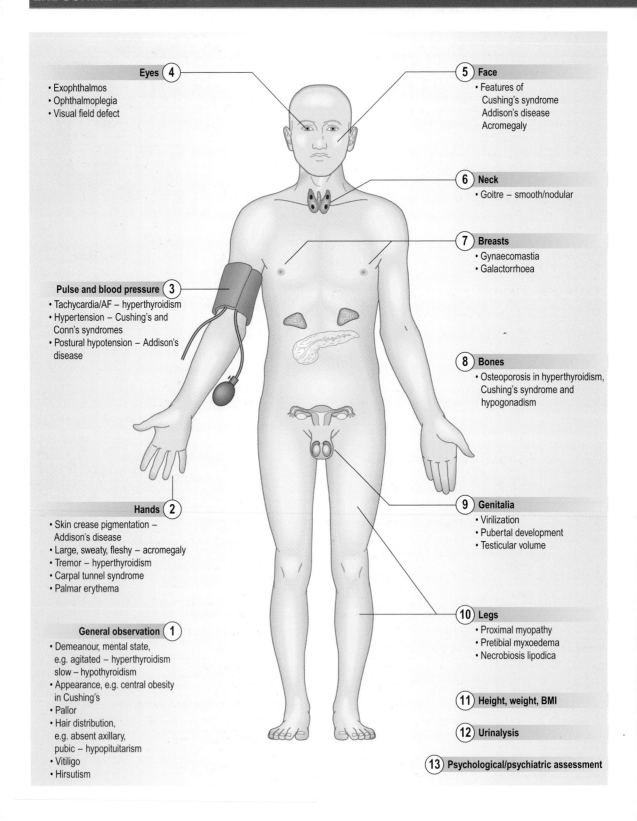

Eyes ④
- Exophthalmos
- Ophthalmoplegia
- Visual field defect

⑤ **Face**
- Features of
  Cushing's syndrome
  Addison's disease
  Acromegaly

⑥ **Neck**
- Goitre – smooth/nodular

⑦ **Breasts**
- Gynaecomastia
- Galactorrhoea

Pulse and blood pressure ③
- Tachycardia/AF – hyperthyroidism
- Hypertension – Cushing's and
  Conn's syndromes
- Postural hypotension – Addison's
  disease

⑧ **Bones**
- Osteoporosis in hyperthyroidism,
  Cushing's syndrome and
  hypogonadism

Hands ②
- Skin crease pigmentation –
  Addison's disease
- Large, sweaty, fleshy – acromegaly
- Tremor – hyperthyroidism
- Carpal tunnel syndrome
- Palmar erythema

⑨ **Genitalia**
- Virilization
- Pubertal development
- Testicular volume

⑩ **Legs**
- Proximal myopathy
- Pretibial myxoedema
- Necrobiosis lipodica

General observation ①
- Demeanour, mental state,
  e.g. agitated – hyperthyroidism
  slow – hypothyroidism
- Appearance, e.g. central obesity
  in Cushing's
- Pallor
- Hair distribution,
  e.g. absent axillary,
  pubic – hypopituitarism
- Vitiligo
- Hirsutism

⑪ **Height, weight, BMI**

⑫ **Urinalysis**

⑬ **Psychological/psychiatric assessment**

ANATOMY

The main endocrine glands are the pituitary, thyroid, parathyroids, pancreas, adrenals and gonads: testes and ovaries (Fig. 5.1). These glands synthesize hormones which are released into the circulation and act at distant sites. Although some endocrine glands, e.g. parathyroid glands and pancreas, respond directly to metabolic signals, most are controlled by hormones released from the pituitary gland. A wide variety of molecules act as hormones:

- peptides, e.g. insulin
- glycoproteins, e.g. thyroid-stimulating hormone (TSH)
- amines, e.g. noradrenaline (norepinephrine)
- steroid hormones, e.g. cortisol
- oestrogen
- triiodothyronine
- vitamin D.

THE PHYSICAL EXAMINATION

Symptoms of endocrine disturbance are frequently varied and non-specific, and affect many body systems (Box 5.1). Endocrine conditions may be picked up by chance: for example, hypothyroidism discovered on blood test screening, goitre found during routine medical examination or acromegaly recognized when

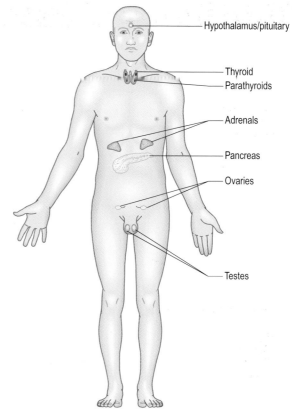

Fig. 5.1 The principal endocrine glands.

5.1 Common clinical features in endocrine disease

Symptom, sign or problem	Differential diagnoses
Weight gain	Hypothyroidism, polycystic ovary syndrome (PCOS), Cushing's syndrome
Weight loss	Hyperthyroidism, diabetes mellitus, adrenal insufficiency
Short stature	Constitutional, non-endocrine systemic disease, e.g. coeliac disease, growth hormone deficiency
Delayed puberty	Constitutional, non-endocrine systemic disease, hypothyroidism, hypopituitarism, primary gonadal failure
Menstrual disturbance	PCOS, hyperprolactinaemia, thyroid dysfunction
Diffuse neck swelling	Simple goitre, Graves' disease, Hashimoto's thyroiditis
Excessive thirst	Diabetes mellitus or insipidus, hyperparathyroidism, Conn's syndrome
Hirsutism	Idiopathic, PCOS, Cushing's syndrome, congenital adrenal hyperplasia
'Funny turns'	Hypoglycaemia, phaeochromocytoma, neuroendocrine tumour
Sweating	Hyperthyroidism, hypogonadism, acromegaly, phaeochromocytoma
Flushing	Hypogonadism (especially menopause), carcinoid syndrome
Resistant hypertension	Conn's syndrome, Cushing's syndrome, phaeochromocytoma, acromegaly, renal artery stenosis
Erectile dysfunction	Primary or secondary hypogonadism, diabetes mellitus, non-endocrine systemic disease
Muscle weakness	Cushing's syndrome, hyperthyroidism, hyperparathyroidism, osteomalacia
Bone fragility and fractures	Cushing's syndrome, hypogonadism, hyperthyroidism
Altered facial appearance	Hypothyroidism, Cushing's syndrome, acromegaly, PCOS

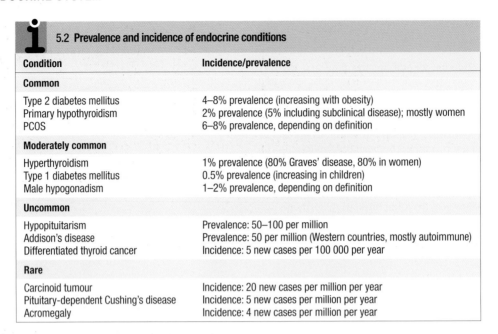

5.2 Prevalence and incidence of endocrine conditions

Condition	Incidence/prevalence
Common	
Type 2 diabetes mellitus	4–8% prevalence (increasing with obesity)
Primary hypothyroidism	2% prevalence (5% including subclinical disease); mostly women
PCOS	6–8% prevalence, depending on definition
Moderately common	
Hyperthyroidism	1% prevalence (80% Graves' disease, 80% in women)
Type 1 diabetes mellitus	0.5% prevalence (increasing in children)
Male hypogonadism	1–2% prevalence, depending on definition
Uncommon	
Hypopituitarism	Prevalence: 50–100 per million
Addison's disease	Prevalence: 50 per million (Western countries, mostly autoimmune)
Differentiated thyroid cancer	Incidence: 5 new cases per 100 000 per year
Rare	
Carcinoid tumour	Incidence: 20 new cases per million per year
Pituitary-dependent Cushing's disease	Incidence: 5 new cases per million per year
Acromegaly	Incidence: 4 new cases per million per year

the doctor meets a patient not seen for several years. Remember that, apart from diabetes mellitus, thyroid disease and some reproductive disorders, endocrine diseases are uncommon; most patients with tiredness or excessive sweating, for example, will not have an underlying endocrine cause (Box 5.2).

Examination sequence

Endocrine disease

◼ Take time at the outset to make some general observations.

◼ The initial handshake may suggest a diagnosis.

◼ Inspect the face for a 'spot' endocrine diagnosis (Figs 5.5A, 5.6A, 5.9A, 5.10A, 5.11A and 5.12A).

◼ Is the patient restless and agitated (hyperthyroidism) or slow and lethargic (hypothyroidism)?

◼ Examine the entire skin surface, looking for abnormal pallor (hypopituitarism), vitiligo, plethora (Cushing's or carcinoid syndrome) or pigmentation (Addison's disease).

◼ If the patient is obese, is the adiposity centrally distributed (Cushing's syndrome and growth hormone deficiency)?

◼ Is the body hair normal in quality and amount? Look for hirsutism in females with menstrual disturbance, especially on the face, chest and abdomen (polycystic ovary syndrome (PCOS)) (Fig. 5.14).

◼ Examine the hands for excessive sweating, soft tissue overgrowth (acromegaly), skin crease pigmentation (Addison's disease) and wasting of the thenar muscles due to carpal tunnel syndrome (hypothyroidism, acromegaly) (Fig. 14.32, p. 379). Patients with Cushing's syndrome often have thin, fragile skin (Fig. 5.11D).

◼ Assess the pulse rate, rhythm and volume. Tachycardia and atrial fibrillation may suggest thyrotoxicosis.

◼ Record the blood pressure. Hypertension is a feature of several endocrine conditions, such as phaeochromocytoma and Conn's syndrome (primary hyperaldosteronism) (Box 5.1). Check for postural hypotension with lying and standing blood pressures if you suspect adrenal insufficiency.

◼ Examine the eyes in all thyroid patients for external inflammation, proptosis, diplopia and visual function. Assess visual acuities and fields in patients with suspected pituitary tumours, to detect bitemporal hemianopia due to compression of the optic chiasm. Examine the fundi for optic atrophy in patients with longstanding optic pathway compression (Fig. 12.32, p. 326).

◼ Examine the neck for goitre. If this is present, record its size, surface and consistency.

◼ Look for gynaecomastia in men (common in Klinefelter's syndrome 47XXY (Fig. 5.13), and for evidence of milk production in a man or non-breastfeeding woman (galactorrhoea). If you suspect galactorrhoea, gently massage the breast tissue in the direction of the nipple to see if milk is expressed. Explain beforehand why you are performing this examination and watch the patient carefully since this may be uncomfortable.

◼ Inspect the axillae for acanthosis nigricans (Fig. 5.8A) or loss of axillary hair (Fig. 5.10B).

◼ Look for a thoracic kyphosis, which may be a sign of osteoporotic vertebral collapse.

◼ Examine the abdomen. Patients with carcinoid syndrome frequently have a palpable, nodular liver, which is sometimes massively enlarged. Adrenal tumours may occasionally be palpable, but be cautious if phaeochromocytoma is suspected, as over-enthusiastic examination may precipitate a hypertensive paroxysm.

◼ Examine the male external genitalia (p. 263). Inspect the amount of pubic hair and make a pubertal staging of all adolescents using Tanner gradings. Record testicular consistency and volume (use an orchidometer; Fig. 15.26, p. 424).

◼ Inspect the legs for evidence of pretibial myxoedema (Graves' disease; Fig. 5.5D), proximal muscle wasting and weakness (Cushing's syndrome and hyperthyroidism).

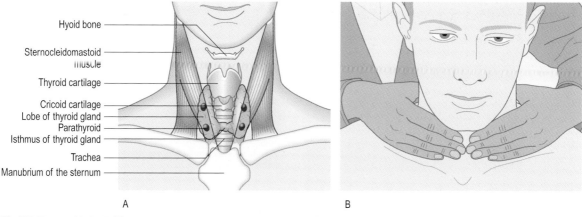

Fig. 5.2 **The thyroid gland. (A)** Anatomy of the gland and surrounding structures. **(B)** Palpating the thyroid gland from behind.

- Measure the patient's height, using a stadiometer in children and adolescents (Fig. 15.23, p. 417), and weight.
- Calculate the body mass index (BMI; p. 59).
- Test the urine for glycosuria (diabetes mellitus) and proteinuria (hypertensive renal damage).
- Formal psychological evaluation may be helpful in selected patients. Two-thirds of patients with Cushing's syndrome have psychological or psychiatric features.

THE THYROID GLAND

Anatomy

The thyroid gland is butterfly-shaped and comprises two symmetrical lobes joined by a central isthmus that normally covers the second and third tracheal rings (Fig. 5.2A). The gland may extend into the superior mediastinum, or may occasionally be entirely retrosternal. Rarely, it is located higher in the neck along the line of the thyroglossal duct. If situated at the back of the tongue (lingual goitre), it may be visible through the open mouth. The normal thyroid gland is palpable in about 50% of women and 25% of men. Goitre is enlargement of the thyroid gland.

◼▶ Examination sequence

The thyroid gland

- Inspect the neck from the front.
- Look for a swelling while the patient swallows a sip of water. The thyroid (or a thyroglossal cyst) moves upwards on swallowing since it is enveloped in the pre-tracheal fascia which is attached to the cricoid cartilage.
- Ask the patient to sit with the neck muscles relaxed and stand behind him.
- Place your hands gently on the front of the patient's neck, with your index fingers just touching (Fig. 5.2B). Ask the patient to swallow a sip of water while you feel over the gland as it moves upwards.

Some patients find neck palpation uncomfortable, so be alert for any signs of distress.
- Note the size, shape and consistency of any goitre and feel for any thrill. Measure any discrete nodules with calipers. With large goitres, record the maximum neck circumference using a tape measure (an objective measurement for long-term follow-up).
- Listen with your stethoscope for a thyroid bruit.

Abnormal findings

Shape and surface

Simple goitres are relatively symmetrical in their earlier stages but often become nodular with time. In Graves' disease the surface of the thyroid gland is usually smooth and diffuse, whereas it is irregular in uninodular or multinodular goitre (Fig. 5.3).

Mobility

Most goitres move upwards with swallowing. Very large goitres may be immobile, and invasive thyroid cancer may fix the gland to surrounding structures.

Consistency

Nodules in the substance of the gland may be large or small, and single or multiple, and are usually benign. A very hard consistency suggests malignant change in the gland. Large, firm lymph nodes near a goitre suggest thyroid cancer (Fig. 5.4).

Tenderness

Diffuse tenderness is typical of viral thyroiditis, whereas localized tenderness may follow bleeding into a thyroid cyst.

Thyroid bruit

This indicates abnormally high blood flow and can be associated with a palpable thrill. It occurs in hyperthyroidism. A thyroid bruit may be confused with other sounds. A bruit arising from the carotid artery or

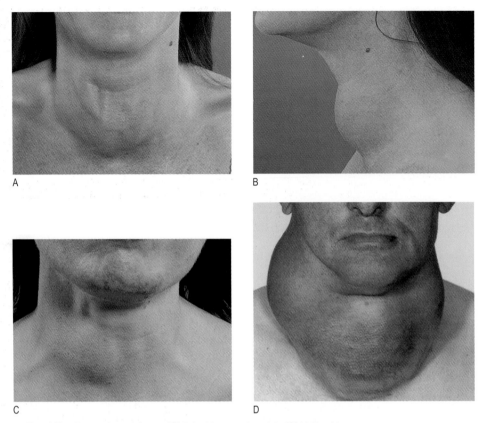

Fig. 5.3 Goitres. (A and **B)** Diffuse — Graves' disease. **(C)** Uninodular — toxic nodule. **(D)** Multinodular.

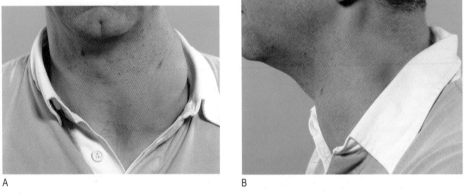

Fig. 5.4 Thyroid cancer. Papillary thyroid cancer with regional cervical lymphadenopathy.

transmitted from the aorta will be louder along the line of the artery. Transient gentle pressure over the root of the neck will interrupt a venous hum from the internal jugular vein.

Thyroid disease

Most hyperthyroidism is due to autoimmune Graves' disease. Look at the patient's face; lid retraction contributes to a rather startled-looking expression (Fig. 5.5A). Patients with Graves' disease may have associated thyroid eye disease, digital acropachy and pretibial myxoedema (Figs 5.5B–D).

Hypothyroidism is usually due to Hashimoto's thyroiditis. The facial appearance may be characteristic, particularly in older patients who usually have marked periorbital myxoedema (Fig. 5.6). Look for cold peripheries, dry skin and hair, bradycardia and delayed muscle relaxation when testing tendon reflexes.

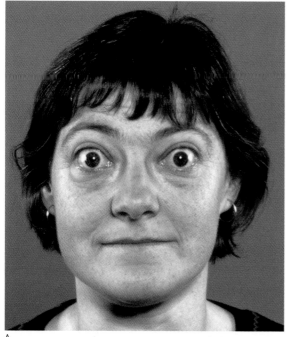

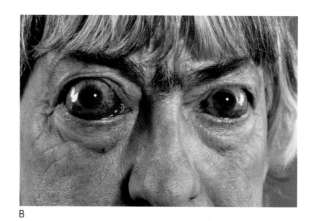

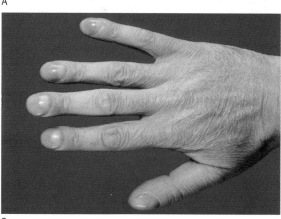

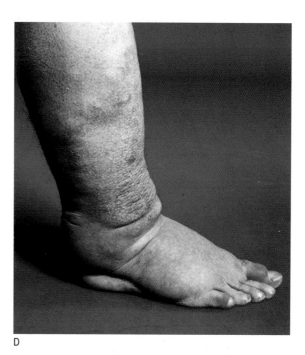

Fig. 5.5 **Graves' hyperthyroidism.** **(A)** Typical facies. **(B)** Severe inflammatory thyroid eye disease. **(C)** Thyroid acropachy. **(D)** Pretibial myxoedema.

THE PARATHYROID GLANDS

There are usually four parathyroid glands which lie posterior to the thyroid (Fig. 5.2A). Each is about the size of a pea and produces parathyroid hormone (PTH), a peptide which increases the level of calcium in the blood.

Parathyroid disease

Parathyroid disease produces few physical signs. A parathyroid tumour is rarely palpable in the neck in patients with hyperparathyroidism. Patients with longstanding disease may have corneal calcification best seen using a slit lamp (Fig. 5.7A). Tender areas of bone fracture deformity ('Brown tumours') may be found (Fig. 5.7B).

Patients with hypoparathyroidism may present with classical carpopedal spasms (tetany). If overt tetany is not present, assess for latent tetany by inflating a blood pressure cuff above arterial pressure for 3 minutes. Carpal muscle spasm should occur within 3 minutes ('main d'accoucheur' or Trousseau's sign).

Patients with autosomal dominant pseudo-hypoparathyroidism are typically short in stature, with round faces and characteristic shortening of some of the metacarpal bones (Figs 5.7C and D).

93

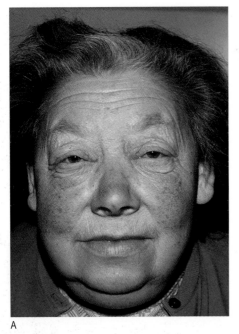 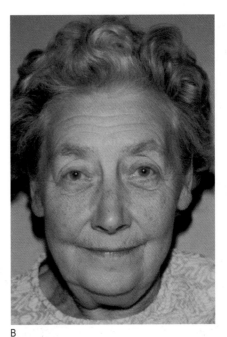

A   B

Fig. 5.6 Hypothyroidism. (A) Before treatment. **(B)** After levothyroxine replacement.

OSCEs 5.3 Examine this patient with weight loss and heat intolerance

1. Shake hands and note excessive warmth and sweating.
2. Look for fine tremor of outstretched hands and acropachy of the fingers (hyperthyroidism).
3. Examine the radial pulse (usually rapid and high-volume unless on a β-blocker). An irregularly irregular pulse is likely to indicate atrial fibrillation.
4. Examine the thyroid and describe its size, surface and consistency. Listen for a thyroid bruit.
5. Look for evidence of thyroid eye disease.
6. Inspect the shins for pretibial myxoedema.

THE PANCREAS

The pancreas lies behind the stomach on the posterior abdominal wall. Its endocrine functions include the production of insulin, glucagon, somatostatin, gastrin and vasoactive intestinal peptide. Its exocrine function is to produce alkaline secretions containing digestive enzymes.

Diabetes mellitus

Diabetes mellitus is characterized by hyperglycaemia due to absolute or relative insulin deficiency. There are two main subtypes:

- type 1: severe insulin deficiency due to autoimmune destruction of the pancreatic islets

- type 2: commonly affects people who are obese and insulin-resistant, although impaired β-cell function is also important.

Microvascular, neuropathic and macrovascular complications of hyperglycaemia (Box 5.4) can occur in patients with any type of diabetes mellitus, and may be present at diagnosis in patients with slow-onset type 2 disease.

Diabetes may present with the classical triad of symptoms:

- polyuria: due to osmotic diuresis caused by glycosuria
- thirst: due to the resulting loss of fluid and electrolytes
- weight loss: due to fluid depletion and breakdown of fat and muscle secondary to insulin deficiency.

Other common symptoms include tiredness, blurred vision (due to glucose-induced changes in lens refraction) and itching of the genitalia (pruritus vulvae in women or balanitis in men) due to *Candida* yeast infection (thrush).

On examination there may be evidence of weight loss and dehydration, and in diabetic ketoacidosis the breath may have the sweet smell of ketones. Skin infections with boils and abscesses are common. Acanthosis nigricans (soft, velvety, brown skin) is a sign of hyperinsulinism and is seen frequently in the axillae and groins of patients with insulin-resistant type 2 diabetes (Fig. 5.8A). Necrobiosis lipoidica, due to collagen degeneration, may occur on the shins of some patients with type 1 diabetes and often causes chronic ulceration (Fig. 5.8B). The causes of diabetic foot ulceration are

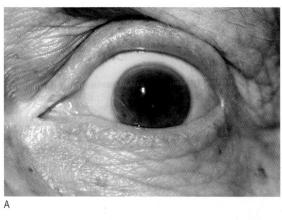

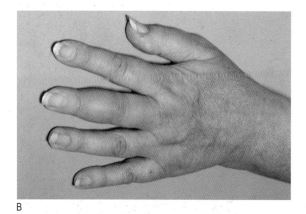

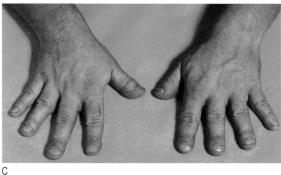

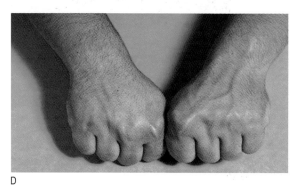

A

B

C

D

Fig. 5.7 Parathyroid disease. (A) Corneal calcification in hyperparathyroidism. **(B)** 'Brown tumour' of the phalanx (middle finger) in hyperparathyroidism. **(C)** Pseudohypoparathyroidism: short metacarpals. **(D)** These are best seen when the patient makes a fist.

5.4 Complications of diabetes mellitus

Microvascular/neuropathic

- Retinopathy, cataract
  Impaired vision
- Nephropathy
  Protein loss, renal failure
- Peripheral neuropathy
  Sensory loss, motor
  weakness

- Autonomic neuropathy
  Postural hypotension,
  vomiting, diarrhoea
- Foot disease
  Ulceration, arthropathy

Macrovascular

- Coronary circulation
  Myocardial ischaemia/
  infarction
- Cerebral circulation
  Transient ischaemic attack
  (TIA), stroke

- Peripheral circulation
  Claudication, gangrene,
  amputation

---

multifactorial, including diabetic neuropathy, arterial insufficiency and increased susceptibility to infection (Fig. 5.8C). Look for xanthomata in all newly presenting diabetic patients; their presence indicates significant hyperlipidaemia (Fig. 5.8D). Examine insulin injection sites for evidence of lipohypertrophy (which may cause unpredictable insulin release), lipoatrophy (now rare) or signs of infection (very rare).

Insulin-dependent patients are particularly susceptible to acute metabolic decompensation due to hypoglycaemia or ketoacidosis, both of which require prompt clinical and biochemical recognition.

THE PITUITARY GLAND

The pituitary gland is enclosed in the sella turcica in the base of the skull beneath the hypothalamus. It is bridged over by a fold of dura mater (diaphragma sellae) with sphenoidal air spaces below and the optic chiasm above. The pituitary has two lobes:

- the anterior pituitary, which secretes several hormones (adrenocorticotrophic hormone (ACTH), prolactin, growth hormone (GH), TSH and gonadotrophins (luteinizing hormone (LH) and follicle-stimulating hormone (FSH))
- the posterior pituitary, an extension of the hypothalamus, which secretes vasopressin (antidiuretic hormone (ADH)) and oxytocin.

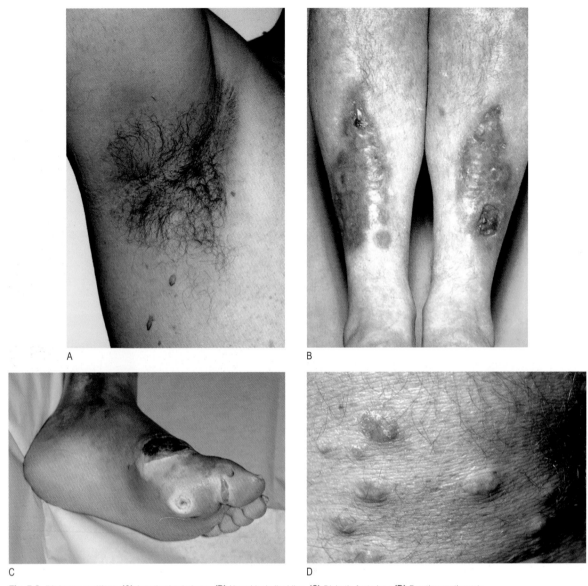

Fig. 5.8 Diabetes mellitus. (A) Acanthosis nigricans. **(B)** Necrobiosis lipoidica. **(C)** Diabetic foot ulcer. **(D)** Eruptive xanthomata.

Acromegaly

Acromegaly is caused by a GH-secreting pituitary tumour. GH stimulates excessive insulin-like growth factor-1 production by the liver, and this hormone is responsible for most of the clinical manifestations. Look for the characteristic facial changes, including coarsening of features, thick greasy skin, enlargement of the nose, prognathism (protrusion of the mandible) and separation of the lower teeth (Figs 5.9A and B). Expansion of the soft tissues of the hands and feet causes tight fitting of rings, gloves and footwear (Figs 5.9C and D). Expansion of the tumour can cause pressure on the optic chiasm, resulting in visual field defects, especially bitemporal hemianopia (Fig. 12.3, p. 309).

Hypopituitarism

Anterior hypopituitarism may be due to compression of the pituitary by a macroadenoma, infarction after childbirth (Sheehan's syndrome), severe head trauma or cranial radiotherapy. Look for extreme skin pallor (a combination of mild anaemia and melanocyte-stimulating hormone deficiency), reduced/absent secondary sexual hair and testicular atrophy (Fig. 5.10). Absence of axillary hair is abnormal after puberty.

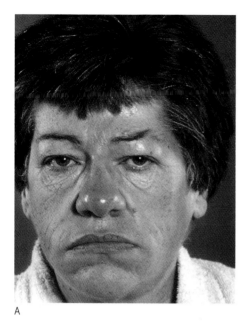

A

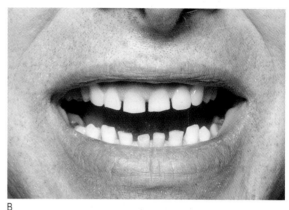

B

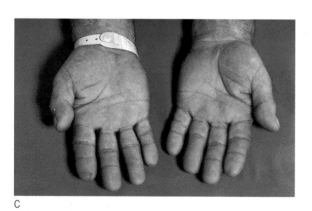

C

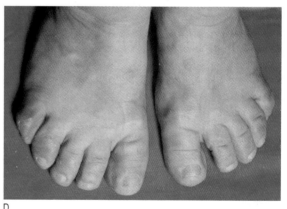

D

Fig. 5.9 Acromegaly. (A) Typical facies. **(B)** Separation of lower teeth. **(C)** Large fleshy hands. **(D)** Widening of the feet.

OSCEs 5.5 Examine this patient with excessive sweating and snoring

1. On greeting the patient, note the large, moist and fleshy hands.

2. Lift a pinch of skin from the dorsum of the hand and note its increased thickness.

3. Look at the face for signs of acromegaly: thick, greasy skin, especially over the forehead, large nose and tongue, prognathism and separation of lower teeth.

4. Inspect feet for increased soft tissues.

5. Look for signs of carpal tunnel syndrome (wasted thenar eminence(s), sensory loss).

6. Check visual fields (possible bitemporal hemianopia).

7. Measure BP (one-third of acromegalics have hypertension).

8. Test the urine for glycosuria (one-third of acromegalics have diabetes mellitus).

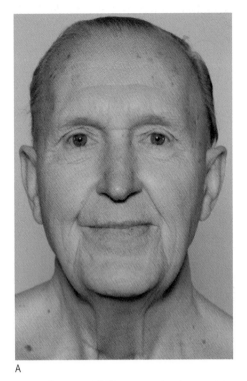
A

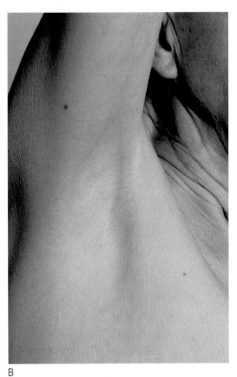
B

Fig. 5.10 Hypopituitarism. (A) Hypopituitarism due to a pituitary adenoma (note the skin pallor). **(B)** Absent axillary hair.

THE ADRENAL GLANDS

The adrenal glands are small pyramidal organs lying immediately above the kidneys on their posteromedial surface.

- The adrenal medulla is part of the sympathetic nervous system and secretes catecholamines
- The adrenal cortex secretes cortisol, mineralocorticoids and androgens.

Cushing's syndrome

Cushing's syndrome is caused by excess exogenous or endogenous corticosteroid exposure. Most cases of Cushing's are iatrogenic, due to side-effects of corticosteroid therapy. 'Endogenous' Cushing's usually results from an ACTH-secreting pituitary microadenoma. Other causes include a primary adrenal tumour or 'ectopic' ACTH secretion.

The catabolic effects of steroids cause widespread tissue breakdown (particularly in skin, muscle and bone) with central accumulation of body fat. Proximal myopathy, fragility fractures, spontaneous purpura, skin thinning and susceptibility to infection are common (Fig. 5.11).

Addison's disease

Addison's disease is due to inadequate secretion of cortisol, usually secondary to autoimmune destruction of the adrenal cortex. The melanocyte-stimulating hormone-dependent brown pigmentation of Addison's disease (primary adrenal insufficiency) is most striking in white Europeans. It is most prominent in surface epithelia subject to trauma: that is, skin creases, pressure areas, buccal mucosa and healing scars (Figs 5.12A–C). Look also for areas of depigmented skin known as vitiligo in patients with Addison's disease (and other autoimmune endocrinopathies; Fig. 5.12D).

THE GONADS

These glands secrete sex hormones (oestrogen and testosterone) in response to gonadotrophins released by the pituitary. They also contain the germ cells.

Reproductive disorders

Klinefelter's syndrome (47XYY) is the most common cause of primary hypogonadism in men (1:600

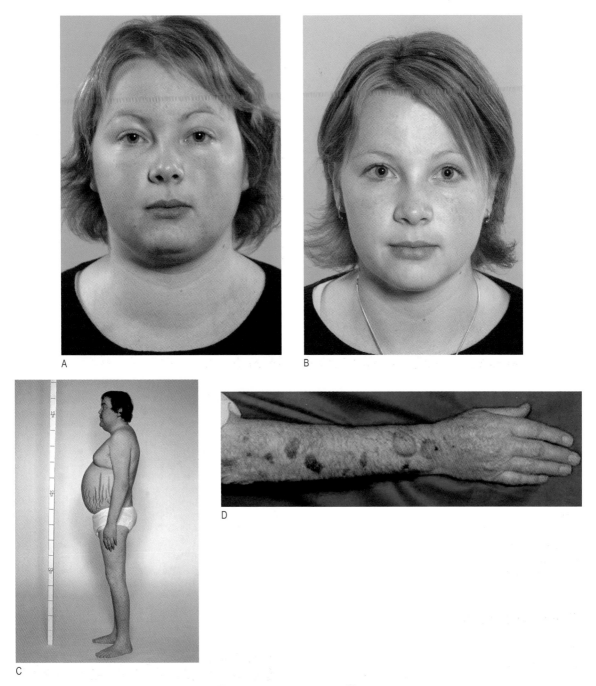

Fig. 5.11 Cushing's syndrome. (A) Cushingoid facies. **(B)** After curative pituitary surgery. **(C)** Typical features: facial rounding, central obesity, proximal muscle wasting and skin striae. **(D)** Skin thinning: purpura caused by wristwatch pressure.

live male births). Diagnosis may be delayed until later life, by which time the features of prolonged testosterone deficiency can be seen. Look for soft, finely wrinkled, hairless facial skin and gynaecomastia and examine the genitalia (pubic hair is often reduced/absent and the testes <3 ml in volume; Fig. 5.13).

Hirsutism (excess body and facial hair) is common in women with PCOS (Fig. 5.14). Examine women with a short history of severe hirsutism for signs of virilization which suggest a possible testosterone-secreting tumour; look for temporal recession of the scalp hair, deepening of the voice, increased muscle bulk and clitoromegaly (Fig. 5.15).

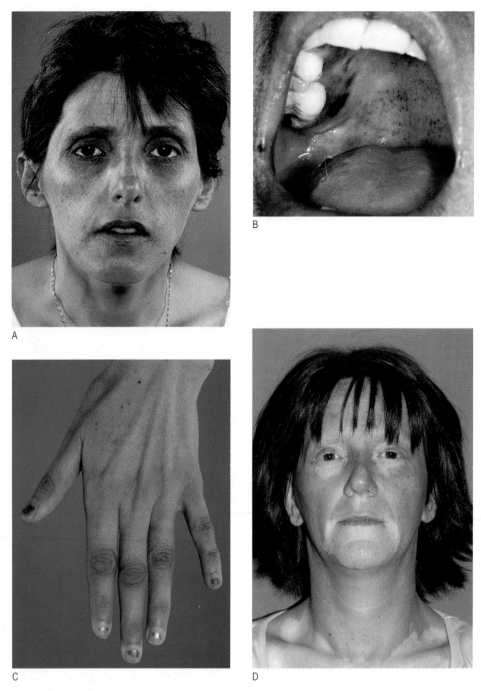

Fig. 5.12 Addison's disease. (A) Facial pigmentation. **(B)** Buccal pigmentation. **(C)** Skin crease pigmentation. **(D)** Vitiligo — particularly striking due to Addisonian pigmentation of the 'normal' skin.

5

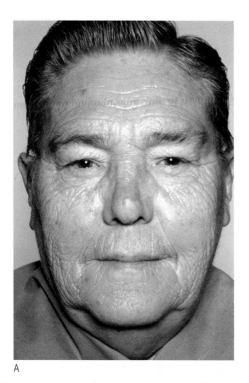

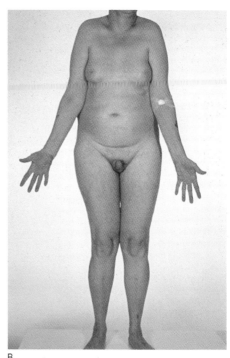

A

B

Fig. 5.13 Klinefelter's syndrome. (A) Hypogonadal facial skin. **(B)** Gynaecomastia, reduced pubic hair and small testes.

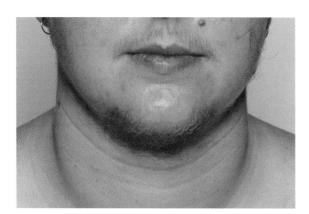

Fig. 5.14 Polycystic ovary syndrome. Facial hirsutism.

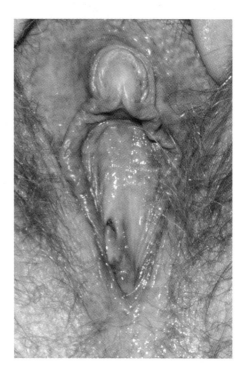

Fig. 5.15 Testosterone-secreting ovarian tumour. Clitoromegaly.

OSCEs 5.6 Examine this patient with tiredness and pallor

1. Look for signs of chronic blood loss or iron deficiency — pallor, angular stomatitis, koilonychia.

2. Look at face for puffiness about the eyes (hypothyroidism) and, in men, poor beard growth (hypopituitarism).

3. Listen to voice — slow, deliberate, croaky (hypothyroidism).

4. Measure BP — hypotension in hypovolaemia, Addison's disease and hypopituitarism.

5. Feel the neck for goitre (hypothyroidism).

6. Palpate abdomen for tenderness, masses and hepatosplenomegaly.

7. Examine for absence of axillary and pubic hair (hypopituitarism).

8. Examine external genitalia — small testes in men (hypopituitarism).

9. Examine visual fields — bitemporal hemianopia (pituitary tumour).

10. Percuss tendon reflexes — delayed relaxation in hypothyroidism.

OSCEs 5.7 Examine this patient with weight loss and a good appetite

1. Observe patient's demeanour — hyperactive, 'staring eyes' (hyperthyroidism).

2. Examine eyes for lid lag and proptosis (thyroid eye disease).

3. Look for signs of dehydration — dry tongue, lack of skin turgor, e.g. diabetes mellitus, coeliac disease.

4. Examine hands for finger clubbing (coeliac disease), warmth, sweating, fine tremor (hyperthyroidism).

5. Examine nails for any onycholysis or thyroid acropachy (hyperthyroidism).

6. Feel pulse — tachycardia in hyperthyroidism, bradycardia in hypothyroidism.

7. Palpate neck for goitre (diffuse or nodular).

8. Look at legs for pretibial myxoedema.

9. Look at optic fundi for diabetic retinopathy.

10. Perform urinalysis for glycosuria (diabetes mellitus).

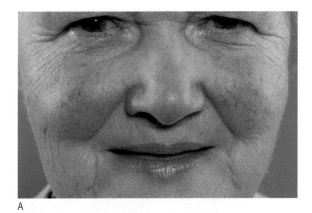

A

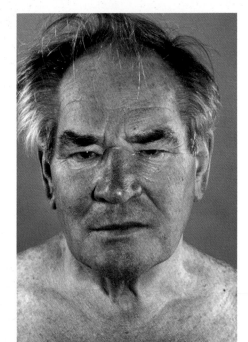

B

Fig. 5.16 Carcinoid syndrome. **(A)** Acute carcinoid flush. **(B)** Chronic telangiectasia.

OTHER ENDOCRINE DISORDERS

Carcinoid syndrome

Liver metastases from mid-gut carcinoid tumours release vasoactive chemicals into the systemic circulation which cause flushing, diarrhoea and bronchospasm. Bending, exercise or even palpation of the enlarged liver may induce typical skin flushing. Permanent facial telangiectasia occurs after many years of carcinoid flushing (Fig. 5.16).

INVESTIGATIONS

Serum hormone levels are measured to assess over- or under-activity. Suppression tests can determine whether hormonal secretion is autonomous. Stimulation tests assess hormonal reserve (or lack of it in deficiency states). Modern imaging enables visualization of small endocrine tumours, sometimes only a few millimetres in diameter (Box 5.8 and Fig. 5.17).

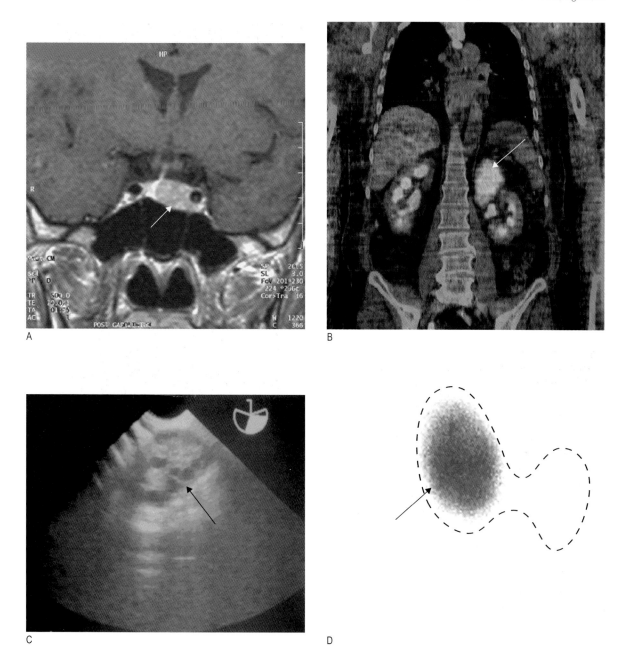

Fig. 5.17 Endocrine imaging. (A) MRI showing pituitary macroadenoma. **(B)** PET-CT showing an adrenal cancer. **(C)** Ultrasound showing polycystic ovary. **(D)** ^{99m}Technetium radionuclide scan confirming unilateral toxic thyroid adenoma (arrowed) — dotted line shows outline of thyroid.

5.8 Investigations in endocrine disease

Investigation	Indication/comment
Bedside	
Urinalysis	Glycosuria in diabetes mellitus Proteinuria in hypertensive renal damage
Capillary blood glucose	High in diabetes mellitus
Blood	
Calcium	High in hyperparathyroidism
Free thyroxine	High in hyperthyroidism Low in hypothyroidism
TSH	Undetectable in hyperthyroidism High in primary hypothyroidism
Serum cortisol	Low in hypoadrenalism, usually with reduced Synacthen response Loss of diurnal rhythm in Cushing's Reduced dexamethasone suppressibility in Cushing's
Gonadotrophins	High in primary hypogonadism in both sexes
Imaging	
Ultrasound	Thyroid, parathyroid, ovary, testis
MRI	Pituitary, pancreas
CT	Pancreas, adrenal
Radionuclide	Thyroid (^{123}I), parathyroid (^{99m}Tc-sesta-MIBI), adrenal (^{123}I-mIBG), neuroendocrine tumours (^{123}I-octreotide)
Positron emission tomography (PET) CT	Thyroid and neuroendocrine tumours
Invasive	
Fine needle aspiration cytology	Thyroid nodule
Inferior petrosal sinus sampling for ACTH	ACTH-dependent Cushing's

5.9 Key points: the endocrine system

- Symptoms of endocrine disturbance are varied and non-specific, and affect many body systems.
- Look carefully at the face for a 'spot' endocrine diagnosis.
- The thyroid gland moves upwards on swallowing (as does a thyroglossal cyst).
- Always palpate the thyroid gland from behind the patient.
- Hyperthyroidism is usually due to autoimmune Graves' disease, which may be associated with thyroid eye disease.
- Periorbital myxoedema is characteristic in primary hypothyroidism.
- Diabetes mellitus may present with the triad of polyuria, thirst and weight loss.
- Diabetic foot ulceration may be due to neuropathy, arterial insufficiency and increased susceptibility to infection.
- Acromegaly presents with characteristic facial features.
- Cushing's syndrome causes tissue breakdown of skin, muscle and bone with central accumulation of fat.
- Addison's disease causes pigmentation of the skin, particularly skin creases, pressure areas, buccal mucosa and healing scars.
- Excess body and facial hair in women (hirsutism) is common in PCOS.

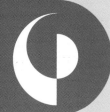

The cardiovascular system

6

CARDIOVASCULAR EXAMINATION

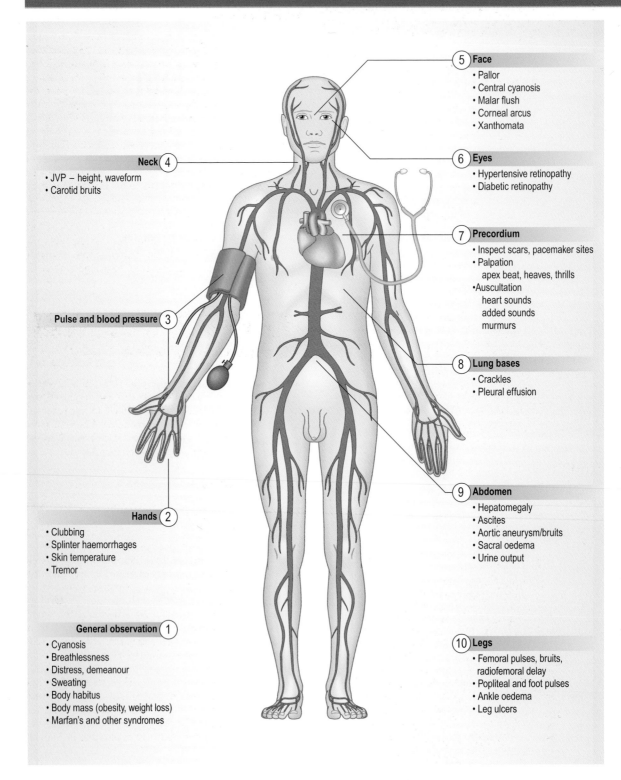

5 Face
- Pallor
- Central cyanosis
- Malar flush
- Corneal arcus
- Xanthomata

6 Eyes
- Hypertensive retinopathy
- Diabetic retinopathy

7 Precordium
- Inspect scars, pacemaker sites
- Palpation
  apex beat, heaves, thrills
- Auscultation
  heart sounds
  added sounds
  murmurs

8 Lung bases
- Crackles
- Pleural effusion

9 Abdomen
- Hepatomegaly
- Ascites
- Aortic aneurysm/bruits
- Sacral oedema
- Urine output

10 Legs
- Femoral pulses, bruits,
  radiofemoral delay
- Popliteal and foot pulses
- Ankle oedema
- Leg ulcers

Neck 4
- JVP – height, waveform
- Carotid bruits

Pulse and blood pressure 3

Hands 2
- Clubbing
- Splinter haemorrhages
- Skin temperature
- Tremor

General observation 1
- Cyanosis
- Breathlessness
- Distress, demeanour
- Sweating
- Body habitus
- Body mass (obesity, weight loss)
- Marfan's and other syndromes

THE HEART

ANATOMY

The heart comprises two muscular pumps working in series, covered in a serous sac (pericardium) which allows free movement with each heart beat and respiration. The heart delivers blood to both pulmonary and systemic circulations (Fig. 6.1). The right heart (right atrium and ventricle) pumps blood returning from the systemic veins into the pulmonary circulation at relatively low pressures. The left heart (left atrium and ventricle) receives blood from the lungs and pumps it round the body to the tissues at higher pressures (Fig. 6.24). The heart muscle (myocardium) is thicker in the ventricles than the atria and in the left heart than the right heart to generate higher pressures.

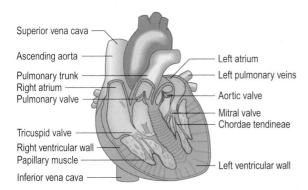

Fig. 6.1 The heart chambers and valves.

Labels:
Superior vena cava
Ascending aorta
Pulmonary trunk
Right atrium
Pulmonary valve
Tricuspid valve
Right ventricular wall
Papillary muscle
Inferior vena cava
Left atrium
Left pulmonary veins
Aortic valve
Mitral valve
Chordae tendineae
Left ventricular wall

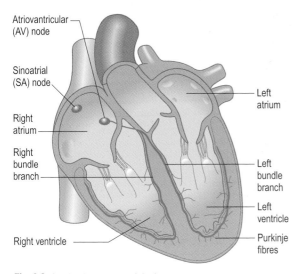

Fig. 6.2 Conducting system of the heart.

Labels:
Atrioventricular (AV) node
Sinoatrial (SA) node
Right atrium
Right bundle branch
Right ventricle
Left atrium
Left bundle branch
Left ventricle
Purkinje fibres

Heart valves

Atrioventricular valves (tricuspid on the right side, mitral on the left) separate the atria from the ventricles. They are attached to papillary muscles in the ventricular myocardium by chordae tendineae (Fig. 6.1) which prevent them from prolapsing into the atria when the ventricle contracts. The pulmonary valve on the right side of the heart and the aortic valve on the left separate the ventricles from the pulmonary and systemic arterial systems respectively. Each has three cusps and, as they are half-moon-shaped, they are called semilunar valves. Cardiac contraction is co-ordinated by specialized groups of cells (Fig. 6.2). The cells in the sinoatrial node normally act as the cardiac pacemaker. The way in which impulses subsequently spread through the heart ensures that atrial contraction is complete before ventricular contraction (systole) begins. At the end of systole the atrioventricular valves open, allowing blood to flow from the atria to refill the ventricles (diastole).

SYMPTOMS AND DEFINITIONS
Chest pain and discomfort

Most chronic cardiac and peripheral vascular diseases are initially asymptomatic, and this silent phase may last for many years. It is important to consider all forms of discomfort, since cardiac problems do not always cause pain. The severity of discomfort does not correlate to the severity of the cardiac problem.

Angina pectoris

Angina pectoris is the most common cardiac pain. It is usually caused by myocardial ischaemia due to obstruction to flow in an epicardial coronary vessel, but can occur in conditions such as aortic stenosis or hypertrophic cardiomyopathy which increase myocardial oxygen demand. Angina is recognized by its character and by its precipitating and relieving factors (Box 6.3). Characteristically it is an ache or dull discomfort, diffusely felt in the centre of the anterior chest, which lasts less than 10 minutes. Patients describe a tight or pressing 'band-like' sensation, similar to a heavy weight, which can be confused with indigestion. It may radiate down one or both arms and into the throat, jaw and teeth (Fig. 6.3). It is unaffected by inspiration, twisting or turning. The severity of the discomfort is a poor guide to prognosis. Anything that increases the force of cardiac contraction, heart rate or blood pressure and increases myocardial oxygen demand may precipitate it. Triggers include:

• exercise
• cold or windy weather (causes peripheral vasoconstriction)

6.1 Common symptoms of heart disease

Symptom	Cardiovascular causes	Other causes
Chest discomfort	Myocardial infarction Angina Pericarditis Aortic dissection	Oesophageal spasm Pneumothorax Musculoskeletal pain
Breathlessness	Heart failure Angina Pulmonary embolism Pulmonary hypertension	Respiratory disease Anaemia Obesity Anxiety
Palpitation	Tachyarrhythmias Ectopic beats	Anxiety Hyperthyroidism Drugs
Syncope/ dizziness	Arrhythmias Postural hypotension Aortic stenosis Hypertrophic obstructive cardiomyopathy Atrial myxoma	Simple faints Epilepsy Anxiety
Oedema	Heart failure Constrictive pericarditis Venous stasis	Nephrotic syndrome Liver disease Drugs Immobility

6.2 Cardiovascular causes of chest pain

Type	Cause	Characteristics
Angina	Coronary artery disease Aortic stenosis Hypertrophic cardiomyopathy	Precipitated by exertion, eased by rest and/or glyceryl trinitrate; characteristic distribution
Myocardial infarction	Coronary artery occlusion	Similar sites to angina; more severe, persists at rest
Pericarditic pain	Pericarditis	Sharp, raw or stabbing; varies with movement or breathing
Aortic pain	Dissection of the aorta	Severe, tearing, sudden onset, radiates to the back

- walking uphill or carrying a heavy load (increases cardiac output and blood pressure)
- exercise following a heavy meal (post-prandial angina) causes redistribution of myocardial blood flow.

6.3 Factors aggravating or relieving angina

Aggravating

- Exertion
- Emotional excitement
- Cold weather
- Exercise after meals

Relieving

- Rest
- Glyceryl trinitrate
- Warm-up before exercise

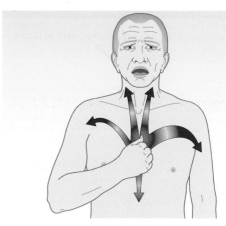

Fig. 6.3 Site and radiation of angina.

Angina is relieved by rest and glyceryl trinitrate (GTN), and is more likely to occur early during exercise. Some patients describe 'walk-through' angina, as peripheral vasodilatation during exercise decreases myocardial workload.

The Canadian Cardiovascular Classification provides an objective assessment of the impact of angina on the patient's lifestyle (Box 6.4).

- Unstable angina is angina of recent onset or increasing severity, duration or frequency. It may occur with minimal exertion or at rest. Unstable angina is a medical emergency, as it may herald myocardial infarction
- Crescendo angina occurs at increasing frequency with decreasing precipitants, but not at rest
- Nocturnal or decubitus angina occurs at night or on lying flat. It is caused by either increased venous return or reducing efficacy of anti-angina drugs, which are often taken in the morning and may wear off overnight. It indicates severe coronary artery disease.

It may be difficult to distinguish between angina pectoris and non-cardiac causes of chest pain, such as oesophageal pain (Box 6.5).

6.4 Canadian Cardiovascular Society: functional classification of stable angina

Grade 1	Ordinary physical activity, such as walking and climbing stairs, does not cause angina. Angina with strenuous or rapid or prolonged exertion at work or recreation
Grade 2	Slight limitation of ordinary activity. Walking or climbing stairs rapidly, walking uphill, walking or stair-climbing after meals, in cold, in wind, or when under emotional stress, or only during the few hours after awakening
Grade 3	Marked limitation of ordinary physical activity. Walking 1–2 blocks on the level and climbing less than one flight in normal conditions
Grade 4	Inability to carry on any physical activity without discomfort; angina may be present at rest

6.6 Differential diagnosis: angina vs myocardial infarction

Factor	Angina	Myocardial infarction
Site	Retrosternal; radiates to arm, epigastrium, neck	Retrosternal; radiates to arm, epigastrium, neck
Precipitated	By exercise or emotion	Often spontaneous
Relieved	By rest, nitrates	Not by rest or nitrates
Anxiety	Absent or mild	Severe
Sympathetic activity	None	Increased
Nausea or vomiting	Unusual	Common

6.5 Differential diagnosis: angina vs oesophageal pain

Factor	Angina	Oesophageal pain
Site	Retrosternal; radiates to arm and jaw	Retrosternal or epigastric; sometimes radiates to arm or back
Precipitated	Usually by exertion	Can be worsened by exertion, but often present at other times
Relieved	Rapidly relieved by rest, nitrates	Not rapidly relieved by rest; often relieved by nitrates
Wakes patient from sleep	Seldom	Often
Relation to heartburn	None (but patients often have 'wind')	Sometimes
Duration	Typically 2–10 minutes	Variable

6.7 Characteristics of pericarditic pain

Factor	Characteristic
Site	Retrosternal; may radiate to left shoulder or back
Prodrome	May be preceded by a viral illness
Onset	No obvious initial precipitating factor; tends to fluctuate in intensity
Nature	May be stabbing or 'raw' — 'like sandpaper'; often described as sharp, rarely as tight or heavy
Made worse	By changes in posture, respiration
Relieved	By analgesics, especially non-steroidal anti-inflammatory drugs (NSAIDs)
Accompanied	By pericardial rub

Myocardial infarction

Symptoms of myocardial infarction are similar to, but more severe and prolonged than, those of angina pectoris (Box 6.6). Other features include restlessness, breathlessness and a feeling of impending death (angor animi). Autonomic stimulation produces sweating, pallor, nausea, vomiting and diarrhoea, particularly in inferior infarction. Pain is absent in up to 30% of patients with myocardial infarction, especially the elderly and those with diabetes mellitus.

Pericardial pain

Pericardial pain is a sharp anterior central chest pain exacerbated by inspiration and movement, particularly leaning forward (Box 6.7). It may be confused with angina but both may co-exist. It is caused by inflammation of the pericardial sac around the heart secondary to myocardial infarction, viral infection, or after surgery, catheter ablation, angioplasty or radiotherapy.

Aortic dissection

A tear in the intima of the wall of the aorta allows blood under high pressure to penetrate into the medial layer, cleaving the aortic wall. This is a dissection. An abrupt, very severe, tearing chest pain occurs which, depending on the origin and extent of the dissection, can radiate to the back (typically interscapular) and be associated with profound autonomic stimulation. If the tear involves the coronary arteries or branches of the aorta, it may cause myocardial infarction, syncope

6

6.8 Characteristics of pain caused by dissection of the thoracic aorta

Factor	Characteristic
Site	Often first felt between shoulder blades and/or behind the sternum
Onset	Usually sudden
Nature	Very severe pain, often described as 'tearing'
Relieved	By nothing, tends to persist; patients often restless with pain
Accompanied	By pallor, sweating, hypertension, asymmetric pulses, unexpected bradycardia, early diastolic murmur, syncope, focal neurological symptoms and signs

and focal neurological signs. Predisposing factors include Marfan's syndrome (Fig. 3.27, p. 63), severe hypertension and trauma (Box 6.8).

Breathlessness

Breathlessness (dyspnoea) is an awareness of increased drive to breathe and is normal on exercise. It is pathological if it occurs at a significantly lower threshold than expected. Breathlessness is a non-specific symptom and may be caused by cardiac, respiratory, neuromuscular and metabolic conditions, or by toxins or anxiety. Other cardiovascular causes of acute breathlessness include pulmonary embolism and arrhythmias.

Breathlessness due to ischaemic heart disease has identical precipitants to angina, may occur with it and may be relieved by GTN. Breathlessness in heart failure may be associated with extreme fatigue. Accumulation of fluid in the alveoli (pulmonary oedema) occurs with left heart failure because increased left atrial end-diastolic pressure leads to elevated pressure in the pulmonary veins and capillaries (Box 6.9). Patients with acute pulmonary oedema usually prefer to be upright, while those with pulmonary embolism are often more comfortable lying flat and may faint (syncope) if made to sit upright. Use the New York Heart Association (NYHA) grading system to assess the degree of symptomatic limitation caused by exertional breathlessness (Box 6.10).

Orthopnoea

Orthopnoea is dyspnoea on lying flat and is a sign of advanced heart failure. Lying flat increases venous return to the heart and in patients with a failing left ventricle may precipitate pulmonary venous congestion and pulmonary oedema. The severity can be graded by the number of pillows the patient uses before feeling comfortable ('three-pillow orthopnoea').

6.9 Some mechanisms and causes of heart failure

Mechanism	Cause
Reduced ventricular contractility (systolic dysfunction)	Myocardial ischaemia Myocardial infarction Cardiomyopathy Myocarditis Drugs with negative inotropic actions, e.g. β-blockers
Impaired ventricular filling (diastolic dysfunction)	Left ventricular hypertrophy Constrictive pericarditis
Increased metabolic and cardiac demand	Pregnancy* Anaemia* Fever* Thyrotoxicosis Arteriovenous fistulae Paget's disease
Arrhythmia	Tachycardia, especially atrial fibrillation Bradycardia
Valvular or structural cardiac lesions	Mitral and/or aortic valve disease Tricuspid and/or pulmonary valve disease (rare) Ventricular septal defect Hypertrophic obstructive cardiomyopathy
Fluid overload	Excessive IV infusion Drugs, e.g. NSAIDs, steroids
Other	Intercurrent non-cardiac illness in patients with cardiac disease

*Aggravating factors which rarely cause heart failure alone.

6.10 New York Heart Association classification of heart failure symptom severity

Class I	No limitations. Ordinary physical activity does not cause undue fatigue, dyspnoea or palpitation (asymptomatic left ventricular dysfunction)
Class II	Slight limitation of physical activity. Such patients are comfortable at rest. Ordinary physical activity results in fatigue, palpitation, dyspnoea or angina pectoris (symptomatically 'mild' heart failure)
Class III	Marked limitation of physical activity. Less than ordinary physical activity will lead to symptoms (symptomatically 'moderate' heart failure)
Class IV	Symptoms of congestive heart failure are present, even at rest. With any physical activity increased discomfort is experienced (symptomatically 'severe' heart failure)

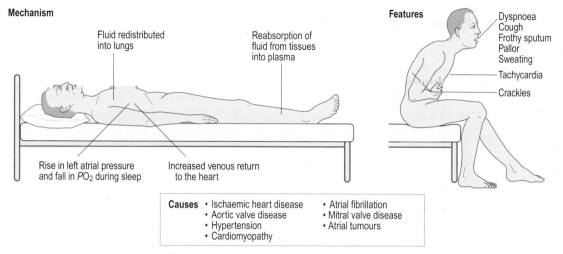

Fig. 6.4 **Paroxysmal nocturnal dyspnoea.**

Paroxysmal nocturnal dyspnoea

Paroxysmal nocturnal dyspnoea is sudden breathlessness which wakes the patient from sleep choking or gasping for air (Fig. 6.4). It has a similar mechanism to orthopnoea and is caused by the gradual accumulation of alveolar fluid during sleep. Patients may sit on the edge of the bed and open windows in an attempt to relieve their distress. It may be confused with asthma, which can also cause night-time symptoms, as it causes wheeze, but patients with heart failure often also produce frothy, bloodstained, sputum.

Palpitation

Palpitation is an unexpected awareness of the heart beating in the chest. Patients experience a rapid, forceful or irregular cardiac impulse and describe this as thumping, pounding, fluttering, jumping, racing or skipping. Ask them to tap out the pattern with their fingers to clarify its rate and rhythm.

Palpitation may occur in sinus rhythm with anxiety, with intermittent irregularities of the heartbeat, e.g. extrasystoles, or with an abnormal rhythm (arrhythmia). Most patients do not have a sustained arrhythmia and not all patients with arrhythmia experience palpitation; for example, atrial fibrillation commonly causes an irregular heartbeat in the elderly but rarely causes palpitation. The history helps distinguish different types of palpitation (Box 6.11). Ask about:

- onset and termination (abrupt or gradual)
- precipitating factors (exercise, alcohol, caffeine, recreational or other drugs)
- frequency and duration of episodes
- character of the rhythm (ask the patient to tap it out).

6.11 Descriptions of arrhythmias

Arrhythmia	Patient's description
Ventricular or atrial extrasystoles	'Heart misses a beat' Heart 'jumps' or 'flutters'
Atrial fibrillation	Heart 'jumping about' or 'racing' Associated breathlessness May be unnoticed
Supraventricular tachycardia	Heart racing or fluttering Associated polyuria
Ventricular tachycardia	Heart racing or fluttering Associated breathlessness May present as syncope rather than as palpitation

Healthy people are occasionally aware of their heart beating when they have normal (sinus) rhythm. This is often related to physical or psychological stress: for example, after exercise, or when waiting for an interview or examination. It is more common in bed at night when external visual and auditory inputs are minimal and visceral sensations more prominent. Slim people may notice it when lying on their left side. Palpitation can also be brought on by excessive caffeine intake (tea, coffee, cola) and by nicotine from smoking. Patients with carotid artery disease may notice an intermittent whooshing noise (bruit) heard 'inside' the affected side of their head.

Common irregularities of the heartbeat

Ectopic beats (extrasystoles) are a benign cause of palpitation at rest and are abolished by exercise. Patients may describe 'missed beats', sometimes followed by a particularly strong heartbeat. This occurs because the ectopic beat produces a small stroke volume and an impalpable impulse due to incomplete left ventricular filling. The subsequent compensatory pause leads to ventricular overfilling and a forceful contraction with the next beat.

Palpitation due to sustained arrhythmias

Pathological rapid heartbeat (tachyarrhythmia) starts suddenly, lasts for minutes or hours, and is not usually triggered by anxiety or stress.

Ask about:

- family history of premature coronary artery disease or sudden death
- past history of rheumatic fever, previous heart attacks or other heart disease
- smoking habit, daily caffeine and weekly alcohol consumption (p. 20)
- any drugs being taken: prescribed, over-the-counter or recreational
- symptoms of recent ill health suggesting an unusual cause, e.g. infective endocarditis

If the attacks are paroxysmal note:

- precipitating factors, e.g. exercise, anxiety or stress
- relieving factors, e.g. breath-holding, exercise
- high-risk features suggesting a malignant ventricular arrhythmia, e.g. presyncope, syncope, extreme chest discomfort or breathlessness.

Patients with coronary artery disease or cardiomyopathy are at particular risk of ventricular arrhythmias. Urgently investigate patients with palpitation or syncope, as they may have a malignant but treatable arrhythmia.

Syncope and dizziness

Syncope is a faint with loss of consciousness. Patients who say they are dizzy are often describing vertigo or light-headedness. Clarify exactly what they mean and differentiate vertigo, light-headedness and syncope (p. 271). Vertigo is rarely caused by heart disease. Light-headedness, syncope or a feeling of impending loss of consciousness (presyncope) may be cardiovascular in origin. There are four main causes:

- postural hypotension
- neurocardiogenic syncope
- arrhythmias
- mechanical obstruction to cardiac output.

Patients with vascular disease affecting the carotid and/or vertebral arteries may present with non-focal cerebral symptoms due to hypoperfusion of the cortex. Common precipitating factors include head-turning,

getting up quickly from sitting or lying, and starting or increasing antihypertensive drugs.

Postural hypotension

Postural hypotension is a fall of >20 mmHg in systolic blood pressure on standing. It is commonly caused by hypovolaemia, antihypertensive drug therapy, especially diuretics and vasodilators (Box 6.12). It is also a symptom of autonomic neuropathy.

Neurocardiogenic syncope

This is a group of conditions caused by abnormal autonomic reflexes. Fainting results from sudden slow heart rate (bradycardia) and/or vasodilatation. It occurs in healthy people forced to stand for a long time in a warm environment or subject to painful or emotional stimuli, e.g. the sight of blood. These patients often give a prior history of fainting with a prodrome of light-headedness, tinnitus, a darkening of vision from the periphery as the retinal blood supply (the most oxygen-sensitive part of the nervous system) is reduced, nausea, sweating and facial pallor. The person then slides to the floor as they lose consciousness. If the person is held upright by misguided bystanders, continued cerebral hypoperfusion may precipitate an anoxic seizure. If allowed to lie flat to aid cerebral circulation, the person wakes up, often with flushing from vasodilatation and nausea and vomiting due to vagal over-activity.

Frequent fainting caused by trivial stimuli may be due to malignant vasovagal syndrome or hypersensitive carotid sinus syndrome (HCSS). In patients with HCSS, gentle pressure over the carotid sinus may reproduce the patient's symptoms by triggering bradycardia.

6.12 Symptoms related to medication

Symptom	Medication
Dyspnoea	β-blockers in patients with asthma. Exacerbation of heart failure by β-blockers, some calcium channel antagonists, NSAIDs
Dizziness	Vasodilators, e.g. nitrates, α-blockers and angiotensin-converting enzyme (ACE) inhibitors
Angina	Aggravated by thyroxine or drug-induced anaemia, e.g. aspirin or NSAIDs
Oedema	From steroids, NSAIDs, calcium channel antagonists, e.g. nifedipine, amlodipine
Palpitation	Tachycardia and/or arrhythmia from thyroxine, β_2 stimulants, e.g. salbutamol, digoxin toxicity, hypokalaemia from diuretics, tricyclic antidepressants

Arrhythmias

Supraventricular tachyarrhythmias such as atrial fibrillation rarely cause syncope. The most common cause is bradyarrhythmia, due to sick sinus syndrome or to atrioventricular block, i.e. Stokes–Adams attacks. Drugs, including digoxin, β-blockers and rate limiting calcium channel blockers, e.g. verapamil, may aggravate attacks. Ventricular tachyarrhythmias often cause syncope or presyncope, especially in patients with impaired left ventricular function.

Mechanical obstruction to cardiac output

Severe aortic stenosis and hypertrophic cardiomyopathy can obstruct left ventricular outflow. This may cause syncope or presyncope, especially on exertion when cardiac output fails to meet the increased metabolic demand. Pulmonary embolism can obstruct outflow from the right ventricle, and is a frequently overlooked cause of recurrent syncope. Atrial myxoma, other cardiac tumours, and blockage or failure of artificial heart valves are rare causes of syncope.

Oedema

Oedema is excess fluid in the interstitial space, and in peripheral sites it causes tissue swelling. Oedema is usually dependent and is especially seen in the ankles, in the lower limbs, or over the sacrum in patients lying in bed. Common causes include heart failure and vasodilator medications, but not all oedema is cardiac in origin (Box 6.13 and Box 3.14, p. 64). In general, if the jugular venous pressure (JVP) is not elevated, then oedema is not cardiogenic.

6.13 Causes of unilateral and bilateral leg oedema

Unilateral

- Deep vein thrombosis
- Soft tissue infection
- Trauma
- Immobility, e.g. hemiplegia
- Lymphatic obstruction

Bilateral

- Heart failure
- Chronic venous insufficiency
- Hypoproteinaemia, e.g. nephrotic syndrome, kwashiorkor, cirrhosis
- Lymphatic obstruction, e.g. pelvic tumour, filariasis
- Drugs, e.g. NSAIDs, nifedipine, amlodipine, fludrocortisone
- Inferior vena caval obstruction
- Thiamine deficiency (wet beriberi)
- Milroy's disease (unexplained lymphoedema which appears at puberty; more common in females)
- Immobility

Other symptoms

Non-cardiac symptoms occur in heart disease (Box 6.14). Infective endocarditis may present with non-specific symptoms including weight loss, tiredness and night sweats, and atrial fibrillation with symptoms and signs of cerebral or systemic embolization (commonly legs, arms or viscera).

6

THE HISTORY

The history is crucial to making a diagnosis. Heart disease commonly occurs without abnormal physical findings; for example, examination is often normal in intermittent arrhythmias between episodes. Examination may confirm a cardiac or peripheral vascular diagnosis, e.g. when examining a patient with a murmur, heart failure or an abdominal aortic aneurysm, but physical signs may be completely absent in serious disease:

- Patients with severe carotid artery disease may have no neck bruit because flow through the stenosis is too slow
- Large abdominal aortic aneurysms can be impalpable in the obese
- Patients with extensive deep vein thrombosis often appear to have normal legs.

Presenting complaint

Establish the frequency, duration and severity of symptoms, and causative and relieving factors. Urgently attend to breathlessness, recent chest or lower limb pain. Many cardiovascular diseases are slowly progressive and the evolution of symptoms guides the timing of investigations and treatment; for example, heart valve surgery is indicated for significantly limiting symptoms and surgery for carotid artery disease is most effective soon after a cerebral event.

6.14 Cardiovascular disease presenting with 'non-cardiac' symptoms

System	Symptom	Cause
Central nervous system	Stroke	Cerebral embolism Endocarditis Hypertension
Gastrointestinal	Jaundice	Liver congestion secondary to heart failure
	Abdominal pain	Mesenteric embolism
Renal	Oliguria	Heart failure

6

Functional impairment

Assess the impact of symptoms on the patient's functional capacity. For chest discomfort or breathlessness establish the intensity of exercise required to induce symptoms.

- Does gentle walking or only strenuous exercise like climbing hills or stairs provoke symptoms?
- Can patients keep up when walking with their partners or friends of the same age?
- What is the extent of domestic, e.g. cooking, cleaning, shopping, social, e.g. mobility, hobbies, sport, and occupational disability?

Light-headedness and syncope may impair confidence, raise fear of physical injury, and have significant implications for patients' safety when driving.

Calf leg pain on walking (intermittent claudication) from lower limb arterial disease is the most common symptom of peripheral vascular disease:

- How far can the patient walk before the pain comes on, and is this on the flat or uphill?

Past history

Ask about rheumatic fever or heart murmurs during childhood and conditions associated with heart disease, including:

- smoking
- hypertension
- diabetes mellitus
- kidney disease
- thyrotoxicosis (atrial fibrillation)
- alcohol intake (arrhythmias and cardiomyopathy)
- Marfan's syndrome (aortic regurgitation or aortic dissection).

In suspected infective endocarditis ask about recent dental work and other potential causes of bacteraemia, e.g. skin infections, intravenous drug use, penetrating trauma. Consider possible links between other organ system diseases and cardiovascular illness: for example, patients with renal failure or disseminated cancer and pericardial effusion; heart failure and cytotoxic drugs; radiotherapy and radiation arteritis in the affected area. Patients with chronic respiratory disease may develop right-sided heart failure (cor pulmonale; p. 166) or atrial fibrillation. Connective tissue diseases such as rheumatoid arthritis are associated with Raynaud's phenomenon (Fig. 6.41) and pericarditis.

Drug history

Drugs may cause or aggravate symptoms such as breathlessness, chest pain, oedema, palpitation or syncope (Box 6.12). Starting thyroxine for hypothyroidism may precipitate or aggravate angina. 'Recreational' drugs such as cocaine and amphetamines can cause arrhythmias, chest pain and even myocardial infarction. Ask about over-the-counter purchases such as NSAIDs and alternative medicine and herbal remedies, as these

| 6.15 Genetically determined cardiovascular disorders |

Single-gene defects

- Hypertrophic cardiomyopathy
- Marfan's syndrome
- Familial hypercholesterolaemia
- Muscular dystrophies
- Long Q–T syndrome

Polygenic inheritance

- Ischaemic heart disease
- Hypertension
- Type 2 diabetes mellitus
- Hyperlipidaemia
- Abdominal aortic aneurysm

may contain ingredients with cardiovascular actions. Beta-blockers may worsen the symptoms of intermittent claudication and any drug that lowers blood pressure tends to impair the peripheral circulation.

Family history

Many cardiac disorders have a genetic component (Box 6.15). Ask about a family history of either premature coronary artery disease in a first-degree relative (<60 years in a female or <55 years in a male) or sudden unexplained death at a young age, raising the possibility of a cardiomyopathy or inherited arrhythmia disorder. Patients with peripheral arterial and venous thrombosis may have inherited thrombophilia, e.g. factor V Leiden deficiency. Familial hypercholesterolaemia is associated with premature cardiac and peripheral arterial disease.

Social history

Smoking is the strongest reversible risk factor for coronary artery disease and peripheral vascular disease. Take a detailed smoking history (p. 20). Alcohol can induce atrial fibrillation, and alcohol excess is associated with obesity, hypertension and dilated cardiomyopathy. Excess alcohol intake with poor nutrition also predisposes to peripheral arterial and venous disease. Intravenous drug use can damage peripheral arteries and veins, most commonly causing an infected false aneurysm of the common femoral artery in the groin: a potential source for infective endocarditis.

Occupational history

Heart disease may impair physical activity and affect employment. This may be a source of anxiety and an indication for treatment. The diagnosis of heart disease has medicolegal consequences in certain occupations, such as commercial drivers and pilots (Box 6.16). Workers exposed to occupational vibration through the use of air-powered tools may develop 'vibration white finger', which presents with vasospastic (Raynaud's phenomenon) and neurosensory (numbness, tingling) symptoms.

6.16 Occupational aspects of cardiovascular disease

Occupational exposure associated with cardiovascular disease

- Organic solvents: arrhythmias, cardiomyopathy
- Vibrating machine tools: Raynaud's phenomenon
- Publicans: alcohol-related cardiomyopathy

Occupational exposure exacerbating pre-existing cardiac conditions

- Cold exposure: angina, Raynaud's disease
- Deep-sea diving: embolism through foramen ovale

Occupational requirements for high standards of cardiovascular fitness

- Pilots
- Public transport/heavy goods vehicle drivers
- Armed forces
- Police

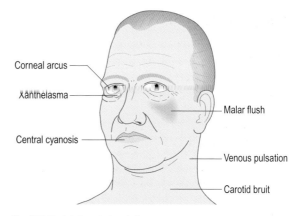

Fig. 6.5 Facial clues to heart disease.

Corneal arcus — Xanthelasma — Central cyanosis — Malar flush — Venous pulsation — Carotid bruit

THE PHYSICAL EXAMINATION

Tailor the sequence and extent of examination to the patient's condition:

- Patients with cardiac or respiratory arrest requiring resuscitation: manage first and examine later (Ch. 17)
- Patients requiring immediate emergency care: rapidly assess and treat first, leaving more detailed examination for later
- Stable patients: examine thoroughly first.

General examination

Look at the patient's general appearance, noting whether he or she:

- looks unwell
- is breathless or cyanosed
- is frightened or distressed.

Look at the hands for signs of tobacco staining (Fig. 7.12, p. 166) and face (Fig. 6.5) for clues to heart disease. Peripheral cyanosis (p. 164) is most commonly seen in healthy patients when the hands are exposed to cold, but may be due to heart failure or rarely congenital heart disease, where it is associated with right-to-left shunting and finger clubbing (Fig. 7.9, p. 165).

Hyperlipidaemia

Hyperlipidaemia is an important risk factor in heart disease and may produce:

- Skin or tendon xanthomata: yellow nodules in the skin or tendons, e.g. patella or Achilles tendon, from deposits of lipid (Fig. 6.6)
- Corneal arcus: a creamy yellow discoloration at the boundary of the iris and cornea caused by precipitation of cholesterol crystals. This can occur

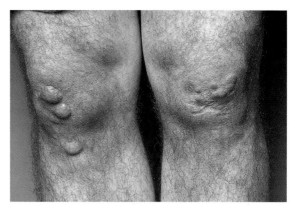

Fig. 6.6 Skin xanthomata over knees.

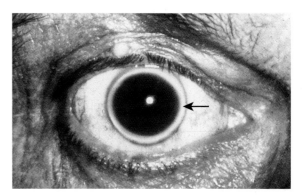

Fig. 6.7 Corneal arcus (arrow).

in those >50 years with no hyperlipidaemia (Fig. 6.7)

- Xanthelasma: yellowish cholesterol plaques around the eyelids and periorbital area (Fig. 6.8).

115

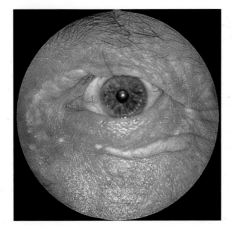

Fig. 6.8 Xanthelasma.

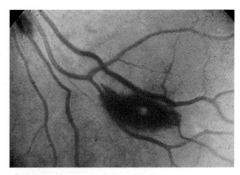

Fig. 6.10 A Roth spot.

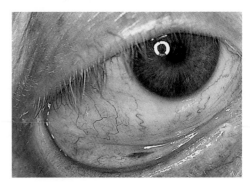

Fig. 6.11 Petechial haemorrhages.

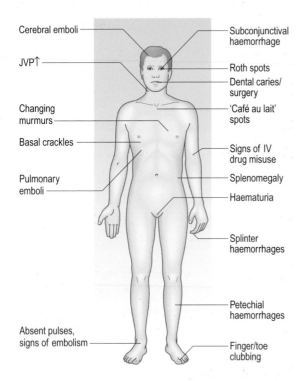

Fig. 6.9 Clinical features of endocarditis.

Cerebral emboli
JVP↑
Changing murmurs
Basal crackles
Pulmonary emboli
Absent pulses, signs of embolism

Subconjunctival haemorrhage
Roth spots
Dental caries/ surgery
'Café au lait' spots
Signs of IV drug misuse
Splenomegaly
Haematuria
Splinter haemorrhages
Petechial haemorrhages
Finger/toe clubbing

Infective endocarditis

Look for (Fig. 6.9):

- Splinter haemorrhages: multiple, linear, reddish-brown marks along the axis of the fingernails and toenails (Fig. 3.16A, p. 54). They are probably due to circulating immune complexes. One or two isolated 'splinters' are common in healthy individuals from trauma

- Roth spots: flame-shaped retinal haemorrhages with a 'cotton-wool' centre seen on ophthalmoscopy (Fig. 6.10). They are caused by a similar mechanism to splinter haemorrhages and can also occur in anaemia or leukaemia
- Multiple capillary haemorrhages (petechiae): found in the skin, most often on the legs and conjunctivae (Fig. 6.11). They are caused by vasculitis and can be confused with the rash of meningococcal disease
- Finger clubbing: a rare feature in chronic bacterial endocarditis
- Microscopic haematuria.

Arterial pulses

Anatomy

As the ventricles eject blood into the arteries (Fig. 6.12) a pressure wave (pulse) is transmitted and can be felt particularly where the arteries are superficial and pass over bone. The pressure wave travels faster than the blood. The pulse waveform depends on the heart rate, stroke volume, peripheral resistance (especially in the arterioles), left ventricular outflow obstruction and the elasticity of peripheral vessels.

Use the larger (brachial, carotid or femoral) pulses to assess the pulse volume and character and in

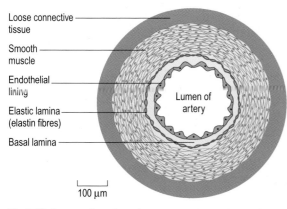

Loose connective tissue

Smooth muscle

Endothelial lining

Elastic lamina (elastin fibres)

Basal lamina

Lumen of artery

100 μm

Fig. 6.12 Cross-section of an artery.

6.17 Surface markings of the arterial pulses

Artery	Surface marking
Radial	At the wrist, lateral to the flexor carpi radialis tendon
Brachial	In the antecubital fossa, medial to the biceps tendon
Carotid	At the angle of the jaw, anterior to the sternocleidomastoid muscle
Femoral	Just below the inguinal ligament, midway between the anterior superior iliac spine and the pubic symphysis (the mid-inguinal point). It is immediately lateral to the femoral vein and medial to the femoral nerve
Popliteal	Lies posteriorly in relation to the knee joint, at the level of the knee crease, deep in the popliteal fossa
Posterior tibial	Located 2 cm below and posterior to the medial malleolus, where it passes beneath the flexor retinaculum between flexor digitorum longus and flexor hallucis longus
Dorsalis pedis	Passes lateral to the tendon of extensor hallucis longus and is best felt at the proximal extent of the groove between the first and second metatarsals. It may be absent or abnormally sited in 10% of normal subjects, sometimes being 'replaced' by a palpable perforating peroneal artery

hypotensive states (Box 6.17). When taking a pulse, characterize the information according to:

- rate
- rhythm
- volume
- character.

Examination sequence

Arterial pulses

If you are in any doubt about whose pulse you are feeling, palpate your own pulse at the same time. If what you are feeling is not synchronous with yours it is the patient's pulse.

Radial pulse

- Place the pads of your three middle fingers over the right radial artery.
- Assess rate, rhythm and volume (Fig. 6.13A).
- Count the pulse rate over 15 s and multiply by 4 to obtain the beats per minute (bpm).
- To detect a collapsing pulse, feel the pulse with the base of your fingers, then raise the patient's hand above his head (Fig. 6.13B).
- Palpate both radial pulses simultaneously, assessing any volume differences.
- Palpate the femoral and radial pulse simultaneously, noting any delay between the two and any difference in pulse volume between them.

Brachial pulse

- This artery lies deeper than the radial, medial to the biceps tendon, so use your thumb to palpate it, with your fingers cupped round the back of the elbow (Fig. 6.13C).
- Assess the character and volume.

Carotid pulse

- Explain to the patient what you are going to do. Never assess both carotid pulses simultaneously.
- Ask the patient to lie semi-recumbent in case you induce a reflex bradycardia.
- Gently place the tip of your thumb between the larynx and the anterior border of the sternocleidomastoid muscle.
- Press your thumb back gently to feel the pulse (Fig. 6.13D).
- Listen for bruits over both carotid arteries, using the diaphragm of your stethoscope while the patient holds his breath.

Femoral pulse

- Ask the patient to lie down and explain what you are going to do.
- With your fingers extended, place the pads of your index and middle fingers over the femoral artery (Fig. 6.13E).
- Check for radiofemoral delay (coarctation of the aorta, Fig. 6.15).
- Listen for bruits over both femoral arteries, using the diaphragm of your stethoscope.

Normal findings

Rate

Assess the pulse rate in the clinical context. A pulse rate of 40 bpm can be normal in a fit, young adult, whereas a pulse rate of 65 bpm may be abnormally low in the setting of acute heart failure. Resting heart rate is normally 60–100 bpm.

- Bradycardia is a pulse rate <60 bpm.
- Tachycardia is a pulse rate of >100 bpm.

Rhythm

Normal rhythm is regular; it is called sinus rhythm, as it originates from the sinoatrial (SA) node (Fig. 6.14A).

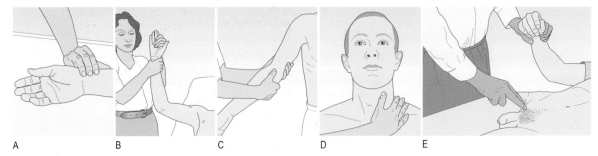

Fig. 6.13 The radial, brachial and carotid pulses. (A) Locating and palpating the radial pulse. **(B)** Feeling for a collapsing radial pulse. **(C)** Assessing the brachial pulse with your thumb. **(D)** Locating the carotid pulse with your thumb. **(E)** Examining the femoral artery, while simultaneously checking for radiofemoral delay.

Sinus rhythm

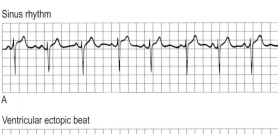

A

Ventricular ectopic beat

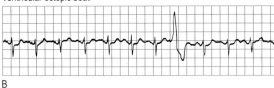

B

Atrial fibrillation

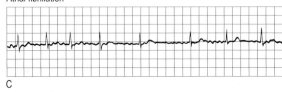

C

Atrial flutter

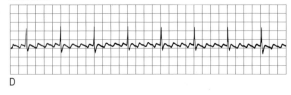

D

Ventricular tachycardia

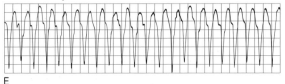

E

Fig. 6.14 ECG rhythm strip. (A) Sinus rhythm. **(B)** Ventricular ectopic beat. **(C)** Atrial fibrillation with 'controlled' ventricular response. **(D)** Atrial flutter: note the regular 'saw-toothed' atrial flutter waves at about 300/min. **(E)** Ventricular tachycardia, with ventricular rate of about 150/min.

i	6.18 Haemodynamic effects of respiration		
		Inspiration	**Expiration**
Pulse/heart rate		Accelerates	Slows
Systolic BP		Falls (up to 10 mmHg)	Rises
JVP		Falls	Rises
Second heart sound		Splits	Fuses

It varies slightly with the respiratory cycle, mediated by the vagus nerve, and is most pronounced in children, young adults or athletes (sinus arrhythmia). During inspiration, parasympathetic tone falls and the heart rate quickens; on expiration, the heart rate falls (Box 6.18).

Volume

Volume means the degree of pulsation and reflects the pulse pressure.

Character

Character means the waveform or shape of the arterial pulse.

Abnormal findings

Rate

The most common causes of bradycardia are:

- medication
- physical conditioning
- disease of the atrioventricular (AV) node (heart block) or SA node, leading to sinus bradycardia or sinus pauses.

SA node and AV node dysfunction can cause syncope (Stokes–Adams attacks) or light-headedness.

Sinus tachycardia occurs in exercise, anxiety, pain or fever. Tachyarrhythmias are abnormal rhythms caused by increased excitability or abnormal conducting pathways in, or between, the atria and ventricles (Box 6.19).

6.19 Causes of a fast or slow pulse

Heart rate	Sinus rhythm	Arrhythmia

Fast (tachycardia, >100/min)	Exercise
	Pain
	Excitement/anxiety
	Fever
	Hyperthyroidism
	Medication:
	  Sympathomimetics
	  Vasodilators
		Atrial fibrillation
		Atrial flutter
		Supraventricular
		tachycardia
		Ventricular
		tachycardia

Slow (bradycardia, <60/min)	Sleep
	Athletic training
	Hypothyroidism
	Medication:
	  β-blockers
	  Digoxin
	  Verapamil,
	  Diltiazem
		Carotid sinus
		hypersensitivity
		Sick sinus
		syndrome
		Second-degree
		heart block
		Complete heart
		block

6.20 Causes of an irregular pulse

- Sinus arrhythmia
- Atrial extrasystoles
- Ventricular extrasystoles
- Atrial fibrillation
- Atrial flutter with variable response
- Second-degree heart block with variable response

6.21 Common causes of atrial fibrillation

- Hypertension
- Heart failure
- Myocardial infarction
- Thyrotoxicosis
- Alcohol-related heart disease
- Mitral valve disease
- Infection, e.g. respiratory, urinary
- Following surgery, especially cardiothoracic surgery

Rhythm

The pulse may be regular or irregular (Box 6.20). If irregular, it may be regularly irregular, due to an ectopic beat occurring at a regular interval. Atrial fibrillation is the most common cause of an irregularly irregular pulse (Box 6.21). The rate depends on the number of beats conducted by the AV node. Untreated, the ventricular rate may be very fast (up to 200 bpm). The variability of the pulse rate (and therefore ventricular filling) explains why the pulse volume varies and there may be a pulse deficit, with some impulses not felt at the radial artery. Calculate the pulse deficit by counting the pulse at the wrist and subtracting this number from the apical heart rate counted by auscultation.

Volume

The heart fills with blood between heartbeats (diastole). With longer intervals, the amount of blood the

6.22 Causes of increased pulse volume

Physiological
- Exercise
- Pregnancy
- Increased environmental temperature
- Advanced age

Pathological
- Peripheral vascular disease
- Hypertension
- Fever
- Thyrotoxicosis
- Anaemia
- Aortic regurgitation
- Paget's disease of bone
- Peripheral AV shunt

ventricles eject with the subsequent contraction (stroke volume) increases. This is one cause of an increase in pulse volume, and explains why the pulse volume (and blood pressure) varies widely with an irregular pulse such as atrial fibrillation, and also why the 'compensatory pause' following a premature ectopic beat is sometimes felt by the patient.

A large pulse volume is a reflection of a large pulse pressure, which can be physiological or pathological (Box 6.22). The most common cause of a large pulse pressure, however, is arteriosclerosis, which is seen in patients with widespread vascular disease, hypertension and advanced age.

A low pulse volume may be due to reduced stroke volume and occurs in left ventricular failure, hypovolaemia or peripheral vascular disease.

- Coarctation is a congenital narrowing of the aorta, usually distal to the left subclavian artery. The clinical signs depend on the location and severity of the narrowing and the age of the patient. In children, the upper limb pulses are usually normal with reduced volume lower limb pulses, which are felt later than the upper limb pulses (radiofemoral delay) (Fig. 6.15). In adults, coarctation usually presents with hypertension and heart failure
- Pulsus alternans is a beat-to-beat variation in pulse volume with a normal rhythm. It is rare and occurs in advanced heart failure
- Pulsus paradoxus is an exaggeration of the normal variability of pulse volume with the respiratory cycle. Pulse volume normally increases in expiration and decreases during inspiration due to intrathoracic pressure changes affecting venous return to the heart. If ventricular interdependence is increased, e.g. pericardial effusion leading to tamponade, or intrathoracic pressure is significantly decreased, e.g. acute severe asthma, these respiration-based changes are exaggerated. In extreme cases the peripheral pulse may disappear completely on inspiration. Assess pulsus paradoxus by measuring the systolic blood pressure during inspiration and expiration. A decrease in systolic blood pressure >15 mmHg with inspiration is pathological.

6

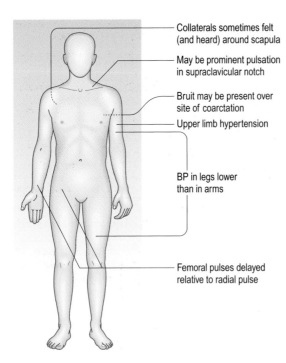

Collaterals sometimes felt (and heard) around scapula

May be prominent pulsation in supraclavicular notch

Bruit may be present over site of coarctation

Upper limb hypertension

BP in legs lower than in arms

Femoral pulses delayed relative to radial pulse

Fig. 6.15 Features of coarctation of the aorta.

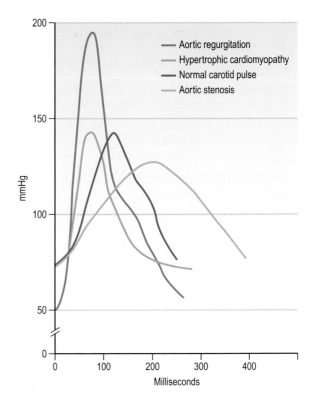

- Aortic regurgitation
- Hypertrophic cardiomyopathy
- Normal carotid pulse
- Aortic stenosis

Fig. 6.16 Pulse waveforms.

Character

- A collapsing pulse is when the peak of the pulse wave arrives early and is followed by a rapid descent. This rapid fall imparts the 'collapsing' sensation and is exaggerated by raising the patient's arm above the level of the heart (Fig. 6.13B). It occurs in severe aortic regurgitation
- A slow-rising pulse has a gradual upstroke with a reduced peak occurring late in systole, and is a feature of severe aortic stenosis
- A bisferiens pulse has two systolic peaks separated by a distinct midsystolic dip and occurs in mixed aortic stenosis and regurgitation (Fig. 6.16).

Blood pressure

Blood pressure (BP) is a measure of the force that the circulating blood exerts against the arterial wall. The systolic BP is the maximal pressure that occurs during ventricular contraction (systole). During ventricular filling (diastole), arterial pressure is maintained, but at a lower level, by the elasticity and compliance of the vessel wall. The lowest value (diastolic BP) occurs immediately before the next cycle.

BP is usually measured by means of a sphygmomanometer cuff (Fig. 6.17). In certain situations, such as the intensive care unit, it is measured invasively using

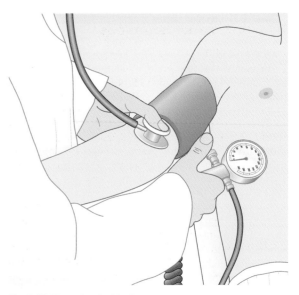

Fig. 6.17 Measuring the blood pressure.

an indwelling intra-arterial catheter connected to a pressure sensor.

BP is measured in mmHg and recorded as systolic pressure/diastolic pressure, together with where, and

6.23 British Hypertension Society classification of blood pressure levels		
Blood pressure	**Systolic BP (mmHg)**	**Diastolic BP (mmHg)**
Optimal	<120	<80
Normal	<130	<85
High normal	130–139	85–89
Hypertension		
Grade 1 (mild)	140–159	90–99
Grade 2 (moderate)	160–179	100–109
Grade 3 (severe)	>180	>110
Isolated systolic hypertension		
Grade 1	140–159	<90
Grade 2	>160	<90

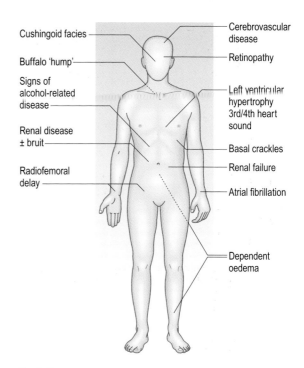

Fig. 6.18 Physical signs associated with hypertension.

how, the reading was taken, e.g. BP: 146/92 mmHg, right arm, supine.

BP is an important guide to cardiovascular risk and provides vital information on the haemodynamic condition of acutely ill or injured patients. BP constantly varies and rises with stress, excitement and environment. 'White-coat hypertension' occurs in patients only when a patient is seeing a healthcare worker. Ambulatory monitoring, where a portable device measures the BP at a regular programmable interval, is a better determinant of cardiovascular risk.

Symptoms and definitions

Hypertension

Hypertension is abnormal elevation of BP and has been defined by the British Hypertension Society (Box 6.23). Normal BP can be defined as <130/85 mmHg. Hypertension is extremely common, being present in 20–30% of the adult population with even higher rates in Black Africans. It is associated with significant morbidity and mortality from vascular disease (heart failure, ischaemic heart disease, cerebrovascular disease and renal failure). The risk of mortality and morbidity rises progressively with increasing systolic and diastolic pressure; for example, isolated grade 1 systolic hypertension is associated with a 2–3-fold risk of cardiac mortality. Lowering BP lowers vascular risk regardless of the starting value. Hypertension is asymptomatic, although rarely in severe hypertension, headaches and visual disturbances occur (Fig. 6.18).

Essential hypertension, in which there is no readily identifiable cause, occurs in >90% of patients with hypertension.

Secondary hypertension is rare, occurring in <1% of the hypertensive population. Causes of secondary hypertension include:

- Renal artery stenosis: suspect if there is other evidence of peripheral vascular disease
- Phaeochromocytoma: a tumour of the adrenal medulla that secretes catecholamines, and often also causes headaches, sweating and palpitation
- Conn's syndrome: a tumour of the adrenal cortex that secretes aldosterone
- Cushing's syndrome: a microadenoma of the pituitary that secretes adrenocorticotrophic hormone (ACTH)
- Coarctation of the aorta
- Polycystic kidney disease (p. 230).

Korotkoff sounds

These noises are produced from under the distal half of the BP cuff between systole and diastole because the artery collapses completely and reopens with each heartbeat. As the artery wall rapidly opens it causes a snapping or tapping sound (like the sail of a boat snapping in the wind). As the cuff pressure falls below the diastolic pressure, the sound disappears as the vessel wall no longer collapses but gently expands with each beat. The first appearance of the sound (phase 1) indicates systole. As the pressure is reduced, the sounds muffle (phase 4) and then disappear (phase 5). Inter-observer agreement is better for phase 5 and this is recorded as diastolic BP. Occasionally muffled sounds persist (phase 4) and do not disappear; in this case, record phase 4 as the diastolic pressure (Fig. 6.19).

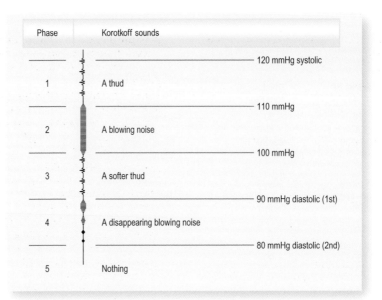

Phase	Korotkoff sounds	
		— 120 mmHg systolic
1	A thud	
		— 110 mmHg
2	A blowing noise	
		— 100 mmHg
3	A softer thud	
		— 90 mmHg diastolic (1st)
4	A disappearing blowing noise	
		— 80 mmHg diastolic (2nd)
5	Nothing	

Fig. 6.19 Korotkoff sounds.

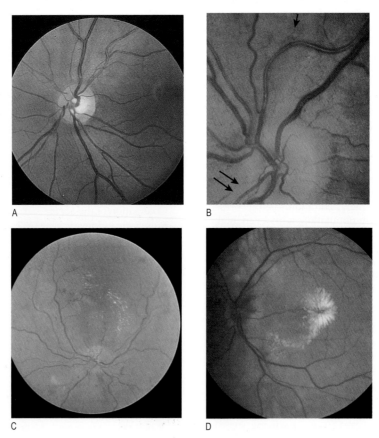

Fig. 6.20 Hypertensive retinopathy. (A) Grade 1: early changes: increased tortuosity of a retinal vessel and increased reflectiveness (silver wiring) of a retinal artery, are seen at 1 o'clock. **(B)** Grade 2: increased tortuosity and silver wiring (double arrow) with 'nipping' of the venules at arteriovenous crossings (single arrow). **(C)** Grade 3: similar to grade 2 plus flame-shaped retinal haemorrhages and soft 'cotton-wool' exudates. **(D)** Grade 4: swelling of the optic disc (papilloedema), retinal oedema, and hard exudates around the fovea, producing a 'macular star'.

Assessment of the hypertensive patient aims to identify:

- any underlying cause
- end-organ damage
    - cardiac — heart failure
    - renal — chronic kidney disease
    - eye — hypertensive retinopathy — 4 grades (Fig. 6.20)
- overall risk of vascular disease, i.e. of stroke, myocardial infarction, heart failure.

◼▸ Examination sequence

Blood pressure

Rest the patient for 5 minutes.

Use either arm unless one arm is known to record a higher pressure. If that is the case, use this arm.

With the patient seated or lying down, support his arm comfortably at about heart level, ensuring that no tight clothing constricts the upper arm. You can measure over thin clothing, as it makes no difference to the result.

The usual sphygmomanometer cuff has a bladder width of 12.5 cm and length of 3–35 cm. Apply the cuff to the upper arm, with the centre of the bladder over the brachial artery.

Palpate the brachial pulse.

Inflate the cuff until the pulse is impalpable. Note the pressure on the manometer; this is a rough estimate of systolic pressure.

Inflate the cuff another 30 mmHg and listen through the diaphragm of the stethoscope placed over the brachial artery.

Deflate the cuff slowly (2–3 mmHg/s) until you hear a regular tapping sound (phase 1 Korotkoff sounds). Record the reading to the nearest 2 mmHg. This is the systolic pressure.

Continue to deflate the cuff slowly until the sounds disappear.

Record the pressure at which the sounds completely disappear as the diastolic pressure (phase 5). Occasionally, muffled sounds persist (phase 4) and do not disappear, in which case the point of muffling is the best guide to the diastolic pressure.

Common problems in BP measurement

- BP different in each arm: A difference >10 mmHg suggests peripheral vascular disease and raises the possibility of renal artery stenosis as the cause of hypertension. Record the highest pressure and treat this
- Wrong cuff size: A cuff of 12.5 × 23 cm is suitable for only 60% of Europeans. The bladder should encircle between 80% and 100% of the arm. In obese patients with large arms a normal-sized cuff will over-estimate BP and the error is greater when the centre of the cuff is not over the brachial artery. Therefore for obese patients a larger cuff must be used. Using too large a cuff produces only a small under-estimation of BP (2–3 mm in systolic BP)
- Auscultatory gap: Up to 20% of elderly hypertensive patients have phase 1 Korotkoff sounds which begin at systolic pressure but then disappear for varying lengths of time, reappearing before diastolic

pressure. If the first appearance of the sound is missed, the systolic pressure will be recorded at a falsely low level. Avoid this by palpating the systolic pressure first

- Excess pressure of stethoscope: Excess pressure can artificially lower the diastolic reading by 10 mmHg. The systolic pressure is not usually affected
- Patient's arm at the wrong level: The patient's elbow should be level with his heart. Hydrostatic pressure effects mean that if the arm is 7 cm higher, both systole and diastole pressures will be 5 mmHg lower. If the arm is 7 cm lower than the heart, they will be about 6 mm higher
- Terminal digit preference: The true reading should be recorded rather than rounding BP to the nearest 0 or 5
- Postural change: When a healthy person stands, the pulse increases by about 11 bpm and stabilizes after 1 min. The BP stabilizes after 1–2 min. Check the BP after a patient has been standing for 2 min; a drop of ≥20 mmHg on standing is postural hypotension
- Abnormal pulse pressure: The pulse pressure is the difference between the systolic and diastolic pressures. A pulse pressure of ≥80 mmHg suggests aortic regurgitation, while a low pulse pressure may occur in aortic stenosis.

OSCEs 6.24 Examine this patient with high blood pressure

1. Check the pulse rate — irregularly irregular suggests atrial fibrillation.
2. Measure the blood pressure in both arms.
3. Check for radiofemoral delay (coarctation of the aorta).
4. Examine the optic fundi for hypertensive retinopathy.
5. Look for features of Cushing's syndrome or virilization.
6. Palpate the abdomen for renal enlargement (adult polycystic kidney disease) and for the abnormal pulsation of an abdominal aortic aneurysm.
7. Listen for bruits over the renal arteries (renal artery stenosis).
8. Examine the heart for the heave of left ventricular hypertrophy and for a fourth heart sound.
9. Look for evidence of heart failure (raised JVP, basal lung crackles, ankle oedema).
10. Perform microscopic examination of the urine, looking for red cell casts.

Jugular venous pressure (JVP) and waveform

Anatomy

The internal jugular vein enters the neck behind the mastoid process. It runs deep to the sternocleidomastoid muscle before entering the thorax between the sternal and clavicular heads and can only be examined when the neck muscles are relaxed. Although the vein itself cannot be seen, a diffuse pulsation is visible when the pressure in the internal jugular vein is elevated.

The external jugular vein is more superficial, prominent and generally easier to see. Although it can be obstructed as it traverses the deep fascia of the neck, this rarely presents a problem. If it is visible, pulsatile and not obstructed, it can be used to assess JVP. Due to the anatomy of the innominate veins, the JVP is best examined on the patient's right side.

Symptoms and definitions

The JVP can be estimated by observing the level of blood in either the internal or external jugular veins. Both veins have valves but, as blood flow is towards the heart, they do not affect this and may even make the waveform easier to see. The normal waveform has 2 peaks per cycle, which helps distinguish it from the carotid arterial pulse (Box 6.25).

The JVP reflects central venous or right atrial pressure (normally <7 mmHg/9 cmH$_2$O) and, indirectly, right ventricular function. The sternal angle is approximately 5 cm above the right atrium, so the normal JVP should be no more than 4 cm above this angle when the patient lies at 45°. If the JVP is low, the patient may have to lie flat for it to be seen; if high, the patient may need to sit upright (Fig. 6.21).

6.25 Differences between carotid and jugular pulsation

Carotid	Jugular
Rapid outward movement	Rapid inward movement
One peak per heartbeat	Two peaks per heartbeat (in sinus rhythm)
Palpable	Impalpable
Pulsation unaffected by pressure at the root of the neck	Pulsation diminished by pressure at the root of the neck
Independent of respiration	Height of pulsation varies with respiration
Independent of position of patient	Varies with position of patient
Independent of abdominal pressure	Rises with abdominal pressure

▶ Examination sequence

JVP and waveform

▶ Position the patient so that he is reclining supine comfortably until the waveform is clearly visible (start at 45°).

▶ Rest the patient's head on a pillow to ensure that the neck muscles are relaxed.

▶ Look across the neck from the right side of the patient (Fig. 6.22A).

▶ Identify the jugular vein pulsation.

▶ If you are not certain, use the abdomino-jugular reflux or occlusion to confirm it is the JVP.

▶ The JVP is the vertical height in centimetres between the top of the venous pulsation and the sternal angle, whether they are sitting at 45° or not (Fig. 6.22B).

▶ Identify the timing and form of the pulsation and note any abnormality.

Aids to differentiate the jugular venous waveform from arterial pulsation

• Abdomino-jugular reflux: Gently press over the abdomen for 10 seconds. This increases venous return to the right side of the heart temporarily and the JVP normally rises. This rise may take 15 seconds to decrease in congestive heart failure

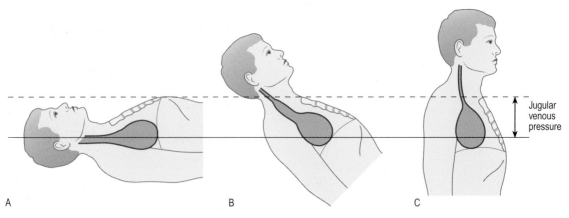

Fig. 6.21 Jugular venous pressure in a healthy subject. (A) Supine: jugular vein distended, pulsation not visible. **(B)** Reclining at 45°: point of transition between distended and collapsed vein can usually be seen to pulsate just above the clavicle. **(C)** Upright: upper part of vein collapsed and transition point obscured.

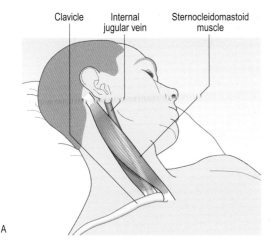

A

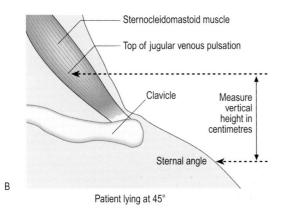

B

Patient lying at 45°

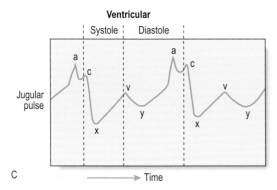

C

Fig. 6.22 Jugular venous pressure. **(A)** Inspecting the jugular venous pressure from the side (the internal jugular vein lies deep to the sternocleidomastoid muscle). **(B)** Measuring the height of the JVP. **(C)** Form of the venous pulse wave tracing from the internal jugular vein: a = atrial systole; c = closure of the tricuspid valve; v = peak pressure in right atrium immediately prior to opening of tricuspid valve; a–x = descent, due to downward displacement of the tricuspid ring during systole; v–y = descent at commencement of ventricular filling.

- Changes with respiration: Normally the JVP falls with inspiration as the decrease in intrathoracic pressure is transmitted to the right atrium
- Waveform: The normal JVP waveform has two distinct peaks per cardiac cycle:

  The 'a' wave corresponds to right atrial contraction and occurs just before the first heart sound. In atrial fibrillation the 'a' wave is lost in the absence of coordinated atrial contraction

  The 'v' wave is caused by atrial filling during ventricular systole when the tricuspid valve is closed

  A third peak ('c' wave) is due to closure of the tricuspid valve but is rarely seen (Fig. 6.22C)
- Occlusion: The JVP waveform is obliterated by gently occluding the vein at the base of the neck with your finger.

Abnormal findings

The JVP and its waveform are affected by certain arrhythmias and cardiac conditions. The JVP is elevated in fluid overload, most characteristically in heart failure. Although it can be elevated in biventricular failure, it is primarily a sign of right ventricular failure. It is elevated in conditions such as acute pulmonary embolism and chronic obstructive pulmonary disease (COPD) with right heart dilatation (cor pulmonale). Mechanical obstruction of the superior vena cava (most often caused by lung cancer) may cause extreme elevation of the JVP. In these circumstances the JVP no longer reflects right atrial pressure and the abdomino-jugular reflux will be absent (Box 6.26).

- Küssmaul's sign: a paradoxical rise of JVP on inspiration. It is seen in pericardial constriction or tamponade, severe right ventricular failure and restrictive cardiomyopathy
- Prominent 'a' wave: seen in any condition with delayed or restricted right ventricular filling, e.g. pulmonary hypertension or tricuspid stenosis

6.26 Abnormalities of the jugular venous pulse

Condition	Abnormalities
Heart failure	Elevation, sustained abdominojugular reflux
Pulmonary embolism	Elevation
Pericardial effusion	Elevation, prominent 'y' descent
Pericardial constriction	Elevation, Küssmaul's sign
Superior vena caval obstruction	Elevation, loss of pulsation
Atrial fibrillation	Absent 'a' waves
Tricuspid stenosis	Giant 'a' waves
Tricuspid regurgitation	Giant 'v' waves
Complete heart block	'Cannon' waves

- Cannon waves: giant 'a' waves which occur when the right atrium contracts against a closed tricuspid valve. Irregular cannon waves are seen in complete heart block and are due to atrioventricular dissociation. Regular cannon waves occur during junctional bradycardias and some ventricular and supraventricular tachycardias
- 'cv' wave: a characteristic fusion of the 'c' and 'v' waves resulting in an increased wave and associated with a pulsatile liver. It is seen in tricuspid regurgitation.

The precordium

The precordium is the area on the front of the chest which relates to the surface anatomy of the heart (Fig. 6.23).

Learn the surface anatomy of the heart to understand how and where the sounds and murmurs radiate and basic cardiac physiology to appreciate their timing (Figs 6.23 and 6.24). The auscultatory areas (aortic, pulmonary, mitral and tricuspid) do not correspond with the surface markings of the heart valves, but are where transmitted sounds and murmurs are best heard (Box 6.27, Fig. 6.25).

Symptoms and definitions

'Funnel chest' (pectus excavatum), a posterior displacement of the lower sternum, and 'pigeon chest' (pectus carinatum) may displace the heart and affect palpation and auscultation (Fig. 7.18, p. 169).

A midline sternotomy scar usually indicates previous coronary artery bypass surgery or aortic valve replacement. A left submammary scar is usually the result of mitral valvotomy. Infraclavicular scars are seen after pacemaker implantation, and the bulge of the pacemaker may be obvious in thin subjects.

Apex beat

The apex beat is the most lateral and inferior position where the cardiac impulse can be felt. The cardiac

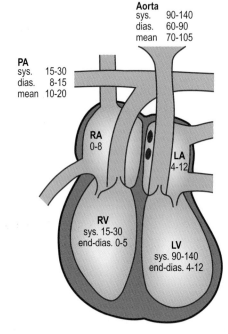

Fig. 6.24 Normal resting pressures (mmHg) in the heart and great vessels.

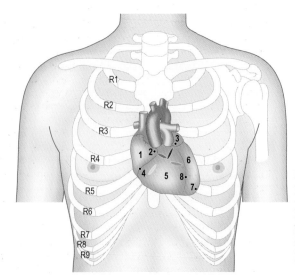

Fig. 6.23 Surface anatomy of the chambers and valves of the heart.

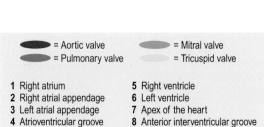

= Aortic valve   = Mitral valve
= Pulmonary valve   = Tricuspid valve

1 Right atrium
2 Right atrial appendage
3 Left atrial appendage
4 Atrioventricular groove
5 Right ventricle
6 Left ventricle
7 Apex of the heart
8 Anterior interventricular groove

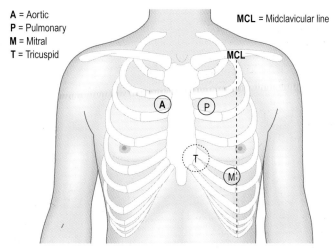

A = Aortic
P = Pulmonary
M = Mitral
T = Tricuspid

MCL = Midclavicular line

MCL

Fig. 6.25 Sites for auscultation. Sites at which murmurs from the relevant valves are usually, but not preferentially, heard.

6.27 Cardiac auscultation: the best sites for hearing abnormality

Site	Sound
Cardiac apex	First heart sound Third and fourth heart sounds Mid-diastolic murmur of mitral stenosis
Lower left sternal border	Early diastolic murmurs of aortic and tricuspid regurgitation
Upper left sternal border	Second heart sound Opening snap of mitral stenosis Pulmonary valve murmurs Pansystolic murmur of ventricular septal defect
Upper right sternal border	Systolic ejection (outflow) murmurs, e.g. aortic stenosis, hypertrophic obstructive cardiomyopathy
Left axilla	Radiation of the pansystolic murmur of mitral regurgitation
Below left clavicle	Continuous 'machinery' murmur of a persistent patent ductus arteriosus

impulse results from the heart rotating, moving forward and striking the chest wall during systole. The apex beat is normally in the 5th left intercostal space (the space below the 5th rib) at, or medial to, the midclavicular line. Count the rib spaces down from the sternal angle, which is at the junction of the sternum and second rib. The midclavicular line is halfway between the suprasternal notch and the acromioclavicular joint.

A normal apical impulse briefly lifts the palpating fingers and is localized. It may be impalpable in overweight or muscular people, or in patients with asthma or emphysema because the chest is hyperinflated. Very occasionally, the heart may be on the right side (dextrocardia).

Displacement

Left ventricular dilatation, as can occur with aortic stenosis, severe hypertension and dilated cardiomyopathy, diffusely displaces the apex beat inferiorly and laterally. This can also occur in chest deformity, or mediastinal shift due to intrathoracic disorders, e.g. massive pleural effusion or tension pneumothorax. In these situations the trachea may also be deviated.

Character of the apical impulse

A heave is a palpable impulse that lifts your hand noticeably. Left ventricular hypertrophy due to hypertension and aortic stenosis produce a forceful, undisplaced apical impulse. This thrusting apical 'heave' is quite different from the diffuse impulse of left ventricular dilatation. A pulsation over the left parasternal area (right ventricular heave) is usually abnormal in adults and indicates right ventricular hypertrophy or dilatation, e.g. pulmonary hypertension. The 'tapping' apex beat in mitral stenosis represents a palpable first heart sound, and is not usually displaced. A double apical impulse is characteristic of hypertrophic obstructive cardiomyopathy.

A thrill is the tactile equivalent of a murmur and feels similar to a mobile telephone vibrating. The most common thrill is that of aortic stenosis which may be palpable at the apex, at the lower sternum or in the neck. The thrill caused by a ventricular septal defect is best felt at the left and right sternal edges. Diastolic thrills are very rare.

6

Heart sounds

The bell and diaphragm of the stethoscope accentuate sounds of different pitches. The bell emphasizes low-pitched sounds such as normal heart sounds and the diastolic murmur of mitral stenosis. The diaphragm filters these sounds and helps to identify high-pitched sounds such as the early diastolic murmur of aortic regurgitation or a pericardial friction rub.

Normal heart valves make a sound when they close but not when they open. The classic 'lub-dub' sounds are caused by closure of the atrioventricular (mitral and tricuspid) valves followed by the outlet (aortic and pulmonary) valves. Develop a routine for auscultation so that you do not overlook subtle abnormalities. Identify and describe the following:

- the first and second heart sounds
- extra heart sounds (third and fourth, heard in diastole)
- additional sounds, e.g. clicks and snaps
- pericardial rubs
- murmurs in systole and/or diastole.

Normal findings

First heart sound

The first heart sound (S_1), 'lub', is caused by closure of the mitral and tricuspid valves at onset of ventricular systole and is best heard at the apex.

Second heart sound

The second heart sound (S_2), 'dup', is caused by closure of the pulmonary and aortic valves at the end of ventricular systole and is best heard at the left sternal edge. It is louder and higher-pitched than the first sound, and the aortic component is normally louder than the pulmonary one. Physiological splitting of the second heart sound occurs because left ventricular contraction slightly precedes that of the right ventricle so that the aortic valve closes before the pulmonary valve. This splitting increases at end-inspiration because the increased venous filling of the right ventricle further delays pulmonary valve closure. This separation disappears on expiration (Fig. 6.26). Splitting of the second sound is best heard at the left sternal edge. On auscultation, you hear 'lub d/dub' (inspiration) 'lub-dub' (expiration).

Third heart sound

A third heart sound (S_3) is a low-pitched early diastolic sound best heard with the bell at the apex. It coincides with rapid ventricular filling immediately after opening of the atrioventricular valves and is therefore heard after the second as 'lub-dub-dum'. A third heart sound is a normal finding in children, in young adults and during pregnancy.

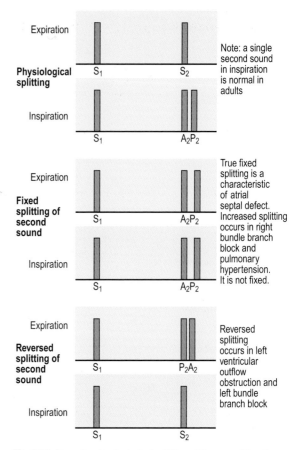

Fig. 6.26 Normal and pathological splitting of the second heart sound.

Abnormal findings

First heart sound

In mitral stenosis the intensity of the first heart sound is increased due to the elevated left atrial pressure (Box 6.28).

Second heart sound

The aortic component of the second heart sound is sometimes quiet or absent in calcific aortic stenosis and reduced in aortic regurgitation (Box 6.29). The aortic component is loud in systemic hypertension, and the pulmonary component is increased in pulmonary hypertension.

Wide splitting of the second heart sound, but with normal respiratory variation, occurs in conditions which delay right ventricular emptying, e.g. right bundle branch block. Fixed splitting, i.e. no variation with respiration of the second heart sound, is a feature of atrial septal defect (Fig. 6.27). In this condition the right ventricular stroke volume is larger than the left, and the splitting is fixed because the defect equalizes the pressure between the two atria throughout the respiratory cycle.

6

6.28 Abnormalities of intensity of the first heart sound

Quiet

- Low cardiac output
- Poor left ventricular function
- Long P–R interval (first-degree heart block)
- Rheumatic mitral regurgitation

Loud

- Increased cardiac output
- Large stroke volume
- Mitral stenosis
- Short P–R interval
- Atrial myxoma (rare)

Variable

- Atrial fibrillation
- Extrasystoles
- Complete heart block

6.29 Abnormalities of the second heart sound

Quiet

- Low cardiac output
- Calcific aortic stenosis
- Aortic regurgitation

Loud

- Systemic hypertension (aortic component)
- Pulmonary hypertension (pulmonary component)

Split

- Widens in inspiration (enhanced physiological splitting):
  Right bundle branch block
  Pulmonary stenosis
  Pulmonary hypertension
  Ventricular septal defect
- Fixed splitting (unaffected by respiration):
  Atrial septal defect
- Widens in expiration (reversed splitting):
  Aortic stenosis
  Hypertrophic cardiomyopathy
  Left bundle branch block
  Ventricular pacing

In reversed splitting the two components of the second heart sound occur together on inspiration and separate on expiration. This occurs when left ventricular emptying is delayed so that the aortic valve closes after the pulmonary valve. Examples include left bundle branch block and right ventricular pacing.

Third heart sound

A third heart sound is usually pathological after the age of 40 years (Box 6.30). The most common causes are left ventricular failure, when it is an early sign, and mitral regurgitation. In heart failure S_3 occurs with a tachycardia and S_1 and S_2 are quiet (lub-da-dub).

Fourth heart sound

A fourth heart sound (S_4) is less common. It is soft and low-pitched, best heard with the bell of the stethoscope at the apex. It occurs just before the first sound (da-lub-dub). It is always pathological and is caused by forceful atrial contraction against a non-compliant or stiff ventricle. A fourth heart sound is most often heard with left ventricular hypertrophy (due to hypertension, aortic stenosis or hypertrophic obstructive cardiomyopathy). It cannot occur when there is atrial fibrillation.

Both a third and a fourth heart sound cause a 'triple' or 'gallop' rhythm.

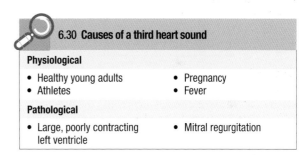

6.30 Causes of a third heart sound

Physiological

- Healthy young adults
- Athletes
- Pregnancy
- Fever

Pathological

- Large, poorly contracting left ventricle
- Mitral regurgitation

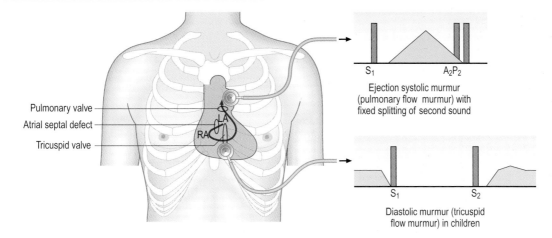

Fig. 6.27 Atrial septal defect.

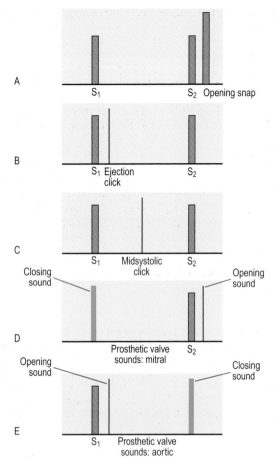

A

S_1 S_2 Opening snap

B

S_1 Ejection click S_2

C

S_1 Midsystolic click S_2

Closing sound   Opening sound

D

Prosthetic valve sounds: mitral S_2

Opening sound   Closing sound

E

S_1 Prosthetic valve sounds: aortic

Fig. 6.28 'Added sounds' on auscultation.

Added sounds

- An opening snap is commonly heard in mitral (rarely tricuspid) stenosis. It results from sudden opening of a stenosed valve and occurs early in diastole, just after the second heart sound (Fig. 6.28A). The opening snap of mitral stenosis is best heard at the apex
- Ejection clicks occur early in systole just after the first heart sound, in patients with congenital pulmonary or aortic stenosis (Fig. 6.28B). The mechanism is similar to that of an opening snap. Ejection clicks do not occur in calcific aortic stenosis because the cusps are rigid
- Midsystolic clicks occur in mitral valve prolapse (Fig. 6.28C) and may be associated with a late systolic murmur. They are high-pitched and best heard at the apex
- Mechanical heart valves can make a sound when they close and open. The closure sound is normally louder, especially with modern valves. The sounds are high-pitched, 'metallic' and often palpable, and

may be heard without a stethoscope. A mechanical mitral valve replacement makes a metallic first heart sound and a sound like a loud opening snap (Fig. 6.28D). Mechanical aortic valves have loud, metallic second heart sounds and an opening sound like an ejection click (Fig. 6.28E). They usually also cause a flow murmur.

Pericardial rub

A pericardial friction rub is a coarse scratching sound which often has systolic and diastolic components. It is best heard using the diaphragm with the breath held in expiration. It may be audible over any part of the precordium but is often localized. It is most often heard in acute viral pericarditis and sometimes 24–72 hours after myocardial infarction. Pericardial rubs vary in intensity over time, and with the position of the patient. A pleuro-pericardial rub is a similar sound that occurs in time with the cardiac cycle but is also influenced by respiration and is pleural in origin. Occasionally a 'crunching' noise can be heard caused by air in the pericardium (pneumopericardium).

Murmurs

Heart murmurs are produced by turbulent flow across an abnormal valve, septal defect or outflow obstruction, or by increased volume or velocity of flow through a normal valve. Murmurs may occur in a healthy heart. These 'innocent' murmurs occur when stroke volume is increased, e.g. during pregnancy, and in athletes with resting bradycardia or children with fever.

Timing

To determine the timing of a murmur, identify the first and second heart sounds. You may find it helps to palpate the patient's carotid pulse with your thumb while you are listening to the precordium.

First determine whether the murmur is systolic or diastolic:

- Systole begins with the first heart sound (mitral and tricuspid valve closure). This occurs when left and right ventricular pressures exceed the corresponding atrial pressures. For a short period all four heart valves are closed (pre-ejection period). Ventricular pressures continue to rise until they exceed those of the aorta and pulmonary artery, and then the aortic and pulmonary valves open. Systole ends with the closure of these valves, producing the second heart sound
- Diastole is the interval between the second and the first heart sound. Physiologically it is divided into three phases:
  - Early diastole (isovolumic relaxation): the time from the closure of the aortic and pulmonary valves until the opening of the mitral and tricuspid valves
  - Mid-diastole: the period of passive ventricular filling
  - Presystole: coinciding with atrial systole.

Murmurs of aortic (and pulmonary) regurgitation start in early diastole and extend into mid-diastole. The murmurs of mitral or tricuspid stenosis cannot start before mid-diastole. Likewise, third heart sounds occur in mid-diastole and fourth heart sounds in presystole.

Duration

The murmurs of mitral and tricuspid regurgitation start concurrent with the first heart sound, sometimes muffling or obscuring it, and continue throughout systole (pansystolic) (Fig. 6.29). The murmur produced by mitral valve prolapse does not begin until the mitral valve leaflet has prolapsed during systole, producing a late systolic murmur. The ejection systolic murmur of aortic or pulmonary stenosis begins after the first heart sound, reaches maximal intensity in midsystole, then fades, stopping before the second heart sound (Fig. 6.30).

Character and pitch

The quality of a murmur is subjective, but terms such as harsh, blowing, musical, rumbling, high- or low-pitched help. High-pitched murmurs often correspond with high-pressure gradients, so the diastolic murmur of aortic regurgitation is higher-pitched than that of mitral stenosis.

Intensity

Six grades of intensity are used to describe murmurs (Box 6.31). The intensity of the murmur does not correlate with the severity of valve dysfunction; for instance the murmur of critical aortic stenosis can be quiet and occasionally inaudible. Changes in intensity with time are important, as they denote progression of a valve lesion. Rapidly changing murmurs are sometimes heard with infective endocarditis because of valve destruction. Diastolic murmurs are rarely louder than grade 3.

Location

Record the site(s) where you hear the murmur best. This helps to differentiate diastolic murmurs (mitral stenosis at the apex, aortic regurgitation at the left sternal edge), but is less helpful with systolic murmurs, which are often loud over all the precordium (Fig. 6.25).

Radiation

Murmurs radiate in the direction of the blood flow to specific sites outside the precordium. Differentiate this from location. The pansystolic murmur of mitral regurgitation radiates towards the left axilla, the murmur of ventricular septal defect towards the right sternal edge, and that of aortic stenosis to the aortic area and the carotid arteries.

Abnormal findings

Systolic murmurs

Ejection systolic murmur

Ejection systolic murmurs are caused by increased stroke volume (flow murmur), or stenosis of the aortic or pulmonary valve (Box 6.32). An ejection murmur is also a feature of hypertrophic obstructive cardiomyopathy and is accentuated by exercise. Aortic flow murmurs can be caused by pregnancy, fever, severe anaemia or bradycardia. Atrial septal defect is characterized by a pulmonary flow murmur during systole.

The murmur of aortic stenosis is often audible all over the precordium (Fig. 6.30). It is harsh, high-pitched and musical, and radiates to the upper right sternal edge and carotids. It is usually loud and there may be a thrill (a palpable murmur).

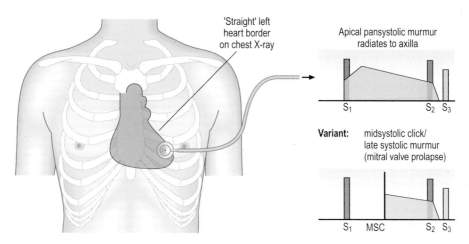

Fig. 6.29 Mitral regurgitation. The murmur begins at the moment of valve closure and may obscure the first heart sound. It varies little in intensity throughout systole. In mitral valve prolapse, the murmur begins in mid- or late systole and there is often a midsystolic click (MSC).

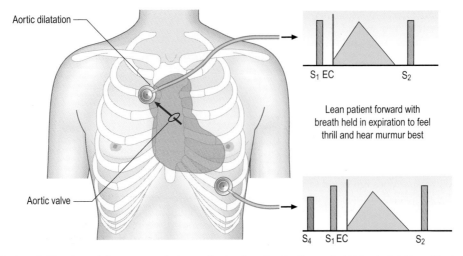

Fig. 6.30 **Aortic stenosis.** There is a systolic pressure gradient across the stenotic aortic valve. The resultant high-velocity jet (arrow) impinges on the wall of the aorta, and is best heard with the diaphragm placed near to this on the chest. Alternatively, the bell may be placed in the suprasternal notch. The diagrammatic representation of the phonocardiogram shows the ejection systolic murmur preceded by an ejection click (EC). A fourth heart sound may be heard at the apex.

6.31 Grades of intensity of murmur	
Grade 1	Heard by an expert in optimum conditions
Grade 2	Heard by a non-expert in optimum conditions
Grade 3	Easily heard; no thrill
Grade 4	A loud murmur, with a thrill
Grade 5	Very loud, often heard over wide area, with thrill
Grade 6	Extremely loud, heard without stethoscope

6.32 Causes of systolic murmurs

Ejection systolic murmurs

- Increased flow through normal valves
  'Innocent systolic murmur': fever, athletes (bradycardia → large stroke volume), pregnancy (cardiac output maximum at 15 weeks)
  Atrial septal defect (pulmonary flow murmur)
  Severe anaemia
- Normal or reduced flow though stenotic valve
  Aortic stenosis
  Pulmonary stenosis
- Other causes of flow murmurs
  Hypertrophic obstructive cardiomyopathy (obstruction at subvalvular level)
  Aortic regurgitation (aortic flow murmur)

Pansystolic murmurs

- All caused by a systolic leak from a high- to a lower-pressure chamber
  Mitral regurgitation
  Tricuspid regurgitation
  Ventricular septal defect
  Leaking mitral or tricuspid prosthesis

Pansystolic murmur

A pansystolic murmur is usually caused by mitral regurgitation. The murmur is often loud and blowing in character, best heard at the apex and radiating to the axilla. With mitral valve prolapse, regurgitation may begin in midsystole, producing a late systolic murmur (Fig. 6.29). The murmur of tricuspid regurgitation is heard at the lower left sternal edge; if significant, it is associated with a 'v' wave in the JVP and a pulsatile liver.

A ventricular septal defect also causes a pansystolic murmur. Small congenital defects produce a loud murmur audible at the left sternal border, radiating to the right sternal border and often associated with a thrill. Rupture of the interventricular septum can complicate myocardial infarction and produces a harsh pansystolic murmur. Other murmurs heard after myocardial infarction include acute mitral regurgitation due to rupture of a papillary muscle or functional mitral regurgitation caused by left ventricular dilatation.

Diastolic murmurs

Early diastolic murmur

The term early diastolic murmur is misleading because the murmur usually lasts throughout diastole, but it is loudest in early diastole. Early diastolic murmurs are

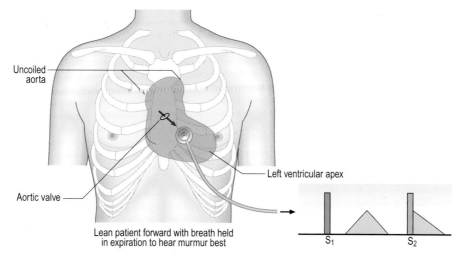

Fig. 6.31 Aortic regurgitation. The pulse pressure is usually increased; the jet from the aortic valve is directed inferiorly towards the left ventricular outflow tract (arrow) during diastole, producing a high-pitched murmur which is best heard with the diaphragm. The diagrammatic representation of the phonocardiogram also shows the associated systolic murmur, which is common because of the increased flow through the aortic valve in systole.

usually caused by aortic regurgitation (Fig. 6.31), are best heard at the left sternal edge and are most obvious in expiration with the patient leaning forward. Since the regurgitant blood volume must be ejected during the subsequent systole, significant aortic regurgitation leads to increased stroke volume and is almost always associated with a systolic flow murmur.

Pulmonary regurgitation is uncommon. It may be caused by pulmonary artery dilatation in pulmonary hypertension (Graham Steell murmur) or to a congenital defect of the pulmonary valve.

Mid-diastolic murmur

A mid-diastolic murmur is usually caused by mitral stenosis. This is a low-pitched, rumbling sound which may follow an opening snap (Fig. 6.32). It is best heard with the bell of the stethoscope at the apex with the patient rolled to the left side. The murmur can be accentuated by listening after exercise. The whole cadence sounds like 'lup-ta-ta-rru' where 'lup' is the loud first heart sound, 'ta-ta' the second sound, and opening snap and 'rru' the mid-diastolic murmur. If the patient is in sinus rhythm, left atrial contraction increases the blood flow across the stenosed valve leading to pre-systolic accentuation of the murmur. The murmur of tricuspid stenosis is similar but rare.

An Austin Flint murmur is a mid-diastolic murmur that accompanies aortic regurgitation. It is caused by the regurgitant jet striking the anterior leaflet of the mitral valve, restricting inflow to the left ventricle.

Continuous murmur

Continuous murmurs are rare in adults. The most common cause is a patent ductus arteriosus, which connects the upper descending aorta and pulmonary artery in the fetus and normally closes just after birth. The murmur is best heard at the upper left sternal border and radiates over the left scapula. Its continuous character is described as 'machinery-like' (Fig. 6.33).

Examination sequence
The precordium and the heart sounds

▪▪ Explain that you wish to examine the chest and ask the patient to remove clothing above the waist. Keep female patients' chest covered with a sheet as far as possible.

▪▪ Inspect the precordium with the patient sitting at a 45° angle with shoulders horizontal. Look for surgical scars, visible pulsations and chest deformity.

▪▪ Lay your whole hand flat over the precordium to obtain a general impression of the cardiac impulse (Fig. 6.34A).

▪▪ Locate the apex beat by laying your fingers on the chest parallel to the rib spaces; if you cannot feel it, ask the patient to roll on to his left side (Fig. 6.34B).

▪▪ Assess the character of the apex beat and note its position.

▪▪ Feel for a heave of the right ventricle, using the heel of your hand applied firmly to the left parasternal position. Ask the patient to hold his breath in expiration (Fig. 6.34C).

▪▪ Palpate for thrills at the apex and both sides of the sternum using the flat of your fingers.

▪▪ Listen with your stethoscope over the precordium. The earpieces should be angled slightly forward and should fit comfortably. The tubing should be about 25 cm long and thick enough to reduce external sound. Make sure the room is quiet when you are auscultating.

▪▪ Listen at the apex, lower left sternal border, and upper right and left sternal borders with the bell then with the diaphragm. Then listen over the carotid arteries and the left axilla.

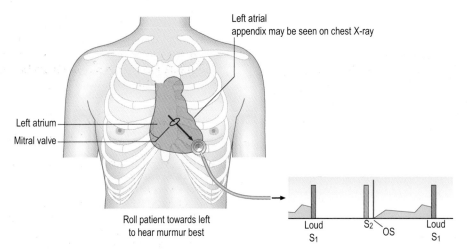

Left atrial appendix may be seen on chest X-ray

Left atrium

Mitral valve

Roll patient towards left to hear murmur best

Loud S₁   S₂ OS   Loud S₁

Fig. 6.32 Mitral stenosis. There is a pressure gradient across the mitral valve; in this example it continues throughout diastole. This causes a sharp movement of the tethered anterior cusp of the mitral valve at the time when the flow commences, and the opening snap (OS) results. The jet through the stenotic valve (arrow) strikes the endocardium at the cardiac apex.

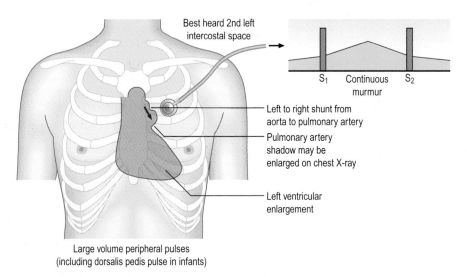

Best heard 2nd left intercostal space

S₁   Continuous murmur   S₂

Left to right shunt from aorta to pulmonary artery

Pulmonary artery shadow may be enlarged on chest X-ray

Left ventricular enlargement

Large volume peripheral pulses (including dorsalis pedis pulse in infants)

Fig. 6.33 Persistent patent ductus arteriosus. A continuous murmur is heard because aortic pressure always exceeds pulmonary arterial pressure, resulting in continuous ductal flow. The pressure difference is greatest in systole, producing a louder systolic component to the murmur.

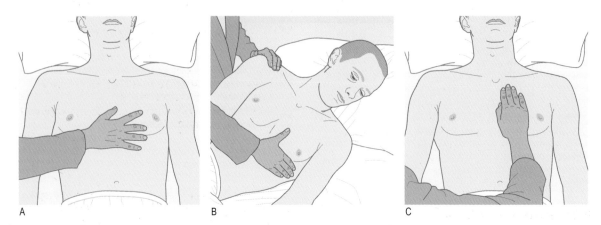

A   B   C

Fig. 6.34 Palpating the heart. (A) Use your hand to palpate the cardiac impulse. **(B)** Localize the apex beat with your finger (roll the patient, if necessary, into the left lateral position). **(C)** Palpate from apex to sternum for parasternal pulsations.

6

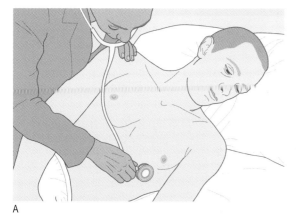

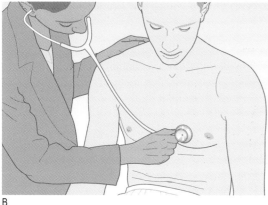

Fig. 6.35 Auscultating the heart. (A) Listen for the murmur of mitral stenosis with the lightly applied bell with the patient in the left lateral position. **(B)** Listen for the murmur of aortic regurgitation with the diaphragm with the patient leaning forward.

- At each site identify the first and second heart sounds. Assess their character and intensity; note any splitting of the second heart sound. Feel the carotid pulse with your thumb to time any murmur. The first heart sound barely precedes the upstroke of the carotid pulsation, while the second heart sound is clearly out of phase with it.
- Concentrate in turn on systole (the interval between S_1 and S_2) and diastole (the interval between S_2 and S_1). Listen for added sounds and then for murmurs. Soft diastolic murmurs are sometimes described as the 'absence of silence'.
- Roll the patient on to his left side. Listen at the apex using light pressure with the bell, to detect the mid-diastolic and presystolic murmur of mitral stenosis (Fig. 6.35A).
- Ask the patient to sit up and lean forwards, then to breathe out fully and hold his breath (Fig. 6.35B). Listen over the right second intercostal space and over the left sternal edge with the diaphragm for the murmur of aortic regurgitation.
- Note the character and intensity of any murmur heard.

Interpreting findings

Auscultation remains an important clinical skill despite the ready availability of echocardiography. You must

OSCEs 6.33 Examine this patient with sudden-onset central chest pain

1. Feel the pulse for bradycardia (heart block), tachycardia (supraventricular tachycardia, ventricular tachycardia) and irregularity (atrial fibrillation, multiple ventricular extrasystoles).
2. Palpate carotid and femoral pulses (may be weak or absent in aortic dissection).
3. Measure the BP.
4. Look for the JVP — raised in heart failure.
5. Examine the trachea and cardiac apex beat for mediastinal shift (tension pneumothorax).
6. Palpate the epigastrium for tenderness (gastro-oesophageal reflux, peptic ulcer, oesophagitis).
7. Listen to the heart for extra heart sounds or gallop rhythm (heart failure), pansystolic murmur radiating to the left axilla (mitral regurgitation due to papillary muscle rupture post-myocardial infarction), pansystolic murmur at the left sternal edge (ventricular septal defect post-myocardial infarction) and pericardial friction rub (pericarditis).

OSCEs 6.34 Examine this patient with sudden loss of consciousness

1. Feel the pulse for bradycardia (faint or syncope; heart block or Stokes–Adams attack), (supraventricular tachycardia or ventricular tachycardia; sinus tachycardia after seizure) and irregularity (sudden-onset atrial fibrillation).
2. Measure the BP for hypotension (septicaemia, acute myocardial infarction).
3. If possible, measure the BP erect and supine (postural fall of >20 mmHg systolic BP).
4. Check temperature — raised in meningitis and subarachnoid haemorrhage.
5. Listen for structural heart disease (valvular heart disease, ventricular septal defect post-myocardial infarction, cardiac tamponade).
6. Listen to the carotids for bruits (embolic cerebrovascular accident).
7. Examine for focal neurological signs (post-epileptic seizure, cerebral haemorrhage).
8. Inspect the tongue for lacerations and check for urinary incontinence (post-epileptic seizure).
9. Assess level of consciousness (epileptic seizure, subarachnoid haemorrhage, intracranial lesion).

be able to detect abnormal signs to prompt appropriate investigation. Auscultatory signs, e.g. third or fourth heart sounds and pericardial friction rubs, have no direct equivalent on echocardiography but are diagnostically important. Some patients, especially those with rheumatic

6

6.35 Investigations in cardiac disease

Investigation	Indication/Comment
Blood tests	
FBC and ESR	Anaemia unmasking angina and connective tissue disease
U & E	Renal function
Blood glucose	Hypertension more common in diabetes
Lipids	Hyperlipidaemia
Cardiac enzymes	Troponins rise after MI
Serology	Connective tissue disease, streptococcal infection
Blood culture	Infective endocarditis
Electrophysiology	
ECG	Cardiac rhythm, conduction, e.g. left bundle branch block Myocardial infarction and ischaemia (usually normal in angina) Assess left ventricular hypertrophy
Exercise ECG	Ischaemia, prognosis post myocardial infarction

Investigation	Indication/Comment
Ambulatory ECG monitoring	Confirms if palpitation coincides with arrhythmia
Radiology	
Chest X-ray	Cardiothoracic ratio (maximum width of the cardiac silhouette/widest part of lung fields) increased in heart failure and valve disease
Echocardiography (transoesophageal echocardiogram more sensitive)	Quantifies valvular defects; assesses left ventricular function (heart failure); valve vegetations in infective endocarditis
Radionuclide studies	Left ventricular function; myocardial ischaemia; pulmonary embolism
Invasive tests	
Cardiac catheterization	Coronary angiography (angina) determines therapy, prior to surgery in valve disease to assess coronary anatomy, and severe heart failure for cardiac transplantation

heart disease, have multiple heart valve defects, and the interpretation of more subtle physical signs is important. For example, a patient with mixed mitral stenosis and regurgitation will probably have dominant stenosis if the first heart sound is loud, but dominant regurgitation if there is a third heart sound.

INVESTIGATIONS IN HEART DISEASE

Electrocardiography (ECG)

The standard 12-lead ECG (Fig. 6.36) uses recordings made from six precordial electrodes (V_1–V_6) and six different recordings from the limb electrodes (left arm, right arm and left leg). The right leg electrode is used as a reference.

Ambulatory ECG monitoring

Ambulatory recordings make a continuous ECG recording that can be analysed by computer and checked by a cardiac technician. A typical recording lasts 24–48 hours. Patient-activated recorders capture occasional arrhythmias and are activated only when symptoms occur (Fig. 6.37).

Exercise ECG

Patients with stable angina may only develop an abnormal ECG during stress. An exercise ECG may unmask evidence of coronary artery disease. Severe ECG abnormalities, or changes that occur during minor exertion, are of prognostic significance and may prompt invasive investigation with cardiac angiography.

Chest X-ray

An enlarged heart, as judged by the cardiothoracic ratio (Fig. 7.27, p. 178), is common in valvular heart disease and heart failure. In heart failure this is often accompanied by distension of the upper lobe pulmonary veins, diffuse shadowing within the lungs due to pulmonary oedema and the finding of Kerley B lines (horizontal engorged lymphatics at the periphery of the lower lobes) (Fig. 6.38). A widened mediastinum may indicate a thoracic aneurysm.

6

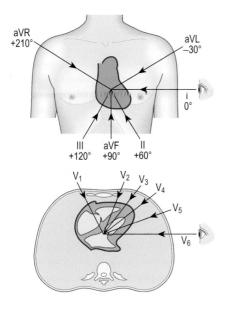

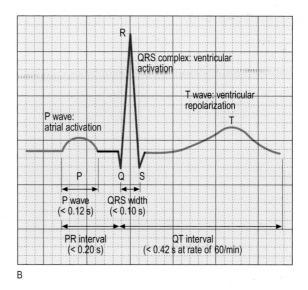

A

B

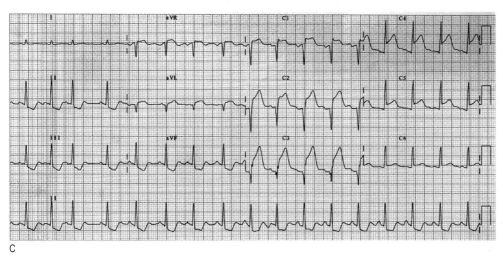

C

Fig. 6.36 Electrocardiography. (A) Diagram to show the directions from which the 12 standard leads 'look at the heart'. The transverse section is viewed from below like a CT scan. **(B)** Normal PQRST complex. **(C)** Acute anterior myocardial infarction. Note ST elevation in leads V_1–V_6 and aVL, and 'reciprocal' ST depression in leads II, III and aVF.

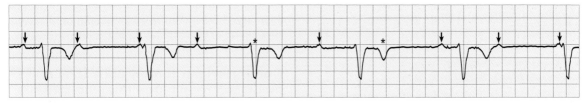

Fig. 6.37 Printout from 24-hour ambulatory ECG recording: showing complete heart block. Arrows indicate visible P waves; at times these are masked by the QRS complex or T wave (*).

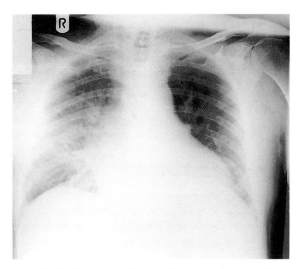

Fig. 6.38 Chest X-ray in heart failure. This shows cardiomegaly with prominent upper lobe veins extending from the hilum and patchy changes of interstitial oedema.

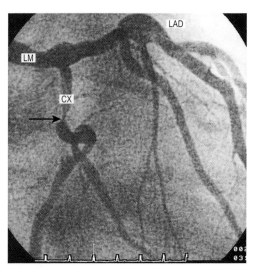

Fig. 6.40 Coronary angiography. The arrow indicates a severe discrete stenosis in the circumflex coronary artery. LM, left main; LAD, left anterior descending; CX, circumflex.

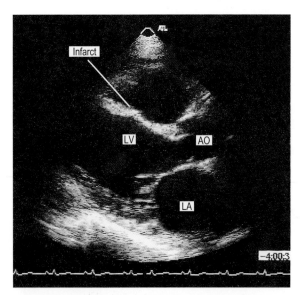

Fig. 6.39 Transthoracic echocardiogram in parasternal long axis view. This shows thinning of the interventricular septum, which has an irregular shape and bright echoes indicating fibrous scarring. This is the site of an old infarct. LA, left atrium; LV, left ventricle; AO, aortic root.

Echocardiography

Echocardiography uses high-frequency sound waves to evaluate valve abnormalities, left ventricular function and blood flow (Doppler echocardiography). Most scans are performed through the anterior wall of the chest (transthoracic) (Fig. 6.39). Transoesophageal echocardiography (TOE) requires formal sedation, but gives high resolution of posterior structures, e.g. left atrium, tricuspid valve and descending aorta.

Radionuclide studies

Technetium-99 is injected intravenously and detected using a gamma camera to assess left ventricular function. Thallium and sesta-MIBI are taken up by myocardial cells and indicate myocardial perfusion at rest and exercise.

Cardiac catheterization

A fine catheter is introduced under local anaesthetic via a peripheral artery (usually the radial or femoral) and advanced to the heart under X-ray guidance. Although measurements of intracardiac pressures and therefore estimates of valvular and cardiac function are possible, the primary application of this technique is coronary artery imaging, using contrast medium. This is performed before revascularization, by either angioplasty or bypass grafting (Fig. 6.40).

Computerized tomography (CT) and magnetic resonance imaging (MRI)

Advances in technology have overcome the problem of motion artifact caused by cardiac contraction. CT,

6.36 Key points: the heart

- Heart disease may be asymptomatic for many years prior to presentation.
- Cardiac discomfort rarely causes severe pain (with the exception of aortic dissection and rarely myocardial infarction). Mild discomfort may still signify a serious problem.
- Systemic disease may exacerbate or expose an underlying cardiac condition. Exclude co-existing anaemia, infection or thyroid disease.
- Lying flat increases venous return to the heart, and in patients with a failing left ventricle may precipitate pulmonary venous congestion and pulmonary oedema (orthopnoea).
- The most common cause of an irregularly irregular pulse is atrial fibrillation. Rarer causes include multifocal ventricular ectopic beats and supraventricular tachycardia with variable AV block.
- Always ask a patient to sit quietly for 5 minutes before taking the BP.
- Obese patients require a larger sphygmomanometer cuff for measurement of BP.
- The JVP is best examined on the patient's right side.
- If the JVP is not elevated in a patient with peripheral oedema, the cause is unlikely to be heart failure.
- While a third heart sound may be physiological in children and young adults, a fourth heart sound is always pathological.
- When listening to the heart, it is helpful to time the cardiac cycle by palpating the carotid artery with a thumb.
- Very severe aortic stenosis may not produce a murmur.
- Look for evidence of aortic outflow obstruction (aortic stenosis, hypertrophic obstructive cardiomyopathy) in any patient with unexplained syncope.
- In a patient with acute myocardial infarction listen for a third or fourth heart sound (impending heart failure), a pansystolic murmur (due to either mitral regurgitation following papillary muscle rupture, or acute ventricular septal defect) and a pericardial friction rub (pericarditis).

with its superior temporal resolution of the coronary arteries, has particular applications in excluding disease in low-risk populations, but these indications are likely to expand significantly.

MRI provides superior tissue resolution and is the imaging modality of choice for the investigation of heart muscle disease.

PERIPHERAL VASCULAR SYSTEM

ANATOMY

SYMPTOMS AND DEFINITIONS

Around 25% of patients over the age of 60 in 'developed' countries have peripheral artery disease (PAD) but only a quarter are symptomatic. In the majority the underlying pathology is atherosclerosis affecting large and medium-sized vessels. Identifying patients with peripheral arterial disease is important because:

- PAD, even if asymptomatic, is a powerful marker for premature vascular death
- the first manifestation of PAD may be a life- or limb-threatening complication, e.g. stroke, acute limb ischaemia or ruptured abdominal aortic aneurysm, if it is not recognized
- modifying vascular risk factors dramatically improves outcomes
- PAD may affect medical and surgical treatment for a range of other conditions, e.g. prescription of a β-blocker may precipitate intermittent claudication.

There are four major ways in which peripheral arterial disease patients may present:

- limb symptoms
- neurological symptoms
- abdominal symptoms
- vasospastic symptoms.

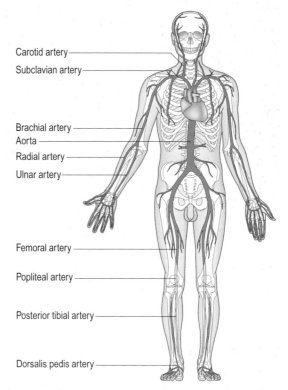

Carotid artery

Subclavian artery

Brachial artery

Aorta

Radial artery

Ulnar artery

Femoral artery

Popliteal artery

Posterior tibial artery

Dorsalis pedis artery

Fig. 6.41 The arterial system.

139

6

Limb symptoms

The legs are eight times more commonly affected than the arms because:

- arterial supply to the legs is less well developed in relation to the muscle mass
- the lower limb is more frequently affected by atherosclerosis.

There are four stages of lower limb lack of blood supply (ischaemia) (Box 6.37).

Asymptomatic ischaemia

Haemodynamically significant lower limb ischaemia is defined as an ankle:brachial pressure index of <0.8 at rest. Most of these patients are asymptomatic, either because they choose not to walk very far, or because their exercise tolerance is limited by other pathology. They have as high a risk from 'vascular' complications as those with symptoms and should be assessed and treated as if they have intermittent claudication.

Intermittent claudication (IC)

IC is pain felt in the legs on walking due to arterial insufficiency. It is the most common symptom of PAD. The pain typically occurs in the calf secondary to femoropopliteal disease but may be felt in the thigh and/or buttock if proximal (aorto-iliac) obstruction to blood flow is present. Patients describe a tightness or 'cramp-like' pain which develops after a relatively constant distance, which is shorter if walking uphill. The pain disappears completely within a few minutes of rest but recurs on walking. The claudication distance is how far patients say they can walk before pain starts. Patients often underestimate this.

Neurogenic claudication

This is leg pain on walking due to neurological and musculoskeletal disorders of the lumbar spine.

Venous claudication

This is pain due to venous outflow obstruction from the leg following extensive deep vein thrombosis.

6.37 Classification of lower limb ischaemia	
I	Asymptomatic
II	Intermittent claudication
III	Night/rest pain
IV	Tissue loss (ulceration/gangrene)

Neurogenic and venous claudication is much less common than arterial claudication, and can be distinguished on history and examination (Box 6.38).

Night/rest pain

The patient goes to bed and falls asleep but is woken 1–2 hours later by severe pain in the foot, usually in the instep. This occurs because the beneficial effects of gravity on lower limb perfusion are lost on lying down. Sleep is also associated with a reduction in heart rate, blood pressure and cardiac output. Patients often obtain relief by hanging the leg out of bed or by getting up and walking around but, when they return to bed, symptoms recur. The pain and sleep disturbance may be so debilitating that they sleep in a chair. This leads to dependent oedema, the increased interstitial tissue pressure causing further reduction in tissue perfusion and more pain.

Rest pain usually indicates severe, multi-level arterial disease. In diabetic patients with rest pain it may be difficult to differentiate between an arterial cause and diabetic neuropathy since both may be worse at night. Neuropathic pain is not, however, usually confined to the foot, is associated with burning and tingling, is not relieved by dependency and is associated with pain or uncomfortable sensations (dysaesthesia) sometimes described as burning, tingling or numbness. Many patients cannot even bear the pressure of bedclothes on their feet.

Tissue loss (ulceration and/or gangrene)

In patients with critical limb ischaemia, trivial injuries do not heal, allowing bacteria to enter, leading to gangrene and/or ulceration. Without revascularization, the ischaemia rapidly progresses, leading to amputation and/or death.

Chronic lower limb ischaemia

Ischaemic changes may be present, including absence of body hair on the legs, dorsum of the feet and toes. Other clinical features of arterial claudication are described in Box 6.38. In many patients the pedal pulses are absent or diminished. The presence of pedal pulses does not, however, exclude significant lower limb PAD. If the history is convincing, ask the patient to walk until the onset of pain. Recheck the pulses because, if the patient's symptoms are vascular in origin, the pulses may disappear. Patients with critical limb ischaemia (rest pain, tissue loss) typically have an ankle blood pressure <50mmHg and a positive Buerger's test.

Acute limb ischaemia

The features of acute limb ischaemia are known as the 6 Ps (Box 6.39). Of these, loss of motor (ability to wiggle the toes/fingers) and/or sensory function (light touch over the forefoot/dorsum of the hand) are the most important and indicate severe nerve ischaemia. A limb

6.38 The clinical features of arterial, neurogenic and venous claudication

	Arterial	Neurogenic	Venous
Pathology	Stenosis or occlusion of major lower limb arteries	Lumbar nerve root or cauda equina compression (spinal stenosis)	Obstruction to the venous outflow of the leg due to iliofemoral venous occlusion
Site of pain	Muscles, usually the calf but may involve thigh and buttocks	Ill-defined. Whole leg. May be associated with numbness and tingling	Whole leg. 'Bursting' in nature
Laterality	Unilateral if femoropopliteal, and bilateral if aorto-iliac disease	Often bilateral	Nearly always unilateral
Onset	Gradual after walking the 'claudication distance'	Often immediate on walking or standing up	Gradual, from the moment walking starts
Relieving features	On stopping walking, the pain disappears completely in 1–2 minutes	Bending forwards and stopping walking. May sit down for full relief	Leg elevation
Colour	Normal or pale	Normal	Cyanosed. Often visible varicose veins
Temperature	Normal or cool	Normal	Normal or increased
Oedema	Absent	Absent	Always present
Pulses	Reduced or absent	Normal	Present but may be difficult to feel owing to oedema
Straight leg raising	Normal	May be limited	Normal

with these features will become irreversibly damaged unless the circulation is restored within a few hours. Muscle tenderness is a grave sign indicating impending muscle infarction. The common causes of acute limb ischaemia are:

- embolic: usually cardiac in origin in association with atrial fibrillation
- thrombotic: with occlusion of a narrowed atherosclerotic arterial segment
- compartment syndrome: there is increased pressure in a fascial compartment, often following trauma which compromises the perfusion and viability of the compartmental structures (Box 6.40).

Acute arterial occlusion is associated with intense spasm in the arterial tree distal to the blockage and the limb appears 'marble white'. Over a few hours, the spasm relaxes and the skin microcirculation fills with deoxygenated blood, leading to mottling which is light blue or purple, has a fine reticular pattern and blanches on pressure. As ischaemia progresses, blood coalescing in the skin produces a coarser pattern which is dark purple, almost black, and does not blanch. In the final stage large patches of fixed staining lead to blistering and liquefaction. Fixed mottling of an anaesthetic, paralysed limb, in association with muscle rigidity and turgor, indicates irreversible ischaemia; amputation is the only option (Fig. 6.42).

6.39 Signs of acute limb ischaemia

Soft signs

- **P**ulseless
- **P**allor
- **P**erishing cold

Hard signs (indicating a threatened limb)

- **P**araesthesia
- **P**aralysis
- **P**ain on squeezing muscle

Neurological symptoms

A stroke is a focal central neurological deficit of vascular cause. Approximately 80% of strokes are ischaemic rather than haemorrhagic. Transient ischaemic attack (TIA) describes a stroke in which symptoms resolve within 24 hours. The term stroke is reserved for those events in which symptoms last for more than 24 hours.

Carotid artery territory

Up to half of all strokes and TIAs are due to embolism from an atheromatous plaque at the common carotid bifurcation. A bruit may arise from stenosis in the external or internal carotid arteries but is an unreliable

6.40 Acute limb ischaemia: embolus vs thrombosis in situ

	Embolus	Thrombosis
Onset and severity	Acute (seconds or minutes), ischaemia profound (no pre-existing collaterals)	Insidious (hours or days), ischaemia less severe (pre-existing collaterals)
Embolic source	Present (usually atrial fibrillation)	Absent
Previous claudication	Absent	Present
Pulses in contralateral leg	Present	Often absent
Diagnosis	Clinical	Angiography
Treatment	Embolectomy and anticoagulation	Medical, bypass surgery, thrombolysis

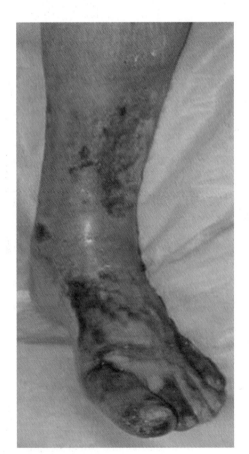

Fig. 6.42 Gangrene of the foot.

sign of the presence or severity of internal carotid artery stenosis. There may be so little blood flow through a critical internal carotid artery stenosis that no bruit is audible. The clinical features vary according to the cerebral area involved but can include motor deficit, visual field defect, e.g. homonymous hemianopia (Fig. 12.3, p. 309), or difficulty with speech (dysphasia, p. 276).

Vertebrobasilar artery territory

TIAs and strokes in this territory cause giddiness, collapse with or without loss of consciousness, transient occipital blindness or complete loss of vision in both eyes. Subclavian artery stenosis or occlusion proximal to the origin of the vertebral artery may cause vertebrobasilar symptoms as part of the 'subclavian steal' syndrome. This happens when the arm is exercised. The increased blood supply requirement in the arm is met by blood travelling up the carotid arteries and then, via the circle of Willis, down the vertebral artery into the arm, so 'stealing' blood from the posterior cerebral circulation. Signs of this include asymmetry of the pulses and blood pressure in the arms, sometimes with a bruit over the subclavian artery in the supraclavicular fossa.

Abdominal symptoms

Visceral ischaemia

Two of the three major visceral arteries (coeliac axis, superior and inferior mesenteric arteries) must be critically stenosed or occluded before a patient develops symptoms and signs of chronic mesenteric arterial insufficiency because of the rich collateral circulation in the gut. Severe central abdominal pain (mesenteric angina) typically develops 10–15 minutes after eating. The patient is scared of eating and significant weight loss is a universal finding. Diarrhoea may be a feature and visceral ischaemia may mimic a whole range of gastrointestinal pathologies. The patient may have had numerous investigations, even laparotomy, before the clinical diagnosis is made and confirmed by angiography.

Acute mesenteric ischaemia is a surgical emergency. The patient presents with severe abdominal pain, shock, bloody diarrhoea and profound metabolic acidosis. Rarely, renal angle pain occurs from renal infarction or ischaemia, and is associated with microscopic or macroscopic haematuria.

Abdominal aortic aneurysm (AAA)

AAA is an abnormal dilatation of the aorta (Fig. 6.43). It is present in 5% of men aged >65 years and is three times more common in men than women. Smoking and hypertension further increase these figures. Most patients are asymptomatic until the aneurysm ruptures, although they may present with abdominal and/or back pain or an awareness of abdominal pulsation.

The aortic bifurcation is at the level of the umbilicus, so feel in the epigastrium for a palpable AAA. A pulsatile mass below the umbilicus suggests an iliac aneurysm. In thin patients a tortuous but normal-diameter aorta can feel aneurysmal. If the abdominal girth exceeds 96–102 cm, even experts can miss a large AAA. Ultrasound studies show that clinical examination is unreliable in establishing the presence or size of an AAA. Assessment whether or not pulsation is expansile is inaccurate and should be avoided. If you are in any doubt, obtain an ultrasound scan.

A ruptured AAA can be difficult to diagnose because many patients do not have the classical features of abdominal and/or back pain, pulsatile abdominal mass and hypotension. The most common misdiagnosis is renal colic (a man, >60 years, presenting with 'renal colic' has a ruptured AAA until proved otherwise).

Embolism of atheromatous material (atheroembolism) and associated platelet debris and thrombotic material may arise from an AAA and cause the 'blue toe syndrome', characterized by purple discoloration of the toes and forefoot with a full set of pedal pulses.

VASOSPASTIC SYMPTOMS

Raynaud's phenomenon is digital ischaemia induced by cold and emotion and has three phases (Fig. 6.44):

- pallor: due to digital artery spasm and/or obstruction
- cyanosis: due to deoxygenation of static venous blood (this phase may be absent)
- redness: due to reactive hyperaemia.

Raynaud's phenomenon may be primary (Raynaud's disease) and due to idiopathic digital artery vasospasm, or secondary (Raynaud's syndrome) (Box 6.41).

Assume that patients >40 years old presenting with unilateral Raynaud's phenomenon have underlying PAD unless proven otherwise, especially if they have risk factors.

THE HISTORY

Ask about risk factors for atheroma (smoking, hypercholesterolaemia, hypertension, diabetes mellitus) and any family history of premature arterial disease. Enquire specifically about diabetes because it is associated with the early development of widespread atheroma which progresses rapidly.

The impact of claudication relates to the patient's age and lifestyle. A postman/postwoman who can walk only 400 m has a serious problem, but an elderly person who simply wants to cross the road to the shops may cope well. Rather than focusing upon absolute

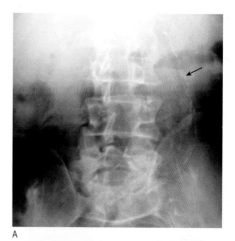

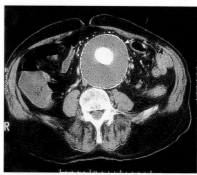

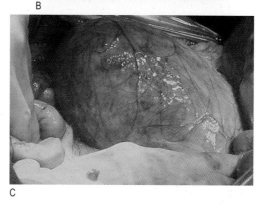

Fig. 6.43 Abdominal aortic aneurysm. (A) Abdominal X-ray showing calcification (arrow). **(B)** CT scan of the abdomen showing an AAA (arrow). **(C)** At laparotomy the aorta is seen to be grossly and irregularly dilated.

distances, ask specific questions like:

- Can you walk to the clinic from the bus stop or car park without stopping?
- Can you do your own shopping?
- What can't you do because of the pain?

Ask about the patient's other medical conditions. There is little point in subjecting patients with intermittent claudication to the risks of vascular surgery, only to find that they are then equally limited by osteoarthritis of the hip, angina or severe breathlessness.

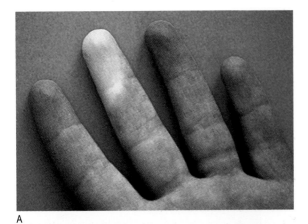

A

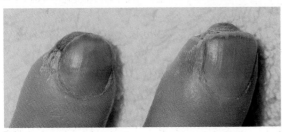

B

Fig. 6.44 Raynaud's syndrome. (A) The acute phase, showing severe blanching of the tip of one finger. **(B)** Primary Raynaud's syndrome occasionally progresses to finger-tip ulceration or even gangrene.

 6.41 Diseases associated with secondary Raynaud's syndrome

- Connective tissue syndromes, e.g. systemic sclerosis, CREST (Calcinosis, Raynaud's phenomenon, oEsophageal dysfunction, Sclerodactyly, Telangiectasia) and SLE
- Atherosclerosis/embolism from proximal source, e.g. subclavian artery aneurysm
- Drug-related, e.g. nicotine, β-blockers, ergot
- Thoracic outlet syndrome
- Malignancy
- Hyperviscosity syndromes, e.g. Waldenström's macroglobulinaemia, polycythaemia
- Vibration-induced disorders (power tools)
- Cold agglutinin disorders

Male patients with buttock (gluteal) claudication due to internal iliac disease invariably cannot achieve or maintain an erection. Enquire into sexual activity (p. 12), as many patients are extremely concerned by this symptom yet too embarrassed to mention it.

THE PHYSICAL EXAMINATION

Follow the routine described for the heart, looking for evidence of anaemia or cyanosis, signs of heart failure,

6.42 Signs suggesting vascular disease

SIGN	IMPLICATION
Hands and arms	
Tobacco stains	Smoking
Purple discoloration of the finger tips	Atheroembolism from a proximal subclavian aneurysm
Pits and healed scars in the finger pulps	Secondary Raynaud's syndrome
Calcinosis and visible nail-fold capillary loops	Systemic sclerosis and CREST
Wasting of the small muscles of the hand	Thoracic outlet syndrome
Face and neck	
Corneal arcus and xanthelasma	Hypercholesterolaemia
Horner's syndrome	Carotid artery dissection or aneurysm
Hoarseness of the voice and 'bovine' cough	Recurrent laryngeal nerve palsy from a thoracic aortic aneurysm
Prominent veins in the neck, shoulder and anterior chest	Axillary/subclavian vein occlusion
Abdomen	
Epigastric/umbilical pulsation	Aorto-iliac aneurysm
Mottling of the abdomen	Ruptured AAA or saddle embolism occluding aortic bifurcation
Evidence of weight loss	Visceral ischaemia

and direct or indirect evidence of vascular disease (Box 6.42). Then perform a detailed examination of the arterial pulses. Abnormally prominent pulsation in the neck of an elderly person is rarely of clinical significance and is normally caused by tortuous arteries rather than a carotid aneurysm or carotid body tumour. However, if in any doubt, arrange for a duplex ultrasound scan.

Record individual pulses as:

- normal   +
- reduced   ±
- absent   −
- aneurysmal   + +

Examination of pulses

If you are in any doubt about whose pulse you are feeling, palpate your own pulse at the same time. If it is not synchronous with yours, it is the patient's.

Buerger's test

With the patient lying supine, stand at the foot of the bed. Raise the patient's feet and support the legs at 45° to the horizontal for 2–3 minutes.

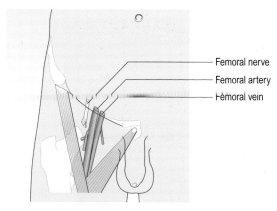

Fig. 6.45 Femoral triangle: vessels and nerves.

Then ask the patient to sit up and hang his or her legs over the edge of the bed. Watch the patient's feet for another 2–3 minutes. Pallor on elevation (with emptying or 'guttering' of the superficial veins), followed by reactive hyperaemia (rubor) on dependency, is a positive test and implies significant PAD.

Examination sequence

Peripheral vascular system

- Start at the patient's head and work down the body, using the sequence and principles of inspection, palpation and auscultation for each area.

The arms

- Examine the radial, brachial and carotid pulses (Fig. 6.13).
- Measure the BP in both arms. Many patients with PAD have asymptomatic subclavian artery disease. A difference of up to 10 mmHg in systolic pressure between the two arms is normal. If the discrepancy is greater than this, then the higher value is the true pressure.

The abdomen

- Look for obvious pulsation.
- Palpate and listen over the abdominal aorta. If the aorta is easily palpable, consider the possibility of an AAA. If in any doubt, arrange a duplex ultrasound scan.

The legs

- Inspect and feel the legs and feet for changes of ischaemia, including temperature and colour changes.
- Note scars from previous vascular or non-vascular surgery and the position, margin, depth and colour of any ulceration.
- Look specifically between the toes and at the heels for ischaemic changes.

Femoral pulse (Figs 6.45 and 6.46A)

- Ask the patient to lie down and explain what you are going to do.
- With your fingers extended, place the pads of your index and middle fingers over the femoral artery. It can be difficult to feel in the obese.
- Check for radiofemoral delay (p. 119).

- Listen for bruits over both femoral arteries, using the diaphragm of your stethoscope.

Popliteal pulse (Fig. 6.46B)

- Ask the patient to lie on a firm comfortable surface and to relax.
- Flex the patient's knee to 30°,
- With your thumbs in front of the knee and your fingers behind, press firmly in the midline over the popliteal artery. It is sometimes difficult to feel.
- Slide your fingers 2–3 cm below the knee crease and try to compress the artery against the back of the tibia as it passes under the soleal arch.
- If the popliteal artery is especially easy to feel, consider the possibility of an aneurysm.

Posterior tibial pulse (Fig. 6.46C)

- Feel 2 cm below and 2 cm behind the medial malleolus, using the pads of your index, middle and ring fingers.

Dorsalis pedis pulse (Fig 6.46D)

- Using the pads of your index, middle and ring fingers, feel in the middle of the dorsum of the foot just lateral to the tendon of extensor hallucis longus.
- Perform Buerger's test.

INVESTIGATIONS IN PERIPHERAL VASCULAR DISEASE

Ankle:brachial pressure index (ABPI)

Use a hand-held Doppler and a sphygmomanometer. The probe is held in turn over the three pedal arteries (posterior tibial, dorsalis pedis, perforating peroneal) while inflating a blood pressure cuff round the ankle. The pressure at which the Doppler signal disappears is the systolic pressure in that artery as it passes under the cuff. The ratio of the highest pedal artery pressure to the highest brachial artery pressure is the ABPI.

Normally the ABPI is >1.0 when the patient is supine. Typical values in claudication and critical limb ischaemia are <0.8 and <0.4 respectively. Absolute values may be less informative than the trend over time.

Patients with severe lower limb ischaemia, particularly those with diabetes mellitus, may have incompressible, calcified crural arteries. This produces falsely elevated pedal pressures and ABPI. In such circumstances, an alternative is to use a Doppler ultrasound probe to detect (isonate) the artery with the hand-held Doppler while elevating the foot. The Doppler signal disappears at a height above the bed (in cm) that is approximately equal to the perfusion pressure in mmHg.

Other tests

Choose further tests to provide the most information at the least risk to the patient and at least expense. In most situations ultrasound techniques have replaced angiography (Box 6.44).

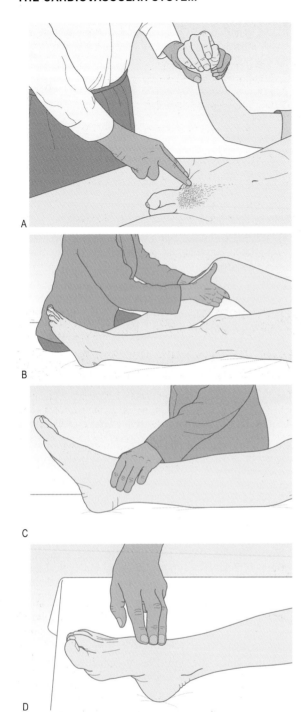

Fig. 6.46 Examination of the femoral, popliteal, posterior tibial and dorsalis pedis arteries. (A) Examine the femoral artery, while simultaneously checking for radiofemoral delay. **(B)** Feel the popliteal artery with the finger tips, having curled both hands into the popliteal fossa. **(C)** Examination of the posterior tibial artery. **(D)** Examination of the dorsalis pedis artery.

1. Feel the radial pulse for irregularity, e.g. atrial fibrillation.
2. Look for evidence of tobacco staining on fingers.
3. Measure the blood pressure in both arms — unequal in aortic dissection.
4. Listen to the heart — early diastolic murmur may indicate aortic regurgitation due to aortic dissection.
5. Feel the abdomen for pulsation of abdominal aortic aneurysm.
6. Auscultate the abdomen for bruits of aorto-iliac disease.
7. Look at the feet for discoloration: marbled in complete acute ischaemia due to embolus; fine reticular blanching/mottling in early stages; coarse, more fixed mottling in late stages.
8. Palpate the femoral and popliteal pulses and feel for popliteal aneurysms.
9. Squeeze the calves — tenderness suggests muscle infarction.
10. Compare the warmth of both feet with the back of your hand.
11. Palpate for the dorsalis pedis and posterior tibial pulses in both feet.
12. Ask the patient to wiggle the toes, and test fine sensation — both motor and sensory function are absent in limb-threatening ischaemia.
13. If acute ischaemia is suspected, refer urgently to a vascular surgeon.

6.44 Investigations in peripheral arterial disease

Investigation	Indication/Comment
Blood tests	
FBC and ESR	Anaemia unmasking symptoms and connective tissue disease
U & E	Renal function
Blood glucose	Hypertension more common in diabetes
Serology	Connective tissue disease
Microbiology	
Bacteriology	Swab base of ulcer
Radiology	
Doppler ultrasound	Ankle pressure, ABPI, pulse waveform analysis
B-mode ultrasound	AAA, popliteal artery aneurysm
Duplex ultrasound	Carotid artery stenosis, vein bypass graft surveillance
CT	AAA, detection of cerebral infarct/haemorrhage
MRI	Arteriovenous malformations, carotid artery stenosis
Angiography	Acute and chronic limb ischaemia, carotid artery stenosis

6.45 Key points: the peripheral arterial system

- Widespread PAD may be asymptomatic for years and then present with life-threatening complications.
- Acute limb ischaemia and chronic arterial insufficiency causing rest pain and/or tissue loss needs urgent assessment.
- Use the ABPI to assess the severity of chronic lower limb ischaemia.
- Patients with hemispheric or ocular TIAs need urgent carotid ultrasound to detect significant carotid stenosis.
- In a large patient, even a sizeable (>6 cm diameter) AAA may be undetectable clinically.
- AAA causes a pulsatile mass in the epigastrium. A pulsatile mass below the umbilicus is likely to be an iliac artery aneurysm.
- Actively exclude AAA as a cause of abdominal pain, especially in men >65 years.
- 'Renal colic' presenting for the first time in a patient >60 yrs is a ruptured AAA until proven otherwise.
- Unilateral Raynaud's phenomenon in patients >40 yrs is often associated with PAD.
- Subclavian artery disease may present with apparent vertebrobasilar insufficiency. A systolic BP difference >15 mmHg between the arms suggests the diagnosis.
- Rest pain of arterial origin in diabetic patients may be misdiagnosed as the pain of diabetic neuropathy.
- Visceral ischaemia is a frequently overlooked cause of 'unexplained' abdominal pain and weight loss. Consider the diagnosis, especially in patients who have had multiple negative gastrointestinal investigations.
- An aneurysmal popliteal artery suggests widespread vascular disease.
- If one popliteal artery is unexpectedly easy to palpate, consider abdominal ultrasonography to exclude an AAA.

6

VENOUS SYSTEM

ANATOMY

The venous system is a low-pressure system. Venous blood drains from the head and neck, assisted by gravity when a person is upright. The lower limbs cannot drain passively and the veins here are divided into superficial and deep veins, separated by one-way valves and connected by perforating veins which also have valves. Muscle contraction during normal activities 'massages' the blood into the deep veins and helps to drive it towards the heart. Backward (retrograde) flow is prevented by the valves.

- In the leg, the long (great) saphenous vein passes anterior to the medial malleolus at the ankle, up the medial aspect of the calf to behind the knee, then up the medial aspect of the thigh to join the common femoral vein in the groin at the saphenofemoral junction (Fig. 6.47)
- The short (lesser) saphenous vein passes behind the lateral malleolus at the ankle and up the posterior aspect of the calf. It commonly joins the popliteal vein at the saphenopopliteal junction, which usually lies 2 cm above the posterior knee crease. There are many intercommunications between the long and short saphenous systems, and the venous anatomy of the leg is highly variable.

Venous disease is most common in the legs and presents in one of four ways:

- varicose veins
- superficial thrombosis
- deep vein thrombosis
- chronic venous insufficiency and ulceration.

SYMPTOMS AND DEFINITIONS

The severity of symptoms and signs may bear little relationship to the gravity of the underlying pathology and the physical signs. Life-threatening deep vein thrombosis may be asymptomatic, while apparently trivial varicose veins may be associated with significant complaints.

There are four cardinal symptoms of lower limb venous disease:

- pain
- swelling
- discoloration
- ulceration.

Pain

Patients with uncomplicated varicose veins (dilated, tortuous veins from incompetent valves in the vein) may have an aching discomfort in the leg, itching and a feeling of swelling. Symptoms are aggravated by prolonged standing and towards the end of the day. The pain of established deep vein thrombosis is deep-seated and associated with swelling below the level of obstruction. Superficial venous thrombophlebitis produces a red, painful area overlying the vein involved. Varicose ulceration may be painless; if it is painful, this may be relieved by limb elevation.

Swelling

Swelling (or oedema) may be associated with varicose veins, deep venous reflux and deep vein thrombosis.

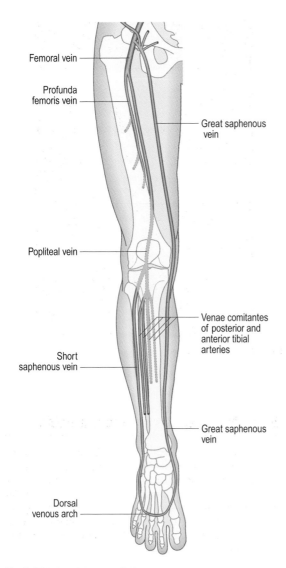

Femoral vein

Profunda
femoris vein

Great saphenous
vein

Popliteal vein

Venae comitantes
of posterior and
anterior tibial
arteries

Short
saphenous vein

Great saphenous
vein

Dorsal
venous arch

Fig. 6.47 Veins of the lower limb.

Discoloration

Chronic venous insufficiency causes pigmentation due to deposition of haemosiderin (from breakdown of extravasated blood) in the skin, leading to lipodermatosclerosis. This varies in colour from deep blue/black to purple or bright red. It affects the medial aspect of the lower third of the leg, but may be lateral if superficial reflux predominates in the short saphenous veins.

Ulceration

Venous ulceration is usually seen above the medial malleolus. It only occurs with severe venous disease

6.46 Features of deep vein thrombosis of the lower limb

Clinical feature	Non-occlusive thrombus	Occlusive thrombus
Pain	Often absent	Usually present
Calf tenderness	Often absent	Usually present
Swelling	Absent	Present
Temperature	Normal or slightly increased	Increased
Superficial veins	Normal	Distended
Pulmonary embolism	High risk	Low risk

6.47 Risk factors for deep vein thrombosis

- Recent bed rest or operations (especially to the leg, pelvis or abdomen)
- Recent travel, especially long flights
- Previous trauma to the leg, especially long bone fractures, plaster of Paris splintage and immobilization
- Pregnancy or features to suggest pelvic disease
- Malignant disease
- Previous deep vein thrombosis
- Family history of thrombosis
- Recent central venous catheterization, injection of drugs, etc.

and patients may not seek medical attention for years. Venous ulceration is always associated with lipodermatosclerosis.

Deep vein thrombosis (DVT)

The leg

The clinical features of DVT depend upon its site, extent and whether it is occlusive or not (Box 6.46). So-called 'classical' features of DVT are of little value and relate to well-established occlusive thrombus. Most patients who die from pulmonary embolus have non-occlusive thrombosis and the leg is normal on clinical examination. Non-occlusive thrombus poses the greatest threat of pulmonary embolus, as the clot lies within a flowing stream of venous blood, is more likely to propagate, and has not yet induced an inflammatory response in the vein wall to anchor it in place. Risk factors for DVT are listed in Box 6.47.

The arm

DVT can occur as a primary event due to repetitive trauma of the axillary or subclavian vein, e.g. thoracic outlet

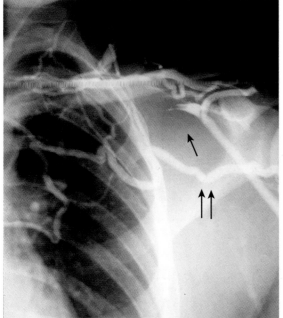

A

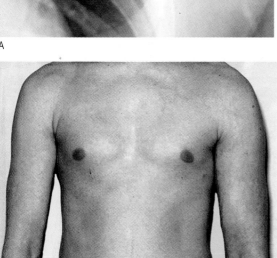

B

Fig. 6.48 Axillary vein thrombosis. (A) Angiogram. Single arrow shows site of thrombosis. Double arrows show dilated collateral vessels. **(B)** Clinical appearance with swollen left arm and dilated superficial veins.

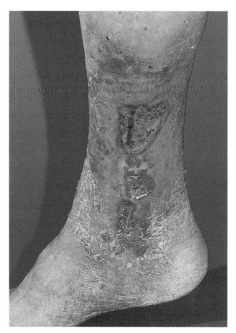

Fig. 6.49 Venous ulceration.

Superficial venous thrombophlebitis

Inflammation of superficial veins is associated with intraluminal, usually sterile, thrombosis. It affects up to 10% of patients with severe varicose veins and is more common during pregnancy. Recurrent superficial thrombophlebitis may be associated with underlying malignancy. Superficial venous thrombophlebitis at, or near, the saphenofemoral junction may be associated with pulmonary embolism.

Chronic venous insufficiency

This produces skin changes in the lower leg (varicose eczema, lipodermatosclerosis, ulceration) due to sustained venous hypertension, which in turn is due to reflux (90%) and/or obstruction (10%) in the superficial and/or deep veins.

Chronic leg ulceration

This is caused by venous and/or arterial disease in developed countries (Fig. 6.49). Other causes include pyoderma gangrenosum, syphilis, tuberculosis, leprosy, sickle cell disease and tropical conditions; 1 in 5 patients with a venous ulcer will have significant arterial disease (Box 6.48). Bandaging for a leg ulcer is contraindicated unless there is documented evidence of adequate arterial circulation. Do this by feeling the pulses or by measuring the ABPI.

syndrome. This may follow strenuous unaccustomed use of the arm. It is more common in body-builders, perhaps because of associated anabolic steroid use and also in injecting drug users. It is a complication of indwelling catheters in the subclavian vein. Symptoms are arm swelling and discomfort, exacerbated by activity, especially when holding the arm overhead.

The arm is swollen and the skin is cyanosed and mottled, especially when dependent. Look for superficial distended veins (acting as collaterals) in the upper arm, over the shoulder region and on the anterior chest wall (Fig. 6.48).

6.48 Clinical features of venous and arterial ulceration

Clinical feature	Venous ulceration	Arterial ulceration
Age	Develops at age 40–45 but may not present for years; multiple recurrences common	First presents in over-60s
Sex	More common in women	More common in men
Past medical history	DVT or suggestive of occult DVT, i.e. leg swelling after childbirth, hip/knee replacement or long bone fracture	Peripheral arterial disease, cardio- and cerebrovascular disease
Risk factors	Thrombophilia, family history, previous DVT	Smoking, diabetes, hypercholesterolaemia and hypertension
Pain	One-third have pain (not usually severe), improves with elevating the leg	Severe pain, except in diabetics with neuropathy; improves on dependency
Site	Gaiter areas; usually medial to long saphenous vein; 20% are lateral to short saphenous vein	Pressure areas (malleoli, heel, 5th metatarsal base, metatarsal heads and toes)
Margin	Irregular, often with neo-epithelium (appears whiter than mature skin)	Regular, indolent, 'punched-out'
Base	Often pink and granulating under green slough	Sloughy (green) or necrotic (black), with no granulation
Surrounding skin	Lipodermatosclerosis always present	No venous skin changes
Veins	Full and usually varicose	Empty with 'guttering' on elevation
Swelling (oedema)	Usually present	Absent
Temperature	Warm	Cold
Pulses	Present, but may be difficult to feel	Absent

THE PHYSICAL EXAMINATION

Examination sequence

Venous system

- Examine the legs with the patient standing and then lying supine.
- Expose the patient's limbs. Inspect the skin for colour changes, swelling and superficial venous dilatation and tortuosity.
- Feel for any differences in temperature.
- Press with your finger tip above the ankle medially for a few seconds (gently, as this can be painful; do not do this near an ulcer) and then see if your finger has left a pit (pitting oedema).
- If the leg is grossly swollen, press at a higher level to establish how far oedema extends.
- If you find oedema, check the JVP (p. 125). If the JVP is raised, this suggests that cardiac disease or pulmonary hypertension is contributing.
- Elevate the limb to about 15° above the horizontal and note the rate of venous emptying.
- If appropriate, perform the Trendelenburg test to detect saphenofemoral junction regurgitation.

The Trendelenburg test

This determines the pattern of venous regurgitation in the leg.

Examination sequence

- Ask the patient to sit on the edge of the examination couch.
- Elevate the limb as far as is comfortable for the patient and empty the superficial veins by 'milking' the leg.
- With the patient's leg still elevated, press with your thumb over the saphenofemoral junction (2–3 cm below and 2–3 cm lateral to the pubic tubercle). A high thigh tourniquet can be used instead of digital pressure.
- Ask the patient to stand while you maintain pressure over the saphenofemoral junction.
- If saphenofemoral junction regurgitation is present, the patient's varicose veins will not fill until your digital pressure, or the tourniquet, is removed.

OSCEs 6.49 **Examine this patient with tiredness and low blood pressure**

1. Look for signs of dehydration, e.g. prolonged diarrhoea.
2. Look for pigmentation in skin creases, scars and buccal mucosa (Addison's disease).
3. Look for signs of blood loss — pallor and postural hypotension.
4. Look for signs of iron deficiency — angular stomatitis, koilonychia.
5. Look for vitiligo (autoimmune disorders).
6. Feel pulse for bradycardia (heart block, Stokes–Adams attack) or tachycardia (supraventricular tachycardia, ventricular tachycardia) and irregularity (atrial fibrillation).
7. Listen to heart — pansystolic murmur (post-myocardial infarction ventricular septal defect or mitral regurgitation), pericardial friction rub (pericarditis).

6.50 **Key points: the venous system**

- The cardinal symptoms of venous disease are pain or discomfort, swelling of the limb and discoloration with ulceration.
- Life-threatening DVT may be asymptomatic.
- Leg ulceration in the elderly is often multifactorial. The most common single underlying cause is chronic venous insufficiency.
- Superficial thrombophlebitis, especially in the absence of varicose veins and where it is migratory in character, often signifies underlying malignancy.
- Around 1 in 5 patients with a venous ulcer has significant arterial disease. Always confirm that pedal pulses are present and the ABPI is normal before prescribing graduated compression bandaging.
- The red discoloration in lipodermatosclerosis may be mistaken for soft tissue infection, especially if there is venous ulceration. Soft tissue infection, unlike lipodermatosclerosis, is associated with the other features of inflammation.

6

Graham Devereux
Graham Douglas

The respiratory system

7

RESPIRATORY EXAMINATION

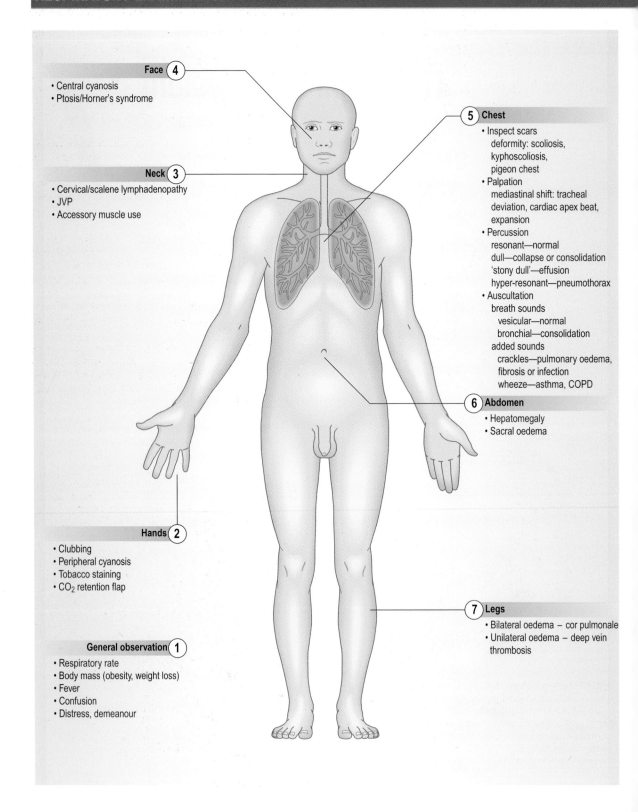

Face (4)
- Central cyanosis
- Ptosis/Horner's syndrome

Neck (3)
- Cervical/scalene lymphadenopathy
- JVP
- Accessory muscle use

(5) **Chest**
- Inspect scars
  deformity: scoliosis,
  kyphoscoliosis,
  pigeon chest
- Palpation
  mediastinal shift: tracheal
  deviation, cardiac apex beat,
  expansion
- Percussion
  resonant—normal
  dull—collapse or consolidation
  'stony dull'—effusion
  hyper-resonant—pneumothorax
- Auscultation
  breath sounds
    vesicular—normal
    bronchial—consolidation
  added sounds
    crackles—pulmonary oedema,
    fibrosis or infection
    wheeze—asthma, COPD

(6) **Abdomen**
- Hepatomegaly
- Sacral oedema

Hands (2)
- Clubbing
- Peripheral cyanosis
- Tobacco staining
- CO_2 retention flap

(7) **Legs**
- Bilateral oedema – cor pulmonale
- Unilateral oedema – deep vein
  thrombosis

General observation (1)
- Respiratory rate
- Body mass (obesity, weight loss)
- Fever
- Confusion
- Distress, demeanour

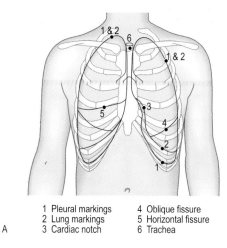

1 Pleural markings   4 Oblique fissure
2 Lung markings   5 Horizontal fissure
3 Cardiac notch   6 Trachea

A

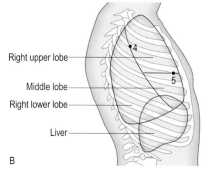

Right upper lobe

Middle lobe

Right lower lobe

Liver

B

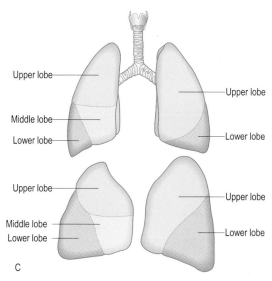

Upper lobe — — Upper lobe

Middle lobe

Lower lobe — — Lower lobe

Upper lobe — — Upper lobe

Middle lobe
Lower lobe — — Lower lobe

C

Fig. 7.1 Surface anatomy of the thorax. (A) Surface markings of the lungs and pleura, trachea and bronchi. The trachea is normally central. The bifurcation of the trachea corresponds on the anterior chest wall with the sternal angle, the transverse bony ridge at the junction of the sternum and manubrium sternum. Count the ribs downwards from the second costal cartilage at the level of the sternal angle. **(B)** Surface markings of the right lung and underlying viscera. **(C)** Lobes of the lungs: anterior view (upper) and lateral view (lower).

ANATOMY

The respiratory system consists of the upper airway from the nose and mouth, larynx, trachea and two lungs. The left lung is smaller than the right lung, containing approximately 45% of the surface area available for gas exchange, because of the presence of the heart within the left side of the chest. The right lung is made up of three lobes (upper, middle and lower) and the left of two lobes (upper and lower) (Fig. 7.1).

Within the lungs the airways (bronchi) transport air with oxygen to the alveoli on inspiration and carry waste gases, e.g. carbon dioxide, away on expiration. The acinus is the gas exchange unit of the lung and consists of branching respiratory bronchioles leading to clusters of alveoli (Fig. 7.2). Alveoli are tiny air sacs lined by flattened epithelial cells (type I pneumocytes) and covered in capillaries where gas exchange occurs. Because the alveoli and capillaries have extremely thin walls and come into very close contact (the alveolar–capillary membrane), carbon dioxide and oxygen readily diffuse between them. There are approximately 300 million alveoli in each lung with a total surface area for gas exchange of 40–80 m^2.

The lung has two blood supplies: the bronchial arteries, which arise from the aorta and supply oxygenated blood to the bronchial walls, and the pulmonary arteries, which circulate deoxygenated blood to the capillaries surrounding the alveoli.

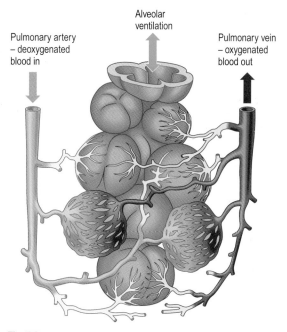

Fig. 7.2 The acinus: the basic gas exchange unit of the lung.

7

7

SYMPTOMS AND DEFINITIONS

The mode of onset, duration, progression and predominance of symptoms vary according to the cause.

Cough

Cough is a forced expulsive manœuvre against an initially closed glottis, causing a characteristic sound. Acute cough is defined as lasting less than 3 weeks, chronic cough more than 8 weeks. The most common cause of acute cough in primary care is acute viral upper respiratory tract infection. Usually acute cough is self-limiting and benign, but it may occur in more serious conditions, which are suggested by 'red flag' symptoms (Box 7.1). Causes of cough are listed in Box 7.2.

Sound

Patients with severe asthma or chronic obstructive pulmonary disease (COPD) have prolonged wheezy coughing. Sometimes the raised intrathoracic pressure impairs venous return to the heart, reducing cardiac

7.1 'Red flag' symptoms associated with cough that should prompt a chest X-ray

- Haemoptysis
- Breathlessness
- Fever
- Chest pain
- Weight loss

7.2 Causes of cough

	Normal chest X-ray	Abnormal chest X-ray
Acute cough (<3 weeks)	Viral respiratory tract infection Bacterial infection (acute bronchitis) Inhaled foreign body Inhalation of irritant dusts/fumes	Pneumonia Inhaled foreign body Acute extrinsic allergic alveolitis
Chronic cough (>8 weeks)	GORD Asthma Postviral bronchial hyper-reactivity Rhinitis/sinusitis Cigarette smoking Drugs, especially ACE inhibitors Irritant dusts/fumes	Lung tumour Tuberculosis Interstitial lung disease Bronchiectasis

output and causing cough syncope. A feeble non-explosive 'bovine' cough with hoarseness suggests lung cancer invading the left recurrent laryngeal nerve and causing paralysis of the left vocal cord, but may occur with respiratory muscle weakness due to neuromuscular disorders. Coughs from laryngeal inflammation, infection and tumour are harsh, barking or painful and associated with hoarseness and the rasping or croaking inspiratory sound of stridor.

A moist cough suggests secretions in the upper and larger airways from bronchial infection and bronchiectasis. A persistent moist 'smoker's cough' first thing in the morning is typical of chronic bronchitis. Smokers often consider this 'normal' but any change in this cough may indicate lung cancer.

Tracheitis and pneumonia typically cause dry, centrally painful and non-productive cough. Patients with asthma may have a paroxysmal dry cough after a viral infection that may last several months (bronchial hyper-reactivity). Chronic dry cough occurs in interstitial lung disease, e.g. idiopathic pulmonary fibrosis, formerly known as fibrosing alveolitis.

Timing and associated features

Nocturnal cough disrupting sleep is common in asthma. Occupational asthma and exposure to dusts and fumes cause a chronic cough that lessens during weekends and holidays. Occult gastro-oesophageal reflux disease (GORD) and chronic sinus disease with associated postnasal drip cause daytime cough. Angiotensin-converting enzyme (ACE) inhibitors cause a dry cough, particularly in women. Coughing during and after swallowing liquids suggests neuromuscular disease of the oropharynx.

Sputum production

Expectorated sputum is always abnormal but patients often find it difficult to discuss or they may swallow it, so specifically ask about this. There are four main types of sputum (Box 7.3).

Amount

How much sputum is coughed up each day? Is it a small (a teaspoonful) or large (a teacupful) amount?
- Bronchiectasis causes large volumes of purulent sputum to be coughed up, varying with posture
- Sudden production of large amounts of purulent sputum on a single occasion suggests rupture of a lung abscess or empyema into the bronchial tree
- Large volumes of watery sputum with a pink tinge in an acutely breathless patient suggest pulmonary oedema, but occurring over weeks (bronchorrhoea) suggest alveolar cell cancer.

7.3 Types of sputum

Type	Appearance	Cause
Serous	Clear, watery Frothy, pink	Acute pulmonary oedema Alveolar cell cancer
Mucoid	Clear, grey White, viscid	Chronic bronchitis/COPD Asthma
Purulent	Yellow	Acute bronchopulmonary infection Asthma (eosinophils)
	Green	Longer-standing infection Pneumonia Bronchiectasis Cystic fibrosis Lung abscess
Rusty	Rusty red	Pneumococcal pneumonia

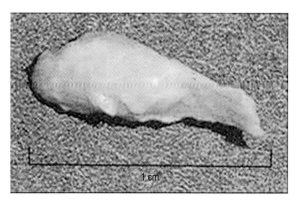

1 cm

Fig. 7.4 Mucus plug from a patient with asthma.

- In early pneumococcal pneumonia sputum may be a rusty red colour, as pneumonic inflammation causes lysis of red cells.

Taste or smell

'Foul' or 'vile'-tasting or -smelling sputum suggests anaerobic bacterial infection, and occurs in bronchiectasis, lung abscess and empyema. In bronchiectasis a change of sputum taste may indicate an infective exacerbation.

Solid material

In asthma and allergic bronchopulmonary aspergillosis viscid secretions can accumulate in airways and be coughed up as 'worm-like' structures that are casts of the bronchi (Fig. 7.4). Other solid matter sometimes coughed up includes necrotic tumour and inhaled foreign bodies, e.g. food, teeth and tablets.

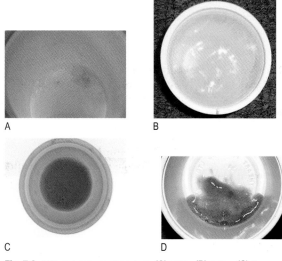

A   B

C   D

Fig. 7.3 Different colours of sputum. **(A)** White. **(B)** Yellow. **(C)** Green. **(D)** Rusty red.

Colour (Fig. 7.3)

- Chronic bronchitis and COPD cause clear or 'mucoid' sputum if there is no active infection
- Yellow sputum occurs in acute lower respiratory tract infection (live neutrophils) and in asthma (eosinophils)
- Green sputum (dead neutrophils) indicates chronic infection in COPD or bronchiectasis
- Purulent sputum is green because of lysed neutrophils which release the green-pigmented enzyme, verdoperoxidase
- The first sputum produced in the morning by a patient with COPD may be green because of nocturnal stagnation of neutrophils

Haemoptysis

Coughing up blood (haemoptysis) is an important presenting symptom of lung cancer (Box 7.4). Clarify whether the blood was coughed up (respiratory tract), vomited (upper gastrointestinal tract) or suddenly appeared in the mouth without coughing (nasopharyngeal). Always investigate haemoptysis.

Amount and appearance

Establish the volume and nature of the blood. Blood-streaked clear sputum or blood clots in sputum for more than a week suggest lung cancer. Haemoptysis with purulent sputum suggests an infective cause. Coughing up large amounts of pure blood is rare but potentially life-threatening; the most frequent causes are lung cancer, bronchiectasis and tuberculosis. Less frequent causes include lung abscess, mycetoma, cystic fibrosis, aorto-bronchial fistula and Wegener's granulomatosis.

7.4 Causes of haemoptysis

Tumour

- Malignant
  Lung cancer
  Endobronchial
  metastases
- Benign
  Bronchial carcinoid

Infection

- Bronchiectasis
- Tuberculosis
- Lung abscess
- Mycetoma
- Cystic fibrosis

Vascular

- Pulmonary infarction
- Arteriovenous malformation

Vasculitis

- Wegener's granulomatosis
- Goodpasture's syndrome

Trauma

- Inhaled foreign body
- Chest trauma
- Iatrogenic
  Bronchoscopic biopsy
  Transthoracic lung
  biopsy
  Bronchoscopic
  diathermy

Cardiac

- Mitral valve disease
- Acute left ventricular failure

Haematological

- Blood dyscrasias
- Anticoagulation

Duration and frequency

- Bronchiectasis causes intermittent haemoptysis associated with respiratory tract infection over years
- Daily haemoptysis for a week or more is a symptom of lung cancer; other causes include tuberculosis and lung abscess
- Single episodes of haemoptysis, if they are large or associated with symptoms, e.g. pleuritic chest pain and breathlessness, suggest pulmonary thromboembolism and infarction, and need immediate investigation.

Pulmonary embolism is an obstruction of part of the pulmonary vascular tree, usually caused by thrombus that has travelled from a distant site, e.g. deep veins in the legs or pelvic veins. Pulmonary embolism is frequently unrecognized and less than a third of patients have symptoms or signs of deep vein thrombosis.

Chest pain

Chest pain can originate from the pleura, the chest wall and mediastinal structures (Box 7.5). The lungs are not a source of pain because their innervation is exclusively autonomic. Characterize pain using SOCRATES (Box 2.10, p. 15).

Pleural pain

Pleuritic pain is sharp, stabbing and intensified by inspiration or coughing. Irritation of the parietal pleura of the upper six ribs causes localized pain. Irritation of

7.5 Causes of chest pain

Non-central

- Pleural
  Infection: pneumonia, bronchiectasis, tuberculosis
  Malignancy: lung cancer, mesothelioma, metastatic
  Pneumothorax
  Pulmonary infarction *PE*
  Connective tissue disease: rheumatoid arthritis, systemic lupus erythematosus (SLE)

- Chest wall
  Malignancy: lung cancer, mesothelioma, bony metastases
  Persistent cough/breathlessness
  Muscle sprains/tears
  Bornholm's disease (Coxsackie B infection)
  Tietze's syndrome (costochondritis)
  Rib fracture
  Intercostal nerve compression
  Thoracic shingles (herpes zoster)

Central

- Tracheal
  Infection
  Irritant dusts
- Cardiac
  Massive pulmonary thromboembolism
  Acute myocardial infarction/ischaemia
- Oesophageal
  Oesophagitis
  Rupture

- Great vessels
  Aortic dissection
- Mediastinal
  Lung cancer
  Thymoma
  Lymphadenopathy
  Metastases
  Mediastinitis

the parietal pleura overlying the central diaphragm innervated by the phrenic nerve is referred to the neck or shoulder tip. The lower six intercostal nerves innervate the parietal pleura of the lower ribs and the outer diaphragm, and pain from these sites may be referred to the upper abdomen. Common causes of pleuritic chest pain are pulmonary embolism, pneumonia, pneumothorax and fractured ribs.

Chest wall pain

Chest wall pain suggests respiratory, cardiac or musculoskeletal disease. Patients with chronic cough or breathlessness often develop a generalized feeling of chest tightness or diffuse pain but rarely mention it as a presenting complaint.

Sudden localized pain after vigorous coughing or direct trauma is characteristic of rib fractures or intercostal muscle injury. Prevesicular herpes zoster and intercostal nerve root compression can cause chest pain in a thoracic dermatomal distribution. Malignant chest wall pain due to direct invasion by lung cancer, mesothelioma or rib metastases is typically dull, aching or gnawing in nature, is unrelated to respiration, progressively worsens and disrupts sleep. Pancoast's tumour of the lung apex eroding the first rib and the brachial plexus causes referred pain down the medial side of the arm.

Mediastinal pain

Mediastinal pain is central, retrosternal and unrelated to respiration or cough. Irritant dusts or infection of the tracheobronchial tree produce a raw, burning retrosternal pain worse on coughing. A dull, aching retrosternal pain that disturbs sleep is a feature of cancer invading mediastinal lymph nodes or an enlarging thymoma. Massive pulmonary thromboembolism increasing right ventricular pressure may produce central chest pain typical of myocardial ischaemia.

Breathlessness

Breathlessness (dyspnoea) is an undue awareness of breathing. It is normal with strenuous physical exercise. Patients use terms such as 'shortness of breath', 'difficulty getting enough air in', 'feeling puffed' or 'tiredness' (Box 7.6).

Mode of onset, duration and progression

Find out if the breathlessness occurred suddenly, progressed rapidly over a few minutes, has occurred gradually and progressed over hours or days, or has occurred gradually and progressed over weeks, months or years (Box 7.7). Breathlessness related to psychogenic factors often occurs suddenly at rest or while talking. The patient often complains of inability to get enough

air into the chest and a need to take deep breaths. Associated symptoms may include a feeling of light-headedness, dizziness, tingling in the fingers and around the mouth, and chest tightness.

7.6 Causes of breathlessness

Non-cardiorespiratory

- Anaemia
- Metabolic acidosis
- Obesity
- Psychogenic
- Neurogenic

Cardiac

- Left ventricular failure
- Mitral valve disease
- Cardiomyopathy
- Constrictive pericarditis
- Pericardial effusion

Respiratory

- Airways
  Laryngeal tumour
  Foreign body
  Asthma
  COPD
  Bronchiectasis
  Lung cancer
  Bronchiolitis
  Cystic fibrosis
- Parenchyma
  Pulmonary fibrosis
  Alveolitis
  Sarcoidosis
  Tuberculosis
  Pneumonia
    Diffuse infections, e.g.
    Pneumocystis jiroveci
    pneumonia
    Tumour (metastatic,
    lymphangitis)
- Pulmonary circulation
  Pulmonary
  thromboembolism
  Pulmonary vasculitis
  Primary pulmonary
  hypertension
- Pleural
  Pneumothorax
  Effusion
  Diffuse pleural fibrosis
- Chest wall
  Kyphoscoliosis
  Ankylosing spondylitis
- Neuromuscular
  Myasthenia gravis
  Neuropathies
  Muscular dystrophies
  Guillain–Barré
  syndrome

7.7 Breathlessness: modes of onset, duration and progression

Minutes

- Pulmonary thromboembolism
- Pneumothorax
- Acute left ventricular failure
- Asthma
- Inhaled foreign body

Hours to days

- Pneumonia
- Asthma
- Exacerbation of COPD

Weeks to months

- Anaemia
- Pleural effusion
- Respiratory
  neuromuscular
  disorders

Months to years

- COPD
- Pulmonary fibrosis
- Pulmonary
  tuberculosis

7.8 Severity of breathlessness: Medical Research Council (MRC) classification	
Grade 1	Breathless when hurrying on the level or walking up a slight hill
Grade 2	Breathless when walking with people of own age or on level ground
Grade 3	Has to stop because of breathlessness when walking on level ground at own pace

Variability and aggravating/relieving factors

The situations or activities which precipitate breathlessness provide clues to the likely cause. Although associated with left ventricular failure, breathlessness when lying flat (orthopnoea) can be a feature of respiratory muscle weakness or any severe lung disease. Breathlessness that wakes the patient from sleep is typical of asthma and left ventricular failure (paroxysmal nocturnal dyspnoea). Patients with asthma typically wake between 3 and 5 a.m. and have associated wheezing. Breathlessness that is worst on waking in the morning is more typical of COPD and may improve after coughing up sputum.

Patients with exercise-induced asthma may notice that their breathlessness continues to worsen for 5–10 minutes after stopping activity. If you suspect asthma, ask about exposure to allergens, smoke, perfumes, fumes, cold air or drugs (aspirin or NSAIDs can trigger breathlessness). Common allergens are house dust mite (shaking bedding, hoovering), animals (cats, dogs, horses) and grass pollens (mowing the lawn, the 'hayfever season') and tree pollens. Breathlessness which improves at the weekend or on holiday suggests occupational asthma or extrinsic allergic alveolitis.

Severity

What effect do symptoms have on how your patient functions? Ask about the effect of work, carrying loads, heavy exertion, walking up hills or walking with contemporaries. Breathlessness while walking on the flat, up gentle inclines and up stairs indicates a more severe degree of breathlessness. Severely breathless patients are dyspnoeic at rest and while walking around the house, getting washed, dressing, eating or doing light housework. Use grading scales for breathlessness (Box 7.8).

How far can the patient walk before stopping to rest? Ask for an estimate of the time taken to walk a distance and the number of stops involved: say, from home to a local shop. How does it affect hobbies such as golf, gardening, dancing, swimming or hill-walking?

Associated symptoms

Box 7.9 outlines some combinations of symptoms in acutely breathless patients.

7.9 Acute breathlessness: commonly associated symptoms	
No chest pain	
• Pulmonary embolism	• Hypovolaemia/shock
• Pneumothorax	• Acute left ventricular failure/pulmonary oedema
• Metabolic acidosis	
Pleuritic chest pain	
• Pneumonia	• Pulmonary embolism
• Pneumothorax	• Rib fracture
Central chest pain	
• Myocardial infarction with left ventricular failure	• Massive pulmonary embolism/infarction
Wheeze and cough	
• Asthma	• COPD

Wheeze

Wheeze is a high-pitched whistling sound produced by air passing through narrowed small airways. Typically, wheeze is limited to expiration, but patients may refer to rattling sounds from secretions in the upper airways or larynx or the inspiratory sound of stridor caused by the partial occlusion of a large airway by tumour or foreign body as wheeze. Wheeze on exercise is a common symptom of asthma and COPD. Night wakening with wheeze suggests asthma, but wheeze after wakening in the morning suggests COPD.

Apnoea

Apnoea means the absence of breathing; hypopnoea is a reduction in airflow or respiratory movements by >50% for 10 seconds or more. Obstructive sleep apnoea/hypopnoea syndrome (OSAHS) is the combination of excessive daytime sleepiness and recurrent upper airway obstruction with sleep fragmentation. Between 2 and 4% of middle-aged men and 1–2% of middle-aged women (Box 7.10) have OSAHS with multiple apnoeas (cessation of airflow for >10 seconds) during sleep when the retropharyngeal airway collapses, obstructing the upper airway.

Ask patients' bed partners about apnoeas, loud snoring, nocturnal restlessness, irritability and personality change. They usually describe loud snoring, then a pause in breathing followed by a grunting noise and restoration of snoring. Snoring is, however, more common than OSAHS, affecting around 40% of middle-aged men and 20% of middle-aged women.

Ask if patients fall asleep at unwanted times, including after meals, in public places, in meetings, in the evening watching television or when reading. A score of >10 on the Epworth Sleepiness Scale (Box 7.11)

7.10 Symptoms of obstructive sleep apnoea/ hypopnoea syndrome (OSAHS)

- Snoring
- Witnessed apnoeas
- Unrefreshing sleep
- Restless sleep
- Nocturia
- Excessive daytime sleepiness
- Impaired concentration
- Choking episodes during sleep
- Irritability/personality change
- Decreased libido

7.11 The Epworth Sleepiness Scale

For each of the situations outlined in recent everyday life, ask the patient to grade the likelihood of dozing off or falling asleep:

0 = Would never doze
1 = Slight chance of dozing
2 = Moderate chance of dozing
3 = High chance of dozing

Situation	Chance of dozing
<ul><li>Sitting and reading</li><li>Watching television</li><li>Sitting inactive in a public place, e.g. a theatre or meeting</li><li>As passenger in a car for 1 hour without a break</li><li>Lying down for a rest in the afternoon when circumstances permit</li><li>Sitting and talking to someone</li><li>Sitting quietly after a lunch without alcohol</li><li>In a car, whilst stopped for a few minutes in traffic</li></ul>	
TOTAL	

7.12 Previous history of illness

History	Current implications
Eczema, hayfever	Allergic tendency relevant to asthma
Childhood asthma	In the past asthma was commonly termed 'wheezy bronchitis'
Recurrent childhood viral-associated wheeze	Relevant to adult-onset (recurrence of) asthma
Whooping cough, measles	Recognized causes of bronchiectasis, especially if complicated by pneumonia
Pneumonia, pleurisy	Recognized cause of bronchiectasis Recurrent episodes may be a manifestation of bronchiectasis
Tuberculosis	Reactivation if not previously treated effectively Respiratory failure may complicate thoracoplasty Mycetoma in lung cavity may present with haemoptysis
Connective tissue disorders, e.g. rheumatoid arthritis	Lung diseases are recognized complications, e.g. pulmonary fibrosis, effusions, bronchiectasis
Previous malignancy	Recurrence, metastatic/pleural disease Chemotherapeutic agents recognized causes of pulmonary fibrosis Radiotherapy-induced pulmonary fibrosis
Recent travel, immobility, cancer	Pulmonary thromboembolism
Recent surgery, loss of consciousness	Aspiration of foreign body, gastric contents Pneumonia, lung abscess
Neuromuscular disorders	Respiratory failure Aspiration

suggests abnormal daytime sleepiness. If the patient drives, ask whether he or she has fallen asleep at the wheel, been involved/nearly involved in accidents because of sleepiness, or stops frequently for catnaps. Urgently investigate patients with daytime sleepiness and drowsiness while driving, especially if the patient has a heavy goods or public service vehicle licence.

THE HISTORY

Past history

Information about previous respiratory and non-respiratory illnesses can help with the diagnosis of the current condition (Box 7.12).

Drug history

Detail the type of inhaler, dose in micrograms (not puffs) and frequency. Note the effectiveness of previously prescribed medications, e.g. corticosteroids and inhalers. Enquire about current and previous medications, if drug-induced respiratory disease is suspected (Box 7.13).

Family history

Cystic fibrosis is the most common severe autosomal recessive disease in Europeans, occurring with a carrier rate of 1 in 25 and an incidence of about 1 in 2500 live births. Alpha-1-antitrypsin deficiency also has recessive inheritance. A family history of asthma, eczema and hayfever increases the chance of a predisposition to form excess IgE in response to allergen (atopy). 'Asthma' in parents or grandparents who were smokers may have been misdiagnosed COPD. A family history of tuberculosis can represent significant past exposure that may reactivate later in life. Patients with asbestos-related disease and no obvious occupational exposure may have had significant exposure through asbestos-contaminated

7.13 Examples of drug-induced respiratory conditions

Respiratory condition	Drug
Bronchoconstriction	β-blockers Opioids NSAIDs
Cough	ACE inhibitors
Bronchiolitis obliterans	Penicillamine
Diffuse parenchymal lung disease	Cytotoxic agents: bleomycin, methotrexate Anti-inflammatory agents: sulfasalazine, penicillamine, gold salts, aspirin Cardiovascular drugs: amiodarone, hydralazine Antibiotics: nitrofurantoin Intravenous drug misuse Radiation
Pulmonary thromboembolism	Oestrogens
Pulmonary hypertension	Oestrogens Dexfenfluramine, fenfluramine
Pleural effusion	Amiodarone Nitrofurantoin Phenytoin Methotrexate Pergolide
Respiratory depression	Opioids Benzodiazepines

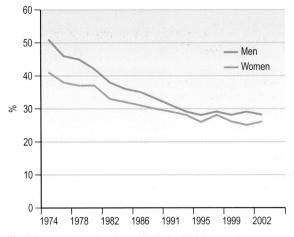

Fig. 7.5 Prevalence of adult smoking in the UK by sex.

work clothes brought home for cleaning by a spouse or parent in a relevant occupation.

Social history

Smoking

Although cigarette smoking has declined in the UK (Fig. 7.5), the current prevalence of COPD and incidence of lung cancer reflect historical smoking patterns. Establish when patients started (and stopped) smoking and average tobacco consumption as cigarettes/day

or ounces/grams of 'roll-up' tobacco/week. Calculate the 'pack year' consumption; smoking 1 pack of 20 cigarettes per day for 1 year equals 1 pack year. Patients with COPD usually have a consumption >20 pack years (p. 21). Stopping smoking before the age of 40 is crucial to improving health; beyond 40 years people lose, on average, 3 months of life expectancy for every further year of continued smoking.

Pets

Ask about exposure to pets because of their association with asthma (dogs, cats, rodents, horses), allergic alveolitis (birds) and psittacosis pneumonia (parrots and parakeets).

Occupational history

Occupation is an important factor in many respiratory disorders. For example, asbestos was widely used in shipyards, building construction and plumbing until the 1970s, and now asbestos-related lung disease, e.g. mesothelioma and asbestosis, is the greatest single cause of work-related death in the UK. Occupation is also particularly important in adult-onset asthma, e.g. baker's asthma due to flour dust, interstitial lung disease, e.g. farmer's lung, or unexplained pleural effusion. Record all occupations, full- and part-time, held since the patient left school and the number of years spent in each job (Box 7.14). Find out exactly what the job entailed and the length of any exposure. Exposure to a recognized hazard helps diagnosis, has implications for current employment, and

7.14 Examples of occupational lung disease

Lung disease	Exposure	Occupation
Pulmonary fibrosis	Asbestos	Shipyard/construction workers, plumbers, boilermakers
	Quartz (silica)	Miners, quarry workers, stone masons
	Coal	Coal miners
	Beryllium	Nuclear, aerospace industries
COPD/emphysema	Coal	Coal miners
Malignancy	Asbestos	Shipyard/construction workers, plumbers, boilermakers
	Radon	Metal miners
Byssinosis	Cotton, flax, hemp	Cotton, flax, hemp manufacturing
Extrinsic allergic alveolitis		
Farmer's lung	Fungal spores of thermophilic actinomycetes or *Micropolyspora faeni*	Farm workers exposed to mouldy hay
Malt worker's lung	*Aspergillus clavatus*	Exposure to whisky maltings
Bird fancier's lung	Bloom on birds' feathers/excreta	Pigeon fanciers, bird owners
Asthma	Animals	Vets, laboratory workers
	Grains, flour	Farmers, bakers, millers
	Hardwood dusts	Joiners, carpenters
	Colophony	Soldering, welders
	Enzymes	Detergent manufacturing, pharmaceuticals
	Isocyanates	Spray painting, varnishing
	Epoxy resins	Adhesives, varnishing
	Drugs	Pharmaceutical industry
	Formaldehyde, paraldehyde, latex	Hospital workers

may be the basis for compensation. Some occupational diseases are worse at the beginning of the working week, e.g. byssinosis and humidifier fever, but occupational asthma is worse at the end of the working week and gets better on holidays away from work.

THE PHYSICAL EXAMINATION

General examination

Observe patients as you first meet them, looking particularly for breathlessness, weight loss, cyanosis and their mental state.

Respiratory rate

Measurement of respiratory rate is essential in the assessment of all patients presenting with acute breathlessness. Tachypnoea is a respiratory rate >15/min and is caused by increased ventilatory drive in fever, acute asthma and exacerbation of COPD, or reduced ventilatory capacity in pneumonia, pulmonary oedema and interstitial lung disease.

Respiratory rate >30/min is the most important prognostic sign associated with death in community-acquired pneumonia (Box 7.15). A slow respiratory rate occurs in opioid toxicity, hypercapnia, hypothyroidism, raised intracranial pressure and hypothalamic lesions.

7.15 Features of severe community-acquired pneumonia (CRB-65)

- **C**onfusion
- **R**espiratory rate >30/min
- **B**lood pressure — diastolic <60 mmHg
- Aged >**65** years

Examination sequence

Note if the patient is breathless at rest and surreptitiously assess chest movements and respiratory rate (breaths/minute) while you feel the pulse.

Breathing patterns

Periodic breathing (Cheyne–Stokes respiration) is cyclically increasing rate and depth of breathing, followed by diminishing respiratory effort and rate, ending in a period of apnoea or hypopnoea.

This relates to altered sensitivity of the respiratory centre to chemical control and delay in circulation time between the lung and chemoreceptors. It is seen most frequently in stroke involving the brainstem and in severe heart failure, but may also occur in the normal elderly.

Hyperventilation is a common response to acute anxiety or emotional distress, and is often associated with respiratory alkalosis with low arterial carbon dioxide tension (p. 181). Breathing is deep, irregular and sighing, and patients describe an inability to fill their lungs completely. When acute hyperventilation is sustained, tetany and occasionally grand mal seizure can occur.

Hyperventilation with deep, sighing respirations (Küssmaul respiration) in response to metabolic acidosis occurs in diabetic ketoacidosis, acute renal failure, lactic acidosis, and salicylate and methanol poisoning (p. 181). Although patients may not be aware of breathlessness, their respiratory rate increases and they appear to have 'air hunger'.

Use of accessory muscles

See if the sternocleidomastoids, platysma and pectoral muscles are being used to increase chest expansion during inspiration. These muscles cause elevation of the shoulders with inspiration and aid respiration by increasing chest expansion. The use of accessory muscles is characteristic of patients with COPD and severe acute asthma.

Most women make more use of the intercostal muscles than of the diaphragm, and therefore respiratory movements are predominantly thoracic. Men rely more on the diaphragm and their respiratory movements are predominantly abdominal.

Stridor

Stridor is a harsh, rasping or croaking inspiratory noise, often aggravated by coughing, and should always be investigated. Causes include foreign body or tumour partially occluding the larynx, trachea or a main bronchus. Ask the patient to cough and then breathe deeply in and out with the mouth wide open. Listen carefully, close to the patient's mouth, for the noise.

Hoarseness

Hoarseness in respiratory disease may be due to damage to the left recurrent laryngeal nerve by lung cancer at the left hilum. The left vocal cord cannot adduct to the midline, causing a prolonged, low-pitched and 'bovine' cough (p. 156).

Cyanosis

Cyanosis is a blue discoloration of the skin and mucous membranes, caused by an absolute concentration of deoxygenated haemoglobin of >50 g/l.

Central cyanosis is arterial hypoxaemia, detected by inspecting the lips and extended tongue in natural light (Fig. 7.6). In patients with a normal haemoglobin concentration, central cyanosis occurs when the arterial oxygen saturation falls below 90%, corresponding to a PaO_2 of approximately 8 kPa (60 mmHg). In anaemic or hypovolaemic patients, cyanosis may not be seen because severe hypoxia is required to produce the necessary concentration of deoxygenated haemoglobin. In contrast, patients with polycythaemia become

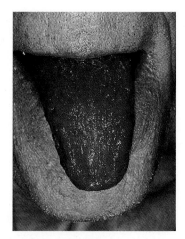

Fig. 7.6 Central cyanosis of the tongue.

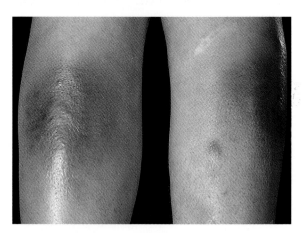

Fig. 7.7 Erythema nodosum on the shins.

cyanosed at higher arterial oxygen tensions. Rarely, central cyanosis is caused by methaemoglobinaemia or sulphhaemoglobinaemia.

Peripheral cyanosis is seen in the fingers and toes and is usually due to circulatory disorders or cold, but can also occur in patients with severe central cyanosis.

Blood pressure

A diastolic pressure of <60 mmHg is associated with increased mortality in community-acquired pneumonia (Box 7.15). In pneumothorax, hypotension may indicate the development of 'tension' with reduction in venous return to the heart and risk of cardiac arrest.

Skin appearances

Erythema nodosum over the shins may herald acute sarcoidosis (Fig. 7.7). Occasionally, raised firm non-tender subcutaneous nodules occur in patients with disseminated cancer (Fig. 7.8).

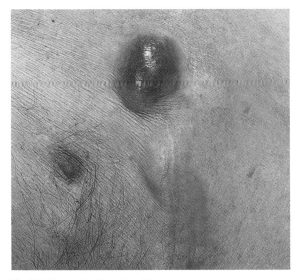

Fig. 7.8 Metastatic skin nodes of lung cancer.

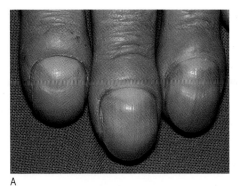

A

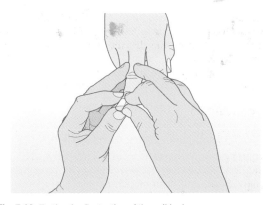

B

Fig. 7.9 Clubbing. **(A)** Anterior view. **(B)** Lateral view.

7.16 Causes of clubbing and hypertrophic pulmonary osteoarthropathy

Familial

Thoracic

- Tumours: benign or malignant
  Lung cancer
  Mesothelioma
  Pleural fibroma
  Oesophageal cancer
  Oesophageal leiomyoma
  Thymoma
  Atrial myxoma
- Interstitial lung disease
  Idiopathic pulmonary fibrosis (fibrosing alveolitis)
  Asbestosis

- Sepsis
  Bronchiectasis
  Empyema
  Lung abscess
  Cystic fibrosis
  Bacterial endocarditis
- Arteriovenous shunting
  AV malformations in the lung
  Cyanotic congenital heart disease

Non-thoracic

- Hepatic cirrhosis
- Coeliac disease
- Ulcerative colitis
- Crohn's disease

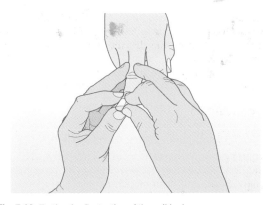

Fig. 7.10 Testing for fluctuation of the nail bed.

Hands

Clubbing

The majority of patients with finger clubbing have thoracic disease but it is also associated with gastrointestinal disorders and can be familial (Box 7.16). Rarely, clubbing develops relatively quickly over several weeks, in empyema.

Clubbing requires (Fig. 7.9):

- loss of the normal angle between the nail and nail bed
- increased nail bed fluctuation
- increased nail curvature in later stages
- increased bulk of the soft tissues over the terminal phalanges.

Examination sequence

- Look across the nail and nail bed at the 'nail bed angle'; this is normally obtuse but disappears in early finger clubbing.
- Place your thumbs under the pulp of the terminal phalanx and attempt to move the nail within the nail bed using your index fingers (Fig. 7.10). A 'spongy feel' confirms nail bed fluctuation.

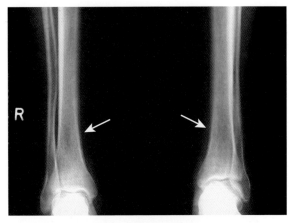

Fig. 7.11 X-ray of the lower legs in hypertrophic pulmonary osteoarthropathy. Arrows show periosteal reaction.

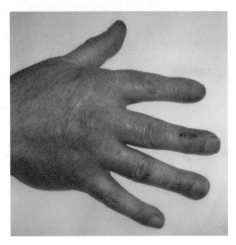

Fig. 7.12 Tobacco 'tar'-stained fingers.

7.17 Causes of asterixis

- Respiratory failure/acidosis (CO_2 retention)
- Liver failure
- Renal failure
- Electrolyte disturbance
    Hypoglycaemia
    Hypokalaemia
    Hypomagnesaemia
- Wilson's disease — hepatolenticular degeneration
- Drugs
    Barbiturates
    Alcohol
    Sodium valproate
    Phenytoin
    Carbamazepine
    Metoclopramide
    Gabapentin
    Ceftazidime
    Opioids
- CNS
    Intracerebral haemorrhage
    Subdural haematoma
    Subarachnoid haemorrhage
    Cerebral ischaemia
    Cerebral lymphoma

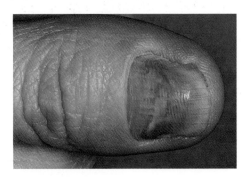

Fig. 7.13 Yellow nail syndrome.

Hypertrophic pulmonary osteoarthropathy

Hypertrophic pulmonary osteoarthropathy (HPOA) is rare and almost always associated with lung cancer, usually squamous cancer. Pronounced clubbing of fingers and toes occurs, with pain and swelling affecting the wrists and ankles. X-rays of the distal forearm and lower legs show subperiosteal new bone formation separate from the cortex of the long bones (Fig. 7.11).

Discoloration of the fingers and nails

A brownish stain on the fingers and nails in cigarette smokers is caused by tar, not nicotine (Fig. 7.12). The rare 'yellow nail syndrome' is associated with lymphoedema and an exudative pleural effusion (Fig. 7.13).

Tremor

A fine finger tremor is caused by excessive use of β-agonist or theophylline bronchodilator drugs. A coarse flapping tremor (asterixis) is seen with severe ventilatory failure and carbon dioxide retention (Box 7.17). This is the result of intermittent failure of parietal mechanisms required to maintain posture.

▶ Examination sequence

▶ Ask the patient to hold out the arms with the hands extended at the wrists (Fig. 7.14). Look for a jerky, flapping tremor.

▶ Alternatively, ask the patient to squeeze your index and middle fingers and maintain this for 30–60 seconds. Patients with a flapping tremor cannot maintain the posture.

Neck

Jugular venous pressure (JVP)

The JVP (Fig. 6.22, p. 125) is raised in right-sided heart failure. Chronic hypoxia in COPD leads to pulmonary

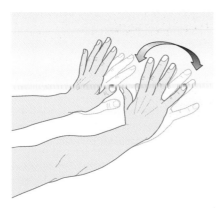

Fig. 7.14 Asterixis. Hand and arm position for observing the 'flapping tremor' of CO_2 retention.

arterial vasoconstriction, pulmonary hypertension, right heart dilatation and elevation of the JVP. This is cor pulmonale. The JVP is also high if the intrathoracic pressure is raised in tension pneumothorax or severe acute asthma. Massive pulmonary embolism may cause the JVP to be so high that the patient has to be sitting upright for it to be seen.

In superior vena caval obstruction (Fig. 7.15A) the JVP is raised and non-pulsatile, and the abdomino-jugular reflex is absent. Most cases are due to lung cancer compressing the superior vena cava. Other causes include lymphoma, thymoma and mediastinal fibrosis.

Neck nodes

Detecting enlargement of the cervical and supraclavicular lymph glands (Fig. 7.16) or scalene lymph nodes

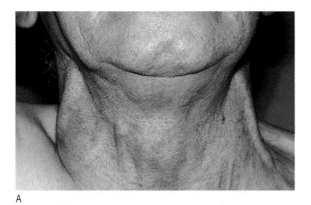

A

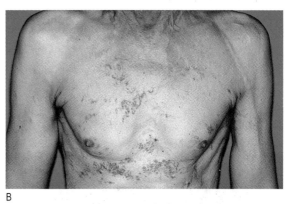

B

Fig. 7.15 Superior vena caval obstruction. (A) Distended neck veins. **(B)** Dilated superficial veins over chest.

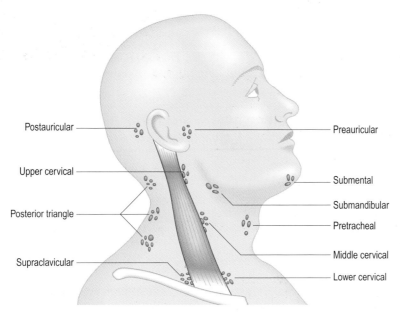

Postauricular

Upper cervical

Posterior triangle

Supraclavicular

Preauricular

Submental

Submandibular

Pretracheal

Middle cervical

Lower cervical

Fig. 7.16 The lymph node groupings in the neck.

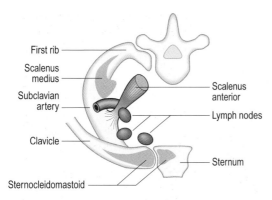

First rib
Scalenus medius
Subclavian artery
Clavicle
Sternocleidomastoid
Scalenus anterior
Lymph nodes
Sternum

Fig. 7.17 Relation of lymph nodes to scalenus anterior.

(Fig. 7.17) is an important part of examination of the respiratory system. Scalene lymph node enlargement may be the first evidence of metastatic lung cancer and localized cervical lymphadenopathy is a common presenting feature of lymphoma.

Examination sequence

Neck nodes

- Ask the patient to sit down and stand behind him.
- Palpate one side of the neck at a time, using the fingers of one hand.
- Feel for scalene nodes above the first rib next to the insertion of the scalenus anterior muscle, with the patient's head slightly tilted to that side (Fig. 3.19B, p. 57).
- Place your index finger between the clavicle and sternocleidomastoid muscle, and press down gently towards the first rib. A palpable scalene node is a soft mobile mass just above the hard first rib.
- Note the size and consistency of any palpable node and whether it is fixed to surrounding structures.

In Hodgkin's disease, the lymph nodes are typically 'rubbery'; in dental sepsis and tonsillitis they are usually tender; in tuberculosis and metastatic cancer they are often 'matted' together to form a mass; and calcified lymph glands feel stony hard. Palpable lymph nodes fixed to deep structures or skin are usually malignant.

Abnormalities in the shape of the chest

Increase in anteroposterior diameter

When the anteroposterior diameter is greater than the lateral diameter, the chest is 'barrel-shaped'. This is associated with lung hyperinflation, as in patients with severe COPD (Fig. 7.18A), although the degree of deformity does not correlate with the severity of airways obstruction.

Kyphosis and scoliosis

Kyphosis is an exaggerated anterior curvature of the spine and scoliosis is lateral curvature. Kyphoscoliosis, involving both deformities (Fig. 7.18B), may be idiopathic or secondary to childhood poliomyelitis or spinal tuberculosis, and may be grossly disfiguring and disabling. It may reduce ventilatory capacity and increase

the work of breathing. These patients develop progressive ventilatory failure with carbon dioxide retention and cor pulmonale at an early age.

Pectus carinatum (pigeon chest)

This is a localized prominence of the sternum and adjacent costal cartilages, often accompanied by indrawing of the ribs to form symmetrical horizontal grooves (Harrison's sulci) above the costal margin (Fig. 7.18C). These result from lung hyperinflation with repeated vigorous contractions of the diaphragm while the bony thorax is in a pliable prepubertal state. The abnormality is most often caused by severe and poorly controlled childhood asthma but can occur in osteomalacia and rickets.

Pectus excavatum (funnel chest)

This developmental deformity is localized depression of the lower end of the sternum (Fig. 7.18D) or, less commonly, of the whole length of the sternum. Patients are usually asymptomatic but concerned about their appearance. In severe cases the heart is displaced to the left and the ventilatory capacity is reduced.

Examination of the thorax

Examine patients with their chest and upper abdomen fully exposed and evenly lit. Ask the patient to sit over the edge of a bed or on a chair if possible.

Inspection

Examination sequence

- Look at the chest; normally it should be symmetrical and elliptical in cross-section.
- Look for scars of previous heart or lung surgery, and for swellings, marks and spots on the skin. Subcutaneous lesions may be visible, including metastatic tumour nodules, neurofibromas and lipomas.
- Look for vascular anomalies, e.g. the dilated venous vascular channels of superior vena caval obstruction (Fig. 7.15B).

Palpation

Position of the mediastinum

Determine the position of the mediastinum by examination of the trachea and cardiac apex beat (Box 7.18).

Examination sequence

- With the patient looking directly forwards, look for any deviation and assess by gently placing the tip of your right index finger into the suprasternal notch and palpating the trachea (Fig. 7.19). This can be uncomfortable; be gentle and explain what you are doing. Slight displacement to the right is common in healthy people.
- Upper mediastinal shift causes deviation of the trachea.

Displacement of the cardiac apex beat indicates shift of the lower mediastinum. Displacement of the cardiac impulse without deviation of the trachea is usually due to left ventricular enlargement but can occur in

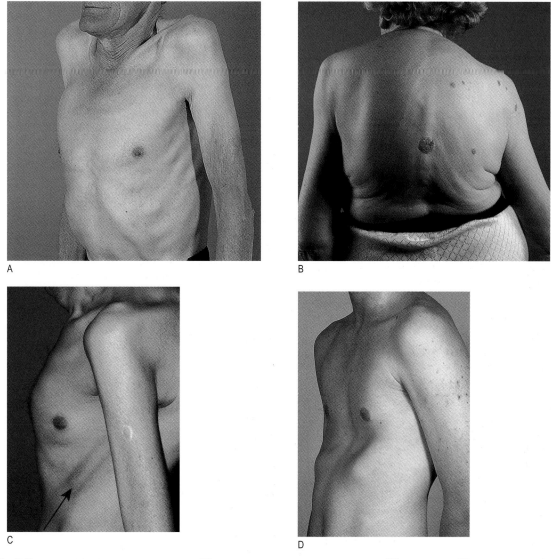

Fig. 7.18 **Abnormalities in the shape of the chest. (A)** Hyperinflated chest with intercostal indrawing. **(B)** Kyphoscoliosis. **(C)** Pectus carinatum with prominent Harrison's sulcus (arrow). **(D)** Pectus excavatum.

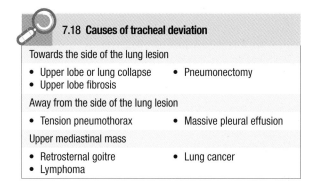

🔍 **7.18 Causes of tracheal deviation**

Towards the side of the lung lesion

- Upper lobe or lung collapse
- Upper lobe fibrosis
- Pneumonectomy

Away from the side of the lung lesion

- Tension pneumothorax
- Massive pleural effusion

Upper mediastinal mass

- Retrosternal goitre
- Lymphoma
- Lung cancer

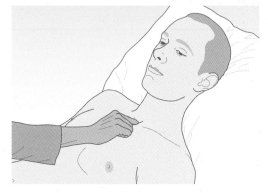

Fig. 7.19 Examining for tracheal shift.

scoliosis, kyphoscoliosis or severe pectus excavatum. The cardiac apex beat may be difficult to localize in obesity, pericardial effusion, poor left ventricular function, or lung hyperinflation as in COPD. The heave of right ventricular hypertrophy, found in severe pulmonary hypertension, is best felt at the left sternal edge (Fig. 6.34C, p. 134).

The distance between the suprasternal notch and cricoid cartilage is normally 3–4 finger breadths; any less suggests lung hyperinflation. A 'tracheal tug' is found in severe hyperinflation; resting on the patient's trachea, your fingers move inferiorly with each inspiration.

Chest expansion

Both sides of the thorax should expand equally during normal (tidal) breathing and maximal inspiration.

![Examination sequence icon] **Examination sequence**

◾ Assess expansion of the upper lobes by observing the clavicles from behind during tidal breathing.
◾ To assess expansion of the lower lobes, place your hands firmly on the chest wall and extend your fingers around the sides of the patient's chest (Fig. 7.20). Your thumbs should almost meet in the midline and hover just off the chest, so that they move with respiration.
◾ Ask the patient to take a deep breath. Your thumbs should move symmetrically, at least 5 cm apart.

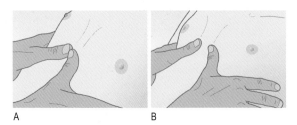

A   B

Fig. 7.20 Assessing chest expansion from the front. (A) Expiration. **(B)** Inspiration.

Reduced expansion on one side indicates abnormality on that side: for example, pleural effusion, lung or lobar collapse, pneumothorax and unilateral fibrosis. Bilateral reduction in chest wall movement is common in severe COPD and diffuse pulmonary fibrosis.

With the patient supine, look for paradoxical inward movement of the abdomen during inspiration. This may indicate diaphragmatic paralysis or, more commonly, severe COPD. Double fracture of a series of ribs or of the sternum allows the chest wall between the fractures to become mobile or 'flail'. Localized indrawing of the chest wall, as it is sucked in with every inspiration and out during expiration, produces paradoxical movement (Fig. 17.7, p. 443).

Subcutaneous emphysema produces a characteristic crackling sensation over gas-containing tissue (Fig. 7.21)

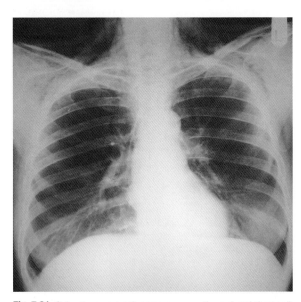

Fig. 7.21 Subcutaneous emphysema seen over the neck and chest wall on chest X-ray.

OSCEs 7.19 Examine this patient with acute breathlessness

1. Assess severity of dyspnoea and record respiratory rate per minute.
2. Look for evidence of weight loss or anaemia.
3. Examine pulse for tachycardia, arrhythmias (cardiac disease) or bradycardia (cardiac disease or severe hypoxia).
4. Measure blood pressure — hypotension found in septicaemia and tension pneumothorax.
5. Examine tongue and lips for central cyanosis (severe hypoxia).
6. Examine JVP — raised in cardiac failure, cor pulmonale, massive pulmonary thromboembolism and tension pneumothorax.
7. Palpate trachea and apex beat for mediastinal shift — displaced away from the lesion in tension pneumothorax or massive pleural effusion; toward the lesion in lobar or lung collapse due to lung cancer.
8. Palpate for chest expansion — unilateral reduction in pleural effusion, consolidation (pneumonia), lung or lobar collapse or pneumothorax.
9. Percuss over the chest — hyper-resonant note may indicate pneumothorax, dull note consolidation (pneumonia), or lung or lobar collapse and a 'stony dull' note pleural effusion.
10. Auscultate the chest — unilateral early inspiratory crackles (bronchial infection or pneumonia), bilateral basal medium crackles (pulmonary oedema), bilateral fine late inspiratory crackles (pulmonary fibrosis), bronchial breathing (pneumonia) and reduced breath sounds (lung or lobar collapse or pleural effusion).
11. Examine lower limb for pitting oedema (bilateral in cor pulmonale or heart failure; unilateral in deep vein thrombosis).

and there may be diffuse swelling of the chest wall, neck and face. It may complicate severe acute asthma, spontaneous or traumatic pneumothorax, or rupture of the oesophagus, and is a complication of intercostal drainage. Mediastinal emphysema occurs if gas tracks into the mediastinum and is associated with a characteristic systolic 'crunching' sound on auscultating the heart (Hamman's sign).

Tenderness over the costal cartilages is found in the costochondritis of Tietze's syndrome. Localized rib tenderness can be found over areas of pulmonary infarction or fracture.

Percussion

Percussion allows you to listen for the pitch and loudness of the percussed note and feel for post-percussive vibrations. It is performed in sequence over corresponding areas on both sides of the chest (Fig. 7.22).

Examination sequence

- Place the palm of your left hand on the chest, with your fingers slightly separated (Fig. 7.23).
- Press the middle finger of your left hand firmly against the chest, aligned with the underlying ribs over the area to be percussed.
- Strike the centre of the middle phalanx of your left middle finger with the tip of your right middle finger, using a loose swinging movement of the wrist and not the forearm.
- Remove the percussing finger quickly so the note generated is not dampened.
- Percuss the lung apices by placing the palmar surface of your left middle finger across the anterior border of the trapezius muscle, overlapping the supraclavicular fossa and percussing downwards.
- Percuss the clavicle directly over the medial third, as percussing laterally is dull over the shoulder muscles.
- To percuss the upper posterior chest ask patients to fold their arms across the front of their chest, thereby moving the scapulae laterally.
- Do not percuss near the midline, as this produces a dull note from the solid structures of the thoracic spine and paravertebral musculature. Map out abnormal areas by percussing from resonant to dull.

Percussing normal lung produces a resonant note (Box 7.21); a pneumothorax produces a hyper-resonant note. Percussion over solid structures, e.g. liver, heart or a consolidated area of lung, produces a dull note. Find the upper level of liver dullness by percussing down the anterior wall of the right chest; in adults the upper level of liver dullness is the 5th rib in the midclavicular

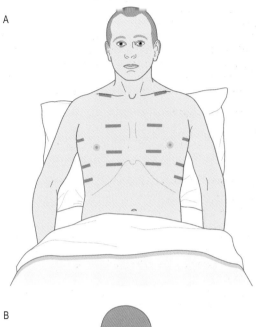

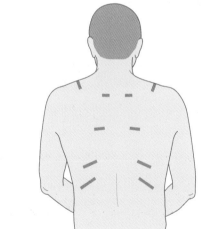

Fig. 7.22 Sites for percussion. (A) Anterior and lateral chest wall. **(B)** Posterior chest wall.

OSCEs 7.20 Examine this patient with haemoptysis

1. General examination, looking for evidence of weight loss, anaemia, iron deficiency and bruising.
2. Examine hands for finger clubbing (lung cancer or bronchiectasis).
3. Feel neck for lymphadenopathy, especially scalene nodes (lung cancer or lymphoma).
4. Inspect chest, e.g. for previous lung resection (lung cancer or bronchiectasis).
5. Palpate trachea and apex beat for mediastinal shift (lung or lobar collapse due to lung cancer).
6. Percuss for dullness — 'stony dullness' in pleural effusion (lung cancer, mesothelioma, tuberculous effusion).
7. Auscultate for crackles persisting on inspiration and expiration (bronchiectasis) or reduced air entry (lung or lobar collapse due to lung cancer; or pleural effusion due to lung cancer or mesothelioma).

line. Resonance below this is a sign of hyperinflation (COPD or severe asthma). The area of cardiac dullness over the left anterior chest may be decreased when the lungs are hyperinflated. Percussion over fluid, e.g.

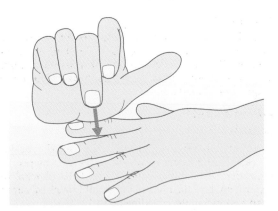

Fig. 7.23 Technique of percussion.

7.21 Percussion note

Type	Detected over
Resonant	Normal lung
Hyper-resonant	Pneumothorax
Dull	Pulmonary consolidation Pulmonary collapse Severe pulmonary fibrosis
Stony dull	Pleural effusion Haemothorax

pleural effusion (Box 7.22), produces an extremely dull (stony dull) note. Basal dullness due to elevation of the diaphragm is easily confused with pleural fluid.

Auscultation

▶ Examination sequence

▪▸ Most sounds reaching the chest wall are low in frequency and best heard with the bell of the stethoscope.

▪▸ Use the diaphragm to locate higher-pitched sounds, such as pleural friction rubs. Stretching the skin and hairs under the diaphragm during deep breathing can produce anomalous noises like crackles, and in thin patients it may be difficult to achieve full contact between the diaphragm and skin of the chest wall.

▪▸ Listen with the patient relaxed and breathing deeply through an open mouth. Avoid asking him to breathe deeply for prolonged periods, as this causes giddiness and even tetany. Auscultate both sides alternately, comparing findings over a large number of equivalent positions to ensure that localized abnormalities are not missed. Listen:
  • anteriorly from above the clavicle down to the 6th rib
  • laterally from the axilla to the 8th rib
  • posteriorly down to the level of the 11th rib.

▪▸ Assess the quality and amplitude of the breath sounds.

▪▸ Identify any gap between inspiration and expiration, and listen for added sounds.

▪▸ Avoid auscultation within 3 cm of the midline anteriorly or posteriorly, as these areas may transmit sounds directly from the trachea or main bronchi.

Vocal resonance

▶ Examination sequence

▪▸ Ask the patient to say 'one, one, one' while you auscultate to assess the quality and amplitude of vocal resonance.

7.22 Causes of pleural effusion based on classic differentiation by pleural fluid protein concentration

	Very common	Less common	Rare
Transudates (pleural fluid protein < 30 g/l)	Left ventricular failure Liver cirrhosis Hypoalbuminaemia Peritoneal dialysis	Hypothyroidism Nephrotic syndrome Mitral stenosis Pulmonary embolism/ infarction (two-thirds are exudates)	Constrictive pericarditis (previous tuberculosis, connective tissue diseases) Ovarian hyperstimulation syndrome Meigs' syndrome — ovarian tumour with right-sided effusion
Exudates (pleural fluid protein >30 g/l)	Malignancy (lung, breast, mesothelioma, metastatic) Parapneumonic (consider subphrenic)	Pulmonary embolism/ infarction (one-third are transudates) Rheumatoid arthritis Autoimmune disease (SLE, polyarteritis) Benign asbestos effusion Pancreatitis Post-myocardial infarction/ cardiotomy syndrome	Yellow nail syndrome Drugs: amiodarone, nitrofurantoin, phenytoin, methotrexate, carbamazepine, penicillamine, bromocriptine, pergolide

- Over normal lung the low-pitched components of speech are heard and high-pitched components attenuated
- Over consolidated lung (pneumonia) the numbers are clearly audible
- Over an effusion or area of collapse the sounds are muffled.

Whispering is not heard over the normal lung, but in consolidation (pneumonia) the sound is transmitted, producing 'whispering pectoriloquy'.

Normal breath sounds

Turbulent flow in large airways causes normal breath sounds heard at the chest wall. Through a stethoscope they have a rustling (vesicular) quality. The larynx makes little contribution in quiet breathing but may accentuate the noise in deep respiration.

The pattern and intensity of breath sounds reflect regional ventilation. Sounds are decreased through normal lungs since the parenchyma transmits sounds poorly. In an upright patient breath sounds are normally loudest at the apex in early inspiration and at the bases in mid-inspiration. During expiration, normal breath sounds rapidly fade as airflow decreases.

The intensity of breath sounds relates to airflow and the tissue through which the sound travels. Diminished vesicular breathing occurs in obesity, pleural effusion, marked pleural thickening, pneumothorax, hyperinflation due to COPD, and over an area of collapse where the underlying major bronchus is occluded (Box 7.23). If breath sounds appear reduced, ask the patient to cough. If the reduced breath sounds are due to bronchial obstruction by secretions, they are likely to become more audible after coughing.

Bronchial breathing

Bronchial breathing is a high-pitched breath sound with a hollow or blowing quality similar to that heard over the trachea and larynx during tidal breathing. The breath sounds are of similar length and intensity in inspiration and expiration, with a characteristic pause between the two phases (Fig. 7.24). Bronchial breath sounds are found whenever normal lung tissue is replaced by uniformly conducting tissue and the underlying major bronchus is patent (Box 7.24), so it tends to exclude the possibility of an obstructing lung cancer. Bronchial breathing and whispering pectoriloquy are heard over pulmonary consolidation from pneumonia, at the top of a pleural effusion and over areas of dense fibrosis.

Aegophony

Aegophony is a bleating or nasal sound heard over consolidated lung or at the upper level of a pleural effusion. It is due to enhanced transmission of high-frequency noise across abnormal lung, with lower frequencies filtered out.

Added sounds

Crackles

Interrupted non-musical sounds are called crackles. Crackles result from peripheral airways collapse on expiration. Air rapidly enters these distal airways on inspiration, and the alveoli and small bronchi abruptly open, producing the crackling noise.

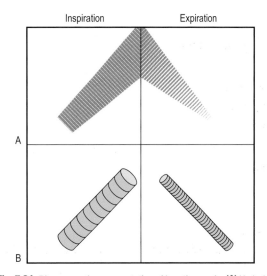

Fig. 7.24 **Diagrammatic representation of breath sounds. (A)** Vesicular. **(B)** Bronchial. Note the gap between inspiration and expiration and change in pitch and the blowing, tubular quality of bronchial breath sounds.

7.23 **Causes of diminished vesicular breathing**	
Reduced conduction	
• Obesity/thick chest wall	• Pneumothorax
• Pleural effusion or thickening	
Reduced air flow	
• Generalized, e.g. COPD	• Localized, e.g. collapsed lung due to occluding lung cancer

7.24 **Causes of bronchial breath sounds**	
Common	
• Lung consolidation (pneumonia)	
Uncommon	
• Localized pulmonary fibrosis	• Collapsed lung (where the underlying major bronchus is patent)
• At the top of a pleural effusion	

7.25 Causes of crackles

Phase of inspiration	Cause
Early	Small airways disease, as in bronchiolitis
Middle	Pulmonary oedema
Late	Pulmonary fibrosis (fine)
	Pulmonary oedema (medium)
	Bronchial secretions in COPD, pneumonia, lung abscess, tubercular lung cavities (coarse)
Biphasic	Bronchiectasis (coarse)

Note when crackles occur within the respiratory cycle (Box 7.25). Early inspiratory crackles suggest small airways disease and can occur in bronchiolitis. In pulmonary oedema crackles occur in mid-inspiration. Fine late inspiratory crackles, which sound similar to rubbing hair between your fingers, are characteristic of pulmonary fibrosis. Bronchiectasis causes crackles throughout inspiration and expiration.

Crackles may be heard when air bubbles through secretions in major bronchi, dilated bronchi in bronchiectasis or in pulmonary cavities. These crackles sound coarse, have a gurgling quality and change if the secretions are dislodged by coughing.

Wheeze

Wheezes have a musical quality caused by continuous oscillation of opposing airway walls. They imply airway narrowing and should be timed in relation to the respiratory cycle. Wheeze tends to be louder on expiration because airways normally dilate during inspiration and narrow on expiration. Inspiratory wheeze implies severe airway narrowing. High-pitched wheeze arises from smaller airways and has a whistling quality. Low-pitched wheeze originates from larger bronchi. It is very important to distinguish wheeze from the harsh rasping sound of stridor, which is only heard on inspiration.

Wheeze is characteristic of asthma and COPD, but is a poor guide to severity of airflow obstruction. In severe airways obstruction wheeze may be absent because of reduced airflow, producing a 'silent chest'. A fixed bronchial obstruction, most commonly due to lung cancer, may cause localized wheeze with a single musical note that does not clear on coughing.

Pleural friction rub

A pleural rub is a creaking sound similar to that produced by bending stiff leather or treading in fresh snow; it is produced when inflamed parietal and visceral pleurae move over one another. It is best heard with the stethoscope diaphragm. It may be heard only on deep breathing at the end of inspiration and beginning of expiration. A pleural

OSCEs 7.26 Examine this patient with pleuritic chest pain

1. General examination, assessing the degree and site of pain.
2. Examine for fever, confusion and raised respiratory rate — all possible in pneumonia.
3. Look for vasculitic skin spots (pulmonary vasculitis).
4. Examine JVP — raised in massive pulmonary embolism.
5. Palpate chest wall for tenderness — found in trauma, fractured rib and sometimes pulmonary embolism.
6. Percuss the chest — dullness is consistent with consolidation (pneumonia) or pleural effusion (pulmonary embolism).
7. Auscultate the chest — bronchial breathing is found over consolidation (pneumonia); reduced air entry over pleural effusion (pulmonary embolism); pleural friction rub heard over consolidation (pneumonia), pulmonary embolism with effusion and sometimes rib fracture.
8. Examine lower legs for signs of deep vein thrombosis (pulmonary embolism).

OSCEs 7.27 Examine this patient with fever and breathlessness

1. Record respiratory rate — >30/min is a sign of severe pneumonia.
2. Assess severity of breathlessness (use MRC scale).
3. Assess mental state and look for confusion — a sign of severe pneumonia.
4. Measure blood pressure — hypotension found in septicaemia; diastolic BP <60 mmHg is a sign of severe pneumonia.
5. Examine tongue and lips for central cyanosis (severe hypoxia).
6. Palpate for chest expansion — unilateral reduction in pleural effusion, empyema or consolidation (pneumonia).
7. Percuss the chest — dull note (consolidation/pneumonia), 'stony dull' note (pleural effusion/empyema).
8. Auscultate the chest — reduced breath sounds (pleural effusion), unilateral inspiratory crackles (bronchial infection or pneumonia), bronchial breathing and whispering pectoriloquy (consolidation/pneumonia).

rub is usually associated with pleuritic pain and may be heard over areas of inflamed pleura in pulmonary infarction, pneumonia or vasculitis. If the pleura adjacent to the pericardium is involved, a pleuropericardial rub may also be heard. Pleural friction rubs disappear if an effusion separates the pleural surfaces.

Pneumothorax click

This rhythmical sound, synchronous with cardiac systole, is produced when there is air between the two layers of pleura overlying the heart.

Mid-expiratory 'squeak'

This is characteristic in obliterative bronchiolitis — a rare complication of rheumatoid arthritis — where small airways are narrowed or obliterated by chronic inflammation and fibrosis.

PUTTING IT ALL TOGETHER

► Examination sequence

Respiratory system

☑ Note the patient's general appearance and demeanour.

☑ Observe the respiratory rate and pattern of breathing, and look for use of accessory muscles.

☑ Listen for hoarseness and stridor.

☑ Look for central cyanosis of the lips and tongue.

☑ Measure the blood pressure.

☑ Examine the skin for rashes and nodules.

☑ Examine the hands for finger clubbing, peripheral cyanosis and tremor.

☑ Examine the neck for raised JVP and cervical lymphadenopathy.

☑ Inspect the chest front and back for abnormalities of shape and scars.

☑ Feel the trachea and cardiac apex beat for evidence of mediastinal shift.

☑ Percuss the chest front and back for areas of dullness or hyper-resonance.

☑ Listen to the chest front and back for altered breath sounds and added sounds.

Certain groups of physical signs are typically associated with particular pathological changes in the lungs (Fig. 7.25).

Pulmonary embolism is an obstruction of part of the pulmonary vascular tree, usually caused by thrombus that has travelled from a distant site, e.g. deep veins in the legs or pelvic veins (Fig. 7.26). Pulmonary embolism is frequently unrecognized. Less than one-third of patients have symptoms or signs of deep vein thrombosis. The most common symptoms are:

- breathlessness (73%)
- pleuritic chest pain (66%), which may be reproduced by palpation over the area
- cough (37%).

The most common signs are:

- tachypnoea (70%), lung crackles (50%), tachycardia (30%), fever (6%) and pleural rub (5%).

Major risk factors for pulmonary embolism include:

- fracture of the hip, pelvis or leg
- hip or knee replacement
- major general surgery
- major trauma
- spinal cord injury
- malignancy.

INVESTIGATIONS

Chest X-ray

The standard chest X-ray is a posteroanterior (PA) view taken with the film in front of the anterior chest and the X-ray source 2 m behind the patient. In an anteroposterior (AP) film the X-ray source is in front of the patient, which tends to enlarge anterior structures such as the heart. A lateral film provides additional information about the nature and site of a pulmonary, pleural or mediastinal abnormality. Always compare an abnormal chest X-ray with previous films to see if abnormalities are resolving or longstanding.

You need knowledge of anatomy, pathology and normal appearances to interpret a chest X-ray (Fig. 7.27).

Systematically check:

- Name, date and orientation of the film: AP films are usually marked as such. Otherwise assume PA
- Lung fields: should be of equal translucency. Identify the horizontal fissure running from the right hilum to the 6th rib in the axillary line
- Lung apices: look specifically for masses, cavitation, consolidation, etc. above and behind the clavicles
- Trachea: confirm this is central, midway between the ends of the clavicles. Look for paratracheal masses, retrosternal goitre
- Heart: check that the heart is of normal shape and the maximum diameter is less than half the internal transthoracic diameter (cardiothoracic ratio). Look specifically for any retrocardiac masses
- Hila: the left hilum should be higher than the right. Compare the shape and density of the two hila; both should appear concave laterally. A convex appearance suggests a mass or lymphadenopathy
- Diaphragms: the right hemidiaphragm should be higher than the left. The anterior end of the right 6th rib should cross the mid-diaphragm. If not, the lungs are hyperinflated
- Costophrenic angles: these should be well-defined, acute angles. Loss of one or both suggests pleural fluid or pleural thickening
- Soft tissues: note the presence of both breast shadows in female patients. Look around the chest wall for any soft tissue masses or subcutaneous emphysema, etc
- Bones: look closely at the ribs, scapulae and vertebrae for fractures and metastatic deposits in each bone

Sputum examination

The normal lung produces about 100 ml of clear sputum each day, which is transported to the oropharynx and swallowed. Coughing up sputum is always abnormal. Inpatients with respiratory symptoms should have a sputum pot for inspection.

Send sputum for cytological examination in patients with unexplained haemoptysis or suspected lung cancer. In lower respiratory tract infection or pneumonia,

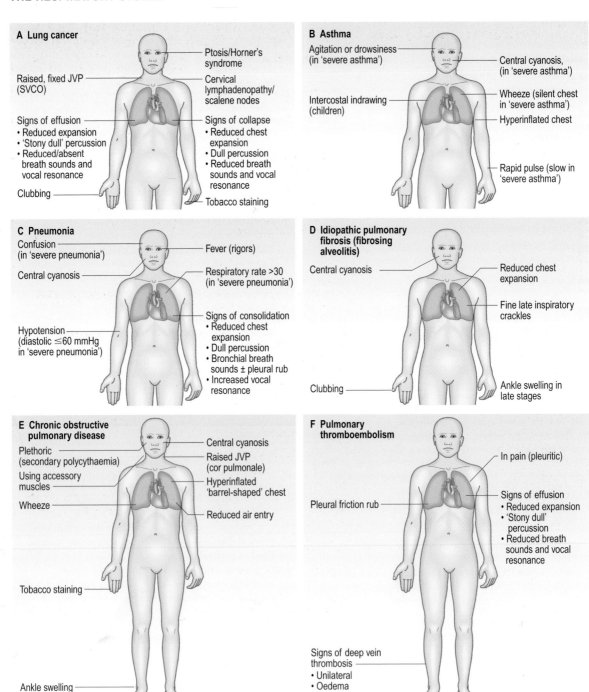

A Lung cancer

Ptosis/Horner's syndrome

Raised, fixed JVP (SVCO)

Cervical lymphadenopathy/ scalene nodes

Signs of effusion
• Reduced expansion
• 'Stony dull' percussion
• Reduced/absent breath sounds and vocal resonance

Signs of collapse
• Reduced chest expansion
• Dull percussion
• Reduced breath sounds and vocal resonance

Clubbing

Tobacco staining

B Asthma

Agitation or drowsiness (in 'severe asthma')

Central cyanosis, (in 'severe asthma')

Intercostal indrawing (children)

Wheeze (silent chest in 'severe asthma')

Hyperinflated chest

Rapid pulse (slow in 'severe asthma')

C Pneumonia

Confusion (in 'severe pneumonia')

Fever (rigors)

Central cyanosis

Respiratory rate >30 (in 'severe pneumonia')

Signs of consolidation
• Reduced chest expansion
• Dull percussion
• Bronchial breath sounds ± pleural rub
• Increased vocal resonance

Hypotension (diastolic ≤60 mmHg in 'severe pneumonia')

D Idiopathic pulmonary fibrosis (fibrosing alveolitis)

Central cyanosis

Reduced chest expansion

Fine late inspiratory crackles

Clubbing

Ankle swelling in late stages

E Chronic obstructive pulmonary disease

Plethoric (secondary polycythaemia)

Central cyanosis

Raised JVP (cor pulmonale)

Using accessory muscles

Hyperinflated 'barrel-shaped' chest

Wheeze

Reduced air entry

Tobacco staining

Ankle swelling (cor pulmonale)

F Pulmonary thromboembolism

In pain (pleuritic)

Pleural friction rub

Signs of effusion
• Reduced expansion
• 'Stony dull' percussion
• Reduced breath sounds and vocal resonance

Signs of deep vein thrombosis
• Unilateral
• Oedema
• Warmth
• Tenderness

Fig. 7.25 Clinical signs of common respiratory conditions.

7.28 Investigations in respiratory disease

Investigation	Indication/Comment
Bedside	
Peak flow rate	Monitoring of asthma/acute asthma
Oximetry	Respiratory failure
	Assessment of oxygen requirements
Blood tests	
White cell count	High in lower respiratory tract infection
Haematocrit	Elevated in polycythaemia
Eosinophil count	High in:
	Allergic asthma
	Pulmonary eosinophilia
	Allergic bronchopulmonary aspergillosis
	Churg–Strauss syndrome
C-reactive protein (CRP)	High in:
	Pneumonia
	Empyema
Serum sodium	Reduced in:
	Small cell lung cancer (inappropriate antidiuretic hormone (ADH) secretion)
	Legionnaire's disease and any severe pneumonia
Blood and urine osmolality	Inappropriate ADH secretion
Serum calcium	Elevated in bony metastases, sarcoidosis and squamous cell lung cancer
Liver function tests	Metastatic liver disease
Immunoglobulins	Deficiencies in bronchiectasis
ACE activity	Elevated in sarcoidosis
Alpha-1-antitrypsin	Deficiency in hereditary panacinar emphysema
Total and specific (radioallergosorbent test) IgE	Atopic status (asthma)
Antinuclear factor	Idiopathic pulmonary fibrosis (fibrosing alveolitis)
Antineutrophil cytoplasmic antibody (ANCA)	
Proteinase 3 (cANCA)	Wegener's granulomatosis
Myeloperoxidase (pANCA)	Microscopic polyangiitis
	Churg–Strauss syndrome
Farmer's lung and avian precipitins	Extrinsic allergic alveolitis
Cold agglutinins (IgM)	*Mycoplasma* infection
Serology (IgG antibodies)	Viral respiratory tract infection, e.g. influenza, respiratory syncytial virus
	Small bacterial infection, e.g. *Mycoplasma*, *Legionella*, *Chlamydia*
D-dimer	Venous thromboembolism
Immunoreactive trypsin	Screening for cystic fibrosis
Complement fixation transmembrane regulator (CFTR) genotyping	Cystic fibrosis
Gamma interferon release assay	Latent infection with *Mycobacterium tuberculosis*
Urine tests	
Pneumococcal capsular antigen	Pneumococcal bacteraemia
Legionella urinary antigen	Legionnaire's disease
Skin tests	
Mantoux test	Exposure to *Mycobacterium tuberculosis*
Allergen skin prick tests	Atopic status (asthma)
Sweat test	Cystic fibrosis in children
Respiratory function	
Arterial blood gas tensions	Respiratory failure, acid–base balance
Spirometry	Diagnosis/monitoring of COPD and asthma
Carbon monoxide gas transfer	Reduced in:
	Interstitial lung disease
	Emphysema/COPD
Flow volume curves	Detection of extra- and intrathoracic large airway obstruction
Maximal mouth pressures	Respiratory neuromuscular disorders
Erect and supine FVC	Respiratory neuromuscular disorders

7

7.28 Continued

Investigation	Indication/Comment
Exercise test	
6 min run	Diagnosis of asthma in children and young adults
6 min walk test	Assessment of disability, e.g. in COPD
Cardiopulmonary exercise test	Peak oxygen consumption (VO_2)
	Differentiates breathlessness due to lung disease from that due to heart disease
Bronchial challenge test	Exclusion of asthma
Bronchial provocation studies	Asthma, especially occupational asthma
Exhaled nitric oxide	Inhaled steroid dosage in asthma
Overnight sleep study	Sleep apnoea/hypopnoea syndrome
Radiology	
CT scan of thorax	Pulmonary or mediastinal mass
	Staging of lung cancer
	Pleural disease
High-resolution CT	Interstitial lung disease
	Bronchiectasis
Isotope VQ lung scan	Pulmonary thromboembolism
CT pulmonary angiogram	Pulmonary thromboembolism
	Pulmonary hypertension
Echocardiogram	Right heart dilatation (cor pulmonale)
Ultrasound of chest wall	Localization of pleural effusion
Positron emission tomography/CT	Staging of lung cancer
Invasive	
Lymph node aspiration	Cervical lymphadenopathy
Bronchoscopy	Suspected lung cancer
	Suspected foreign body inhalation
	Obtaining specimens for microbiology
Transbronchial lung biopsy	Suspected pulmonary sarcoidosis
	Suspected diffuse malignancy
Pleural aspiration and biopsy	Undiagnosed pleural effusion
Percutaneous fine needle lung aspiration	Peripheral lesion/suspected lung cancer
Mediastinoscopy	Staging of lung cancer
	Mediastinal mass
Thoracoscopy	Undiagnosed pleural disease
Lung biopsy (open or video-assisted thoracoscopic surgery)	Interstitial lung disease

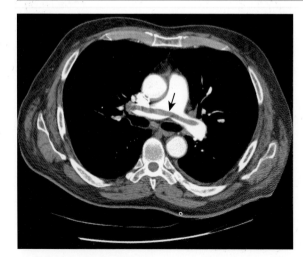

Fig. 7.26 CT pulmonary angiogram showing large embolus within the main pulmonary artery (arrowed).

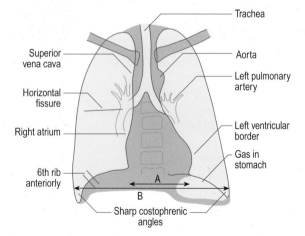

Fig. 7.27 Normal posteroanterior chest X-ray. Note vertebral outlines just seen through the heart shadow. A/B: the cardiothoracic ratio (CTR) should be <50%.

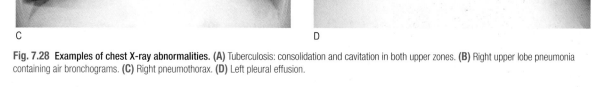

Fig. 7.28 Examples of chest X-ray abnormalities. (A) Tuberculosis: consolidation and cavitation in both upper zones. **(B)** Right upper lobe pneumonia containing air bronchograms. **(C)** Right pneumothorax. **(D)** Left pleural effusion.

send sputum for microbiological culture. Gram stain of sputum helps rapid identification of the causative organism: for example, Gram-positive — pneumococcus or staphylococcus; Gram-negative — *Haemophilus influenzae*. Patients with symptoms and chest X-ray suggesting pulmonary tuberculosis should have several sputum samples sent urgently for auramine staining (screening); if these are positive, a Ziehl–Neelsen stain

should be obtained. Positive samples indicate a high degree of infectivity and the patient must be urgently isolated and treated, and the condition notified.

Pulse oximetry

An oximeter is a spectrophotometric device that measures arterial oxygen saturation (SpO_2) by determining the

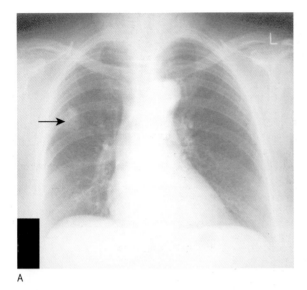

A

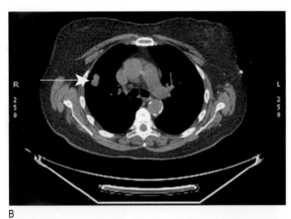

B

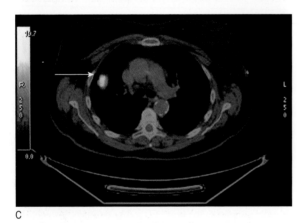

C

Fig. 7.29 Lung cancer in right lung. (A) Chest X-ray. **(B)** CT scan of thorax. **(C)** Positron emission tomography (PET)/CT scan showing increased uptake in tumour.

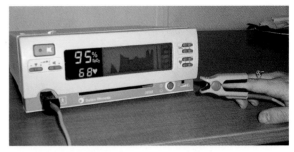

Fig. 7.30 Pulse oximeter with probe on finger.

differential absorption of light by oxyhaemoglobin and deoxyhaemoglobin. Modern oximeters use a probe incorporating a light source and sensor that is attached to a patient's ear or finger (Fig. 7.30).

Oximeters are easy to use, portable, non-invasive and inexpensive. They are widely used for the continuous measurement of SpO_2 and to adjust oxygen therapy. In acutely ill patients with no risk of CO_2 retention, SpO_2 should be maintained at 94–98%. Movement artifact, poor tissue perfusion, hypothermia and nail varnish can lead to spuriously low SpO_2 values. Dark skin pigmentation, and raised levels of bilirubin or carboxyhaemoglobin can result in false increases in SpO_2. Oximetry is less accurate with saturations <75% and unreliable when peripheral perfusion is poor.

Arterial blood gas analysis

Arterial blood gas (PaO_2, $PaCO_2$) and acid–base (pH) status are obtained from heparinized samples of arterial blood from the radial, brachial or femoral artery (Box 7.29). Figure 7.31 shows the relationship of arterial pH (H^+), $PaCO_2$ and bicarbonate with disturbances of acid–base balance.

Respiratory acidosis

An acute rise in $PaCO_2$ caused by alveolar hypoventilation occurs in severe acute asthma, severe pneumonia and exacerbations of COPD, and is associated with a decrease in pH. Elevation of $PaCO_2$ for more than 2–3 days may occur in COPD, respiratory muscle weakness due to neuromuscular disorders and thoracic skeletal deformities, and leads to renal retention of HCO_3^- and normalization of pH. This pattern of reduced PaO_2, raised $PaCO_2$ and normal pH is known as compensated respiratory acidosis. In some patients with COPD low PaO_2 levels drive respiratory effort. Removal of this stimulus by excessive oxygen therapy may result in alveolar hypoventilation with further increase in $PaCO_2$, which can lead to deterioration and death.

Respiratory alkalosis

Hyperventilation occurs with respiratory conditions (asthma, pulmonary thromboembolism, pleurisy), high altitude and acute anxiety. Alveolar hyperventilation leads to decrease in $PaCO_2$ and a consequent increase

7.29 Common causes of acid–base disturbance

Disturbance	pH	CO_2	HCO_3	Cause
Respiratory acidosis	↓	↑	↑	Acute ventilatory failure with: Severe acute asthma Severe pneumonia Exacerbation of COPD Thoracic skeletal abnormality, e.g. kyphoscoliosis Neuromuscular disorders, e.g. muscular dystrophy
Respiratory alkalosis	↑	↓	↓	Hyperventilation due to anxiety/panic Central nervous system causes, e.g. stroke, subarachnoid haemorrhage Salicylate poisoning, early phase
Metabolic acidosis	↓	↓	↓	Increased production of organic acids: Diabetic ketoacidosis Poisoning: alcohol, methanol, ethylene glycol, iron, salicylate Acute renal failure Lactic acidosis, e.g. shock, post-cardiac arrest Loss of bicarbonate: Renal tubular acidosis Severe diarrhoea Addison's disease
Metabolic alkalosis	↑	↑	↑	Loss of acid: Severe vomiting Nasogastric suction Loss of potassium: Excess diuretic therapy Hyperaldosteronism Cushing's syndrome Liquorice ingestion Excess alkali ingestion: milk–alkali syndrome

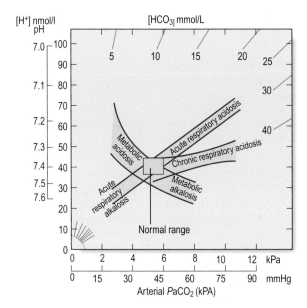

Fig. 7.31 Acid–base diagram. Acid–base nomogram for the interpretation of arterial blood gases. The bands represent 95% confidence limits of acid–base disturbance.

in pH. If hyperventilation persists, as occurs with stays at high altitude, increased renal excretion of HCO_3^- results in normalization of pH, i.e. compensated respiratory alkalosis.

Metabolic acidosis

The primary abnormality of metabolic acidosis is loss of HCO_3^- and decrease in pH. This can occur in acute renal failure, diabetic ketoacidosis and lactic acidosis. The decrease in pH stimulates arterial chemoreceptors, resulting in alveolar hyperventilation with a consequent decrease in $PaCO_2$.

Metabolic alkalosis

The primary abnormality of metabolic alkalosis is retention of HCO_3^-, often related to tubular K^+ depletion or loss of H^+ resulting in an increase in pH. The increase in pH induces alveolar hypoventilation via arterial chemoreceptors, with consequent increase in $PaCO_2$.

Spirometry

Dynamic lung volumes are measured by inhaling to total lung capacity and then exhaling into a spirometer with maximal effort to residual volume. The volume

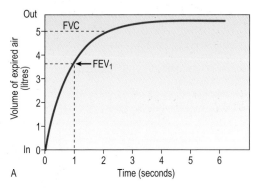
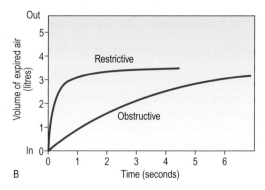

Fig. 7.32 Volume–time curves obtained using a wedge-bellows spirometer. (A) The patient takes a full inspiration and exhales forcibly and fully. Maximal flow decelerates as forced expansion proceeds. **(B)** Obstructive and restrictive patterns. In obstruction, FEV$_1$/FVC is low; in restriction, it is normal or high.

exhaled in the first second is the forced expiratory volume in 1 second (FEV$_1$) and the total volume exhaled is the forced vital capacity (FVC). Normal predictive values for FEV$_1$ and FVC are influenced by age, gender, height and race. In healthy young and middle-aged adults the FEV$_1$/FVC ratio is usually >75%. In the elderly the ratio is usually 70–75%. Reduction in the FEV$_1$/FVC ratio indicates airway obstruction. The severity of obstruction is represented by the absolute FEV$_1$ expressed as a percentage of predicted. Airway obstruction that reverses with inhaled β$_2$-agonist or a trial of oral steroid over 5 days or more (an absolute increase in FEV$_1$ >200 ml that is >15% of baseline) favours a diagnosis of asthma over COPD.

In interstitial lung disorders, e.g. idiopathic pulmonary fibrosis, pulmonary sarcoidosis or extrinsic allergic alveolitis, there is a decrease in FVC with preservation of FEV$_1$/FVC ratio, a restrictive defect (Fig. 7.32).

Peak expiratory flow

Peak expiratory flow (PEF) is measured by inhaling to total lung capacity and exhaling into a peak flow meter with maximal effort. Measurement of PEF is vital in the assessment of acute asthma, in monitoring response to treatment and for the diagnosis of occupational asthma where falls in PEF occur during the working week but improve during weekends and holidays. Early morning falls in PEF of >60 l/min (>20% maximal PEF) are very suggestive of asthma. A >60 l/min fall in PEF (>15% baseline) after exercise is diagnostic of asthma.

7.30 Key points: the respiratory system

- Night-time wakening with cough and wheeze is characteristic of poorly controlled asthma.
- Always consider an occupational cause in adult-onset asthma.
- Consider sleep apnoea in patients who snore and have daytime sleepiness. Ask specifically about driving and occupational risks.
- Chronic cough with a normal chest X-ray is usually caused by smoking, sinusitis, GORD, asthma or ACE inhibitors.
- Patients with severe COPD may lose weight.
- Respiratory rate, blood pressure and mental state are important markers of pneumonia severity.
- Always investigate haemoptysis in a smoker with a chest X-ray and, if appropriate, bronchoscopy.
- 'Bovine cough' or superior vena caval obstruction in a patient with lung cancer indicates that the tumour is inoperable.
- Bronchial breathing is unlikely in lung cancer.
- Distinguish stridor from wheeze, and always investigate its cause.
- Pulmonary thromboembolism usually occurs in the absence of clinical signs of deep vein thrombosis.
- Local chest wall tenderness occurs in costochondritis, rib fracture and pulmonary infarction.
- Always perform pleural biopsy on initial aspiration of an undiagnosed pleural effusion.
- In patients with suspected pulmonary tuberculosis, arrange urgent sputum examination by auramine (screening) and Ziehl–Neelsen staining. If positive, the patient should be isolated and treated, and the disease notified.

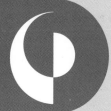

The gastrointestinal system

Michael J. Ford
Alastair MacGilchrist
Rowan W. Parks

8

GASTROINTESTINAL EXAMINATION

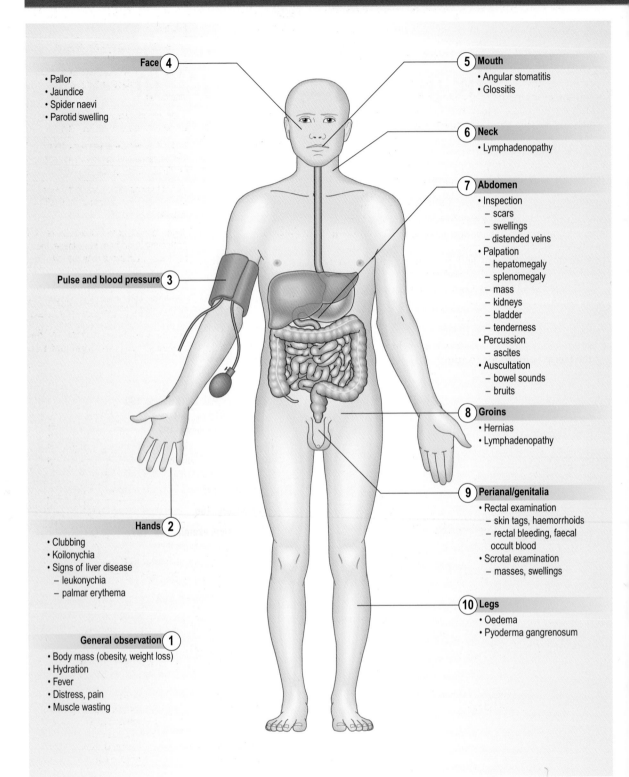

Face (4)
- Pallor
- Jaundice
- Spider naevi
- Parotid swelling

(5) **Mouth**
- Angular stomatitis
- Glossitis

(6) **Neck**
- Lymphadenopathy

(7) **Abdomen**
- Inspection
  - scars
  - swellings
  - distended veins
- Palpation
  - hepatomegaly
  - splenomegaly
  - mass
  - kidneys
  - bladder
  - tenderness
- Percussion
  - ascites
- Auscultation
  - bowel sounds
  - bruits

Pulse and blood pressure (3)

(8) **Groins**
- Hernias
- Lymphadenopathy

(9) **Perianal/genitalia**
- Rectal examination
  - skin tags, haemorrhoids
  - rectal bleeding, faecal occult blood
- Scrotal examination
  - masses, swellings

Hands (2)
- Clubbing
- Koilonychia
- Signs of liver disease
  - leukonychia
  - palmar erythema

(10) **Legs**
- Oedema
- Pyoderma gangrenosum

General observation (1)
- Body mass (obesity, weight loss)
- Hydration
- Fever
- Distress, pain
- Muscle wasting

ANATOMY

The gastrointestinal tract extends from the mouth to the anus and includes the oesophagus, stomach, duodenum, small and large bowel, and rectum (Figs 8.1–8,4),

After swallowing, peristalsis propels the food bolus down the oesophagus to the stomach. Food is retained within the stomach, where it is exposed to gastric acid which starts digestion. Partially digested food then passes into the duodenum and small bowel.

In the fasted state the small bowel has very little muscular activity, but every 1–2 hours a wave of peristaltic activity (the migrating motor complex) occurs. Fluid containing amylase, lipase, colipase and proteolytic enzymes is secreted into the small bowel by the pancreas. Every day the liver secretes 1–2 litres of bile, containing bile acids and phospholipids, into the small bowel. These enzymes and salts aid breakdown of complex sugars, fats and protein, which are then absorbed across the small bowel mucosa.

The large bowel (colon) absorbs water and electrolytes, and is subject to two types of contraction:

- segmentation (ring contraction), which forms stools
- propulsion (peristaltic contraction), which propels the faecal bolus to the rectum.

8.1 Surface markings of the gastrointestinal system

Structure	Position
Liver	Upper border: 5th right intercostal space on full expiration Lower border: at the costal margin in the midclavicular line (MCL) on full inspiration
Spleen	Underlies left ribs 9, 10 and 11, posterior to the mid-axillary line
Gallbladder	At the intersection of the right lateral vertical plane and the costal margin i.e. tip of the 9th costal cartilage
Pancreas	Neck of the pancreas lies at the level of L1; head lies below and right; tail lies above and right
Kidneys	Upper pole lies deep to the 12th rib posteriorly, 7 cm from the midline; the right is 2–3 cm lower than the left

The abdomen

The abdomen can be divided into nine regions by the intersection of imaginary planes: two horizontal and two vertical (Fig. 8.5).

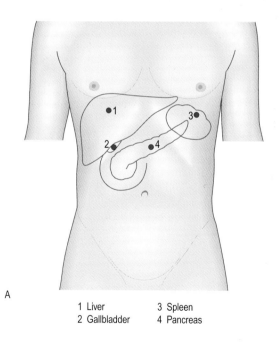

A

1 Liver   3 Spleen
2 Gallbladder   4 Pancreas

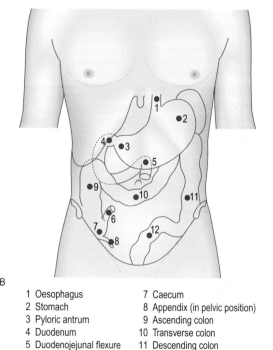

B

1 Oesophagus   7 Caecum
2 Stomach   8 Appendix (in pelvic position)
3 Pyloric antrum   9 Ascending colon
4 Duodenum   10 Transverse colon
5 Duodenojejunal flexure 11 Descending colon
6 Terminal ileum   12 Sigmoid colon

Fig. 8.1 Surface anatomy. (A) Surface markings of non-alimentary tract abdominal viscera. **(B)** Surface markings of the alimentary tract.

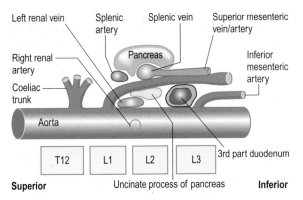

Fig. 8.2 **Longitudinal section at L1 vertebral level:** viewed from the right.

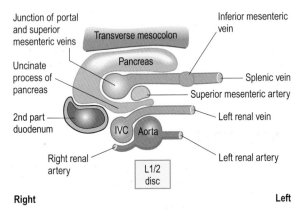

Fig. 8.3 **Axial cross section at L1 vertebral level:** looking towards the head.

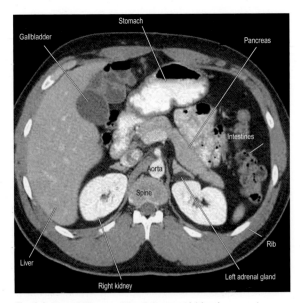

Fig. 8.4 **Normal CT scan of the abdomen at L1 level.**

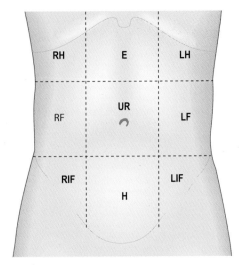

Fig. 8.5 **Regions of the abdomen.** RH, right hypochondrium; RF, right flank or lumbar region; RIF, right iliac fossa; E, epigastrium; UR, umbilical region; H, hypogastrium or suprapubic region; LH, left hypochondrium; LF, left flank or lumbar region; LIF, left iliac fossa.

Normal appearance

The abdomen is normally flat or slightly scaphoid and symmetrical. At rest, respiration is principally diaphragmatic; the abdominal wall moves out and the liver, spleen and kidneys move downwards during inspiration. The umbilicus is usually inverted.

The normal liver is identified as an area of dullness to percussion over the right anterior chest between the 5th rib and the costal margin. The normal spleen is identified as an area of dullness to percussion posterior to the left mid-axillary line beneath the 9th, 10th and 11th ribs.

Normal findings on abdominal palpation may include the following (Fig. 8.1):

- the liver edge may be felt below the right costal margin
- the aorta may be palpable as a pulsatile swelling above the umbilicus
- the lower pole of the right kidney may be palpable in the right flank
- faecal scybala may be palpable in the sigmoid colon in the left iliac fossa
- a full bladder arising out of the pelvis may be palpable in the suprapubic region.

SYMPTOMS AND DEFINITIONS

Anorexia and weight loss

Anorexia is loss of appetite and/or a lack of interest in food. In addition to asking about appetite, ask 'Do you still enjoy your food/meals?'.

8.2 Common gastrointestinal symptoms

Symptom	Definition
General	
Anorexia	Loss of appetite
Weight loss	Significant >3 kg in 6 months
Pain	Midline or lateralized: chest, abdomen or pelvis
Abdominal distension	Localized or generalized
Upper gastrointestinal	
Xerostomia	Dry mouth
Halitosis	Bad breath due to gingival, dental or pharyngeal infection
Painful lips, tongue and mouth	Pain at the angles of the mouth and buccal mucosa
Dysgeusia	Altered taste sensation
Cacageusia	Foul taste sensation, e.g. rotting food
Globus	Sensation of a lump in the throat
Odynophagia	Pain on swallowing
Heartburn	Burning retrosternal discomfort radiating upward
Water brash	Sudden appearance of excessive saliva in the mouth
Dyspepsia	Non-specific epigastric discomfort — 'indigestion'
Early satiety	Premature fullness on eating
Nausea	Feeling sick
Haematemesis	Vomiting fresh or altered blood
Hiccups	Persistent hiccups suggest diaphragmatic disorder
Lower gastrointestinal	
Wind and flatulence	Excessive, offensive flatus
Bloating	Uncomfortable distension
Altered bowel habit	
Diarrhoea	Abnormally soft stools and/or frequent defecation
Constipation	Abnormally firm stools and/or infrequent defecation
Steatorrhoea	Fatty stools, pale, greasy, difficult to flush
Haematochezia	Rectal bleeding
Anismus/dyschezia	Difficulty emptying the rectum despite prolonged straining
Tenesmus	Persistent urge to empty the rectum with the feeling of incomplete evacuation
Melaena	Black, tarry stools indicating bleeding from the upper GI tract
Hepatobiliary	
Jaundice (icterus)	Yellow discoloration of skin and sclerae
Itch (pruritus)	Generalized itch

Weight loss is usually the result of reduced energy intake, not increased energy expenditure (Box 8.3). Reduced energy intake arises from dieting, loss of appetite or malabsorption. Energy loss occurs in uncontrolled diabetes mellitus due to marked glycosuria. Increased energy expenditure occurs in hyperthyroidism, fever or the adoption of a more energetic lifestyle. A net calorie deficit of 1000 kcal per day will produce a weight loss of approximately 1 kg per week (7000 kcal is the equivalent of 1 kg of fat). Greater weight loss during the initial stages of energy restriction arises from salt and water loss and depletion of hepatic glycogen stores, and not from fat loss. Rapid weight loss over days suggests loss of body fluid, such as with vomiting, diarrhoea or diuretic therapy (1 litre of water = 1 kg).

Isolated weight loss is rarely associated with serious organic disease, and loss of <3 kg in the previous 6 months is rarely significant. Confirm subjective assessment of weight loss from ill-fitting clothes and by reviewing documented weights from the case records. Weight loss does not specifically indicate gastrointestinal disease but is common in many upper gastrointestinal disorders, including malignancy and liver diseases. Weight loss with amenorrhoea in an adolescent female suggests anorexia nervosa. However, amenorrhoea is not specific to anorexia nervosa and menstrual irregularity is common in women who lose weight from any cause.

Painful mouth

There are many causes of sore lips, tongue or buccal mucosa, including iron, folate or vitamin B_{12} deficiency, dermatological disorders, e.g. lichen planus, chemotherapy, aphthous ulcers and infective stomatitis (Box 8.4 and Fig. 8.6). Inflammatory bowel disease and gluten enteropathy are associated with mouth ulcers. Aphthous mouth ulcers are suggested by a history of recurrent painful tiny mouth ulcers, onset at the menarche, exacerbations during menstruation and a family history of mouth ulcers.

Dysphagia

Dysphagia (Boxes 8.5 and 8.6) is difficulty swallowing; it should always be investigated. Ask the patient, 'Does food (or drink) stick when you swallow?'. Do not confuse dysphagia with early satiety, the inability to complete a full meal because of premature fullness, or globus, the feeling of a lump in the throat. Globus does not interfere with swallowing and is not related to eating.

Odynophagia is pain on swallowing, often precipitated by drinking hot liquids. It can be present with or without dysphagia and may indicate active oesophageal ulceration from peptic oesophagitis or oesophageal candidiasis. It indicates intact mucosal sensation, making oesophageal cancer unlikely.

Neurological dysphagia resulting from bulbar or pseudobulbar palsies is typically worse for liquids

8

8.3 Energy requirements

Males	2500 kcal/day
Females	2000 kcal/day
Calorie deficit of 500 kcal/day = weight loss of 0.5 kg/week	
No calorie intake at all = weight loss of approximately 2 kg/week	

8.4 Causes of a painful mouth

Idiopathic

- Recurrent aphthous mouth ulcers

Infections

- Candidiasis
- Dental sepsis
- Herpes simplex virus (HSV1 and 2)
- Coxsackie A virus: herpangina, hand-foot-mouth, Vincent's angina (ulcerative gingivitis)

Miscellaneous

- Trauma from teeth/dentures
- Leukoplakia

Associated with systemic disorder

- Drugs allergies, e.g. sulphonamides, gold, cytotoxics
- Iron, folate, vitamin B_{12} deficiency
- Leucopenia, acute leukaemia
- Reactive arthritis, Behçet's disease
- Crohn's disease, ulcerative colitis
- Coeliac disease

Associated with skin disorder

- Lichen planus, erythema multiforme
- Pemphigoid, pemphigus vulgaris

8.5 Causes of dysphagia

Oral

- Painful mouth ulcers
- Tonsillitis, glandular fever, pharyngitis, peritonsillar abscess

Neurological

- Cerebrovascular accident
- Bulbar or pseudobulbar palsy

Neuromuscular

- Achalasia
- Pharyngeal pouch
- Myasthenia gravis
- Oesophageal dysmotility

Mechanical

- Oesophageal cancer
- Peptic oesophagitis
- Other benign strictures, e.g. after prolonged nasogastric intubation
- Extrinsic compression, e.g. lung cancer
- Systemic sclerosis

8.6 Symptom checklist in dysphagia

- Is dysphagia painful or painless?
- Is dysphagia intermittent or progressive?
- How long is the history of dysphagia?
- Is there a previous history of dysphagia or heartburn?
- Is the dysphagia for solids or liquids or both?
- At what level does food stick?
- Is there complete obstruction with regurgitation?

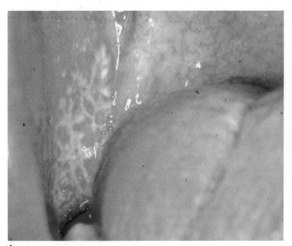

A

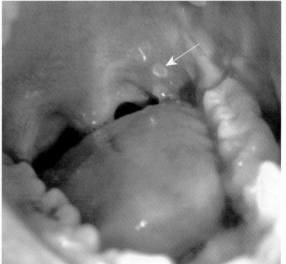

B

Fig. 8.6 Some causes of a painful mouth. (A) Lichen planus. **(B)** Small, 'punched out' aphthous ulcer.

than for solids, and may be accompanied by choking, spluttering and regurgitating fluid from the nose.

Neuromuscular dysphagia, or oesophageal dysmotility, most often presents in middle age. It is worse for solids and may be helped by liquids and sitting upright. Achalasia, when the lower oesophageal sphincter fails to relax normally, leads to progressive oesophageal dilatation above the sphincter. Overflow of secretions and food into the respiratory tract may then occur, especially at night when the patient lies down, and cause aspiration pneumonia. Oesophageal dysmotility can cause oesophageal spasm and central chest pain, and may be confused with cardiac pain.

'Mechanical' dysphagia is often due to oesophageal stricture. With weight loss, a short history and no reflux symptoms, suspect oesophageal cancer. Longstanding dysphagia without weight loss but accompanied by heartburn is more likely to be due to benign peptic stricture. The site at which the patient feels the food sticking is not a reliable guide to the site of oesophageal obstruction. Dysphagia should always be investigated to distinguish between oesophageal cancer and benign stricture.

Heartburn and reflux symptoms

Heartburn is a hot, burning retrosternal discomfort which radiates upwards. When heartburn is the principal symptom, gastro-oesophageal reflux disease (GORD) is the likeliest diagnosis. Regurgitating gastric acid producing a sour taste in the mouth is called acid reflux. Differentiate heartburn from cardiac chest pain by its burning quality, upward radiation, association with acid reflux and its occurrence on lying flat or bending forward. Water brash, the sudden onset of excessive saliva in the mouth due to reflex salivation, is uncommon but may occur in peptic ulcer disease.

Dyspepsia

Indigestion is a term commonly used for ill-defined symptoms from the upper gastrointestinal tract. Dyspepsia is pain or discomfort centred in the upper abdomen. Dyspepsia affects up to 80% of the population at some time. In the majority, no identifiable cause is found (functional dyspepsia). Clusters of symptoms are used to classify dyspepsia:

- reflux-like dyspepsia (heartburn-predominant dyspepsia)
- ulcer-like dyspepsia (epigastric pain relieved by food or antacids)
- dysmotility-like dyspepsia (nausea, belching, bloating and premature satiety).

There is considerable overlap and it is impossible to diagnose functional dyspepsia on history alone, without investigation. Dyspepsia that is worse with an empty stomach and eased by eating is the classical symptom of peptic ulceration. The patient may indicate a single localized point in the epigastrium (pointing sign), and complain of nausea and abdominal fullness which is worse after meals with a high spice or fat content. 'Fat intolerance' is common in all causes of dyspepsia, including gallbladder disease.

Nausea and vomiting

Nausea is the sensation of feeling sick. Vomiting is the expulsion of gastric contents via the mouth. Both are associated with pallor, sweating and hyperventilation. Nausea and vomiting, particularly with abdominal pain or discomfort, suggest upper gastrointestinal disorders. Remember to consider non-gastrointestinal causes of nausea and vomiting, especially adverse drug effects, pregnancy and vestibular disorders (Boxes 8.7 and 8.8).

Dyspepsia causes nausea without vomiting. Peptic ulcers seldom cause painless vomiting unless complicated by pyloric stenosis. Gastric outlet obstruction causes projectile vomiting of large volumes of gastric content that is not bile-stained (green). Obstruction distal to the pylorus produces bile-stained vomit. The more distal the level of intestinal obstruction, the more marked the accompanying symptoms of abdominal distension and intestinal colic.

Vomiting is common in gastroenteritis, cholecystitis, pancreatitis and hepatitis. Vomiting is typically preceded by nausea, but in raised intracranial pressure

8.7 Non-alimentary causes of vomiting

Neurological

- Raised intracranial pressure, e.g. meningitis, brain tumour
- Labyrinthitis and Ménière's disease
- Migraine
- Vasovagal syncope, shock, fear and severe pain, e.g. renal colic, myocardial infarction

Drugs

- Alcohol, opioids, theophyllines, digoxin, cytotoxic agents, antidepressants
- Consider any drug

Metabolic/endocrine

- Pregnancy
- Diabetic ketoacidosis
- Renal failure
- Liver failure
- Hypercalcaemia
- Addison's disease

Psychological

- Anorexia nervosa
- Bulimia

8

8.8 Symptom checklist in vomiting

- What medications has the patient been taking?
- Is vomiting heralded by nausea or does it occur without warning?
- Is vomiting associated with dyspepsia or abdominal pain?
- Is dyspepsia or abdominal pain relieved by vomiting?
- Is vomiting related to meal-times, early morning or late evening?
- Is the vomitus bile-stained, bloodstained or faeculent?

8.9 Symptom checklist in haematemesis and melaena

- Is there a previous history of dyspepsia, peptic ulceration, GI bleeding or liver disease?
- Is there a history of alcohol, NSAID or corticosteroid ingestion?
- Did the vomitus comprise fresh blood or coffee ground-stained fluid?
- Was the haematemesis preceded by intense retching?
- Was bloodstaining of the vomitus apparent in the first vomit?

may occur without warning. Vomiting may be caused by severe pain, e.g. renal or biliary colic, myocardial infarction, or by systemic disease, metabolic disorders and drug therapy.

Anorexia nervosa and bulimia are eating disorders characterized by undisclosed, self-induced vomiting. In bulimia, weight is maintained or increased, unlike in anorexia nervosa where weight loss is obvious. Rumination, the habitual, involuntary, subconscious regurgitation of gastric contents which are then chewed and swallowed, is uncommon.

Haematemesis and melaena

Haematemesis is the vomiting of blood, which can be fresh and red, or degraded by gastric pepsin, when it is dark brown in colour and resembles coffee grounds (Box 8.9). If the source of bleeding is above the gastro-oesophageal sphincter, e.g. from oesophageal varices, fresh blood may well up in the mouth, as well as being actively vomited. With a lower oesophageal mucosal tear due to the trauma of retching (Mallory–Weiss syndrome) the patient vomits forcefully several times and fresh blood only appears after the initial vomit. Melaena results from upper gastrointestinal bleeding; the stool is 'tarry' and shiny black with a characteristic odour. Distinguish this from the matt black stools associated with oral iron or bismuth therapy. Enquire about recent ingestion of aspirin, non-steroidal anti-inflammatory drugs (NSAIDs) and alcohol. Excessive alcohol ingestion may cause haematemesis from erosive gastritis, Mallory–Weiss tear or bleeding oesophageal varices. Peptic ulceration is a common cause of upper gastrointestinal bleeding (Box 8.10). The Rockall score is used to assess the mortality risk associated with upper gastrointestinal bleeding (Box 8.11).

Abdominal pain

Site of pain

Visceral abdominal pain from distension of hollow organs, mesenteric traction or excessive smooth muscle contraction is a deep, poorly localized sensation in the midline. It is conducted via sympathetic splanchnic

8.10 Causes of upper gastrointestinal bleeding

- Gastric or duodenal ulcer
- Mallory–Weiss oesophageal tear
- Oesophagitis, gastritis, duodenitis
- Oesophagogastric varices
- Oesophageal or gastric cancer
- Vascular malformation

8.11 Prediction of the risk of mortality in patients with upper GI bleeding: Rockall score

Criterion	Score
1. Age	
<60 yrs	0
60–79 yrs	1
>80 yrs	2
2. Shock	
None	0
Pulse >100 bpm and	
Systolic BP >100 mmHg	1
Systolic BP <100 mmHg	2
3. Co-morbidity	
None	0
Heart failure, ischaemic heart disease or other major illness	2
Renal failure or disseminated malignancy	3
4. Endoscopic findings	
Mallory–Weiss tear and no visible bleeding	0
All other diagnoses	1
Upper GI malignancy	2
5. Major stigmata of recent haemorrhage	
None	0
Visible bleeding vessel/adherent clot	2
Total score	
Pre-endoscopy (max. score = 7)	Score 4 = 25% mortality pre-endoscopy
Post-endoscopy (max. score = 11)	Score 8+ = 40% mortality post-endoscopy

nerves. Somatic pain from the parietal peritoneum and abdominal wall is lateralized and localized to the area of inflammation. It is conducted via intercostal (spinal) nerves.

Pain arising from foregut structures (stomach, pancreas, liver and biliary system) is localized above the umbilicus (Fig. 8.7). Pain solely from the small intestine, e.g. small intestinal obstruction, is felt around the umbilicus (periumbilical). If the parietal peritoneum is involved, the pain will localize to that area, e.g. right iliac fossa pain in acute appendicitis and in Crohn's disease of the terminal ileum. Colonic pain can be felt either below the umbilicus, e.g. in the left iliac fossa from diverticular disease of the sigmoid colon, or in the upper abdomen, e.g. in the right hypochondrium from disease in the hepatic flexure.

Pain from an unpaired structure, such as the pancreas, is felt in the midline and radiates through to the back. Pain from paired structures is felt on and radiates to the affected side, e.g. renal colic. Boys with abdominal pain may have torsion of the testis (Fig. 10.47, p. 261). In women, consider gynaecological causes, e.g. ruptured ovarian cyst, pelvic inflammatory disease or an ectopic pregnancy. In any patient with acute right iliac fossa pain, consider appendicitis. Radiation of pain to either or both shoulder tips indicates peritoneal inflammation adjacent to the diaphragm, e.g. cholecystitis (Fig. 8.8).

Nature of pain

Ask 'Is the pain constant or does it come and go (colic)?'. Constant pain usually arises from a solid organ, e.g. pancreatitis. Colicky pain lasts for a short period of time (seconds or minutes), eases off and then returns. It arises from hollow structures, e.g. small or large bowel obstruction, or the uterus during labour. Biliary and renal 'colic' are misnamed, as the pain is rarely colicky; pain rapidly increases to a peak intensity and persists over several hours before gradually resolving (Box 8.12).

Speed of onset

In a previously asymptomatic patient, the sudden onset of severe abdominal pain, rapidly progressing to become generalized and constant, suggests perforation of a hollow viscus, a ruptured abdominal aortic aneurysm or mesenteric infarction. Accompanying or preceding symptoms help differentiate the likely cause. Preceding constipation suggests colorectal cancer or diverticular disease as the cause of perforation and prior dyspepsia suggests peptic ulceration. Co-existing

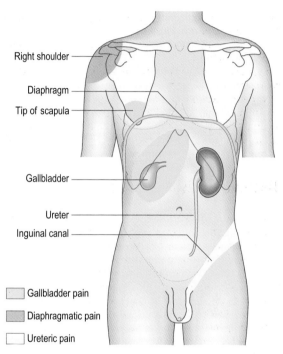

Right shoulder
Diaphragm
Tip of scapula
Gallbladder
Ureter
Inguinal canal

Gallbladder pain
Diaphragmatic pain
Ureteric pain

Fig. 8.8 Characteristic radiation of pain from the gallbladder, diaphragm and ureters.

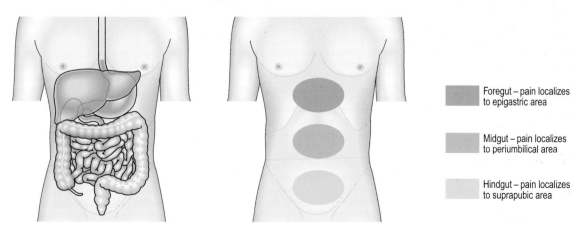

Foregut – pain localizes to epigastric area

Midgut – pain localizes to periumbilical area

Hindgut – pain localizes to suprapubic area

Fig. 8.7 **Abdominal pain.** Perception of visceral pain is localized to the epigastric, umbilical or suprapubic region, according to the embryological origin of the affected organ.

8

8.12 Analysis of abdominal pain

	Disorder			
	Peptic ulcer	**Biliary colic**	**Acute pancreatitis**	**Renal colic**
Site	Epigastrium	Epigastrium/right hypochondrium	Epigastrium/left hypochondrium	Loin
Onset	Gradual	Rapidly increasing	Sudden	Rapidly increasing
Character	Gnawing	Constant	Constant	Constant
Radiation	Into back	Below right scapula	Into back	Into genitalia and inner thigh
Timing Frequency/ periodicity Special times	Remission for weeks/ months Nocturnal and especially when hungry	Able to enumerate attacks Unpredictable	Able to enumerate attacks After heavy drinking	Usually a discrete episode Following periods of dehydration
Duration	½–2 hours	4–24 hours	>24 hours	4–24 hours
Exacerbating factors	Stress, spicy foods, alcohol, NSAIDs	Unable to eat during bouts	Alcohol Unable to eat during bouts	
Relieving factors	Food, antacids, vomiting		Eased by sitting upright	
Severity	Mild to moderate	Severe	Severe	Severe

peripheral vascular disease, hypertension, heart failure or atrial fibrillation may suggest a vascular disorder, e.g. aortic aneurysm or mesenteric ischaemia.

Development of peripheral circulatory failure (shock) following the onset of pain suggests intra-abdominal sepsis or bleeding, e.g. ruptured aortic aneurysm or ectopic pregnancy. Torsion of the testis or ovary produces severe acute abdominal pain and nausea. Torsion of the caecum or sigmoid colon (volvulus) presents with sudden abdominal pain associated with acute intestinal obstruction. Abdominal pain persisting for hours or days suggests an inflammatory disorder, such as acute appendicitis, cholecystitis or diverticulitis.

Symptom progression

During the first hour or two after perforation, a 'silent interval' may occur when abdominal pain resolves transiently. The initial chemical peritonitis may subside before bacterial peritonitis becomes established. In appendicitis, pain is initially localized around the umbilicus (visceral pain) and spreads as the inflammatory response progresses to involve the right iliac fossa (parietal or somatic pain). If the appendix ruptures, generalized peritonitis may develop. Occasionally, a localized appendix abscess develops, with a palpable mass and localized pain in the right iliac fossa.

Change in the pattern of symptoms suggests either that the initial diagnosis was wrong, or that complications have developed. In acute small bowel obstruction, a change from typical intestinal colic to persistent pain with abdominal tenderness suggests intestinal ischaemia,

e.g. strangulated hernia, an indication for urgent surgical intervention.

Accompanying features

Abdominal pain due to irritable bowel syndrome, diverticular disease or colorectal cancer is invariably accompanied by an alteration in bowel habit. Other features such as breathlessness or palpitation suggest non-alimentary causes (Box 8.13).

Wind and flatulence

Belching, excessive or offensive flatus, abdominal distension and borborygmi (audible bowel sounds) are often called 'wind' or flatulence. Clarify exactly what patients mean. Belching is due to air swallowing (aerophagy) and has no medical significance. It may indicate anxiety, but sometimes occurs in an attempt to relieve abdominal pain or discomfort, and accompanies GORD.

Between 200 and 2000 ml of flatus is normally passed per day. Flatus is a mixture of gases derived from swallowed air and from colonic bacterial fermentation of poorly absorbed carbohydrates. Excessive flatus is particularly troublesome in lactase deficiency and intestinal malabsorption. Inability to pass flatus is a feature of intestinal obstruction.

Borborygmi result from movement of fluid and gas along the bowel. Loud borborygmi, particularly if

8.13 Non-alimentary causes of abdominal pain

Disorder	Clinical features
Myocardial infarction	Epigastric pain without tenderness Angor animi (feeling of impending death), hypotension, cardiac arrhythmias
Dissecting aortic aneurysm	Tearing interscapular pain Angor animi, hypotension Asymmetry of femoral pulses
Acute vertebral collapse	Lateralized pain restricting movement Tenderness overlying the involved vertebra
Cord compression	Pain on percussion of thoracic spine Hyperaesthesia in dermatomal distribution Spinal cord signs
Pleurisy	Lateralized pain on coughing Chest signs, e.g. pleural rub
Herpes zoster	Hyperaesthesia in dermatomal distribution Vesicular eruption
Diabetic ketoacidosis	Cramp-like pain, vomiting, air hunger Tachycardia, ketotic breath
Salpingitis or tubal pregnancy	Suprapubic and iliac fossa pain, localized tenderness, nausea, vomiting, fever
Torsion of the testis/ ovary	Lower abdominal pain Nausea, vomiting, localized tenderness

associated with colicky discomfort, suggest small bowel obstruction or dysmotility.

Abdominal distension

Abdominal girth slowly increasing over months or years is usually due to obesity, but in a patient with weight loss it suggests intra-abdominal disease (Box 8.14).

Ascites is an accumulation of fluid in the peritoneal cavity. Exudates from the peritoneal membrane have a higher protein content than transudates and indicate an inflammatory or malignant disease (Fig. 8.9; Box 8.15).

Functional bloating is fluctuating abdominal distension that develops during the day and resolves overnight. It is particularly common in women and is rarely due to organic disease. It usually occurs in irritable bowel syndrome.

Chronic simple constipation rarely produces painful distension, unless associated with the irritable bowel syndrome. Painless abdominal distension in women may be the presenting symptom of ovarian pathology or a concealed pregnancy.

8.14 Causes of abdominal distension

Factor	Consider
Fat	Obesity
Flatus	Pseudo-obstruction, obstruction
Faeces	Subacute obstruction, constipation
Fluid	Ascites, tumours (especially ovarian), distended bladder
Fetus	Check date of the last menstrual period
Functional	Bloating often associated with irritable bowel syndrome

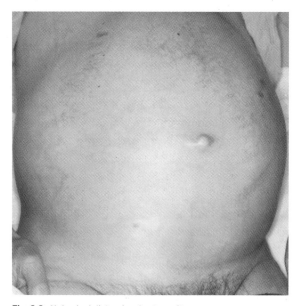

Fig. 8.9 Abdominal distension due to ascites.

8.15 Causes of ascites

Common
Hepatic cirrhosis with portal hypertension
Intra-abdominal malignancy with peritoneal spread
Congestive heart failure
Uncommon
Hepatic or portal vein occlusion
Constrictive pericarditis
Hypoproteinaemia, e.g. nephrotic syndrome, protein-losing enteropathy
Peritonitis, e.g. tuberculosis, pancreatitis

8.16 Symptom checklist in patients with constipation

- Has constipation been life-long or is it of recent onset?
- How often do the bowels empty each week?
- How much time is spent straining at stool?
- Is there associated abdominal pain, anal pain on defecation or rectal bleeding?
- Has the shape of the stool changed, e.g. become pellet-like?
- Has there been any change in drug therapy?

8.17 Causes of constipation

- Lack of fibre in diet
- Irritable bowel syndrome
- Intestinal obstruction (cancer)
- Drugs (opioids, iron)
- Metabolic/endocrine (hypothyroidism, hypercalcaemia)
- Immobility (stroke, Parkinson's disease)

Altered bowel habit

Normal bowel movement frequency ranges from three times daily to once every three days. Diarrhoea is the frequent passage of loose stools. Constipation is the infrequent passage of hard stools. Clarify exactly what patients mean when they use these terms.

Constipation (Box 8.16) may be due to impaired motility in the colon, physical obstruction in the colon, impaired rectal sensation with no normal 'call to stool' or anorectal dysfunction impairing the process of evacuation (anismus) (Box 8.17). Tenesmus is the sensation of needing to defecate, although the rectum is empty and suggests rectal inflammation or tumour.

The principal site of water absorption is the colon. High-volume diarrhoea (>1 litre per day) occurs when stool water content is increased and may be:

- secretory, due to intestinal inflammation, e.g. viral or bacterial infection, or inflammatory bowel disease
- osmotic, due to malabsorption, adverse drug effects or motility disorders (Box 8.18).

If the patient fasts, osmotic diarrhoea stops but secretory diarrhoea persists. Steatorrhoea is diarrhoea associated with fat malabsorption. The stools are greasy, pale and bulky, and they float, making them difficult to flush away.

Low-volume diarrhoea is associated with the irritable bowel syndrome (Box 8.19). The diagnosis of irritable bowel syndrome is based on a pattern of gastrointestinal symptoms (Box 8.20). Abdominal bloating, dyspepsia and often non-alimentary symptoms, including urinary frequency, backache, tiredness, anxiety and depression, commonly accompany irritable bowel symptoms.

Alarm features raise the probability of a serious alternative or co-existent diagnosis (Box 8.21). The risk

8.18 Symptom checklist in patients with diarrhoeal disorders

- Is the diarrhoea acute, chronic or intermittent?
- Is there tenesmus, urgency or incontinence?
- Is the stool watery, unformed or semisolid?
- Is the stool of large volume and not excessively frequent, suggesting small bowel disease?
- Is the stool of small volume and excessively frequent, suggesting large bowel disease?
- Is there blood, mucus or pus associated with the stool?
- Does diarrhoea disturb sleep, suggesting organic disease?
- Is there a history of contact with diarrhoea or of travel abroad?
- Does the sexual history provide a clue ('gay bowel syndrome', HIV)?
- Is there a history of alcohol abuse or relevant drug therapy?
- Is there a past medical history of GI surgery, GI disease or inflammatory bowel disease?
- Is there a family history of GI disorder, e.g. gluten enteropathy, Crohn's?
- Are there any other GI symptoms, e.g. abdominal pain and vomiting?
- Are there symptoms of systemic disease, e.g. rigors or arthralgia?

8.19 Causes of diarrhoea

Acute

- Infective gastroenteritis
- Drugs (esp. antibiotics)

Chronic

- Irritable bowel syndrome
- Inflammatory bowel disease
- Parasitic infestations, e.g. *Giardia lamblia*
- Colorectal cancer
- Autonomic neuropathy (esp. diabetic)
- Laxative abuse and other drug therapies
- Hyperthyroidism
- Constipation and faecal impaction (overflow)
- Small bowel or right colonic resection
- Malabsorption

8.20 Rome III criteria: diagnosis of irritable bowel syndrome

Recurrent abdominal pain, for at least the last 6 months, on at least 3 days per month in the last 3 months, associated with two or more of the following:
- Improvement with defecation
- Onset associated with a change in stool frequency
- Onset associated with a change in form of stool

of serious disease, e.g. colon cancer, increases with age, and patients >50 years should be investigated before a functional bowel disorder, such as irritable bowel syndrome, is diagnosed.

8.21 Gastrointestinal 'alarm features'

- Persistent vomiting
- Dysphagia
- Fever
- Weight loss
- GI bleeding
- Anaemia
- Painless, watery, high-volume diarrhoea
- Nocturnal symptoms disturbing sleep

8.22 Causes of rectal bleeding

- Haemorrhoids
- Anal fissure
- Colorectal polyps
- Colorectal cancer
- Inflammatory bowel disease
- Ischaemic colitis
- Complicated diverticular disease
- Vascular malformation

8.23 Common causes of jaundice

Increased bilirubin production

- Haemolysis (unconjugated hyperbilirubinaemia)

Impaired bilirubin excretion

- Congenital
  Gilbert's syndrome
  (unconjugated)
- Hepatocellular
  Viral hepatitis
  Cirrhosis
  Drugs
  Autoimmune hepatitis
- Intrahepatic cholestasis
  Drugs
  Primary biliary cirrhosis
- Extrahepatic cholestasis
  Gallstones
  Cancer: pancreas,
  cholangiocarcinoma

8

8.24 Urine and stool analysis in jaundice

	Urine			Stools
	Colour	Bilirubin	Urobilinogen	Colour
Unconjugated	Normal	−	+ + + +	Normal
Hepatocellular	Dark	+ +	+ +	Normal
Obstructive	Dark	+ + + +	−	Pale

Rectal bleeding

Fresh rectal bleeding indicates a disorder in the anal canal, rectum or colon (Box 8.22). Blood may be mixed with stool, coat the surface of otherwise normal stool, or be seen on the toilet paper or in the pan. Melaena signifies blood loss from the upper gastrointestinal tract. During severe upper gastrointestinal bleeding, blood may pass through the intestine unaltered, causing fresh rectal bleeding. This may be accompanied by hypovolaemic shock.

Jaundice

Jaundice is a yellowish discoloration of the skin, sclerae (Fig. 8.10) and mucous membranes due to hyperbilirubinaemia (Box 8.23). Levels of bilirubin >50 μmol/l are needed for clinical detection in good light. Unconjugated bilirubin is insoluble and transported in plasma bound to albumin; it is therefore not filtered by the renal glomeruli. In jaundice due to unconjugated hyperbilirubinaemia, the urine is normal in colour (acholuric jaundice; Box 8.24).

In the liver, bilirubin is conjugated to form bilirubin diglucuronide and excreted, giving bile its characteristic green colour (Fig. 8.11). In conjugated hyperbilirubinaemia, the urine is dark brown in colour

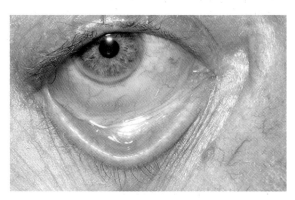

Fig. 8.10 Yellow sclera of jaundice.

due to the presence of bilirubin diglucuronide. In the colon, conjugated bilirubin is metabolized by bacterial flora to stercobilinogen and stercobilin which are excreted in the stool, contributing to the brown colour of stool. Stercobilinogen is absorbed from the bowel and excreted in the urine as urobilinogen, a colourless, water-soluble compound.

Prehepatic jaundice

In haemolytic disorders the accompanying anaemic pallor combined with jaundice may produce a pale lemon complexion. The stools and urine are normal in colour.

195

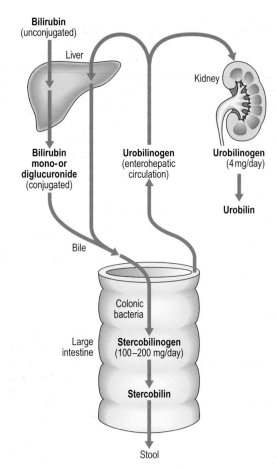

Bilirubin
(unconjugated)

Liver

Kidney

Bilirubin
mono- or
diglucuronide
(conjugated)

Urobilinogen
(enterohepatic
circulation)

Urobilinogen
(4 mg/day)

Urobilin

Bile

Colonic
bacteria

Large
intestine

Stercobilinogen
(100–200 mg/day)

Stercobilin

Stool

Fig. 8.11 Pathway of bilirubin excretion.

8.25 Checklist for the history of jaundice

- Appetite and weight change
- Abdominal pain, altered bowel habit
- Gastrointestinal bleeding
- Pruritus, dark urine, rigors
- Drug and alcohol history
- Past medical history (pancreatitis, biliary surgery)
- Previous jaundice or hepatitis
- Blood transfusions (hepatitis B or C)
- Family history, e.g. congenital spherocytosis, haemochromatosis
- Sexual and contact history (hepatitis B or C)
- Travel history and immunizations (hepatitis A)
- Skin tattooing (hepatitis B or C)

OSCEs 8.26 Examine this patient with jaundice

1. Look for signs of chronic liver disease:
    Finger clubbing, palmar erythema, leukonychia
    Spider naevi: upper trunk, head, neck and arms
    Gynaecomastia in males.
2. Look for signs of liver failure:
    Flapping tremor of outstretched hands
    Sweet smell on breath of fetor hepaticus
    Confusion, diminished mental state.
3. Look for pallor — haemolytic anaemia.
4. Look for signs of weight loss — malignancy with liver metastases.
5. Smell the breath for alcohol.
6. Look for hepatomegaly, splenomegaly, ascites and caput medusae.
7. Look for:
    Needle track marks — evidence of drug misuse (hepatitis B and C)
    Tattoos and body piercing — hepatitis B and C
8. Look for scratch marks (obstructive jaundice).
9. Examine ankles and sacrum for oedema (hypoalbuminaemia).
10. Look at stools — pale in post-hepatic jaundice.
11. Urinalysis — dark urine in hepatic or post-hepatic jaundice.

Gilbert's syndrome is common and causes unconjugated hyperbilirubinaemia. Serum liver enzyme concentrations are normal and jaundice is mild (plasma bilirubin <100 μmol/l) but increases during prolonged fasting or intercurrent febrile illness.

Hepatic jaundice

Hepatocellular disease causes hyperbilirubinaemia that is both unconjugated and conjugated. Urine will be dark and stools normal in colour.

Post-hepatic jaundice

In biliary obstruction, conjugated bilirubin in the bile does not reach the intestine, so the stools are pale. Conjugated bilirubin is soluble and filtered by the kidney, so the urine is dark brown. Obstructive jaundice may be accompanied by generalized itch (pruritus) due to skin deposition of bile salts. Obstructive jaundice with abdominal pain is usually due to gallstones; if fever or rigors also occur (Charcot's triad), ascending cholangitis is likely. Painless obstructive

jaundice suggests malignant biliary obstruction, e.g. cholangiocarcinoma or cancer of the head of the pancreas. Obstructive jaundice can be hepatic as well as post-hepatic intrahepatic cholestasis, e.g. primary biliary cirrhosis (Boxes 8.25 and 8.26).

THE HISTORY

Presenting complaint

Gastrointestinal symptoms are common and are often caused by functional dyspepsia and irritable bowel syndrome. Explore the patient's FIFE (p. 10) to understand the context in which symptoms have arisen.

8.27 Examples of drug-induced gastrointestinal conditions

Symptom	Drug
Weight gain	Oral corticosteroids
Dyspepsia and GI bleeding	Aspirin NSAIDs
Diarrhoea	Antibiotics Proton pump inhibitors
Constipation	Opioids
Jaundice: hepatitis	Paracetamol Pyrazinamide Rifampicin Isoniazid
Jaundice: cholestatic	Flucloxacillin Chlorpromazine Co-amoxiclav
Liver fibrosis	Methotrexate

8.28 Calorie value of some food groups

Food group	Calorific value of food
Dairy products (milk, butter, cheese, yoghurt)	Milk = 500 kcal/l Fat = 9 kcal/g
Wheat (bread, pasta)	Carbohydrates = 4 kcal/g
Meat, fish	Protein = 4 kcal/g
Alcohol	Wine = 500 kcal/70 cl Beer = 400 kcal/l

8.29 Risk factors for viral hepatitis

- Intravenous drug use
- Tattoos
- Foreign travel
- Blood transfusion
- Sex between men or with prostitutes
- Multiple sexual partners

Always investigate 'alarm symptoms', particularly in those >50 years.

Past history

History of a similar problem may suggest the diagnosis: for example, bleeding peptic ulcer or inflammatory bowel disease. Ask about previous abdominal surgery, X-rays, scans and other investigations.

Drug history

Ask about all prescribed medications, over-the-counter medicines and herbal preparations. Many drugs affect the gastrointestinal tract (Box 8.27):

- Aspirin and NSAIDs can cause dyspepsia, gastric erosions or peptic ulcers
- Selective serotonin reuptake inhibitor antidepressants often cause nausea
- Opioid analgesics can cause nausea, vomiting and constipation
- Antibiotics can cause diarrhoea (with or without *Clostridium difficile* infection — pseudomembranous colitis)

Many drugs are hepatotoxic.

Family history

Inflammatory bowel disease is more common in patients with a family history of either Crohn's disease or ulcerative colitis. Colorectal cancer in a first-degree relative increases the risk of colorectal cancer and polyps. Peptic ulcer disease is familial but this may be due to environmental factors, e.g. transmission of *Helicobacter pylori* infection. Gilbert's syndrome is an autosomal dominant condition; haemochromatosis and Wilson's disease are autosomal recessive disorders.

Social history

Take a dietary history and assess the approximate intake of calories and sources of essential nutrients (Box 8.28). Painless diarrhoea may indicate alcohol abuse, lactose intolerance or gluten enteropathy. Patients with irritable bowel syndrome often report specific food intolerances, including wheat, dairy products, fruit and others.

Calculate the patient's alcohol consumption in units (p. 21).

Smokers are at increased risk of oesophageal cancer, colorectal cancer, Crohn's disease and peptic ulcer, while patients with ulcerative colitis are less likely to smoke. Many gastrointestinal disorders, particularly irritable bowel syndrome and dyspepsia, are exacerbated by stress and emotional ill health. Ask about potential sources of stress, including work, home, relationships and finance, as well as about the symptoms of anxiety and depression (Box 2.49, p. 31).

In patients with liver disease, ask about specific risk factors (Box 8.29). Some forms of hepatitis, e.g. B and C, may present with chronic liver disease or cancer decades after primary infection, so enquire about drug use and other risk factors in the distant as well as the recent past. Foreign travel is important in relation to diarrhoeal illnesses.

THE PHYSICAL EXAMINATION

General examination

Nutritional state

Record the height, weight, waist circumference and the patient's body mass index (Fig. 3.23, p. 59). Note whether obesity is truncal or generalized. Look for abdominal striae, which indicate rapid weight gain, previous pregnancy or, rarely, Cushing's syndrome. Loose skin folds signify recent weight loss. Look for stigmata of iron deficiency, including koilonychia (spoon-shaped nails), angular cheilitis (painful hacks at the corners of the mouth) and atrophic glossitis (pale, smooth tongue). The tongue has a beefy, raw appearance in folate and vitamin B_{12} deficiency.

Liver disease

If jaundice is not obvious, ask the patient to look up and retract the lower eyelid to expose the sclera in order to see if it is yellow in natural light (Fig. 8.10). Do not confuse the diffuse yellow sclerae of jaundice with the small yellowish fat pads (pinguecula) sometimes seen at the periphery of the sclerae.

There are several signs which suggest chronic liver disease (Fig. 8.12):

* Palmar erythema and spider naevi suggest the presence of significant liver disease and are due to excess oestrogen associated with reduced breakdown of sex steroids within the liver.

Spider naevi are isolated telangiectases that characteristically fill from a central feeding vessel found in the distribution of the superior vena cava on the upper trunk, arms and face (Fig. 8.13). Women may have up to five spider naevi in health; palmar erythema and numerous spider naevi are normal during pregnancy

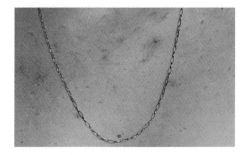

Fig. 8.13 Spider naevi.

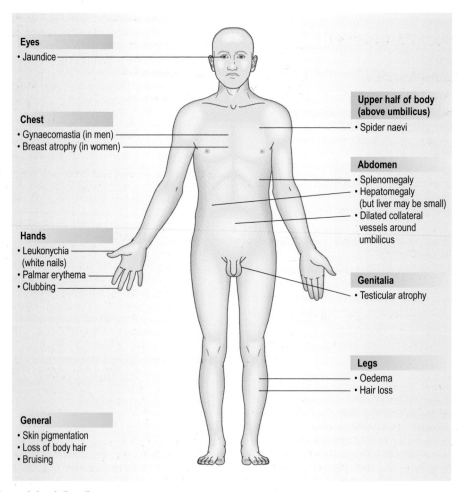

Eyes
• Jaundice

Chest
• Gynaecomastia (in men)
• Breast atrophy (in women)

Hands
• Leukonychia
(white nails)
• Palmar erythema
• Clubbing

General
• Skin pigmentation
• Loss of body hair
• Bruising

**Upper half of body
(above umbilicus)**
• Spider naevi

Abdomen
• Splenomegaly
• Hepatomegaly
(but liver may be small)
• Dilated collateral
vessels around
umbilicus

Genitalia
• Testicular atrophy

Legs
• Oedema
• Hair loss

Fig. 8.12 Features of chronic liver disease.

- Gynaecomastia (breast enlargement) in men may occur, with loss of body hair and testicular atrophy
- Leukonychia (white nails), caused by hypoalbuminaemia, may also occur in protein calorie malnutrition (kwashiorkor), malabsorption due to protein-losing enteropathy e.g. coeliac disease or heavy and prolonged proteinuria (nephrotic syndrome) (Fig. 3.16D, p. 54).
- Finger clubbing may be associated with liver cirrhosis, inflammatory bowel disease and malabsorption syndromes.

Bilateral parotid swelling due to sialoadenosis of the salivary glands may be a feature of chronic alcohol abuse; it is also seen in bulimia associated with recurrent vomiting.

Look at the mouth and throat for aphthous ulcers, which are common in gluten enteropathy and inflammatory bowel disease (Fig. 8.6B).

Examine the cervical, axillary and inguinal lymph nodes; gastric and pancreatic cancer may spread to cause enlargement of the left supraclavicular lymph nodes (Troisier's sign). More widespread lymphadenopathy with hepatosplenomegaly suggests lymphoma.

Examination of the abdomen

Examination sequence

Inspection of the abdomen

- Examine the patient in good light and warm surroundings.
- Position the patient comfortably supine with the head only resting on one or two pillows to relax the abdominal wall muscles.
- Use extra pillows to support a patient with kyphosis or breathlessness.
- Look at the teeth, tongue and buccal mucosa and ask about mouth ulcers.
- Note any smell, e.g. alcohol, fetor hepaticus, uraemia, melaena or ketones.
- Expose the abdomen from the xiphisternum to the symphysis pubis, leaving the chest and legs covered.

Abnormal findings

Skin

In older patients, seborrhoeic warts, ranging from pink to brown or black, and haemangiomas (Campbell de Morgan spots) are common and normal, but note any striae, bruising or scratch marks.

Visible veins

Abnormally prominent veins on the abdominal wall suggest portal hypertension or vena caval obstruction. In portal hypertension, recanalization of the umbilical vein along the falciform ligament produces distended veins which drain away from the umbilicus: the 'caput medusae'. The umbilicus may appear bluish and distended due to an umbilical varix. In contrast, an umbilical hernia is a distended and everted umbilicus

which does not appear vascular and may have a palpable cough impulse. Dilated tortuous veins with blood flow superiorly are collateral veins due to obstruction of the inferior vena cava. Rarely, obstruction of the superior vena cava gives rise to similar distended abdominal veins which all flow inferiorly.

Abdominal distension

Is the abdomen distended? If so, is the distension generalized or localized? In obesity, the umbilicus is usually sunken; in ascites, it is flat or everted. Look tangentially across the abdomen and from the foot of the bed for any asymmetry associated with a localized mass, such as an enlarged liver or bladder.

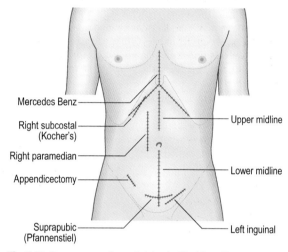

Fig. 8.14 Some commonly used abdominal incisions. The midline and oblique incisions avoid damage to the innervation of the abdominal musculature and the later development of incisional herniae.

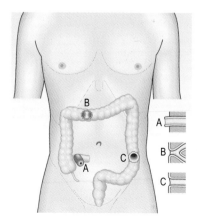

Fig. 8.15 Surgical stomas. (A) An ileostomy is usually in the right iliac fossa and is formed as a spout. **(B)** A loop colostomy may be created by temporary defunctioning of the distal bowel. It is usually in the transverse colon and has afferent and efferent limbs. **(C)** A colostomy may be terminal, i.e. resected distal bowel. It is usually flush and in the left iliac fossa.

8

Abdominal scars and stomas

Note any surgical scars or stomas and clarify what operations have taken place (Figs 8.14 and 8.15). A small infra-umbilical incision is usually the result of previous laparoscopy. Puncture scars from the ports used for laparoscopic surgery may be visible. An incisional hernia at the site of a scar is palpable as a defect in the abdominal wall musculature and becomes more obvious as the patient raises the head off the bed or coughs.

▶ Examination sequence

Palpation of the abdomen

- Ensure that your hands are warm.
- If the bed is low, kneel beside it.
- Ask the patient to show you where the pain is and to report any tenderness elicited during palpation.
- Ask the patient to place the arms by the sides to help relax the abdominal wall.
- Use your right hand, keeping it flat in contact with the abdominal wall.
- Observe the patient's face for any sign of discomfort throughout the examination.
- Begin with light superficial palpation away from any site of pain.
- Palpate each region in turn, then repeat during deeper palpation.
- Test abdominal muscle tone by light, dipping movements with your fingers.

Abnormal findings (Fig. 8.16)

Tenderness

Discomfort during palpation may vary and be accompanied by resistance to palpation. Consider the patient's level of anxiety when assessing the severity of pain and tenderness elicited. Tenderness in several areas on minimal pressure may be due to generalized peritonitis but is more often due to anxiety. Severe superficial pain with no tenderness on deep palpation or pain that disappears if the patient is distracted also suggests anxiety. With these exceptions, tenderness is a useful indication of underlying pathology. Voluntary guarding is the voluntary contraction of the abdominal muscles when palpation provokes pain. Involuntary guarding is the reflex contraction of the abdominal muscles when there is inflammation of the parietal peritoneum. If the whole peritoneum is inflamed (generalized peritonitis) due to a perforated viscus, the abdominal wall no longer moves with respiration; breathing becomes increasingly thoracic and the muscles of the anterior abdominal wall are held rigid (board-like rigidity).

The site of tenderness is important. For example, tenderness in the epigastrium suggests peptic ulcer; in the right hypochondrium, cholecystitis; in the right iliac fossa, appendicitis or Crohn's ileitis. 'Rebound tenderness' is a sign of intra-abdominal disease but not necessarily of parietal peritoneal inflammation (peritonism). Ask the patient to cough or gently percuss the abdomen to elicit

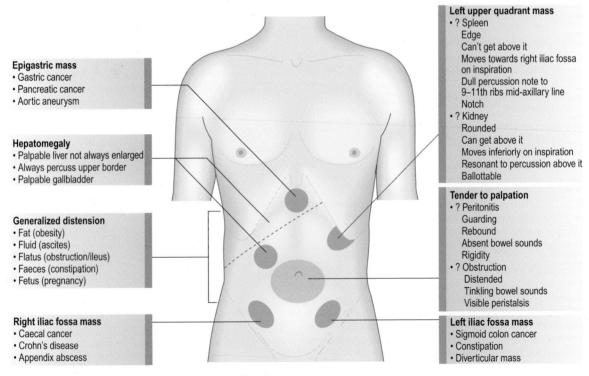

Epigastric mass
- Gastric cancer
- Pancreatic cancer
- Aortic aneurysm

Hepatomegaly
- Palpable liver not always enlarged
- Always percuss upper border
- Palpable gallbladder

Generalized distension
- Fat (obesity)
- Fluid (ascites)
- Flatus (obstruction/ileus)
- Faeces (constipation)
- Fetus (pregnancy)

Right iliac fossa mass
- Caecal cancer
- Crohn's disease
- Appendix abscess

Left upper quadrant mass
- ? Spleen
  Edge
  Can't get above it
  Moves towards right iliac fossa on inspiration
  Dull percussion note to 9–11th ribs mid-axillary line
  Notch
- ? Kidney
  Rounded
  Can get above it
  Moves inferiorly on inspiration
  Resonant to percussion above it
  Ballottable

Tender to palpation
- ? Peritonitis
  Guarding
  Rebound
  Absent bowel sounds
  Rigidity
- ? Obstruction
  Distended
  Tinkling bowel sounds
  Visible peristalsis

Left iliac fossa mass
- Sigmoid colon cancer
- Constipation
- Diverticular mass

Fig. 8.16 Diagram of abdomen showing palpable abnormalities.

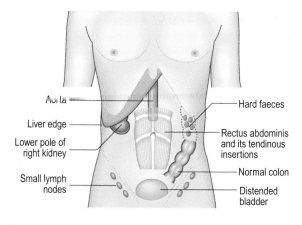

Fig. 8.17 Diagram of abdomen, showing palpable masses which may be physiological as opposed to pathological.

any pain or tenderness. Rapidly removing your hand after deep palpation increases the pain.

Palpable mass (Fig. 8.17)

If the mass seems superficial, it may be within the anterior abdominal wall rather than within the abdominal cavity. Ask the patient to tense the abdominal muscles by lifting the head; an abdominal wall mass will still be palpable, whereas an intra-abdominal mass will not. Is the mass an enlarged abdominal organ or separate from the solid organs? If the latter, is it a tumour or abscess, or just palpable faeces within the colon? Palpable faeces can usually be indented with your fingers and may disappear following defecation.

Describe any mass using the basic principles outlined in Chapter 3 (Box 3.10, p. 58). Describe its site, size, surface, shape and consistency, and note whether it moves on respiration. Is the mass fixed or mobile? A pulsatile mass palpable in the upper abdomen may be normal aortic pulsation in a thin person, a gastric or pancreatic tumour transmitting underlying aortic pulsation, or an aortic aneurysm.

Palpation for enlarged organs

Examine the liver, gallbladder, spleen and kidneys in turn during deep inspiration. Keep your examining hand still and wait for the organ to descend. Do not start palpation too close to the costal margin, missing the edge of the liver or spleen.

Hepatomegaly

Hepatic enlargement can result from chronic parenchymal liver disease from any cause (Boxes 8.30 and 8.31). The liver is enlarged in early cirrhosis but often shrunken in advanced cirrhosis. Fatty liver (hepatic steatosis) can cause marked hepatomegaly. Hepatic enlargement due to metastatic tumour is hard and irregular. An enlarged left lobe may be felt in the epigastrium or even in the left hypochondrium. An audible bruit may be heard over the liver in hepatocellular cancer and sometimes in

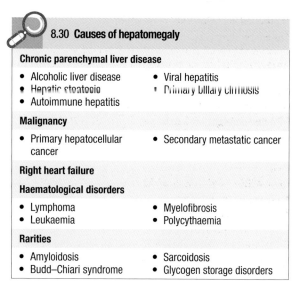

8.30 Causes of hepatomegaly

Chronic parenchymal liver disease

- Alcoholic liver disease
- Hepatic steatosis
- Autoimmune hepatitis
- Viral hepatitis
- Primary biliary cirrhosis

Malignancy

- Primary hepatocellular cancer
- Secondary metastatic cancer

Right heart failure

Haematological disorders

- Lymphoma
- Leukaemia
- Myelofibrosis
- Polycythaemia

Rarities

- Amyloidosis
- Budd–Chiari syndrome
- Sarcoidosis
- Glycogen storage disorders

8.31 Signs of liver failure

- Fetor hepaticus: stale 'mousy' smell of the volatile amine, methyl mercaptan, on the breath
- Flapping tremor of outstretched arms with hands dorsiflexed ('asterixis')
- Mental state varies from
  Drowsiness with day/night pattern reversed,
  through confusion and disorientation,
  to unresponsive coma
- Late neurological features
  Spasticity and extension of the arms and legs
  Extensor plantar responses

8.32 Grading of hepatic encephalopathy (West Haven)

Stage	State of consciousness
0	No change in personality or behaviour No asterixis (flapping tremor)
1	Impaired concentration and attention span Sleep disturbance, slurred speech Euphoria or depression Asterixis present
2	Lethargy, drowsiness, apathy or aggression Disorientation, inappropriate behaviour, slurred speech
3	Confusion and disorientation, bizarre behaviour Drowsiness or stupor Asterixis usually absent
4	Comatose with no response to voice commands Minimal or absent response to painful stimuli

ℹ 8.33 Severity and prognosis in cirrhosis (Child–Pugh classification)

Score	1	2	3
Bilirubin (μmol/l)	<34	34–50	>50
Albumin (g/l)	>35	28–35	<28
Prothrombin time (secs prolonged)	<4	4–6	>6
Ascites	None	Mild	Marked
Encephalopathy	None	Mild	Marked

Child A = score <7; Child B = score 7–9; Child C = score >9.

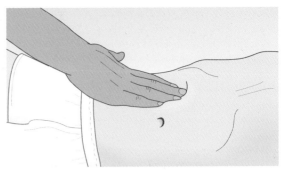

Fig. 8.18 Palpation of the liver.

OSCEs 8.34 Examine this patient who may have chronic liver disease

1. Examine the fingers for white nails (leukonychia) with loss of the lunula (half-moons at the nail base) and ankle oedema — all due to hypoalbuminaemia.
2. Look for spider naevi (upper half of the body), palmar erythema, gynaecomastia and testicular atrophy — all due to oestrogen excess.
3. Look for bruising due to:
   Thrombocytopenia (hypersplenism)
   Reduced hepatic synthesis of coagulation factors (II, VII, IX and X)
   Multiple falls due to alcohol intoxication.
4. Look for muscle wasting from malnutrition and/or liver synthetic failure.
5. Examine for signs of liver failure:
   Look for a coarse flap of the outstretched hands (asterixis) due to metabolic brainstem dysfunction (other causes include heart, renal and respiratory failure)
   Smell the patient's breath to detect fetor hepaticus (a sweetish, musty smell) due to accumulation of the volatile amine, methyl mercaptan
   Check for signs of hepatic encephalopathy (grade 1–4) due to the metabolic changes affecting cerebral function.

alcoholic hepatitis. In right heart failure, the congested liver is usually soft and tender; a pulsatile liver indicates tricuspid regurgitation.

The West Haven grades of hepatic encephalopathy and the Child–Pugh scale of severity and prognosis in cirrhosis are shown in Boxes 8.33 and 8.34.

▶ Examination sequence

Liver and gallbladder

▶ Start in the right iliac fossa. Place your hand flat on the abdomen with your fingers pointing upwards and sensing fingers (index and middle) lateral to the rectus muscle, so that your finger tips lie parallel to rectus sheath (Fig. 8.18).

▶ Keep your hand stationary. Ask the patient to breathe in deeply through the mouth. Feel for the liver edge as it descends on inspiration.

▶ Move your hand progressively up the abdomen, 1 cm at a time, between each breath the patient takes, until you reach the costal margin or detect the liver edge.

▶ If you feel the liver edge, the liver may be enlarged or displaced downwards by hyperinflated lungs (Fig. 8.19A).

▶ Percuss downwards from the right 5th intercostal space in the midclavicular line to locate the upper border of the liver, with the patient's breath held in full expiration. Resonance below the 5th intercostal space suggests emphysema or occasionally the interposition of the transverse colon between the liver and the diaphragm (Chilaiditi's sign). Measure the distance in centimetres below the costal margin in the midclavicular line or from the upper border of dullness to the palpable liver edge.

▶ If you feel a liver edge, describe:
- size
- surface — smooth or irregular
- edge — smooth or irregular
- consistency — soft or hard
- tenderness
- whether it is pulsatile
- any audible bruit.

▶ In cholecystitis, feel for gallbladder tenderness. Ask the patient to breathe in deeply as you gently palpate the right upper quadrant of the abdomen in the midclavicular line. As the liver descends, the inflamed gallbladder contacts the finger tips, causing pain and the sudden arrest of inspiration (Murphy's sign).

▶ Palpable distension of the gallbladder has a characteristic globular shape. It is rare and results from either obstruction of the cystic duct, as in a mucocoele or empyema of the gallbladder, or obstruction of the common bile duct (providing the cystic duct is patent), as in pancreatic cancer. If the gallbladder is palpable in a jaundiced patient, the obstruction is likely to be due to pancreatic cancer or distal cholangiocarcinoma and not gallstones (Courvoisier's law). In gallstone disease the gallbladder may be tender but impalpable because of fibrosis of the gallbladder wall.

Splenomegaly

The spleen has to increase in size threefold before it becomes palpable, so a palpable spleen always indicates splenomegaly. The spleen enlarges from under the left costal margin down and medially towards the umbilicus (Fig. 8.19B). A characteristic notch may be palpable midway along its leading edge, differentiating it from an enlarged left kidney (Boxes 8.35–8.37).

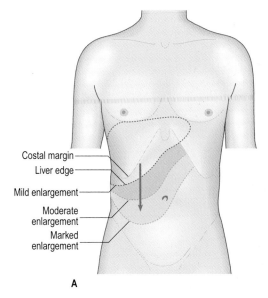

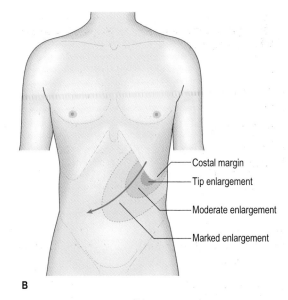

Costal margin
Liver edge
Mild enlargement
Moderate enlargement
Marked enlargement

A

Costal margin
Tip enlargement
Moderate enlargement
Marked enlargement

B

Fig. 8.19 Patterns of progressive enlargement of liver and of spleen. (A) Direction of enlargement of the liver. **(B)** Direction of enlargement of the spleen. The spleen moves downwards and medially during inspiration.

8.35 Causes of splenomegaly

Haematological disorders

- Lymphoma and lymphatic leukaemias
- Myeloproliferative diseases, polycythaemia rubra vera and myelofibrosis
- Haemolytic anaemia, congenital spherocytosis

Portal hypertension

Infections

- Glandular fever
- Malaria, kala azar (leishmaniasis)
- Brucellosis, tuberculosis, salmonellosis
- Bacterial endocarditis

Rheumatological conditions

- Rheumatoid arthritis (Felty's syndrome)
- Systemic lupus erythematosus

Rarities

- Sarcoidosis
- Amyloidosis
- Glycogen storage disorders

8.36 Differentiation of a palpable spleen from the left kidney

Distinguishing feature	Spleen	Kidney
Mass is smooth and regular in shape	More likely	Polycystic kidneys are bilateral irregular masses
Mass descends in inspiration	Yes, travels superficially and diagonally	Yes, moves deeply and vertically
Able to feel deep to the mass	Yes	No
Palpable notch on the medial surface	Yes	No
Bilateral masses palpable	No	Sometimes (e.g. polycystic kidneys)
Percussion resonant over the mass	No	Sometimes
Mass extends beyond the midline	Sometimes	No (except with horse-shoe kidney)

Hypersplenism is pancytopenia (low platelet count, white cell count and haemoglobin concentration) caused by splenic enlargement. Haematological disorders causing splenomegaly commonly, but not invariably, also cause enlargement of the liver. Haemolytic anaemia causes mild splenomegaly without hepatomegaly.

8.37 Causes of hepatosplenomegaly

- Lymphoma
- Myeloproliferative diseases
- Cirrhosis with portal hypertension
- Amyloidosis, sarcoidosis, glycogen storage disease

Examination sequence

Spleen

⬛ Start from the umbilicus. Keep your hand stationary and ask the patient to breathe in deeply through the mouth. Feel for the splenic edge as it descends on inspiration (Fig. 8.20A).

⬛ Move your hand diagonally upwards towards the left hypochondrium 1 cm at a time between each breath the patient takes.

⬛ Feel the costal margin along its length, as the position of the spleen tip is variable.

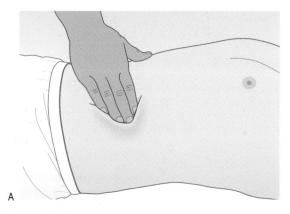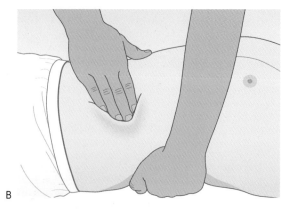

A
B

Fig. 8.20 Palpation of the spleen.

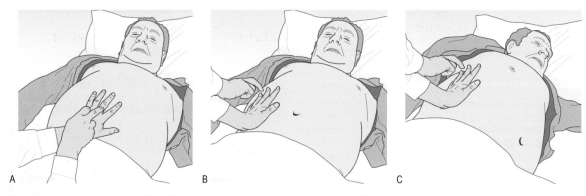

A
B
C

Fig. 8.21 Percussing for ascites. (A and **B)** Percuss towards the flank from resonant to dull. **(C)** Then ask the patient to roll on to his other side. In ascites, the note then becomes resonant.

■➤ If you cannot feel the splenic edge, ask the patient to roll towards you and on to his right side; repeat the above. Palpate with your right hand, placing your left hand behind the patient's left lower ribs, pulling the ribcage forward (Fig. 8.20B).

■➤ Feel along the left costal margin and percuss over the lateral chest wall to confirm or exclude the presence of splenic dullness.

Shifting dullness (ascites)

■➤ **Examination sequence**

Ascites

■➤ With the patient supine, percuss from the midline out to the flanks (Fig. 8.21). Note any change from resonant to dull, along with the areas of dullness and resonance.

■➤ Keep your finger on the site of dullness in the flank and ask the patient to turn on to his opposite side. Pause for at least 10 seconds to allow any ascites to gravitate, then percuss again. If the area of dullness is now resonant, shifting dullness is present, indicating ascites.

Fluid thrill

■➤ If the abdomen is tensely distended and you are not certain whether ascites is present, look for the presence of a fluid thrill.

■➤ Place the palm of your left hand flat against the left side of the abdomen and flick a finger of your right hand against the right side of the abdomen.

■➤ If you feel a ripple against your left hand, ask an assistant to place the edge of their hand on the midline of the abdomen (Fig. 8.22). This prevents transmission of the impulse via the skin rather than through the ascites. If you still feel a ripple against your left hand, a fluid thrill is present (only detected in gross ascites).

■➤ **Examination sequence**

Auscultation of the abdomen

■➤ With the patient lying on his back, place the stethoscope diaphragm to the right of the umbilicus and do not move it. Bowel sounds are gurgling noises from the normal peristaltic activity of the gut. They normally occur every 5–10 seconds, but the frequency varies.

■➤ Listen for up to 2 minutes before concluding that bowel sounds are absent. Absence of bowel sounds implies paralytic ileus or peritonitis. In intestinal obstruction, bowel sounds occur with increased frequency, volume and pitch, and have a high-pitched, tinkling quality.

■➤ Listen above the umbilicus over the aorta for arterial bruits, which suggest an atheromatous or aneurysmal aorta or superior mesenteric artery stenosis.

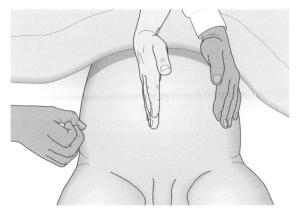

Fig. 8.22 Eliciting a fluid thrill.

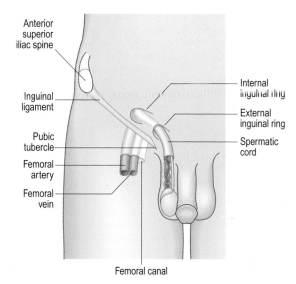

Fig. 8.23 Anatomy of the inguinal canal and femoral sheath.

OSCEs 8.38 Examine this patient with an abdominal swelling

1. Position the patient supine with one pillow beneath the head, not the shoulders.
2. Expose the area to be examined while maintaining the patient's dignity.
3. Look at the shape of the abdomen to clarify the nature of any distension.
4. Note the position of scars and check the nature of any surgery with the patient.
5. Ask the patient about areas of tenderness and ask him to tell you if discomfort arises.
6. Palpate superficially, then more deeply in the abdomen.
7. Palpate and percuss for liver enlargement.
8. Palpate and percuss for splenic enlargement.
9. Percuss the flanks and hypogastric areas for evidence of dullness. If this is present, look for shifting dullness by percussing in the supine, then the left lateral position. If ascites is suspected, look for a fluid thrill. If this is present, ask the patient to place a hand along the midline to exclude cutaneous transmission of a thrill.

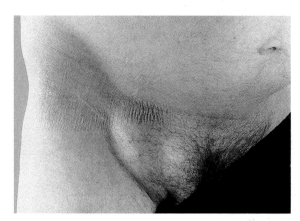

Fig. 8.24 Right inguinal hernia.

▪▪ Now place the stethoscope 2–3 cm above and lateral to the umbilicus and listen for renal artery bruits from renal artery stenosis.

▪▪ Listen over the liver for bruits due to hepatoma or acute alcoholic hepatitis. A friction rub, which sounds like rubbing your dry fingers together, may be heard over the liver (perihepatitis) or spleen (perisplenitis).

▪▪ A succussion splash sounds like a half-filled water bottle being shaken. Explain the procedure to the patient then shake the abdomen by lifting him with both hands under the pelvis. An audible splash more than 4 hours after the patient has eaten or drunk anything indicates delayed gastric emptying, e.g. pyloric stenosis.

Hernias

Anatomy

The inguinal canal extends from the pubic tubercle to the anterior superior iliac spine (Fig. 8.23). It has an internal ring at the mid-inguinal point and an external ring at the pubic tubercle. The mid-inguinal point is midway between the pubic symphysis and the anterior superior iliac spine, and not at the midpoint of the inguinal ligament. The femoral canal lies below the inguinal ligament and lateral to the pubic tubercle.

Abnormal findings

- An indirect inguinal hernia bulges through the internal ring and follows the course of the inguinal canal. It may extend beyond the external ring and enter the scrotum. Indirect hernias comprise 85% of all hernias and are more common in younger men
- A direct inguinal hernia forms at a site of muscle weakness in the posterior wall of the inguinal canal and rarely extends into the scrotum. It is more common in older men and women (Fig. 8.24)
- A femoral hernia projects through the femoral ring and into the femoral canal.

Inguinal hernias are palpable above and medial to the pubic tubercle. Femoral hernias are palpable below the inguinal ligament and lateral to the pubic tubercle.

An external abdominal hernia is an abnormal protrusion of bowel and/or omentum, from the abdominal cavity. Hernias are common and typically occur at openings of the abdominal wall: for example, the inguinal, femoral and obturator canals, the umbilicus and the oesophageal hiatus. They may occur at sites of weakness of the abdominal wall or be related to previous surgical incisions. Internal hernias occur through defects of the mesentery or into the retroperitoneal space and are not visible. External hernias are more obvious when the pressure within the abdomen rises: for example, when the patient is standing, coughing or straining at stool. An impulse can often be felt in the hernia during coughing (cough impulse). Identify a hernia from its anatomical site and characteristics, and attempt to differentiate between direct and indirect inguinal types (Box 8.39).

In a reducible hernia the contents can be returned to the abdominal cavity, spontaneously or by manipulation; if they cannot, the hernia is irreducible. An abdominal hernia has a covering sac of peritoneum and the neck of the hernia is a common site of compression of the contents (Fig. 8.25). If bowel is contained within the hernia, obstruction may occur. If the blood supply to the contents of the hernia (bowel or omentum) is restricted, the hernia is strangulated. It is tense and tender and has no cough impulse; there may be bowel obstruction and later, signs of sepsis and shock. A strangulated hernia is a surgical emergency and, if left untreated, will lead to bowel infarction and peritonitis.

Examination sequence

Hernias

First examine the groin with the patient standing upright. Inspect the inguinal and femoral canals and the scrotum for any lumps or bulges.

Ask the patient to cough; look for an impulse over the femoral or inguinal canals and scrotum.

Identify the anatomical relationships between the bulge, the pubic tubercle and the inguinal ligament to distinguish a femoral from an inguinal hernia.

Palpate the external inguinal ring and along the inguinal canal for possible muscle defects. Ask the patient to cough and feel for a cough impulse.

8.39 Causes of palpable swellings in the groin

- Inguinal hernia: indirect and direct
- Femoral hernia
- Lymph node(s)
- Saphena varix (a varicosity of the long saphenous vein)
- Skin and subcutaneous lumps, e.g. lipoma, sebaceous cyst
- Hydrocoele of spermatic cord
- Undescended testis
- Femoral aneurysm
- Psoas abscess

OSCEs 8.40 Examine this patient with an inguinal hernia

1. With the patient supine, expose the groins and scrotum.
2. Inspect both groins for swelling and scars indicating previous surgery.
3. Ask the patient to point to where the swelling usually appears.
4. Ask the patient to cough and look for the appearance of a swelling.
5. Ask the patient to reduce the lump. If the patient cannot, try to reduce it yourself.
6. Palpate the swelling to check its position relative to the pubic tubercle.
7. If the hernia is reducible, apply pressure over the deep inguinal ring and ask the patient to cough. Does this control the hernia?
8. Examine the other groin to exclude bilateral hernias.
9. In a male patient, examine the scrotum and testes with the patient standing. Does the hernia pass into the scrotum? If it does and it is irreducible, does it transilluminate and are there bowel sounds audible in the hernia?

OSCEs 8.41 Examine this patient for an abdominal hernia

1. Ask the patient to lie flat with arms by the sides.
2. Look at the obvious lump for scars, discoloration and pulsation.
3. Ask the patient to sit up to see if the lump increases with abdominal pressure.
4. Ask the patient if the lump has ever been painful, then palpate the lump.
5. Ask the patient to reduce the lump. If the patient cannot, try to reduce it yourself.
6. Feel for a cough impulse.

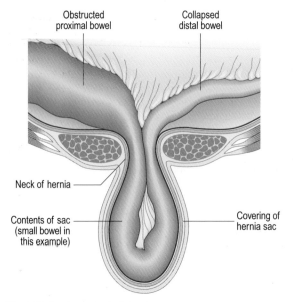

Fig. 8.25 Hernia: anatomical structure.

Obstructed proximal bowel

Collapsed distal bowel

Neck of hernia

Contents of sac (small bowel in this example)

Covering of hernia sac

Ask the patient to lie down and establish whether the hernia reduces spontaneously. If so, press two fingers over the internal inguinal ring at the mid-inguinal point and ask the patient to cough or stand up while you continue to press over the internal inguinal ring. If the hernia re-appears, it is a direct hernia. If it can be prevented from re-appearing, it is an indirect inguinal hernia.

Examine the opposite side to exclude the possibility of asymptomatic hernias.

Rectal examination

Digital examination of the rectum is an important part of the general medical examination (Box 8.42). Do not avoid the examination because you or the patient finds it disagreeable. The normal rectum is usually empty and smooth-walled, with the coccyx and sacrum lying posteriorly. In the male, anterior to the rectum from below upwards, lie the membranous urethra, the prostate and the base of the bladder. The normal prostate is smooth and has a firm consistency, with lateral lobes and a median groove between them. In the female, the vagina and cervix lie anteriorly. The upper end of the anal canal is marked by the puborectalis muscle, which is readily palpable and contracts as a reflex action on coughing or on conscious contraction by the patient. Beyond the anal canal, the rectum passes upwards and backwards along the curve of the sacrum.

Spasm of the external anal sphincter is common in the anxious patient. When associated with local pain, it is probably due to an anal fissure (a tear in the mucosa). If an anal fissure is suspected, use a local anaesthetic suppository 10 minutes beforehand to reduce the pain and spasm and to facilitate satisfactory examination.

8.42 Indications for rectal examination

Alimentary

- Suspected appendicitis, pelvic abscess, peritonitis, lower abdominal pain
- Diarrhoea, constipation, tenesmus or anorectal pain
- Rectal bleeding or iron deficiency anaemia
- Unexplained weight loss
- Bimanual examination of lower abdominal mass for diagnosis or staging
- Malignancies of unknown origin

Genitourinary

- Assessment of the prostate in prostatism or suspected prostatic cancer
- Dysuria, frequency, haematuria, epididymo-orchitis
- Instead of vaginal examination in patients where this would be inappropriate

Miscellaneous

- Unexplained bone pain, backache or lumbosacral nerve root pain
- Pyrexia of unknown origin
- Abdominal, pelvic or spinal trauma

Examination sequence
Rectum

Explain what you are going to do and ask for permission to proceed. Offer a chaperone; if the offer of a chaperone is refused, record the fact. Explain that the examination may be uncomfortable but should not be painful.

Position the patient in the left lateral position with the buttocks at the edge of the couch, the knees drawn up to the chest, and the heels clear of the perineum (Fig. 8.26).

Put on gloves and examine the perianal skin, using an effective light source and looking for evidence of skin lesions, external haemorrhoids and fistulae.

Lubricate your index finger with water-based gel. Place the pulp of the forefinger on the anal margin and with steady pressure on the sphincter push your finger gently through the anal canal into the rectum (Fig. 8.27).

If anal spasm is encountered, ask the patient to breathe in deeply and relax. Use a local anaesthetic suppository before trying again. If pain persists, examination under general anaesthesia may be necessary.

Ask the patient to squeeze your finger with the anal muscles and note any weakness of sphincter contraction.

Palpate systematically around the entire rectum; note any abnormality and examine any mass. Record the percentage of the rectal circumference involved by disease and its distance from the anus (Fig. 8.28).

Identify the uterine cervix in women and the prostate in men; assess the size, shape and consistency of the prostate and note any tenderness.

If the rectum contains faeces and you are in doubt about palpable masses, repeat the examination after the patient has defecated.

Slowly withdraw your finger and examine it for stool colour and the presence of blood or mucus (Box 8.43).

Abnormal findings

Haemorrhoids ('piles', congested venous plexuses around the anal canal) are not palpable unless thrombosed. In patients with chronic constipation the rectum is often loaded with faeces. Faecal masses are often palpable, should be movable and can be indented.

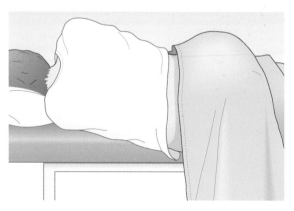

Fig. 8.26 The correct position of the patient before a rectal examination.

In women, a retroverted uterus and the normal cervix are often palpable through the anterior rectal wall and a vaginal tampon may be confusing. Cancer of the lower rectum is palpable as a mucosal irregularity. Obstructing cancer of the upper rectum may produce ballooning of the empty rectal cavity below. Metastases or colonic tumours within the pelvis may be mistaken for faeces and vice versa. Lateralized tenderness suggests pelvic peritonitis. Gynaecological malignancy may cause a 'frozen pelvis' with a hard, rigid feel to the pelvic organs due to extensive peritoneal disease, e.g. radiotherapy or metastatic cervical or ovarian cancer.

Benign prostatic hyperplasia often produces palpable symmetrical enlargement, but not if the hyperplasia is confined to the median lobe. A hard, irregular or asymmetrical gland with no palpable median groove suggests prostate cancer. Tenderness accompanied by a change in the consistency of the gland may be due to prostatitis or prostatic abscess. The prostate is abnormally small in hypogonadism.

Proctoscopy

Always undertake a digital rectal examination before visual examination of the anal canal by proctoscopy. If an examination of the rectal mucosa is required, sigmoidoscopy is indicated rather than proctoscopy.

▶ Examination sequence

Proctoscopy

▶ Place the patient in the left lateral position, as for digital rectal examination.

▶ With gloved hands, separate the buttocks with the forefinger and thumb of one hand: with your other hand, gently insert a lubricated proctoscope with its obturator into the anal canal and rectum in the direction of the umbilicus.

▶ Remove the obturator and examine the rectal mucosa carefully under good illumination, noting any abnormality.

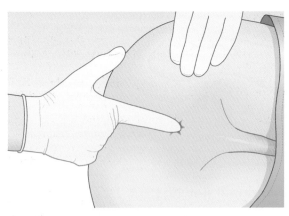

Fig. 8.27 Rectal examination. The correct method to insert your index finger in rectal examination.

🔍 8.43 Causes of abnormal stool appearance

Stool appearance	Cause
Abnormally pale	Biliary obstruction
Pale and greasy	Steatorrhoea
Black and tarry (melaena)	Bleeding from the upper GI tract
Grey/black	Oral iron or bismuth therapy
Silvery	Steatorrhoea plus upper GI bleeding, e.g. pancreatic cancer
Fresh blood in or on stool	Large bowel, rectal or anal bleeding
Stool mixed with pus	Infective colitis or inflammatory bowel disease
Rice-water stool (watery with mucus and cell debris)	Cholera

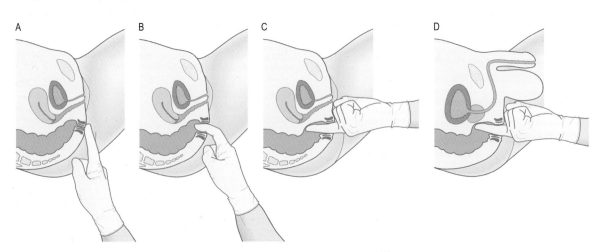

Fig. 8.28 Examination of the rectum. (A and **B)** Insertion of the finger. The hand is then rotated. **(C)** The most prominent feature in the female is the cervix. **(D)** The most prominent feature in the male is the prostate.

8

- Carefully examine the anal canal for fissures, particularly if the patient has experienced pain during the procedure.
- Ask the patient to strain down as the instrument is slowly withdrawn to detect any degree of rectal prolapse and the presence and severity of any haemorrhoids.

Abnormal findings

Proctoscopic examination of the anus and lower rectum can confirm or exclude the presence of haemorrhoids, anal fissures and rectal prolapse. Rectal mucosa appears similar to buccal mucosa, apart from the presence of prominent submucosal veins. During straining, haemorrhoids distend with blood and may prolapse. If the degree of protrusion is more than 3–4 cm, a rectal prolapse may be present.

THE ACUTE ABDOMEN

Patients with an 'acute abdomen' comprise the majority of general surgical emergencies. Causes range from self-limiting conditions to severe life-threatening diseases (Box 8.44). Rapidly evaluate then immediately resuscitate critically ill patients before further assessment and surgical intervention. Give parenteral opioid analgesia early to alleviate severe abdominal pain, as it will help, not hinder, clinical assessment. In patients with undiagnosed acute abdominal pain, regularly re-assess their clinical state,

8.44 Common non-traumatic causes of the acute abdomen

Pathology	Organ	Disease
Inflammation	Appendix	Acute appendicitis
	Gallbladder	Acute cholecystitis
	Colon	Diverticulitis
	Fallopian tube	Salpingitis
	Pancreas	Acute pancreatitis
Obstruction	Intestine	Intestinal obstruction
	Gallbladder/bile duct	Biliary obstruction
	Ureter	Ureteric obstruction
	Urethra/bladder	Urinary retention
Ischaemia	Intestine	Strangulated hernia
		Volvulus
		Thromboembolism
	Ovary	Torsion of ovarian cyst
Perforation	Duodenum	Perforated peptic ulcer
	Stomach	Perforated ulcer/cancer
	Colon	Perforated diverticulum
		Perforated cancer
	Gallbladder	Biliary peritonitis
Rupture	Fallopian tube	Ruptured ectopic pregnancy
	Abdominal aorta	Ruptured aneurysm

investigations and likelihood of surgical intervention before administering repeat analgesia.

Patients may be so occupied by recent and severe symptoms that they forget important details of the history unless questioned directly (Box 8.45). Ask family or friends for additional information if severe pain, shock or altered consciousness makes it difficult to obtain an accurate history from the patient. Note any past history which may be relevant, e.g. acute perforation in a patient with known diverticular disease. Remember that disease outside the abdomen, e.g. myocardial infarction, pneumonia, diabetic ketoacidosis or herpes zoster, may present with acute abdominal pain (Box 8.12). Abdominal signs may be masked in patients taking immunosuppressants or anti-inflammatory drugs, in alcohol intoxication or in altered states of consciousness (Box 8.46).

The history

Pain

Acute abdominal pain is the most common presenting symptom and its site may indicate the likely origin of the pathology.

Pain experienced predominantly in the upper abdomen arises from disorders of foregut structures, e.g. duodenal ulcer, cholecystitis or pancreatitis. Central abdominal pain arises from midgut structures, e.g. small bowel and appendix. Lower abdominal pain arises from hindgut structures, e.g. colon. Gynaecological and testicular pathology also cause lower abdominal pain.

Visceral pain is diffuse, midline and difficult to localize. Somatic pain is accurately localized and felt at the site of the disease process. In acute appendicitis, pain is initially periumbilical (visceral pain) and moves to the right iliac fossa when localized inflammation of the parietal peritoneum becomes established (somatic pain) (Fig. 8.30).

Excruciating pain, poorly relieved by opioid analgesia, suggests an ischaemic vascular event, e.g. bowel infarction or ruptured abdominal aortic aneurysm. Severe pain rapidly eased by potent analgesia is more typical of acute pancreatitis or peritonitis secondary to a ruptured viscus. Biliary or renal colic is usually promptly relieved by parenteral analgesia. Dull, vague and poorly localized pain is more typical of an inflammatory process or low-grade infection. Severe pain of sudden onset is likely to be due to a vascular event or rupture of a viscus. Moderately severe pain of rapid onset is typical of renal or biliary colic, acute pancreatitis or small bowel obstruction. Slowly progressive pain of gradual onset is more characteristic of peritoneal infection or inflammation, e.g. salpingitis, appendicitis or diverticulitis.

Inflammation and obstruction are the principal pathological processes producing acute abdominal

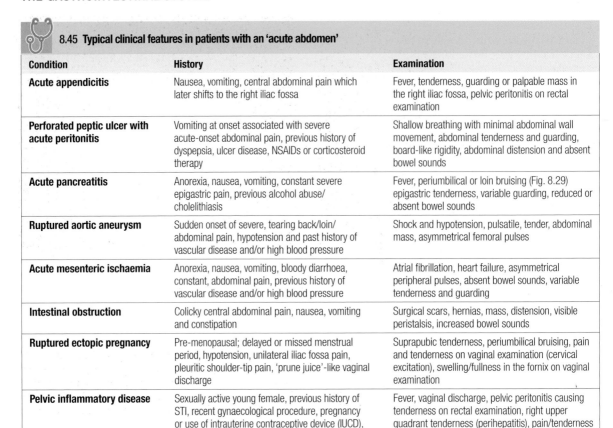

8.45 Typical clinical features in patients with an 'acute abdomen'

Condition	History	Examination
Acute appendicitis	Nausea, vomiting, central abdominal pain which later shifts to the right iliac fossa	Fever, tenderness, guarding or palpable mass in the right iliac fossa, pelvic peritonitis on rectal examination
Perforated peptic ulcer with acute peritonitis	Vomiting at onset associated with severe acute-onset abdominal pain, previous history of dyspepsia, ulcer disease, NSAIDs or corticosteroid therapy	Shallow breathing with minimal abdominal wall movement, abdominal tenderness and guarding, board-like rigidity, abdominal distension and absent bowel sounds
Acute pancreatitis	Anorexia, nausea, vomiting, constant severe epigastric pain, previous alcohol abuse/cholelithiasis	Fever, periumbilical or loin bruising (Fig. 8.29) epigastric tenderness, variable guarding, reduced or absent bowel sounds
Ruptured aortic aneurysm	Sudden onset of severe, tearing back/loin/abdominal pain, hypotension and past history of vascular disease and/or high blood pressure	Shock and hypotension, pulsatile, tender, abdominal mass, asymmetrical femoral pulses
Acute mesenteric ischaemia	Anorexia, nausea, vomiting, bloody diarrhoea, constant, abdominal pain, previous history of vascular disease and/or high blood pressure	Atrial fibrillation, heart failure, asymmetrical peripheral pulses, absent bowel sounds, variable tenderness and guarding
Intestinal obstruction	Colicky central abdominal pain, nausea, vomiting and constipation	Surgical scars, hernias, mass, distension, visible peristalsis, increased bowel sounds
Ruptured ectopic pregnancy	Pre-menopausal; delayed or missed menstrual period, hypotension, unilateral iliac fossa pain, pleuritic shoulder-tip pain, 'prune juice'-like vaginal discharge	Suprapubic tenderness, periumbilical bruising, pain and tenderness on vaginal examination (cervical excitation), swelling/fullness in the fornix on vaginal examination
Pelvic inflammatory disease	Sexually active young female, previous history of STI, recent gynaecological procedure, pregnancy or use of intrauterine contraceptive device (IUCD), irregular menstruation, dyspareunia, lower or central abdominal pain, backache, pleuritic right upper quadrant pain (Fitz-Hugh–Curtis syndrome)	Fever, vaginal discharge, pelvic peritonitis causing tenderness on rectal examination, right upper quadrant tenderness (perihepatitis), pain/tenderness on vaginal examination (cervical excitation), swelling/fullness in the fornix on vaginal examination

8.46 Clinical signs in the 'acute abdomen'

Sign	Disease associations	Examination
Murphy's	Acute cholecystitis Sensitivity 50–97% Specificity 50–80% Likelihood ratio 1.9 if present Likelihood ratio 0.6 if absent	As the patient takes a deep breath in, gently palpate in the right upper quadrant of the abdomen; the acutely inflamed gallbladder contacts the examining fingers, evoking pain with the arrest of inspiration
Rovsing's	Acute appendicitis Sensitivity 20–70% Specificity 40–96% Likelihood ratio 2.5 if present Likelihood ratio 0.7 if absent	Palpation in the left iliac fossa produces pain in the right iliac fossa
Iliopsoas	Retro-ileal appendicitis, iliopsoas abscess, perinephric abscess	Ask the patient to flex the thigh against the resistance of your hand; a painful response indicates an inflammatory process involving the right psoas muscle
Grey–Turner's and Cullen's	Haemorrhagic pancreatitis, aortic rupture and ruptured ectopic pregnancy (Fig. 8.29)	Bleeding into the falciform ligament; bruising develops around the umbilicus (Cullen) or in the loins (Grey–Turner)

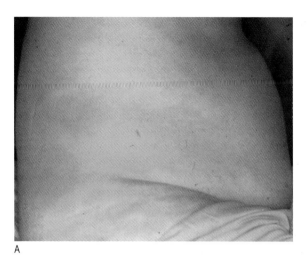

A

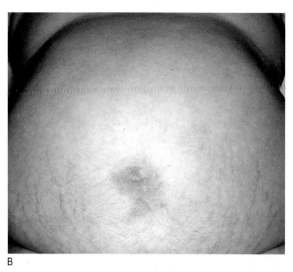

B

Fig. 8.29 Acute pancreatitis. (A) Bruising over the flanks (Grey–Turner's sign). **(B)** Bruising round the umbilicus (Cullen's sign).

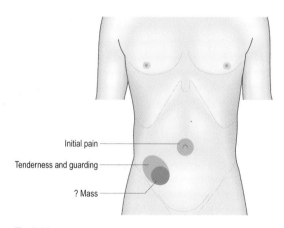

Initial pain —

Tenderness and guarding —

? Mass —

Fig. 8.30 Acute appendicitis.

typical of renal colic. Central upper abdominal pain radiating through to the back, partially relieved by sitting forward, is common in patients with pancreatitis. The combination of severe back and abdominal pain may indicate a ruptured or dissecting abdominal aortic aneurysm.

Anorexia, nausea and vomiting are common but non-specific symptoms reflecting the nature and severity of pain; they may be absent, even in advanced intra-abdominal disease. Severe vomiting without significant pain suggests gastric outlet or proximal small bowel obstruction. Faeculent vomiting, of small bowel contents (not faeces), is a late feature of distal small bowel or colonic obstruction. In peritonitis, the vomitus is usually small in volume but persistent. Severe vomiting with retching may result in laceration at the gastro-oesophageal junction (Mallory–Weiss tear), or oesophageal rupture (Boerhaave's syndrome).

Other features

Ask about prior episodes of pain that were similar, what symptoms and features were present, and what investigations were performed. In women take a menstrual and sexual history, and consider (ectopic) pregnancy. Ask about previous sexually transmitted infection (STI), purulent vaginal discharge and pain on sexual intercourse (dyspareunia), suggesting pelvic inflammatory disease (PID) or endometriosis.

Alteration of bowel function is common in patients with acute abdominal emergencies. Absolute constipation — that is, no gas or bowel movements — suggests intestinal obstruction and is likely to be associated with abdominal pain, vomiting and

pain. Inflammation usually produces constant pain exacerbated by movement or coughing. Patients typically lie still in order not to exacerbate the pain. Obstruction of a viscus produces an intermittent, colicky pain and characteristically patients move around or draw their knees up towards the chest during painful spasms. In contrast, obstruction of the gallbladder, biliary tree or ureter from a stone produces sustained, severe pain unaffected by movement, causing restlessness and an inability to lie still.

Radiation of the pain is often a helpful clinical clue. Pain radiating from the right hypochondrium to the shoulder or interscapular region may reflect irritation of the diaphragm, e.g. in acute cholecystitis. Pain radiating from the loin to the groin and genitalia is abdominal distension. Diarrhoea is a common symptom of both intra- and extra-abdominal disorder, including gastroenteritis, pelvic appendicitis or pneumonia with bacteraemia. Bloody diarrhoea may be due to inflammatory bowel disease, colonic ischaemia or infective gastroenteritis.

The physical examination

◼◥ Examination sequence

Acute abdomen

Inspection

◼◥ Does the patient look unwell, with pallor, sweating and reluctance to move? Critically ill patients may be confused, with an altered state of consciousness.

◼◥ Record the temperature, heart rate, blood pressure and respiratory rate regularly.

◼◥ Examine the cardiovascular and respiratory systems, as myocardial infarction, pneumonia and shingles may present with acute abdominal pain.

Palpation, percussion and auscultation

◼◥ Examine the abdomen, then the back, groins, perineum and genitalia.

◼◥ Perform a rectal examination unless the patient is to be seen imminently by the surgeon, who may wish to perform a rectal examination.

◼◥ Gently percuss the abdomen to localize and assess rebound tenderness and to check for fluid in the peritoneal cavity. Diminished or absent liver dullness to percussion may be present in patients with perforation of a hollow viscus and air under the diaphragm.

◼◥ Absent bowel sounds on auscultation may indicate diffuse peritonitis. Increased peristalsis produces frequent, high-pitched 'tinkling' bowel sounds characteristic of intestinal obstruction, gastroenteritis or severe inflammatory bowel disease.

INVESTIGATIONS

Stool

Test the stool for the presence of faecal occult blood (FOB test). A positive FOB is produced by any cause of gastrointestinal haemorrhage, e.g. bleeding peptic ulcer, colorectal cancer and inflammatory bowel disease. FOB tests are sensitive but not specific; false positive tests occur after vigorous tooth brushing or after eating rare steak or other red meat. False negative tests occur in patients with proven colorectal or gastric cancers, chronic upper gastrointestinal haemorrhage and inflammatory bowel disease.

Urine

Test the urine for bilirubin and urobilinogen to confirm jaundice and point to its cause (Box 8.23). Urinalysis may also be useful in diagnosing non-surgical causes of acute abdominal pain, e.g. diabetes mellitus and porphyria, by demonstrating glycosuria and the presence of porphobilinogen respectively.

Radiography

Chest X-ray and plain film of the abdomen are essential in the assessment of the acute abdomen. Perforated peptic ulcers can cause pneumoperitoneum with air under the diaphragm on chest X-ray, while plain film of the abdomen can reveal many abnormalities, such as dilated small bowel due to intestinal obstruction, dilated large bowel due to toxic dilatation, and twisted and dilated bowel (volvulus) (Fig. 8.33).

Ascitic fluid

Obtain a sample of fluid for inspection and analysis from all patients with ascites. Use either iliac fossa at a point one-third of the distance from the anterior superior iliac spine to the umbilicus, avoiding any previous surgical scars. Insert a needle using strict aseptic technique and aspirate up to 20 ml into a syringe. This procedure is called a diagnostic ascitic tap or abdominal paracentesis.

Ascitic fluid is usually clear and straw-coloured. Uniformly bloodstained fluid suggests intra-abdominal malignancy. Turbid fluid may indicate a high cell count due to infection, or high protein content. Occasionally, ascitic fluid may be chylous, with a milky appearance due to a high lipid content usually indicating lymphatic obstruction. Analyse the fluid for protein content. Protein concentration $<25\,g/l$, or a gradient between the serum and ascitic albumin concentration $>11\,g/l$ indicates a transudate. This is seen in heart failure, in cirrhosis with portal hypertension and in other hypoalbuminaemic states, e.g. nephrotic syndrome. Protein concentration $>25\,g/l$, or a gradient $<11\,g/l$, indicates an exudate and suggests malignancy or infection. Send the fluid for cell count and culture, cytology for malignant cells, and measurement of amylase (raised in pancreatic ascites) and glucose (low in tuberculous ascites) (Box 8.15).

8.47 Investigations in gastrointestinal and hepatobiliary disease

Investigation	Indication/Comment	Investigation	Indication/Comment
Radiology		CT colonography	Unexplained GI bleeding or pain Useful in colon cancer screening, in the frail, sick patient and if colonoscopy is unsuccessful
Chest X-ray	Acute abdomen, perforated viscus, subphrenic abscess Pneumonia, free air beneath diaphragm, pleural effusion, elevated diaphragm		
		Video capsule endoscopy	Unexplained GI bleeding, small bowel diseases Vascular malformations, inflammatory bowel disease
Abdominal X-ray	Intestinal obstruction, perforation, renal colic Fluid levels, air above the liver, urinary tract stones	MR cholangiopancreatography (MRCP)	Obstructive jaundice, acute and chronic pancreatitis Diagnostic role only
Barium meal	Dysphagia, dyspepsia if gastroscopy is not possible Oesophageal obstruction (endoscopy preferable, especially if previous gastric surgery)	Endoscopic retrograde cholangiopancreatography (ERCP)	Obstructive jaundice, acute and chronic pancreatitis Diagnostic and therapeutic role Stenting strictures and removing stones
Small bowel barium follow-through or MR enteroclysis	Malabsorption, subacute obstruction, unexplained GI bleeding Duodenal diverticulosis, Crohn's disease, lymphoma	Abdominal CT scan (Fig. 8.32)	Acute abdomen, suspected pancreatic or renal mass, tumour staging, abdominal aortic aneurysm Useful to confirm or exclude metastatic disease and leaking from aortic aneurysm
Large bowel barium enema or CT colonography	Altered bowel habit, iron deficiency anaemia, rectal bleeding if colonoscopy is not possible Colon cancer, inflammatory bowel disease, diverticular disease	Laparoscopy	Acute abdomen, chronic pelvic pain, suspected ovarian disease, peritoneal and liver disease Appendicitis, hepatic cirrhosis, ectopic pregnancy, ovarian cysts, endometriosis, pelvic inflammatory disease
Upper abdominal ultrasound scan (Fig. 8.31)	Biliary colic, jaundice, pancreatitis, malignancy Gallstones, liver metastases, cholestasis, pancreatic calcification, subphrenic abscess		
		Guided aspiration cytology and biopsy	Liver metastases, intra-abdominal or retroperitoneal tumours Tissue biopsy guided by ultrasound scanning
Pelvic ultrasound scan	Pelvic masses, inflammatory diseases, ectopic pregnancy, polycystic ovary syndrome Pelvic structures and abnormalities Ascitic fluid	Liver biopsy	Parenchymal disease of liver Tissue biopsy by percutaneous, transjugular or laparoscopic route
Invasive		**Others**	
Upper GI endoscopy	Dysphagia, dyspepsia, GI bleeding, gastric ulcer, malabsorption Gastric and/or duodenal biopsies are useful	Pancreatic function tests	Suspected pancreatic exocrine failure Stool elastase Pancreolauryl test
Lower GI endoscopy (colonoscopy)	Rectal bleeding, unexplained GI bleeding, inflammatory bowel disease Biopsy to confirm presence and type of colitis		

8

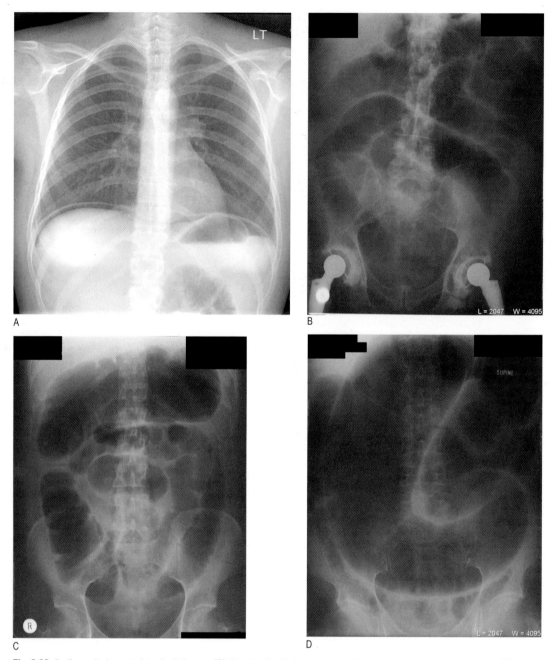

Fig. 8.33 Radiography in gastrointestinal disease. (A) Air under the diaphragm on chest X-ray due to perforated duodenal ulcer. **(B)** Dilated small bowel due to acute intestinal obstruction. **(C)** Dilated large bowel due to toxic megacolon. **(D)** Dilated loop of large bowel due to sigmoid volvulus.

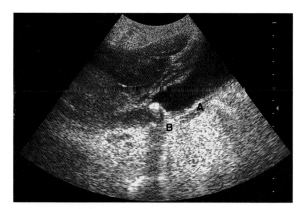

Fig. 8.31 Ultrasound scan showing thick-walled gallbladder (A) containing gallstones with posterior acoustic shadowing (B).

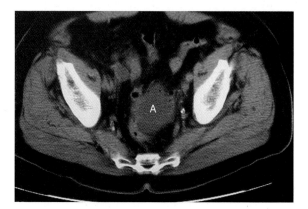

Fig. 8.32 CT scan of pelvis showing diverticular abscess (A).

8.48 Key points: the gastrointestinal system

- Common conditions such as GORD and irritable bowel syndrome can be diagnosed on the history alone.
- Diagnose irritable bowel syndrome positively from the pattern of symptoms and the absence of alarm features; do not use 'irritable bowel' as a label for 'medically unexplained gastrointestinal symptoms'. Remember that patients with irritable bowel syndrome may also have other significant additional gastrointestinal disease.
- Renal and biliary 'colic' are characterized by sustained pain not 'colicky' pain.
- In hepatomegaly, the left lobe often enlarges to a greater degree than the right lobe; look for evidence of a palpable liver edge in the epigastrium.
- In patients with hepatosplenomegaly, look for other signs of chronic liver disease and lymphadenopathy.
- A palpable spleen is always pathological; a palpable liver may be a normal liver displaced downwards.
- Always consider (ectopic) pregnancy and pelvic inflammatory disease as a cause of abdominal pain in women of child-bearing age.
- Always consider acute appendicitis in the differential diagnosis of acute abdominal pain.
- Pelvic peritonitis is often best elicited by rectal examination.
- Assess all patients with gastrointestinal bleeding for evidence of hypovolaemia.

8

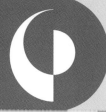

Allan Cumming
Stephen Payne

The renal system

9

RENAL EXAMINATION

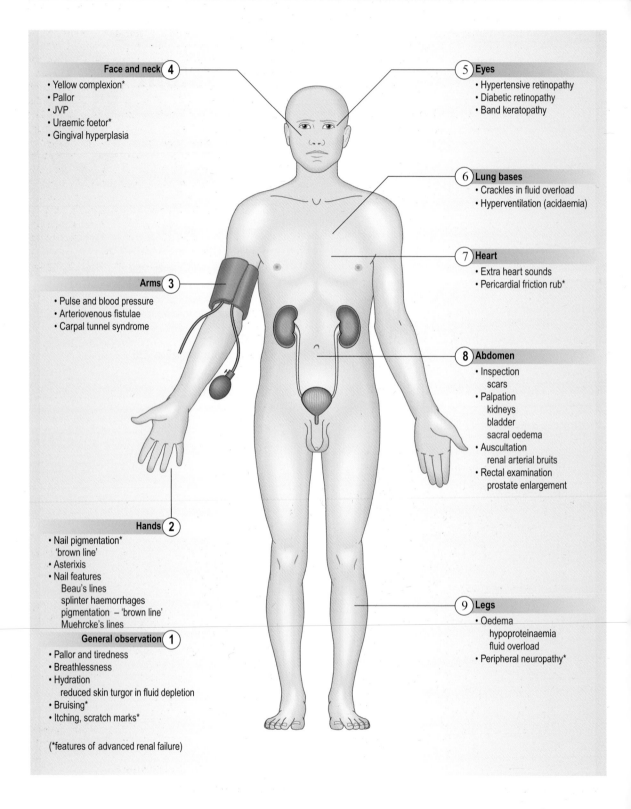

Face and neck ④
- Yellow complexion*
- Pallor
- JVP
- Uraemic foetor*
- Gingival hyperplasia

Eyes ⑤
- Hypertensive retinopathy
- Diabetic retinopathy
- Band keratopathy

Lung bases ⑥
- Crackles in fluid overload
- Hyperventilation (acidaemia)

Heart ⑦
- Extra heart sounds
- Pericardial friction rub*

Arms ③
- Pulse and blood pressure
- Arteriovenous fistulae
- Carpal tunnel syndrome

Abdomen ⑧
- Inspection
  scars
- Palpation
  kidneys
  bladder
  sacral oedema
- Auscultation
  renal arterial bruits
- Rectal examination
  prostate enlargement

Hands ②
- Nail pigmentation*
  'brown line'
- Asterixis
- Nail features
  Beau's lines
  splinter haemorrhages
  pigmentation – 'brown line'
  Muehrcke's lines

General observation ①
- Pallor and tiredness
- Breathlessness
- Hydration
  reduced skin turgor in fluid depletion
- Bruising*
- Itching, scratch marks*

Legs ⑨
- Oedema
  hypoproteinaemia
  fluid overload
- Peripheral neuropathy*

(*features of advanced renal failure)

ANATOMY

The kidneys are retroperitoneal and lie on either side of the spine at the T12–L3 level (Fig. 9.1). Normal kidneys are 11–14 cm long. The right kidney lies 1.5 cm lower than the left because of the liver. Each kidney contains about one million nephrons, comprising a glomerulus, proximal tubule, loop of Henle, distal tubule and collecting duct (Fig. 9.2).

The primary function of the kidneys is to excrete waste products of metabolism, e.g. urea, maintain the body's water and electrolyte homeostasis, and regulate blood pressure via the renin–angiotensin system. They also have endocrine functions in erythropoiesis and vitamin D metabolism.

The kidneys produce urine, which is passed to the bladder by peristaltic waves in the smooth muscle of the ureters. Together, the kidneys receive ~25% of the cardiac output. The T10–12/L1 roots innervate the renal capsule and ureter, and pain from these structures is felt in these dermatomes (Fig. 11.30, p. 298). The bladder acts as a reservoir and, when empty, is shaped like a tetrahedron. As it fills, it becomes ovoid, and rises out of the pelvis in the midline towards the umbilicus, adjacent to the anterior abdominal wall. The bladder wall contains a layer of smooth muscle, the detrusor. The conscious desire to urinate occurs when the bladder holds about 250–350 ml of urine. The detrusor contracts under parasympathetic control, allowing urine to pass through the urethra (micturition). The urethra runs from the bladder to the external meatus. The male urethra runs from the bladder to the tip of the penis and has three parts: prostatic, membranous and spongiose

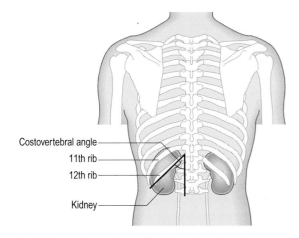

Fig. 9.1 The surface anatomy of the kidneys from the back.

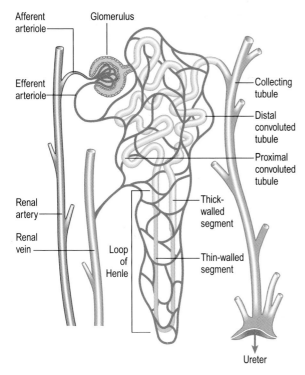

Fig. 9.2 A single nephron.

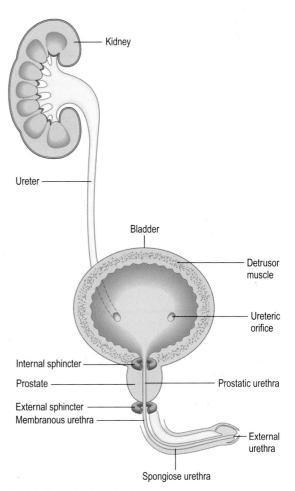

Fig. 9.3 The male urinary tract.

9

219

9

(Fig. 9.3). The female urethra is much shorter, with the external meatus situated anterior to the vaginal orifice and behind the clitoris (Fig. 10.17, p. 243). Two muscular rings acting as valves (sphincters) control micturition:

- The internal sphincter is at the bladder neck and is involuntary
- The external sphincter surrounds the membranous urethra and is under voluntary control; it is innervated by the pudendal nerves (S2, 3 and 4).

SYMPTOMS AND DEFINITIONS

Even severe renal disease may be asymptomatic or have non-specific symptoms, such as tiredness or breathlessness from renal failure or associated anaemia. Ask about the following symptoms, but always test urine and blood to confirm a diagnosis and assess renal function (Box 9.1).

Pain

Pain may arise from the kidney (loin pain), the ureter (ureteric colic) or the bladder (suprapubic pain or pain on passing urine — voiding).

Renal angle (between the 12th rib and the spine) or loin pain is due to stretching of the renal capsule or renal pelvis. Causes include infection, inflammation or mechanical obstruction. Constant loin pain, with systemic upset, fever, rigors and pain on voiding, suggests infection of the upper urinary tract and kidney (acute pyelonephritis). Chronic dull, aching loin discomfort may occur with chronic renal infection and scarring from vesico-ureteric reflux, adult polycystic kidney disease (APKD) or chronic urinary tract obstruction. Chronic obstruction may be pain-free. Dull, non-localized loin pain occurs in renal stone disease and some forms of glomerulonephritis, e.g. IgA nephropathy, and can mimic musculoskeletal conditions.

Renal or ureteric colic is caused by acute obstruction with distension of the renal pelvis and ureter by a stone, blood clot or, rarely, a necrotic renal papilla. The pain is of sudden onset, severe and sustained, and may radiate to the iliac fossa, the groin and the genitalia, especially the testis. The patient is restless and nauseated, and often vomits. Once the obstructing pathology reaches the bladder, symptoms may resolve.

In the loin pain–haematuria syndrome patients complain of chronic unilateral or bilateral loin discomfort of varying severity. They characteristically have microscopic haematuria and occasionally frank (macroscopic) haematuria.

Voiding pain (dysuria) is pain during or immediately after passing urine, often described as a 'burning' sensation felt at the urethral meatus or suprapubically and associated with a desire to pass urine more often (frequency). The most common cause is infection and/or inflammation of the bladder (cystitis). Prostatitis and urethritis produce similar symptoms. Prostatitis causes perineal and rectal pain at the same time. Pain localized

9.1 Common symptoms	
Symptom	**Definition/Comments**
Kidneys upper urinary tract	
Pain	Usually felt in lumbar regions
Swelling	Usually of feet/ankles and/or around eyes
Macroscopic haematuria	Blood visible in urine with naked eye
Lower urinary tract	
Voiding pain	Pain passing urine
Frequency	Passing urine more often than usual
Urgency	An uncontrollable need to pass urine
Nocturia	Waking to pass urine during the night
Hesitancy	Delay in initiating urine flow; seen in bladder outlet obstruction
Poor flow	A reduction in the urinary stream
Post-micturition dribbling	Dribbling of urine after voiding; usually due to bladder outlet obstruction
Stress incontinence	Involuntary passage of urine related to increased intra-abdominal pressure
Urge incontinence	Involuntary passage of urine related to abnormal detrusor function
General	
Polyuria	Passing a larger volume of urine than normal
Oliguria	Passing a smaller volume of urine than normal
Anuria	Total absence of urine output
Haematuria	Blood in the urine
Pneumaturia	Gas in the urine
Urethral discharge	Purulent material from urethra, suggesting sexually acquired infection

to the penis indicates local pathology, such as stricture, stone or, rarely, tumour.

Testicular and epididymal pain may be felt primarily in the groin and lower abdomen. Distinguish tenderness and swelling of the testis from a strangulated hernia or acute epididymo-orchitis; in pubertal boys and young men consider torsion of the testis (pp. 205 and 261).

Voiding symptoms

Lower urinary tract symptoms occur:

- during the storage phase of micturition
- during the voiding phase of micturition
- after micturition
- with incontinence.

Storage symptoms

- Frequency is increased micturition with no increase in the total urine output
- Urgency is a sudden strong need to pass urine and may cause incontinence if there is no opportunity to urinate. Urgency is due either to overactivity in the detrusor muscle or abnormal stretch receptor activity from the bladder
- Nocturia means being wakened once, or more, at night to void.

Storage symptoms are usually associated with bladder, prostate or urethral problems, e.g. lower urinary tract infection, tumour, urinary stones or urinary tract obstruction, or are a consequence of neurological disease.

Voiding phase symptoms

Hesitancy is difficulty or delay in initiating urine flow. In men over 40 this is commonly due to bladder outlet obstruction by prostatic enlargement (Box 9.3). In women these symptoms suggest urethral obstruction due to stenosis or genital prolapse.

After micturition

Dribbling and incomplete emptying are caused by obstruction but, with associated storage symptoms, indicate abnormalities of detrusor function.

Incontinence

Involuntary release of urine may occur with a need to void (urge incontinence), be related to an increase in intra-abdominal pressure (stress incontinence), or be a combination of both (mixed incontinence) (Boxes 9.4–9.6). Urge incontinence occurs when the detrusor is overactive. Stress incontinence occurs in women and is due to weakness of the pelvic floor following

9.3 Features of bladder outlet obstruction due to prostatic hyperplasia

- Slow flow
- Hesitancy
- Incomplete emptying (the need to pass urine again within a few minutes of micturition)
- Dribbling after micturition
- Frequency and nocturia (due to incomplete bladder emptying)
- A palpable bladder

9.4 Urinary incontinence: points to cover in the history

- Age at onset and frequency of wetting
- Ever dry at night?
- Number of pads used. Are they damp, wet or soaked?
- Occurrence during sleep (enuresis)
- Any other urinary symptoms
- Provocative factors, e.g. coughing, sneezing, exercising
- Past medical, obstetric and surgical histories
- Impact on daily living

9.5 Causes of urinary incontinence

- Degenerative brain diseases and stroke
- Spinal cord damage
- Neurological diseases, e.g. multiple sclerosis
- Pelvic floor weakness following childbirth
- Bladder outlet obstruction
- Urinary tract infection
- Childbirth, pelvic surgery or radiotherapy
- Detrusor instability

OSCEs 9.2 Examine this patient with loin pain

1. Measure temperature — raised in urinary infection.
2. Measure blood pressure — elevated in renovascular disease and chronic kidney disease.
3. Look at optic fundi for hypertensive retinopathy.
4. Examine abdomen for tenderness (renal or ureteric stones or other causes of obstruction, renal infection or inflammation).
5. Examine abdomen for enlarged, palpable kidneys:
   Unilateral in renal cancer, urinary tract obstruction
   Bilateral in adult polycystic kidney disease.
6. Look for evidence of non-renal causes of loin pain, e.g. spinal or other locomotor disease.
7. Examine urine for haematuria and proteinuria — haematuria alone is non-specific; presence of both suggests renal inflammation.

9

9.6 Functional assessment of lower urinary tract function

Frequency/volume chart

- Use to monitor micturition patterns, including nocturia, and fluid intake
- The patient collects his/her urine, measures each void, and charts it against time over 3–5 days

Urine flow rate

- The patient voids into a special receptacle that measures the rate of urine passage
- A low flow does not differentiate between poor detrusor contractility and bladder outlet obstruction

Urodynamic tests

- Invasive tests, necessitating insertion of bladder and rectal catheters to measure total bladder pressure and abdominal pressure and to allow bladder filling
- Filling studies determine detrusor activity and compliance
  Low detrusor pressures with low urine flow suggest detrusor function problems
  High detrusor pressures with a low flow suggest bladder outlet obstruction

9.7 International Prostate Symptom Score (IPSS)

Symptom	Not at all	Less than 1 time in 5	Less than half the time	About half the time	More than half the time	Almost always	Score
Incomplete emptying							
Over the past month, how often have you had a sensation of not emptying your bladder completely after you finish urinating?	0	1	2	3	4	5	
Frequency							
Over the past month, how often have you had to urinate again less than 2 hours after you finished urinating?	0	1	2	3	4	5	
Intermittency							
Over the past month, how often have you found you stopped and started again several times when you urinated?	0	1	2	3	4	5	
Urgency							
Over the last month, how difficult have you found it to postpone urination?	0	1	2	3	4	5	
Weak stream							
Over the past month, how often have you had a weak urinary stream?	0	1	2	3	4	5	
Straining							
Over the past month, how often have you had to push or strain to begin urination?	0	1	2	3	4	5	
Nocturia	None	1 time	2 times	3 times	4 times	5 times or more	
Over the past month, now many times did you most typically get up to urinate from the time you went to bed until the time you got up in the morning?	0	1	2	3	4	5	
Quality of life due to urinary symptoms	Delighted	Pleased	Mostly satisfied	Mixed about equally satisfied and dissatisfied	Mostly dissatisfied	Unhappy	Terrible
If you were to spend the rest of your life with your urinary condition the way it is now, how would you feel about that?	0	1	2	3	4	5	6

Total IPSS score: 0–7 mildly symptomatic; 8–19 moderately symptomatic; 20–35 severely symptomatic.

childbirth. Continual incontinence implies a fistula between the bladder and either the urethra or the vagina due to complications of obstetric delivery, pelvic surgery, radiotherapy, tumour or trauma. Enuresis is incontinence at night and is common and normal in childhood. It indicates bladder outlet obstruction or abnormalities of the wakening mechanism in adults.

Use the International Prostate Symptom Score (IPSS) in men to determine the severity of lifestyle intrusion from bladder outlet obstruction (Box 9.7).

Abnormalities in urine volume and composition

Healthy adults produce 2–3 litres of urine per day, equivalent to their fluid intake minus insensible fluid losses through the skin and respiratory tract (500–800 ml per day).

Polyuria

Polyuria is an abnormally large volume of urine, most commonly from excessive fluid intake. Rarely, this is a manifestation of psychiatric disease (psychogenic polydipsia), when the patient may pass up to 12 litres of urine daily. Polyuria also occurs when the kidneys cannot concentrate urine appropriately. Causes may be extrarenal: e.g. diuretic drugs, hyperglycaemia with glycosuria in diabetes mellitus causing an osmotic diuresis; lack of antidiuretic hormone (ADH) from the pituitary gland in cranial diabetes insipidus, or failure of aldosterone secretion by the adrenal gland in Addison's disease. Renal causes occur when the kidney tubules fail to reabsorb water appropriately in response to ADH. This impaired concentrating ability occurs in nephrogenic diabetes insipidus, which is usually due to genetic mutation in the tubular ADH receptor. It may also reflect chronic tubulo-interstitial damage, reflux nephropathy, analgesic nephropathy and other drugs, e.g. lithium.

Oliguria

Oliguria, a reduction in urine volume to <800 ml/day, may be appropriate with a very low fluid intake, but may also indicate loss of kidney function. The minimum urine volume needed to excrete the daily solute load varies with diet, physical activity and metabolic rate, but is not <400 ml/day. Acute renal failure is usually associated with oliguria, although 20% of patients have non-oliguric acute renal failure.

Anuria

Anuria, the total absence of urine production, suggests lower urinary tract obstruction when bladder neck or urethral obstruction causes acute urinary retention. Spinal injury may cause this through neurological damage.

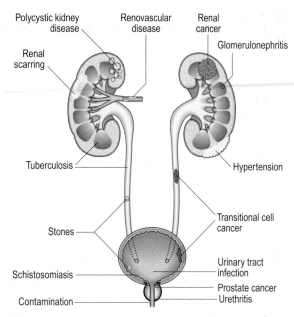

Fig. 9.4 Principal sources of haematuria.

Pneumaturia

Pneumaturia, passing gas bubbles in the urine, is rare. It may be associated with faecuria, in which faeces are voided. It suggests a fistula between the bladder and the colon, from a diverticular abscess, cancer or Crohn's disease.

Haematuria

Haematuria, red blood cells in the urine from the kidneys or urinary tract, may be microscopic (detected on urinalysis) or macroscopic (visible to the naked eye). Microscopic haematuria is a common feature of renal or urinary tract disease, especially if associated with proteinuria, hypertension, raised serum creatinine or reduced estimated glomerular filtration rate (eGFR). It may be a solitary and benign finding if these are all normal. Painless macroscopic haematuria must be investigated, as it may be due to cancer of the kidney, bladder or prostate.

Distinguish haematuria from contamination of the urine by blood from the female genital tract during menstruation. Free haemoglobin in the urine due to haemolysis, myoglobin in rhabdomyolysis, and other abnormalities of urine colour may mimic haematuria (Box 9.12). Confirm haematuria by urinalysis and urine microscopy (Fig. 9.4 and Box 9.8).

Proteinuria

Proteinuria is usually asymptomatic and detected by simple urinalysis; it usually indicates kidney disease (Boxes 9.10 and 9.11). Proteinuria up to 2 g/24h is non-specific. Values greater than this indicate a glomerular abnormality, most commonly glomerulonephritis or diabetic nephropathy. Radioimmunoassay techniques can detect albumin excretion rates as low as 30 mg/day.

9.8 Causes of haematuria

Painless

- Glomerulonephritis
- Tumours of the kidney, ureter, bladder or prostate*
- Tuberculosis*
- Schistosomiasis*
- Hypertensive nephrosclerosis
- Interstitial nephritis (unless very acute/severe)

- Acute tubular necrosis
- Renal ischaemia (renovascular disease)
- Distance running or other severe exercise
- Coagulation disorders, anticoagulant therapy

Painful

- Urinary tract infection
- Renal stones with obstruction

- Loin pain–haematuria syndrome

May be either

- Urinary tract infection
- Reflux nephropathy and renal scarring

- Adult polycystic kidney disease
- Renal stones without obstruction

*Painless provided there is no acute obstruction of the urinary tract.

OSCEs 9.9 Examine this patient with frank haematuria

1. Measure temperature — raised in urinary tract infection, connective tissue disease, endocarditis with renal involvement.
2. Look for bruising or purpura (coagulation disorder, Henoch–Schönlein purpura, vasculitis).
3. Examine nails for splinter haemorrhages (bacterial endocarditis with renal involvement).
4. Measure blood pressure — elevated in renovascular and chronic kidney disease.
5. Look at optic fundi for hypertensive retinopathy.
6. Examine abdomen for renal tenderness (renal or ureteric stones or other causes of obstruction, renal infection or inflammation).
7. Examine abdomen for enlarged, palpable kidneys — unilateral in renal cancer, urinary tract obstruction; bilateral in polycystic kidney disease.
8. Palpate suprapubically for palpable bladder (benign prostatic enlargement, prostate or bladder cancer).
9. Assess peripheral pulses and listen for renal artery or other bruits (renovascular disease).
10. In men, perform rectal examination to assess enlargement of prostate — irregular in prostate cancer.
    In women, consider a pelvic examination to assess reproductive organs.

9.10 Causes of proteinuria

Renal disease

- Glomerulonephritis
- Diabetes mellitus
- Amyloidosis
- Systemic lupus erythematosus

- Drugs, e.g. gold, penicillamine
- Malignancy, e.g. myeloma
- Infection

Non-renal disease

- Fever
- Severe exertion
- Severe hypertension

- Burns
- Heart failure
- Orthostatic proteinuria*

*Occurs when a patient is upright but not lying down; the first morning sample will not show proteinuria.

9.11 Causes of transient proteinuria

- Cold exposure
- Vigorous exercise
- Febrile illness

- Orthostatic (postural) proteinuria
- Abdominal surgery
- Congestive heart failure

Rates of 30–300 mg/day (microalbuminuria) occur in early diabetic nephropathy.

Proteinuria may occur in normal patients with febrile illness. Proteinuria <1 g/l which disappears when lying supine (orthostatic proteinuria) is occasionally found in healthy young subjects in whom protein is not detected in the first urine passed after sleeping recumbent overnight, but is present during the day.

Severe proteinuria may produce frothy urine. If it lowers the plasma albumin concentration enough to reduce the plasma oncotic pressure, the patient develops generalized oedema: the nephrotic syndrome.

THE HISTORY

Past history

Ask about any previous history of renal system disease, specifically:

- hypertension (which may cause or result from renal disease)
- diabetes mellitus (associated with diabetic nephropathy and renovascular disease)

- vascular disease at other sites (which makes renovascular disease more likely)
- past history of urinary tract stones or surgery
- recurrent infections (particularly urinary — associated with renal scarring, and upper respiratory — associated with glomerulonephritis and/or vasculitis)
- anaemia.

Growth retardation is common with chronic renal failure in childhood. Pruritus (itch) is prominent with chronic renal failure at any age. Other symptoms include tiredness, breathlessness, poor appetite, sleep disturbance, restless legs particularly at night, muscle twitching due to hypocalcaemia and, in advanced renal failure, vomiting, diarrhoea, confusion and altered consciousness.

Drug history

Renal failure affects drug metabolism and pharmacokinetics, and drugs may affect renal function or damage the kidneys.

Drugs which accumulate in renal failure include digoxin, lithium, aminoglycosides, opioids and water-soluble β-blockers, e.g. atenolol. Drugs which may affect renal function include angiotensin-converting enzyme (ACE) inhibitors, angiotensin receptor antagonists and non-steroidal anti-inflammatory drugs (NSAIDs). These drugs do not affect normal kidneys, but reduce glomerular filtration when the kidneys are underperfused. Ask about over-the-counter NSAIDs, which can dramatically reduce renal function in systemic infection or hypovolaemia. Aminoglycosides, amphotericin, lithium, ciclosporin, tacrolimus and, in overdose, paracetamol are toxic to normal kidneys. Some drugs indirectly cause renal failure: for example, rhabdomyolysis and myoglobinuria cause acute renal failure in intravenous drug users.

Family history

Note any family members with renal disease. The most common inherited conditions are APKD (autosomal dominant) and Alport's syndrome (X-linked dominant) (Box 9.13). APKD is associated with subarachnoid haemorrhage from intracranial berry aneurysms; Alport's syndrome is associated with high-tone sensineural deafness. Some patients with type 1 diabetes mellitus have a genetically increased susceptibility to diabetic nephropathy.

9.12 Abnormalities of urine colour

Orange-brown

- Conjugated bilirubin
- Rhubarb, senna
- Concentrated normal urine, e.g. very low fluid intake

Red-brown

- Blood, myoglobin, free haemoglobin, porphyrins
- Beetroot, blackberries
- Drugs: rifampicin, metronidazole, warfarin

Brown-black

- Conjugated bilirubin
- Drugs: L-dopa
- Homogentisic acid (in alkaptonuria or ochronosis)

Blue-green

- Drugs/dyes, e.g. propofol, fluorescein

9.13 Some hereditary and congenital conditions affecting the kidneys and urinary tract

Name	Principal findings	Commonly associated abnormalities	Most common form of inheritance
Adult polycystic kidney disease	Bilateral enlarged kidneys, sometimes massive, with nodular surface	Liver cysts Intracranial berry aneurysms Mitral or aortic valve abnormalities	Autosomal dominant
Alport's syndrome	Haematuria, proteinuria, renal failure	Nerve deafness Lens and retinal abnormalities	X-linked dominant
Medullary sponge kidney	Tubular dilatation; renal stones	Other congenital abnormalities, e.g. hemihypertrophy, cardiac valve abnormalities, Marfan's syndrome	Congenital, rarely familial
Nail–patella syndrome	Proteinuria Renal failure (30%)	Nail dysplasia, patellar dysplasia or aplasia	Autosomal dominant
Cystinosis	Tubular dysfunction; renal failure	Rickets, growth retardation, retinal depigmentation and visual impairment	Autosomal recessive
Tuberous sclerosis complex	Renal cysts Renal angiolipomata	Seizures, mental retardation, facial angiofibromata, retinal lesions	Autosomal dominant
Prune-belly syndrome	Dilated bladder and urinary tract; urinary infection and renal failure	Absent abdominal wall musculature	Sporadic mutation

Social, environmental and occupational histories

End-stage renal failure requiring dialysis and/or transplantation has major implications for lifestyle, employment and relationships. Incontinence has major implications for daily living. Find out about your patients' feelings, ideas, functioning and expectations (FIFE; p. 10).

Smoking is a risk factor for atheromatous renal vascular disease, for nephropathy in diabetic patients and in urothelial cancers. Excess alcohol consumption is associated with hypertensive renal damage and increased incidence of IgA nephropathy.

Take a dietary history in patients with renal stones: intake of water, calcium, e.g. milk and dairy products, and oxalate, e.g. chocolate, rhubarb, spinach and soya. Assess dietary protein intake in patients with chronic renal failure. Ask about sodium intake in patients with hypertension and renal disease.

Occupation may be relevant. Living and working in hot conditions with more concentrated urine may increase renal stones (Box 9.14). Exposure to organic solvents may cause glomerulonephritis. Aniline dye and rubber workers have an increased incidence of urothelial cancer. Long-term exposure to lead and cadmium may cause chronic renal damage.

Some renal conditions are found in particular ethnic groups: for example, Balkan nephropathy (interstitial nephritis and urinary tract tumours, probably caused by fungal toxins in grain), systemic lupus erythematosus (SLE) with nephritis in the Far East, and severe hypertension or diabetes mellitus with renal failure in patients of African origin.

THE PHYSICAL EXAMINATION

Physical examination may be normal, even with significant kidney disease.

General examination

Examination sequence
General
- Assess the patient's general appearance and conscious level. Is he well or ill?
- Look for fatigue, pallor, breathlessness, uraemic complexion, Cushingoid appearance and hirsutism.
- Measure the temperature.
- Measure the blood pressure.
- Look at the eyes for the conjunctival pallor of anaemia and calcification at the junction of the iris and conjunctiva (limbic calcification).
- Note any bruising or excoriation.
- Examine the hands for nail changes.
- Ask the patient to hold out the arms and fully extend the hands. Look for a coarse flapping tremor (asterixis) developing after a few seconds (Fig. 7.14, p. 167).
- Smell the breath for uraemic fetor and look at the teeth and gums.
- Assess the state of hydration by checking skin turgor and eyeball tone (p. 62).

Abnormal findings

In untreated end-stage renal failure there may be altered consciousness and asterixis.

Chronic renal failure causes a lemon-yellow coloration of the skin (uraemic complexion; Fig. 9.5), and bruising and excoriation secondary to pruritus (Fig. 9.6). These patients are often anaemic and have a urine-like smell on the breath (uraemic fetor). Nail changes include a brownish discoloration of the distal nail bed (Fig. 9.7), leukonychia (white nails), Muehrcke's nails (leukonychia striata; band-like pale discolorations) and Beau's lines (transverse grooves or furrows on the nail plate) in chronic hypoalbuminaemia (Fig. 3.16C, p. 54).

There may be a surgically created arteriovenous (AV) fistula at the wrist or elbow to allow vascular access for haemodialysis.

Drug treatment may cause general examination abnormalities: for example, Cushing's disease with steroid therapy, hirsutism and gum hypertrophy related to ciclosporin, and warts and skin cancers with immunosuppression in patients with a renal transplant.

9.14 Kidney stones: predisposing factors

Environmental and dietary
- Low urine volumes: high ambient temperature, low fluid intake
- Diet: high protein intake, high sodium, low calcium
- High sodium excretion
- High oxalate excretion
- High urate excretion
- Low citrate excretion

Other medical conditions
- Hypercalcaemia of any cause
- Ileal disease or resection (leads to increased oxalate absorption and urinary excretion)
- Renal tubular acidosis type I (distal), e.g. in Sjögren's syndrome

Congenital and inherited conditions
- Familial hypercalciuria
- Medullary sponge kidney
- Cystinuria
- Renal tubular acidosis type I (distal)
- Primary hyperoxaluria

9

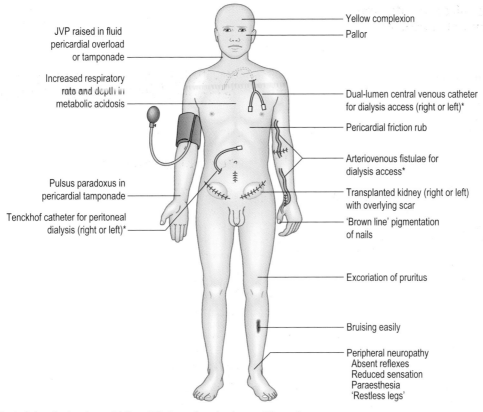

- JVP raised in fluid pericardial overload or tamponade
- Increased respiratory rate and depth in metabolic acidosis
- Pulsus paradoxus in pericardial tamponade
- Tenckhof catheter for peritoneal dialysis (right or left)*
- Yellow complexion
- Pallor
- Dual-lumen central venous catheter for dialysis access (right or left)*
- Pericardial friction rub
- Arteriovenous fistulae for dialysis access*
- Transplanted kidney (right or left) with overlying scar
- 'Brown line' pigmentation of nails
- Excoriation of pruritus
- Bruising easily
- Peripheral neuropathy
  Absent reflexes
  Reduced sensation
  Paraesthesia
  'Restless legs'

Fig. 9.5 Physical signs in chronic renal failure. (* Features of renal replacement therapy.)

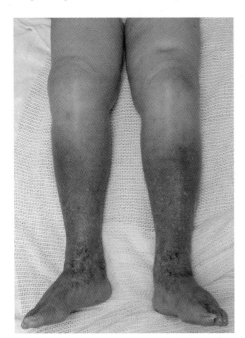

Fig. 9.6 Pruritus/excoriation in chronic renal failure.

Cardiovascular examination

◢ Examination sequence

Cardiovascular

- ◢ Look for pitting oedema in the ankles, the sacrum and the back of the thighs in recumbent patients (Fig. 9.8).
- ◢ Measure the pulse and blood pressure (not on the arm with an AV fistula; Fig. 9.9).
- ◢ Check the jugular venous pulse (JVP) (Fig. 6.22, p. 125).
- ◢ Palpate the apex beat (p. 127).
- ◢ Auscultate for:
  - a midsystolic 'flow' murmur
  - third or fourth heart sounds
  - pericardial friction rub.

Abnormal findings

In the nephrotic syndrome, although oedema is present, the JVP is not usually raised and there are no added heart sounds, as the intravascular volume is normal or reduced. Consider pericardial tamponade in a patient with a raised JVP and low blood pressure in end-stage renal failure. The blood pressure is often elevated in renal disease, but may be low with a postural drop in

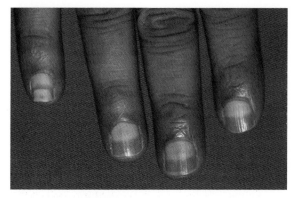

Fig. 9.7 Brown nail banding.

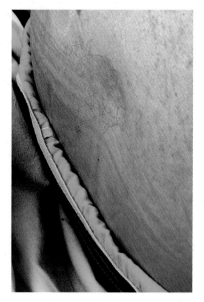

Fig. 9.8 Sacral oedema showing pitting.

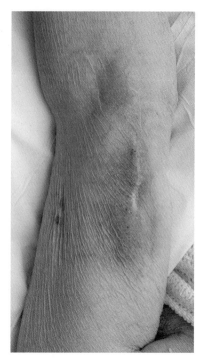

Fig. 9.9 Arteriovenous fistula showing sites of needle cannulation for haemodialysis.

Respiratory examination

▶ Examination sequence

Respiratory

- Measure the respiratory rate (p. 163)
- Percuss the chest to detect pleural effusions.
- Auscultate for bilateral basal lung crackles indicating fluid overload or heart failure.

Abnormal findings

In renal failure, respiratory compensation for the associated metabolic acidosis leads to increase in respiratory rate and deep sighing respirations (Küssmaul respiration; p. 164). Fluid overload and the nephrotic syndrome may cause pleural effusions.

Abdominal examination

Ask patients to lie flat with their head on a pillow and their arms by their side to relax the abdominal muscles. Expose the abdomen fully.

▶ Examination sequence

Abdomen

Inspection

- Look for distension (from the enlarged kidneys of polycystic kidney disease, or occasionally in obstructive uropathy). Gross bladder distension causes suprapubic swelling.

patients with tubulo-interstitial disease who lose sodium and water inappropriately because of impaired tubular reabsorption. Pulsus paradoxus (p. 119) may be present with pericardial tamponade due to uraemic pericarditis.

The apex beat may be displaced in fluid overload and heart failure, or heaving in patients with left ventricular hypertrophy or secondary to hypertension. 'Flow' murmurs are common in patients with 'renal' anaemia, particularly if the cardiac output is increased because of an AV fistula. Added heart sounds occur in fluid overload and/or heart failure, and a pericardial friction rub may be present due to uraemic pericarditis.

Patients having dialysis for end-stage renal failure may have temporary or permanent catheters placed in internal jugular, subclavian or femoral veins. Where these veins have been accessed repeatedly or chronically, they may become permanently occluded.

Look for scars in the loins of renal tract surgery and in the iliac fossae of transplant surgery. A catheter for peritoneal dialysis may be present, or may have left small scars in the midline and hypochondrium.

Palpation

Use the fingers of your right hand. Start in the right lower quadrant and palpate each area systematically (Fig. 0.5, p. 100). A distended bladder is felt as a smooth firm mass arising from the pelvis which disappears after urethral catheterization. Polycystic kidneys have a distinctive nodular surface.

To detect lesser degrees of kidney enlargement, place your left hand behind the patient's back below the lower ribs and your right hand anteriorly over the upper quadrant just lateral to the rectus muscle (Fig. 9.10). Firmly, but gently, push your hands together as the patient breathes out. Ask the patient to breathe in deeply; feel for the lower pole of the kidney moving down between your hands. If this happens, gently push the kidney back and forwards between your two hands to demonstrate its mobility. This is ballotting, and confirms that this structure is the kidney.

If the kidney is palpable, assess its size, surface and consistency.

Ask the patient to sit up. Palpate the renal angle firmly but gently. If this does not cause the patient discomfort, firmly (but with moderate force only!) strike the renal angle once with the ulnar aspect of your closed fist after warning the patient what to expect (Fig. 9.11).

Percussion

Percussion of the kidneys is unhelpful. Percuss for the bladder over a resonant area in the upper abdomen in the midline and then down towards the symphysis pubis. A change to a dull percussion note indicates the upper border of the bladder.

Auscultation

Auscultate to detect bruits arising from the renal arteries. Listen carefully over both loins posteriorly and in the epigastrium, using the stethoscope diaphragm. Renal artery bruits cannot be distinguished from those in adjacent vessels, e.g. the mesenteric arteries, but any abdominal bruits, diminished or absent femoral artery pulses and bruits increase the probability of co-existent atheromatous renal artery disease.

Test for ascites (p. 193), which may be found in nephrotic syndrome or in patients having peritoneal dialysis.

In men examine the external genitalia and perform a rectal examination (pp. 207 and 263) to assess the prostate for benign or malignant change. In female patients, if you suspect malignant disease involving the pelvis, ureters or bladder, perform a vaginal examination (p. 248).

Abnormal findings

The kidneys are normally mobile and may move up to 3 cm inferiorly on inspiration. It is usually easier to feel the right kidney, as it is lower than the left. Minor degrees of kidney enlargement are difficult to assess. In very thin subjects the lower pole of a normal right kidney may be palpable, but even very large kidneys may be impossible to feel in obese subjects. When the liver is markedly enlarged it may be difficult to differentiate from the right kidney, especially if polycystic kidney disease is associated with cystic disease of the liver.

Enlargement of one kidney may result from compensatory hypertrophy due to renal agenesis, hypoplasia or atrophy, or surgical removal of the other kidney. It may also be due to a renal tumour or

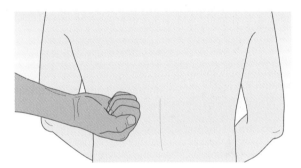

Fig. 9.11 Assessing tenderness over the renal angles.

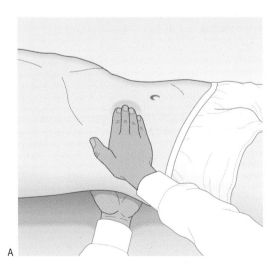

A

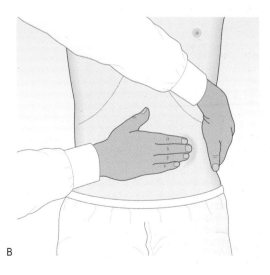

B

Fig. 9.10 Palpation of the kidney. (A) Right kidney. **(B)** Left kidney.

hydronephrosis. Enlargement of both kidneys occurs in polycystic kidney disease, amyloidosis and in acute glomerulonephritis. A transplanted kidney is palpable as a smooth mass in either iliac fossa with an overlying scar.

Polycystic kidneys have an irregular nodular surface and may vary in size from moderately enlarged to filling the whole of one side of the abdomen. Kidneys containing tumours are usually firm and irregular, and sometimes tethered to surrounding structures. Enlarged obstructed or hypertrophic kidneys have a smooth surface.

Renal tenderness is most often due to acute pyelonephritis or acute urinary obstruction.

Examination of the nervous system

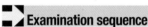**Examination sequence**

Nervous system

▶ Assess level of consciousness.

▶ Test sensation and the tendon reflexes. Peripheral neuropathy occurs in chronic renal failure.

▶ Examine the optic fundi (p. 325).

Abnormal findings

Retinal infarcts are seen in severe vasculitis or SLE, and retinopathy is an important finding in diabetes mellitus.

INVESTIGATIONS

Examine the urine in all patients. Urine abnormalities may reflect:

- abnormally high levels of a substance in the blood exceeding the capacity for normal tubular reabsorption, e.g. glucose, ketones, conjugated bilirubin and urobilinogen
- altered kidney function, e.g. proteinuria, failure to concentrate urine

---

OSCEs 9.15 Examine this patient with newly diagnosed renal failure

1. Look for pallor, uraemic complexion, excoriation, bruising, uraemic fetor, asterixis (features of chronic renal failure). Look for hyperventilation (Kussmaul respiration), suggesting metabolic acidosis.
2. Examine skin for signs of cutaneous vasculitis, or purpura (Henoch–Schönlein disease). Look for the nail-bed pigmentation of chronic renal failure.
3. Assess skin turgor and eyeball tone as possible indicators of severe salt and water depletion causing renal failure.
4. Look for limbic calcification (chronic renal failure).
5. Look at optic fundi for hypertensive or diabetic retinopathy, or retinal infarcts in systemic vasculitis or systemic lupus erythematosus.
6. Measure blood pressure (elevated in chronic renal failure; may be low with postural drop if the patient is fluid-deplete).
7. Listen for heart murmurs, especially an early diastolic murmur or other manifestations to suggest subacute bacterial endocarditis.
8. Examine abdomen for enlarged, smooth kidneys or bladder (obstructive uropathy).
9. Palpate for large cystic kidneys in adult polycystic kidney disease.
10. Auscultate for epigastric and femoral bruits, and assess peripheral pulses (may suggest generalized vasculopathy with renal artery stenosis).
11. Look for peripheral oedema.
12. Assess peripheral nerve function (peripheral neuropathy of chronic renal failure or diabetic neuropathy).
13. Examine urine for haematuria, proteinuria, casts, crystals, white cells and bacteria.

OSCEs 9.16 Examine this patient with oedema

1. Assess extent and degree of oedema present, e.g. facial, flanks, abdominal wall, sacral, genitalia, thighs, ankles and pedal.
2. Look for nail changes associated with hypoproteinaemia (leukonychia, Muehrcke's nails, Beau's lines).
3. Examine optic fundi for diabetic or hypertensive retinopathy.
4. Measure blood pressure (may be elevated, but may be low with postural drop if plasma volume reduced due to severe hypoproteinaemia).
5. Assess JVP (may be high-heart failure; but may be low if plasma volume reduced due to severe hypoproteinaemia).
6. Auscultate for heart murmurs, especially a pansystolic mitral murmur to indicate dilatation of the left ventricle.
7. Listen for extra heart sounds to indicate fluid overload and/or heart failure.
8. In the lungs, look for signs of pleural effusions (nephrotic syndrome) or crackles indicating pulmonary oedema.
9. Examine the abdomen for enlarged, smooth kidneys (renal amyloidosis causing nephrotic syndrome).
10. Test for ascites (nephrotic syndrome).
11. Assess peripheral nerve function (peripheral neuropathy seen in diabetes mellitus and amyloidosis).
12. Examine urine for haematuria, proteinuria, casts and crystals.

OSCEs 9.17 Perform urinalysis

1. The urine specimen should be <4 hours old.
2. Wear a disposable apron and gloves.
3. Examine the specimen for smell, colour, clarity and other abnormalities.
4. Use a watch that indicates seconds.
5. Dip the reagent strip into the urine specimen, making sure all the test areas are covered. Remove the strip after 2 seconds.
6. Tap the edge of the strip against the rim of the container to remove excess urine.
7. Hold the strip horizontally with test areas upward. Hold as close to the colour chart as possible and compare the test areas, reading each reagent at the time specified.
8. Dispose of test strip, apron and gloves into a clinical waste bag; wash hands.
9. Document the results in the patient's clinical record.

9.20 Uses of urinalysis

Use	Indication	Of value in
Screening	Random	Diabetes mellitus Asymptomatic bacteriuria
	Selective	Antenatal care Hypertensive patients
Diagnosis	Primary renal disease	Glomerulonephritis
	Secondary renal disease	Bacterial endocarditis
	Non-renal disorders	Diabetes mellitus
Monitoring	Disease progression	Diabetic nephropathy
	Drug toxicity	Gold therapy
	Drug compliance	Rifampicin therapy
	Illicit drug use	Opioids, benzodiazepines

OSCEs 9.18 Perform microscopy on this urine specimen

1. Centrifuge 10 ml of fresh urine for 5 minutes at 3000 rpm.
2. Remove the supernatant, leaving 0.5 ml of urine and the deposit.
3. Mix the sediment gently and place one drop on a clean slide using a pipette.
4. Overlay a cover slip and examine under the microscope with low illumination and low-power magnification.
5. Examine under high-power magnification to clarify abnormalities seen.
6. Dispose of sample, slide and pipette safely and wash hands.
7. Document the findings in the patient's record.

- abnormal contents, e.g. blood entering at any point from the kidney to the urethra.

Normal fresh urine is clear but varies in colour. Phosphates and urates may precipitate out of normal clear urine left to stand and make it cloudy. Cloudy fresh urine is usually due to the presence of pus cells (pyuria), often with bacteria. An unusually strong fishy smell suggests urinary infection. Some foods, e.g. asparagus, impart a characteristic smell to the urine.

Measure the 24-hour urine volume to confirm oliguria or polyuria. In critically ill patients, hourly urine flow is a good dynamic indicator of organ perfusion.

Investigations in renal disease are outlined in Boxes 9.20–9.24.

OSCEs 9.19 Obtain a midstream urine sample from this patient

1. Give the patient a sterile urine container (a tray for a female patient).
2. Ask the patient to start passing urine before collecting 10–20 ml in the container.
3. Wash hands, put on gloves, and transfer urine from the tray to the laboratory container (female patient).
4. Label the container with time, date and patient's name.
5. Send to the laboratory without delay. If delay is unavoidable, place the sample in a fridge (not freezer) until transport is available.
6. In children or non-compliant adults, consider suprapubic aspiration and samples obtained via a urethral catheter.

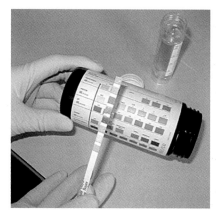

Fig. 9.12 Stix testing of urine.

9.21 Urine dipstick test*

Investigation	Comment
Specific gravity	Reflects urine solute concentration. Varies between 1.002 and 1.035; ↑ when kidneys actively reabsorb water, e.g. fluid depletion or renal failure due to reduced perfusion. Abnormally low values indicate failure of the renal tubules to concentrate urine
pH	Normally 4.5–8.0. In renal tubular acidosis pH never falls <5.3
Glucose	Small amounts may be excreted by normal kidneys producing a colour between the −ve and 5.5 mmol/l blocks
Ketones	Test is specific for aceto-acetate and does not detect other ketones, e.g. β-OH butyrate, acetone. False +ve may occur with highly concentrated urine Ketonuria occurs in diabetic ketoacidosis, starvation, alcohol use and very low carbohydrate diets
Protein	Readings > 'trace' (300 mg/l) indicate significant proteinuria. Proteinuria >2 g/day suggests glomerular disease False +ve occurs with phenothiazines, contamination with detergents, chlorhexidine and alkalis. False −ve occurs in acid preservative contamination and Bence Jones proteinuria (Ig light chains) in myeloma
Blood	Intact erythrocytes cause green spots, and free haemoglobin a green colour, on the reagent area. The test does not differentiate between haemoglobin and myoglobin. If you suspect rhabdomyolysis, measure myoglobin with specific laboratory test False +ve occurs in contamination with bleach (hypochlorite) and stale urine, and blood of non-renal origin, e.g. menstruation
Bilirubin and urobilinogen	Bilirubin is not normally present. False +ve occurs with phenothiazines, and false −ve with vitamin C intake Urobilinogen may be up to 33 μmol/l in health. False +ve occurs with sulphonamides and salicylates, and false −ve with formalin contamination. Abnormalities of bilirubin and urobilinogen require investigation for possible haemolysis or hepatobiliary disease
Leucocytes	Seen in urinary inflammation, stone disease and urothelial cancers
Nitrite	Most Gram −ve bacteria convert urinary nitrate (from diet) to nitrite. A +ve result indicates bacteriuria, but a −ve result does not exclude its presence

*Use freshly passed urine (Fig. 9.12).

9.22 Urine microscopic and microbiological investigations

Investigation	Indication/Comment
Microscopy (Fig. 9.13)	Distinguishes true haematuria from haemoglobinuria and myoglobinuria. Look for bacteria with unstained films at low power, and use higher magnification to distinguish cells, yeasts and crystals. Cytological examination of early morning urine specimens may demonstrate malignant cells in cancers of the bladder, ureter or kidney
Red blood cells	Seen as small round cells without a nucleus. Red cells which have passed through glomeruli are mostly dysmorphic (irregular in size and shape). Those originating from elsewhere in the urinary tract have normal morphology
White blood cells	Have lobed nuclei and granular cytoplasm. White cells with no bacterial growth on standard culture (sterile pyuria) suggest renal tuberculosis Renal tubular epithelial cells are larger and have oval nuclei. They are seen in infection, inflammatory conditions, e.g. tubulo-interstitial nephritis, and glomerulonephritis. Bladder epithelial cells are similar, even larger, and of no clinical significance
Urinary casts	Casts are cylindrical structures formed in the renal tubules Hyaline casts are relatively clear, homogeneous cylindrical structures, consisting principally of Tamm–Horsfall mucoprotein secreted by tubular cells. ↑ numbers are non-specific and seen with severe exercise, fever and chronic renal disease Granular casts are hyaline casts containing granules of albumin and immunoglobulin; they may also contain cellular debris. They are found in disorders associated with significant proteinuria, e.g. glomerulonephritis and diabetic nephropathy Red cell casts indicate haematuria of glomerular origin and are most often seen in acute disease, e.g. acute diffuse proliferative glomerulonephritis White cell casts suggest renal infection or inflammation
Crystals	Urate crystals are seen in gout or urate nephropathy, oxalate crystals in hyperoxaluric stone disease, cystine crystals in cystinosis
Microbiology	For suspected bacterial infections use a fresh, clean-voided, midstream urine sample (MSU). If tuberculosis is suspected, send at least three early morning urine samples for specific mycobacterial culture

9.23 Biochemical and serological investigations

Investigation	Indication/comment
Plasma urea/creatinine	Levels generally ↑ as GFR ↓, but values are affected by diet and muscle mass and do not measure renal function accurately
Creatinine clearance	Gives a good measurement of GFR, but requires a 24 h urine collection and a blood sample

Estimated glomerular filtration rate (eGFR)	Calculate the eGFR from the equation:
	$eGFR = 186 \times (\text{plasma creatinine}/88.4)^{-1.154} \times (\text{age})^{-0.203} \times (0.742 \text{ if female}) \times (1.210 \text{ if black})$
	Normal eGFR is ~100 ml/min/1.73m^2
	Values: 60–89 — mildly reduced function
	           30–59 — moderately reduced function
	           15–29 — severely reduced function
	             <15 — very severe/end-stage renal failure

Plasma electrolytes	↑ potassium (↓ excretion) occurs in acute, and advanced chronic, renal failure ↓ bicarbonate (↓ H$^+$ excretion) common in acute and chronic renal failure ↓ calcium (impaired renal vitamin D$_3$ activation) and ↑ phosphate (↓ excretion) in chronic renal failure ↑ urate common in chronic renal failure (but seldom associated with gout)
Urine osmolality	The definitive measurement of renal concentrating ability. In unexplained hyponatraemia, test for the syndrome of inappropriate ADH secretion (SIADH) by simultaneous measurement of plasma and urine osmolality. If the plasma osmolality is low, the urine osmolality should be lower still (<150 mOsm/kg); in the absence of hypovolaemia, any other finding is consistent with SIADH In patients with unexplained polyuria, test the concentrating ability of the kidneys by an overnight fluid deprivation test. In healthy subjects, urinary osmolality should rise to >800 mOsm/kg; any other finding suggests lack of ADH or renal tubular unresponsiveness to ADH
Alkaline phosphatase and parathyroid hormone	↑ in secondary hyperparathyroidism related to ↓ calcium and ↑ phosphate levels
Antinuclear factor and antineutrophil cytoplasmic antibodies	Systemic lupus erythematosus and vasculitis may affect the kidney

9.24 Imaging and biopsy investigations

Investigation	Indication/Comment
Plain abdominal X-ray	Assesses renal outline/size, stones (>90% are radio-opaque), gas in the urinary collecting system
Ultrasound scan	Assesses kidney size/shape/position; evidence of obstruction; renal cysts or solid lesions; stones; ureteric urine flow; gross abnormality of bladder, post-micturition residual volume Used to guide kidney biopsy
Doppler ultrasound of renal vessels	Assesses renovascular disease, renal vein thrombosis Arterial resistive index may indicate obstruction
IV urography	Haematuria, renal colic, renal mass; renal, ureteric or bladder stones, cysts, tumours, hydronephrosis, other diseases
CT scan	Stone disease, renal mass, ureteric obstruction, tumour staging, renal, retroperitoneal or other tumour masses or fibrosis
Angiography/CT MR angiography	Hypertension ± renal failure, renal artery stenosis; angioplasty and/or stenting
Isotope scan	Suspected renal scarring, e.g. reflux nephropathy, obstruction Assessment of GFR Renal uptake and excretion of radio-labelled chemicals
Renal biopsy	Used to diagnose parenchymal renal disease Performed under ultrasound guidance; complication rates are low but include haemorrhage and arteriovenous fistulae formation Contraindications include markedly reduced kidney size, absence or inadequate function of the contralateral kidney, uncontrolled hypertension, severe obesity and clotting abnormality

9

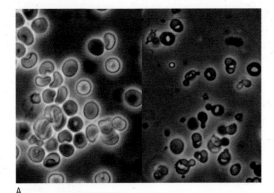

A

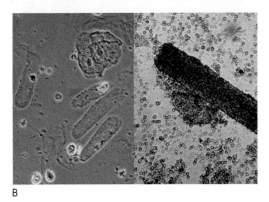

B

Fig. 9.13 Urine microscopy. (A) Phase contrast images of RBCs
(×400). Right, glomerular bleeding with many dysmorphic forms including
acanthocytes (teardrop forms). Left, bleeding from lower in the urinary tract.
(B) Right, numerous red cells and a large red cell cast in acute glomerular
inflammation (×100, not phase contrast). Left, phase contrast images show
hyaline casts, a normal feature of urine (×160).

9.25 Key points: the renal system

- Advanced renal failure occurs without specific symptoms or physical signs. Always check blood tests to exclude renal dysfunction in patients with non-specific symptoms, e.g. tiredness.
- Haematuria combined with significant proteinuria (++ or more) usually indicates glomerular disease.
- Painless haematuria (microscopic or macroscopic) is an important presenting symptom of urothelial cancer. Cystoscopy is essential.
- Differentiate the oedema of nephrotic syndrome from heart failure by testing the urine for protein; a 3–4+ positive result confirms nephrotic syndrome.
- Nephrotic syndrome may be associated with underlying cancer, particularly in the elderly.
- Renovascular disease is an important cause of hypertension and renal failure. Examine for atheromatous vascular disease elsewhere — cerebral, cardiac or peripheral; listen for abdominal bruits.
- Look for features of diabetes mellitus.
- Consider systemic vasculitis in patients with multisystem or atypical symptoms and signs. Symptoms and signs of systemic vasculitis can mimic those of subacute bacterial endocarditis.
- Dipstick the urine of patients concerned about its colour or frothy nature to exclude proteinuria.
- Even patients with early chronic kidney disease have an increased risk of cardiovascular complications and require active management of this.

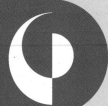

The reproductive system

10

THE BREAST

Anatomy

The breasts are modified sweat glands. Pigmented skin covers the areola and the nipple, which is erectile tissue. The openings of the lactiferous ducts are seen near the apex of the nipple. The nipple is in the 4th intercostal space in the midclavicular line, but accessory breast/nipple tissue may develop anywhere down the nipple line (axilla to groin) (Fig. 10.1).

The adult breast is divided into the nipple, the areola and four quadrants, upper and lower, inner and outer, with an axillary tail projecting from the upper outer quadrant (Fig. 10.2).

The size and shape of the breasts are influenced by age, hereditary factors, sexual maturity, phase of the menstrual cycle, parity, pregnancy, lactation and general state of nutrition. Fat and stroma surrounding the glandular tissue determine the size of the breast, except during lactation, when enlargement is mostly glandular. The breast responds to fluctuations in oestrogen and progesterone levels. Swelling and tenderness are more common in the premenstrual phase. The amount of glandular tissue reduces and fat increases with age, so that the breasts are softer and more pendulous. Lactating breasts are swollen and engorged with milk, and are best examined after breastfeeding.

SYMPTOMS AND DEFINITIONS

Breast lump

Breast cancer

In the UK, this common malignancy affects 1 in 9 women. The incidence increases with age, but women regard any mass as potentially malignant and so should you until proven otherwise. Cancer of the male breast is uncommon and has a strong genetic factor.

Cancers are solid masses with an irregular outline. They are usually, but not always, painless, firm and hard, contrasting in consistency with the surrounding breast tissue. The cancer may extend directly into the overlying tissues such as skin, pectoral fascia and pectoral muscle, or metastasize to regional lymph nodes or the systemic circulation.

Fibrocystic changes

Fibrocystic changes or irregular nodularity of the breast are common, especially in the upper outer quadrant in young women. The tissue is usually rubbery in texture and is most prominent premenstrually. The changes are usually bilateral and benign, but any new focal change in young women which persists after menstruation should be investigated.

Fibroadenomas

These benign lumps are an overgrowth of parts of the terminal duct lobules. They are smooth, mobile, discrete and rubbery, and are the second most common cause of a breast mass in women under 35 years old.

Breast cysts

These are smooth fluid-filled sacs, most common in women aged 35–50. They may be soft and fluctuant when the pressure in the sac is low, but hard and painful if the pressure is high. Cysts may occur in multiple clusters. Most are benign, but any cyst in which the aspirate is bloodstained or there is a residual mass following aspiration, or which recurs after aspiration, should be investigated.

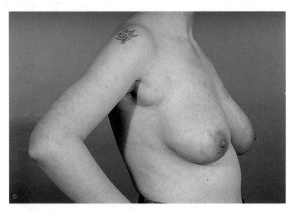

Fig. 10.1 Accessory breast tissue in the axilla.

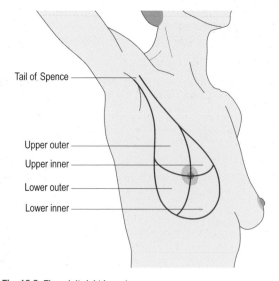

Tail of Spence

Upper outer

Upper inner

Lower outer

Lower inner

Fig. 10.2 The adult right breast.

Breast abscesses

There are two types:

- Lactational abscesses in women who are breastfeeding, usually peripheral
- Non-lactational abscesses, which occur as an extension of periductal mastitis. They are usually found under the areola and are often associated with nipple inversion. They usually occur in young female smokers. Occasionally, a non-lactating abscess may discharge spontaneously through a fistula, classically at the areolocutaneous border (Fig. 10.3).

Breast pain

At some time in their life, most women suffer cyclical mastalgia (Box 10.1). Pain from the chest wall may be confused with breast pain.

Skin changes

These may take various forms:

- Simple skin dimpling; the skin remains mobile over the cancer (Fig. 10.4)
- Indrawing of the skin; the skin is fixed to the cancer
- Lymphoedema of the breast; the skin is swollen between the hair follicles and looks like the peel of an orange (peau d'orange; Fig. 10.5). This is caused by infection and accompanied by redness, warmth and tenderness. Investigate any 'infection' which does not respond to one course of antibiotics to exclude an inflammatory cancer. These are aggressive tumours with a poor prognosis
- Eczema of the nipple and areola; this may be part of a generalized skin disorder. If it affects the true nipple, it may be due to Paget's disease (Fig. 10.6), or invasion of the epidermis by an intraductal cancer.

10.1 Characteristics of mastalgia

Cyclical mastalgia

- Related to the menstrual cycle; usually worse in the latter half of the cycle and relieved by the period

Non-cyclical mastalgia

- No variation

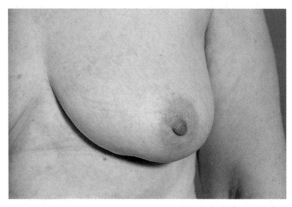

Fig. 10.4 Skin dimpling due to underlying malignancy.

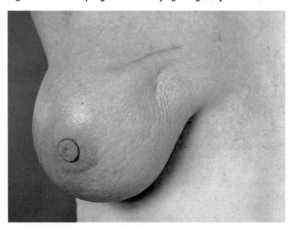

Fig. 10.5 Peau d'orange of the breast.

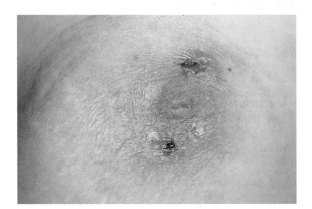

Fig. 10.3 Mamillary fistulae at the areolocutaneous border.

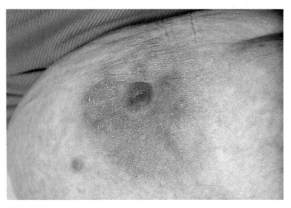

Fig. 10.6 Paget's disease of the nipple.

10

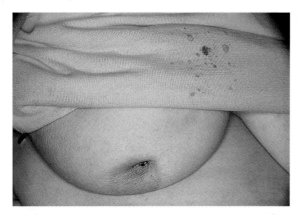

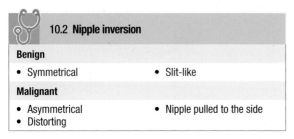

Fig. 10.7 Breast cancer presenting as indrawing of the nipple. Note the bloody discharge on the underclothing.

10.2 Nipple inversion

Benign

- Symmetrical
- Slit-like

Malignant

- Asymmetrical
- Nipple pulled to the side
- Distorting

Nipple changes

Nipple inversion

Retraction of the nipple is common (Fig. 10.7 and Box 10.2).

Nipple discharge

A small amount of fluid may be expressed from multiple ducts by massaging the breast. It may be clear, yellow, white or green in colour. Investigate persistent single duct discharge or bloodstained (macroscopic or microscopic) discharge to exclude duct ectasia, periductal mastitis, intraduct papilloma or intraduct cancer.

Galactorrhoea

Galactorrhoea is a milky discharge from multiple ducts in both breasts due to hyperprolactinaemia. It often causes hyperplasia of Montgomery's tubercles, small rounded projections covering areolar glands.

Gynaecomastia

Gynaecomastia is enlargement of the male breast and often occurs in pubertal boys. In chronic liver disease gynaecomastia is caused by high levels of circulating oestrogens which are not metabolized by the liver. Many drugs can cause breast enlargement (Box 10.3 and Fig. 10.8).

10.3 Causes of gynaecomastia

Drugs, including

- Cannabis
- Oestrogens used in treatment of prostate cancer
- Spironolactone
- Cimetidine
- Digoxin

Decreased androgen production

- Klinefelter's syndrome

Increased oestrogen levels

- Chronic liver disease
- Thyrotoxicosis
- Some adrenal tumours

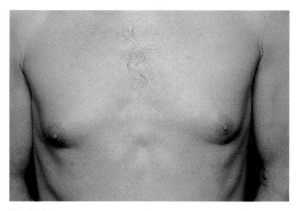

Fig. 10.8 Drug-induced gynaecomastia caused by cimetidine.

10.4 Indicators of breast cancer risk*

- Female gender
- Increasing age
- Family history, esp. if associated with:
  Early age of onset
  Multiple cases of breast cancer
  Ovarian cancer
  Male breast cancer
- Early menarche
- Nulliparity or late age of first child
- Late menopause
- Prolonged HRT use
- Postmenopausal obesity
- Mantle irradiation for Hodgkin's disease, esp. at young age (<30 years)

*The role of the oral contraceptive pill as a major risk factor for breast cancer is still debated.

THE HISTORY

Not all patients have symptoms. Women may have an abnormality on screening mammography; asymptomatic women may present with concerns about their family history. Remember, too, that men may present with gynaecomastia.

Benign and malignant conditions cause similar symptoms but benign changes are more common.

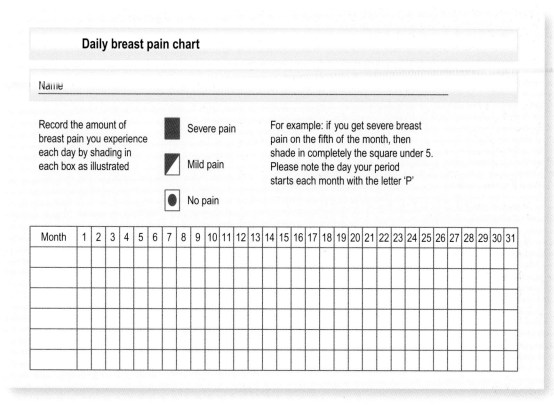

Daily breast pain chart

Name

Record the amount of breast pain you experience each day by shading in each box as illustrated

Severe pain

Mild pain

No pain

For example: if you get severe breast pain on the fifth of the month, then shade in completely the square under 5. Please note the day your period starts each month with the letter 'P'

Month	1	2	3	4	5	6	7	8	9	10	11	12	13	14	15	16	17	18	19	20	21	22	23	24	25	26	27	28	29	30	31

Fig. 10.9 Breast pain chart.

Explore the patient's FIFE (p. 10). Women are often worried that they have breast cancer.

Presenting complaint

Ask:

- How long have symptoms been present?
- What changes have occurred?
- Is there any relationship to the menstrual cycle?
- Does anything make it better or worse?

Breast cancer may present with symptoms of metastatic disease.

Evaluate potential risk factors (Box 10.4) and menopausal status. Use a pain chart to establish the timing of symptoms (Fig. 10.9).

THE PHYSICAL EXAMINATION

Offer a chaperone and record the person's name; make a note of the fact if the patient refuses to have someone present. Male doctors must always have a chaperone.

Examination sequence

Breast

- Ask the patient to undress to the waist and sit upright on a well-illuminated chair or the side of a bed.
- Ask her to rest her hands on the thighs to relax the pectoral muscles (Fig. 10.10A).
- Face the patient and look at the breasts for:
  - asymmetry
  - local swelling
  - skin changes
  - nipple changes.
- Ask the patient to press her hands firmly on the hips to contract the pectoral muscles and repeat the inspection (Fig. 10.10B).
- Ask her to raise her arms above the head and then to lean forward to expose the whole breast and exacerbate skin dimpling (Figs. 10.10C and D).
- Ask the patient to lie with her head on one pillow and her hand under the head on the side to be examined. Ask her to do this on both sides at the same time (Fig. 10.11).
- Hold your hand flat to the skin and palpate the breast tissue, using the palmar surface of your middle three fingers. Compress the breast tissue firmly against the chest wall.

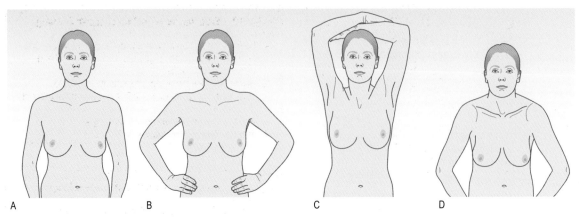

Fig. 10.10 Positions for inspecting the breasts. (A) Hands resting on thighs. **(B)** Hands pressed onto hips. **(C)** Arms above head. **(D)** Leaning forward with breasts pendulous.

▶ View the breast as a clock face. Examine each 'hour of the clock' from the outside towards the nipple, including under the nipple (Fig. 10.12). Compare the texture of one breast with the other. Examine all the breast tissue. The breast extends from the clavicle to the upper abdomen, and from the midline to the anterior border of latissimus dorsi (posterior axillary fold). Define the characteristics of any mass (Box 3.10, p. 58).

▶ Elevate the breast with your hand to uncover dimpling overlying a tumour which may not be obvious on inspection.

▶ Is the mass fixed underneath? With the patient's hands on her hips, hold the mass between your thumb and forefinger. Ask her to contract and relax the pectoral muscles alternately by pushing into her hips. As the pectoral muscle contracts, note whether the mass moves with it and if it is separate when the muscle is relaxed. Infiltration suggests malignancy.

▶ Examine the axillary tail between your finger and thumb as it extends towards the axilla.

▶ Palpate the nipple by holding it gently between your index finger and thumb. Try to express any discharge. Massage the breast towards the nipple to uncover any discharge. Note the colour and consistency of any discharge, along with the number and position of the affected ducts. Test any nipple discharge for blood using urine-testing sticks.

▶ Palpate the regional lymph nodes, including the supraclavicular group. Ask the patient to sit facing you, and support the full weight of her arm at the wrist with your opposite hand. Move the flat of your other hand high into the axilla and upwards over the chest to the apex. This can be uncomfortable for patients, so warn them beforehand and check for any discomfort. Compress the contents of the axilla against the chest wall. Assess any palpable masses for:

- size
- consistency
- fixation.

▶ Examine the supraclavicular fossa, looking for any visual abnormality. Palpate the neck from behind and systematically review all cervical lymphatic chains (Boxes 10.5 and 10.6).

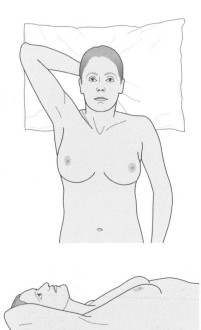

Fig. 10.11 Position for examination of the right breast.

INVESTIGATIONS

Accurate diagnosis of breast lesions depends on clinical assessment, backed up by mammography and/or breast ultrasound and pathological diagnosis, either by fine needle aspiration cytology or core biopsy ('triple assessment') (Box 10.7). Up to 5% of malignant lesions require excision biopsy for the diagnosis to be made. In the UK there are specific guidelines for the appropriate referral of patients with breast symptoms to specialist units where this assessment is carried out.

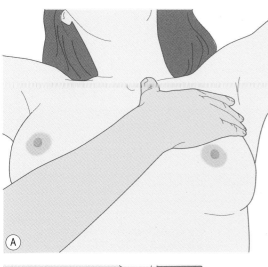
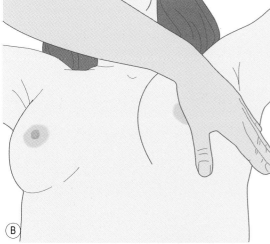
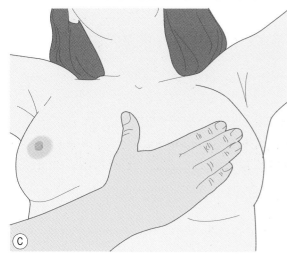

Fig. 10.12 Clinical examination of the breast: palpating clockwise to cover all of the breast.

OSCEs 10.5 Examine this patient with a nipple discharge

1. Look for visible abnormalities with the patient sitting, first with her hands on her thighs and then above her head.
2. Palpate for any masses.
3. Gently massage the breast and identify any nipple discharge, noting colour, position, laterality and number of ducts affected.
4. Examine the axilla if you detect any lumps.
5. Test the discharge for blood with Microstix.

OSCEs 10.6 Examine this patient with a breast lump

1. Look for signs of swelling, skin changes (dimpling, erythema, peau d'orange) and nipple change (asymmetric pull, Paget's disease).
2. Examine the breast for a mass and record site, size, consistency, position, tethering and fixation to chest wall or skin.
3. Check for bloodstained nipple discharge.
4. Examine regional nodes in axilla and supraclavicular fossa. Comment on size, consistency and fixation.

10.7 Investigation of breast lumps

Investigation	Indication/comment
Ultrasound (Fig. 10.13)	Lump
Mammography (Fig. 10.14)	Not in women under 35 unless there is a strong suspicion of cancer
MRI (Fig. 10.15)	Dense breasts/ruptured implant
Fine needle aspiration	Aspirate lesion using a 21 or 23 G needle
Core biopsy	To differentiate invasive or in situ cancer
Large core vacuum-assisted core biopsy	
Open surgical biopsy	

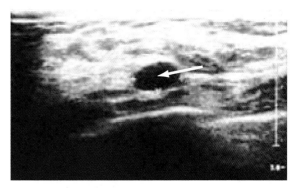

Fig. 10.13 Ultrasound of a breast cyst: showing a characteristic smooth-walled hypoechoic lesion (arrow).

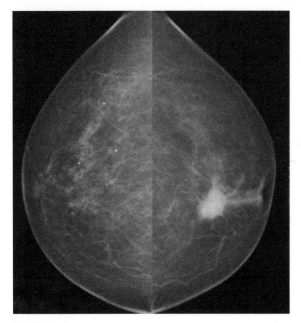

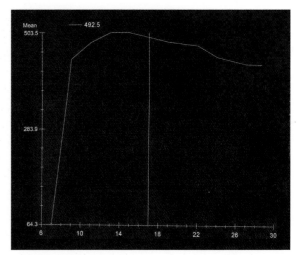

Fig. 10.15 Magnetic resonance image of a breast cancer. The characteristic uptake and washout pattern of signalling following gadolinium enhancement.

Fig. 10.14 Digital mammogram: demonstrating a spiculate opacity characteristic of a cancer.

10.8 Key points: the breast examination

- Breast cancer is very common — 1 in 9 women have a lifetime risk.
- Breast cancer risk increases with age.
- Regard any breast lump as potentially malignant until proven otherwise.
- Always inspect the breast in various positions.
- Follow this by systematic palpation of the gland and of the regional lymph nodes.
- Urgently refer women over 35 with a discrete breast lump to a specialist breast unit.

THE GYNAECOLOGICAL EXAMINATION

ANATOMY

The internal female genitalia comprise the uterus, Fallopian tubes, ovaries and vagina. These lie in the pelvis, posterior to the bladder and anterior to the rectum (Fig. 10.16).

The external female genitalia, the vulva, includes the labia majora, labia minora, vaginal opening or introitus, urethra and clitoris (Fig. 10.17).

The uterus

This is a pear-shaped, muscular organ with a central cavity and a rounded top (fundus; Fig. 10.18). The cervix (neck of the uterus) lies within the upper vagina

and the body of the uterus sits above it. The uterus is 'anteverted' if angled forward from the axis of the vagina and 'retroverted' when it tips backwards (Fig. 10.19). The muscular uterine wall is the myometrium, lined by the endometrium.

The uterine adnexa

The Fallopian tubes, along with the ovaries and their attachments, make up the uterine adnexa. The Fallopian tubes lead from the upper outer aspects of the uterus (the cornua) and curve round to meet the ovaries. Each opens into a trumpet-shaped infundibulum. Each ovary is oval in shape, measuring about $3 \times 2 \times 2\,cm$, and rests on the side wall of the pelvis.

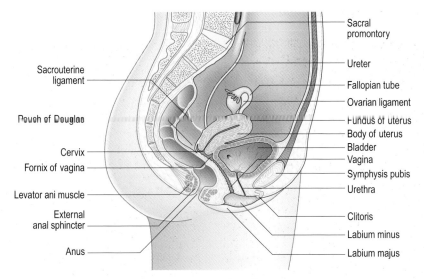

Fig. 10.16 **Lateral view of the female internal genitalia:** showing the relationship to the rectum and bladder.

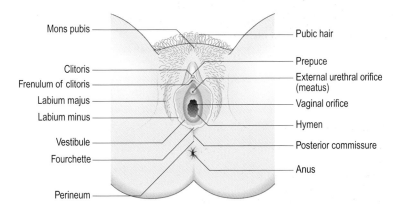

Fig. 10.17 **The external female genitalia.**

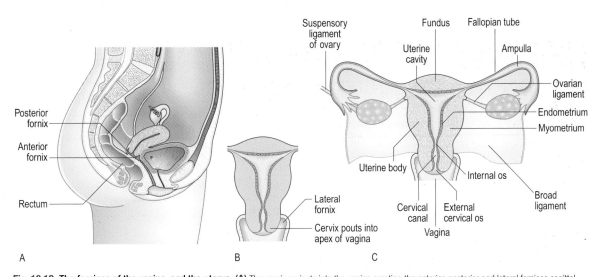

Fig. 10.18 **The fornices of the vagina, and the uterus. (A)** The cervix projects into the vagina creating the anterior, posterior and lateral fornices sagittal section. **(B)** Lateral fornices; coronal section. **(C)** Section through the pear-shaped, muscular uterus (showing the cervix, body (corpus) and fundus) and the fallopian tubes, showing the ligamentous attachments of the ovary. The uterine mucosa is the endometrium. The cervical canal has an internal and an external os.

The vagina

This flattened tube, 8–10cm long, passes upwards and back from the vulva to the cervix. At the top, the cervix divides the upper vaginal vault into anterior, posterior and lateral compartments or fornices (Fig. 10.18).

The vulva

The size and shape of the labia differ widely, resulting in the variable appearance of the normal vulva. The labia minora demarcate the vulval vestibule, containing the urethral opening and the vaginal orifice. The clitoris is usually obscured by a prepuce or hood. The perineum lies between the vagina and the anus.

The pelvic floor

The muscular base of the pelvis supports the pelvic organs and helps maintain continence of the urinary and anal sphincters.

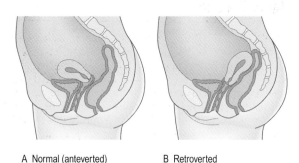

A Normal (anteverted) B Retroverted

Fig. 10.19 The different anatomical positions of the uterine body within the pelvis.

SYMPTOMS AND DEFINITIONS

Menstruation

Menstrual bleeding ('the period') normally occurs every 22–35 days, and lasts 3–7 days. Total monthly blood loss is around 35 ml. The length of one cycle is calculated from day 1 of bleeding to day 1 of bleeding in the next period. For example, a woman who bleeds for 5 days every 29 days is recorded as 5/29 (Box 10.9).

Dyspareunia

This is pain during intercourse, which may be felt around the entrance to the vagina (superficial) or

	10.9 Common menstrual terms and symptoms	
Term/symptom	**Definition**	**Comment**
Menarche	Age when periods commence	Average age is 12 years in Western countries but is often later when girls are less well nourished
Primary amenorrhoea	No periods by the age of 16 years	Investigate
Secondary amenorrhoea	No periods for 3 months or more in a woman who previously menstruated regularly	Investigate only after 6 months; menstruation often resumes spontaneously. Exclude pregnancy
Oligomenorrhoea	Periods occurring at intervals longer than 35 days and/or being particularly light	As above
Heavy menstrual bleeding (previously called menorrhagia)	Excessive blood loss	If affecting quality of life then investigate
Flooding	Episodes of very heavy menstrual blood loss	Embarrassing as may soak clothes, bedding or chairs. Passing clots simply indicates very heavy bleeding
Painful menstrual bleeding or dysmenorrhoea	Pain prior to or during the period	Usually felt in the lower abdomen, the back or the upper thighs
Menopause	The final spontaneous menstrual period. Only known for certain after no further bleeding for 1 year	Occurs on average at 51 years of age with a normal range 45–55 years
Perimenopause	Time around the menopause when periods become erratic and menopausal symptoms (hot flushes and sweats) occur	Lasts 2–5 years on average
Postmenopausal bleeding	Spontaneous vaginal bleeding more than 1 year after the final menstrual period	Requires urgent investigation to exclude cancer in the genital tract

within the pelvis. Pain due to involuntary spasm of muscles at the vaginal entrance (vaginismus) may make intercourse impossible. Persistent deep dyspareunia suggests underlying pelvic pathology. Dyspareunia can occur due to vaginal dryness following the menopause.

Vaginal discharge

A variable amount of a white or clear discharge is normal in women of reproductive age. Ask about the colour, smell, heaviness, duration and associated symptoms, such as itching or soreness. A vaginal infection may or may not be sexually transmitted.

- Thrush. The most common non-sexually transmitted infection (caused by *Candida* species) gives a thick, white, curdy discharge often associated with marked vulval itching
- Bacterial vaginosis (BV) This common non-sexually acquired infection, usually caused by *Gardnerella vaginalis*, produces a watery, fishy-smelling discharge. The pH of normal vaginal secretions is usually <4.5 but in BV it is >5
- Sexually transmitted infections (STIs). Vaginal discharge, vulval ulceration or pain, dysuria, lower abdominal pain and general malaise can all be caused by STIs. They also occur in asymptomatic women.

Pelvic masses

- A pregnant uterus. This is the most common cause of a mass arising from the pelvis in a woman of

reproductive age. Other masses could be uterine or ovarian, and may need ultrasound examination to determine the diagnosis
- Uterine fibroids. These common benign tumours of the uterine wall often cause heavy menstrual bleeding and may become very large
- Ovarian masses. Benign ovarian cysts and ovarian cancer can present as pelvic masses. They may grow very large (Fig. 10.20).

10

Incontinence

Involuntary and inappropriate voiding or leakage of urine or faeces is most frequent in women who have borne children. Weakness of the pelvic floor causes stress incontinence with urinary leakage on coughing, sneezing or sudden exertion. If the detrusor muscle of the bladder is unstable, this causes a strong desire to pass urine even when the bladder is not full (urgency) and leakage (urge incontinence) (Box 9.4, p. 221).

Prolapse

The structures in the pelvis may drop down and cause discomfort if the pelvic floor muscles are weak after childbirth. Women report this feels like 'something coming down' particularly when they are standing. The anterior and posterior vaginal walls or cervix can bulge through the vaginal opening and, in extreme cases, the entire uterus can prolapse externally (Fig. 10.21).

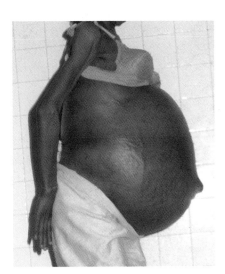

Fig. 10.20 Massive ovarian cyst.

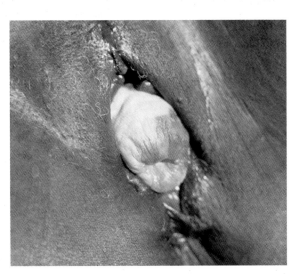

Fig. 10.21 External prolapse of the uterus.

THE HISTORY

Presenting complaint

Clarify the woman's presenting complaint along with her FIFE (p. 10). She may have no specific problems and has come to the surgery for a routine cervical smear; alternatively, she may think she is pregnant and wish to discuss her options. People often find it difficult to discuss sexual problems but this may be the underlying reason for the consultation (Box 10.10).

Past history

Note any previous similar problems and endocrine or autoimmune conditions which may affect menstrual function.

Drug history

Check what medications, both prescribed and over-the-counter, the patient is taking. Ask about contraception (Box 10.11). If the patient is menopausal, note current or past use of hormone replacement therapy and duration of use.

Family history

A history of ovarian or breast cancer may be relevant. Age of menopause may be familial but menstrual problems are not usually familial.

Social history

Note how the patient's current symptoms affect her family life, work and current relationship.

10.11 Methods of contraception

- Condoms
- Combined oral contraceptive pill (or combined transdermal patch)
- Progestogen-only pill ('mini pill')
- Depot progestogen injection (Depo-Provera®)
- Progestogen implant (Implanon®)
- Copper intrauterine device (IUD or coil)
- Progestogen-releasing intrauterine system (IUS or Mirena®)
- Female barrier method: diaphragm, cervical cap or female condom
- Natural methods: rhythm method, Persona®, lactational amenorrhoea
- Sterilization: vasectomy or female sterilization

10.10 Menstrual history checklist

Ask about	Information to obtain	Comment
Menarche	Age at which periods began	Not essential in older women with children
Last menstrual period	Date of the first day of the last period	If the period is late, exclude pregnancy. If the patient is menopausal, record the age at which periods stopped
Length of period	Number of days the period lasts	Normal 4–7 days
Amount of bleeding	How heavy the bleeding is each month (light, normal or heavy). Any episodes of flooding or passed clots	If heavy, how many sanitary pads and tampons are used? Does the patient get up at night to change her sanitary protection? How many times?
Regularity of periods	Number of days between each period. Is the pattern regular or irregular?	Normal 22–35 days. Around the menopause, cycles lengthen until they stop altogether
Erratic bleeding	Bleeding between periods or after intercourse	May indicate serious underlying disease
Pain	Association with menstruation. Does the pain precede or occur during the period?	Common in early adolescence; usually no underlying pathology. Painful periods starting in older women may be associated with underlying disease
Pregnancies	Record any births, miscarriages or abortions	Some women may not disclose an abortion or baby given up for adoption
Infertility	Is the patient trying to become pregnant?	How long has she been trying to conceive?
Contraception	Record current and previous methods. Note that the patient's partner may have had a vasectomy or she may be in a same sex relationship	Hormonal and intrauterine contraception can affect menstrual bleeding patterns
Lifestyle	Ask about weight, dieting and exercise	Rapid or extreme weight loss and excessive exercise often cause oligo-amenorrhoea. Obesity causes hormonal abnormalities, menstrual changes and infertility. Acne and hirsutism may be signs of an underlying hormonal disorder

Sexual history

Sexual problems are common and distressing. The patient may find it embarrassing and difficult to discuss them, so put her at ease and be comfortable yourself about these issues. Use a simple pattern of questioning, and be straightforward and unambiguous (Box 10.12). The exact questions will depend on her individual answers but, if the consultation is about a gynaecological problem, contraception or an STI, explain why you need to ask these types of question.

Partner notification

The sexual partners of women with STIs must be informed and treated to prevent further transmission of the infection or re-infection of the treated person. Confidentiality is paramount, so do not give information to a third party.

THE PHYSICAL EXAMINATION

This can be an embarrassing and uncomfortable experience for women, so be particularly sensitive. Explain what you are going to do and why this is needed. Offer a chaperone and record that person's name; record the fact if the woman declines.

Abdominal examination

Examine the abdomen to elicit any tenderness and to detect any masses arising from the pelvis. Look for any lymphadenopathy in the inguinal regions (Fig. 3.20C, p. 57) (Boxes 10.13 and 10.14).

Vaginal examination

If a woman has never had penetrative sexual intercourse, do not carry out a vaginal examination (Box 10.15).

10.12 Taking a sexual history

- Are you currently in a relationship?
- How long have you been with your partner?
- Is it a sexual relationship?
- Is your partner a man or a woman?
- When did you last have sex with:
    Your partner?
    Anyone else?
- Are you concerned about any sexual issues?

Use a good movable light and an examination couch that can be mechanically raised or lowered and that is positioned away from the wall to allow the patient's knees to fall out to the side. The woman should have an empty bladder. Ask her to remove her clothing from the waist downwards and use a modesty sheet to cover her abdomen and lower part of her body. Leave her to undress in privacy. She should lie back on the couch with a pillow for her head. Ask her to bend up both knees and, either with her heels together in

OSCEs 10.13 Examine this patient with acute pelvic pain

1. Look for signs of shock: pallor, low blood pressure and weak rapid pulse (acute blood loss or sepsis).
2. Record the temperature.
3. Feel the lower abdomen for tenderness, guarding, rebound and any masses arising from the pelvis.
4. Inspect the vulva for signs of bleeding.
5. Pass a vaginal speculum and look for bleeding or vaginal discharge.
6. Take endocervical swabs for chlamydia or gonorrhoea and a high vaginal swab.
7. Perform bimanual examination to assess the size of the uterus and any adnexal masses, and to elicit any tenderness of the pelvic organs.
8. Perform rectal examination if you suspect appendicitis.
9. Perform a pregnancy test in any woman of reproductive age. Measure serum beta human chorionic gonadotrophin if the pregnancy test is negative and you suspect ectopic pregnancy.
10. Consider further investigations, including pelvic ultrasound scan and diagnostic laparoscopy.

OSCEs 10.14 Examine this patient with postmenopausal bleeding

1. Look for evidence of weight loss or anaemia.
2. Feel the abdomen to detect any mass arising from the pelvis.
3. Inspect the vulva for possible malignancy.
4. Pass a vaginal speculum and inspect:
    the vaginal walls for atrophic change or, rarely, vaginal cancer
    the cervix for cancer or a cervical polyp.
5. Take a cervical smear if this is due or the cervix looks abnormal.
6. Perform bimanual examination and assess uterine size and any adnexal mass.
7. Consider further investigations, e.g. endometrial biopsy, transvaginal ultrasound scan, examination under anaesthetic, diagnostic curettage, colposcopy and cervical biopsy.

10.15 Reasons to carry out a vaginal examination

- To take a cervical smear
- To assess the size of a pregnant uterus (<12 weeks' gestation)
- In the presence of:
    Suspected infection
    Menstrual bleeding problems
    Lower abdominal pain or dyspareunia
    Urogenital prolapse
    Early pregnancy problems
    A mass arising from the pelvis

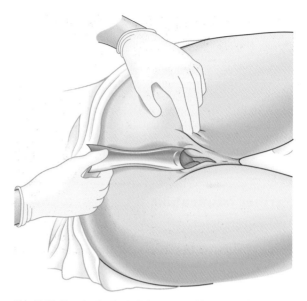

Fig. 10.23 Examination in the left lateral position using a Sim's speculum.

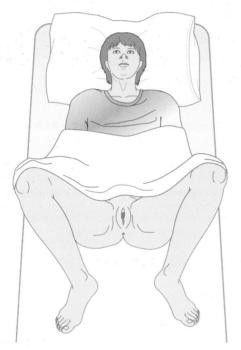

Fig. 10.22 Position for examination.

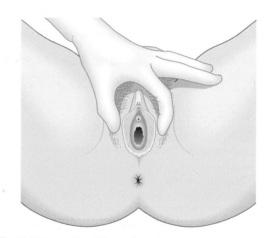

Fig. 10.24 Inspection of the vulva.

the middle or separated, let her knees drop apart (Fig. 10.22).

Women dislike having their legs 'put up in stirrups' and this is not required for a routine smear or examination. Leg supports or foot stirrups are helpful if the examination is prolonged or for minor procedures.

Use the left lateral position to examine for prolapse (Fig. 10.23). The patient lies on her left side, with her knees drawn up slightly towards her chin.

▰▱ Examination sequence

Vagina

▰▱ Wash your hands and put on gloves. Look at the vulval area before separating the labia with the forefinger and thumb of your left hand (Fig. 10.24). Inspect the vaginal opening and urethra.

▰▱ Look for discharge, inflammation, atrophy or ulceration. Check for any swelling of the Bartholin's glands: pea-sized mucus glands lying deep to the posterior margins of the labia minora which can become infected or blocked (Fig. 10.25). Ask the patient to cough or strain down, and look for prolapse of the vaginal walls. Note the position and extent of prolapse and any uterine descent. Watch for involuntary leakage of urine (stress incontinence).

Speculum examination

▰▱ Use a vaginal speculum (Fig. 10.26) to see the cervix and the vaginal walls, to carry out a cervical smear and to take swabs. Specula are metal or plastic and come in various sizes and lengths. A woman who has been pregnant will need a larger or longer speculum if the cervix is very posterior. Metal specula may be sterilized and re-used. Plastic specula are always disposable. A metal speculum is cold, so warm it under the hot tap. Most

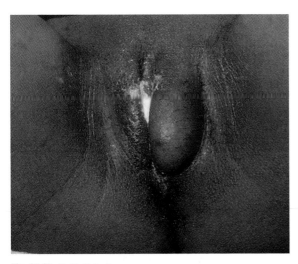

Fig. 10.25 Bartholin's abscess.

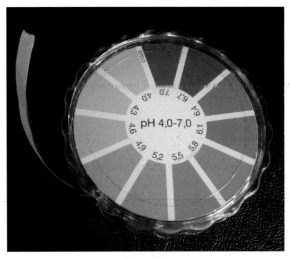

Fig. 10.27 pH paper for vaginal discharge.

10

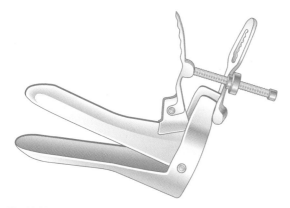

Fig. 10.26 Bivalve speculum.

women find a speculum examination mildly uncomfortable, so put a small amount of lubricating gel on the tip of each blade, even if you are carrying out a cervical smear.

▪◣ Part the labia with your left hand. Take the speculum in your right hand with the blades closed and the handles positioned towards the woman's left leg. Gently insert the speculum to its full length into the vaginal opening and, as you do so, rotate it through 90°, bringing the handles anteriorly. This avoids manipulating around the perianal region, which women may dislike. (If the procedure is being performed under general anaesthetic in theatre, the handles are positioned posteriorly.) If a woman finds the speculum examination difficult, ask her to insert the speculum herself.

▪◣ Gently open the blades of the speculum and identify the cervix. Vaginal squamous epithelium and the endocervical columnar epithelium meet on the cervix. The position of this squamo-columnar junction varies throughout reproductive life and so the cervix can look very different in individual women. Look for any polyps, or a malignancy which would appear vascular and irregular in appearance. If you do not see the cervix immediately, withdraw the speculum slightly, close the blades and press the

speculum slightly deeper at a different angle before re-opening the blades. Use pH paper to check the pH of any discharge (Fig. 10.27).

▪◣ Take swabs or a cervical smear before performing a bimanual vaginal examination to avoid removing cellular material from the cervix. Remove the speculum and offer tissues and privacy for the woman to tidy herself up. Discuss your findings with her after she is dressed.

Taking a cervical smear

There are two ways of taking a smear:

* using a microscope slide
* using liquid-based cytology.

Liquid-based cytology allows smears to be processed more efficiently and gives a smaller percentage of inadequate smears. Always label the microscope slide (in pencil) or the vial of cytological medium with the woman's details before examining her so you do not mix up specimens (Fig. 10.28).

▪◣ Examination sequence

Taking a cervical smear

▪◣ Label the microscope slide or cytological medium.
▪◣ Clearly visualize the entire cervix.
▪◣ For a conventional smear, insert the longer blade of the spatula into the cervical os.
▪◣ Rotate the spatula through 360°.
▪◣ Spread once across the glass slide.
▪◣ Place the slide immediately into fixative (methylated spirits) for 3–4 minutes.
▪◣ Leave to dry in air.
▪◣ Insert the centre of the plastic broom into the cervical os.

A Using a spatula

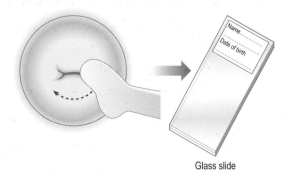

Glass slide

B Liquid-based cytology

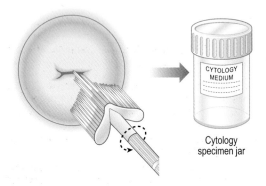

CYTOLOGY
MEDIUM

Cytology
specimen jar

Fig. 10.28 Taking a cervical smear.

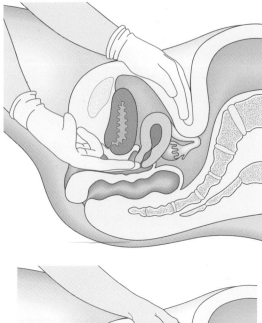

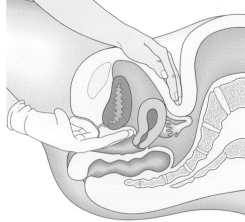

B

Fig. 10.29 Bimanual examination of the uterus. (A) Use your vaginal fingers to push the cervix back and upwards, and feel the fundus with your abdominal hand. **(B)** Then move your vaginal fingers into the anterior fornix and palpate the anterior surface of the uterus, holding it in position with your abdominal hand.

- Rotate the broom five times through 360°.
- Push the brush ten times against the bottom of the specimen container.
- Twirl five times through 360° to dislodge the sample.
- Firmly close the lid.

Bimanual examination

Examination sequence

Bimanual examination of the uterus

- Apply lubricating gel to your right index finger, and as you insert it into the vagina, turn your palm upwards. If the woman is tense or experiences discomfort, only use this one finger. Use your index and middle finger in women who are relaxed to enable you to feel more deeply (Fig. 10.29A).
- Feel for the cervix in the upper vagina. This points down and feels firm like the tip of the nose. Move the cervix from side to side and note any tenderness (cervical excitation). This can be a sign of infection.

- With your fingers posterior to the cervix, place your left hand flat on the lower abdomen above the pubic symphysis (Fig. 10.29B).
- Move your vaginal fingers to push the cervix upwards and feel the fundus of the uterus with your left hand. Identify the size, position and surface characteristics of the uterus and any tenderness. If you cannot feel the uterus, it may be retroverted. Put your fingers in the posterior vaginal fornix and try again.
- Put your fingers in each lateral vaginal fornix in turn, bringing your right hand up towards your left hand on the abdomen, to assess enlargement or tenderness of the ovaries or Fallopian tubes (Fig. 10.30).

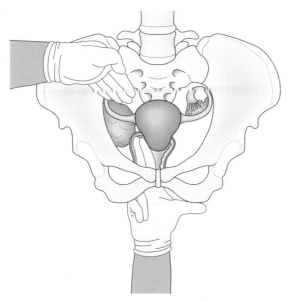

Fig. 10.30 Palpation of an ovarian mass.

OSCEs 10.16 Examine this patient with secondary amenorrhoea

1. Measure the body mass index.
2. Consider hyperthyroidism — palpate the thyroid gland, look for exophthalmos, check the pulse and examine for tremor.
3. Look for acne or excess body hair affecting the patient's face (upper lip and chin) or the nipple area, or extending up to the umbilicus from the pubic hair, suggesting possible polycystic ovary syndrome (PCOS).
4. Examine the nipples and check for galactorrhoea (hyperprolactinaemia).
5. Examine the abdomen for any masses arising from the pelvis. Consider pregnancy.
6. Use a speculum to examine the cervix then carry out a bimanual pelvic examination to assess uterine size.
7. Perform a pregnancy test.
8. Check the full blood count and thyroid function. Check hormone profile: FSH and LH (↑ if the patient is menopausal; ↓ if she has anorexia/weight loss, is stressed or exercises excessively), prolactin and testosterone (↑ in the presence of PCOS).
9. Further investigations as appropriate, e.g. pelvic ultrasound scan of the ovaries if PCOS is suspected.

OSCEs 10.17 Examine this patient with urinary incontinence

1. Examine the abdomen for any large mass arising from the pelvis.
2. Examine the vulva.
3. Inspect the urethral orifice. Ask the woman to cough and look for urine leaking.
4. Look for prolapse of the vaginal walls or descent of the cervix outside the vaginal orifice.
5. Carry out a bimanual examination to assess enlargement of the pelvic organs.
6. Dipstick the urine for glucose, protein and blood to exclude diabetes and urinary tract infection.
7. Arrange urodynamic assessment tests to differentiate between stress and urge incontinence.

OSCEs 10.18 Examine this patient with very heavy menstrual bleeding

1. Look for evidence of iron deficiency (smooth tongue, angular stomatitis, koilonychia) and anaemia.
2. Examine the patient's abdomen for any mass arising from the pelvis.
3. Perform a speculum examination to check the cervix for any polyps or prolapsing fibroid.
4. Carry out a bimanual pelvic examination to assess the size, position and surface characteristics of the uterus, looking for fibroids.
5. Check haemoglobin concentration and serum ferritin.
6. Arrange a pelvic ultrasound scan.
7. If the patient is >45 years, arrange an endometrial biopsy. Consider a diagnostic hysteroscopy if the ultrasound suggests the presence of an endometrial abnormality.

10.19 Key points: the gynaecological examination

- Employ particular care and sensitivity when taking a gynaecological history and performing a vaginal examination.
- Always offer the patient a chaperone.
- Pregnancy is the most common cause of amenorrhoea and/or a pelvic mass in a woman of reproductive age.
- If a patient finds speculum examination difficult, offer her the chance to insert the speculum herself.
- Women who have never been sexually active do not need a cervical smear.
- STIs are often asymptomatic in women.
- One-third of women in their late forties have uterine fibroids. Most are asymptomatic.
- Urgently investigate any vaginal bleeding more than 1 year after the menopause to exclude an underlying malignancy.
- Ovarian cancer often presents at an advanced stage with a large pelvic mass.

10

10.20 Investigations in gynaecological disease

Investigation	Indication/Comment
Vaginal pH	pH of vaginal secretions is normally <4.5
Urinary pregnancy test	Amenorrhoea or symptoms of pregnancy
Full blood count	Anaemia with heavy periods
Thyroid function	Amenorrhoea (thyrotoxic) Heavy, prolonged periods (hypothyroid)
Serum beta human chorionic gonadotrophin (β-HCG)	Elevated in very early pregnancy, useful in ectopic pregnancy
Serum oestradiol, progesterone, follicle-stimulating hormone (FSH), luteinizing hormone (LH), prolactin, testosterone	Amenorrhoea, premature menopause, infertility, hirsutism, galactorrhoea
Ovarian tumour markers, CA 125 and carcino-embryonic antigen	Ovarian cancer
Endocervical and high vaginal swabs	STIs
Abdominal or transvaginal ultrasound (Figs 10.31 and 10.32)	Early pregnancy, pelvic mass, abnormal menstrual bleeding, postmenopausal bleeding
Endometrial biopsy	Abnormal menstrual bleeding or postmenopausal bleeding
Diagnostic hysteroscopy	Abnormal menstrual bleeding or postmenopausal bleeding
Diagnostic laparoscopy	Chronic or acute pain, infertility

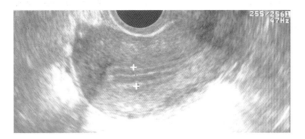

Fig. 10.31 Transvaginal ultrasound scan: showing longitudinal view of uterus with cursors demarcating endometrial thickness.

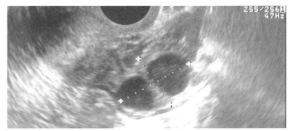

Fig. 10.32 Transvaginal ultrasound scan: showing left ovary measuring 2.9 × 2.1 cm with two small follicles.

THE OBSTETRIC EXAMINATION

Examining a pregnant patient differs from examining other patients because two individuals are assessed simultaneously. Work closely with the midwife and make sure communication between all parties is excellent by applying the principles discussed in Chapter 2.

Symptoms and definitions

Length of pregnancy

A normal pregnancy lasts 266 days (38 weeks) from the date of conception and 280 days (40 weeks) from the last menstrual period in a regular 28-day menstrual cycle.

Expected date of delivery

Add 1 year 7 days and subtract 3 months from the first day of your patient's last period, assuming she has a regular 28-day cycle. In longer cycles, ovulation is delayed because the interval between ovulation and the first day of menstruation is always 14 days; so for a 35-day cycle, the expected date of delivery is 7 days later than the date calculated for a 28-day cycle. Check that the last menstrual period was normal, lasted the usual length of time and occurred after the usual interval. Bleeding from implantation of the fertilized ovum can mimic a period, but is usually lighter and shorter, and the expected date of delivery will be 4 weeks earlier than anticipated. If the period occurred on stopping the oral contraceptive pill, ovulation may be delayed and the expected date of delivery will be

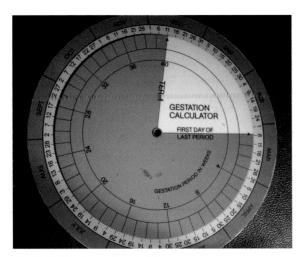

Fig. 10.33 Wheel gestation calculator.

10.21 Examples of gravidity and parity

A women who	Gravida	Para
Is not pregnant, has had a single live birth, one miscarriage and one termination	3	1 + 2
Has had two previous pregnancies resulting in a live birth and a stillbirth	3	2 + 0
Is pregnant with a singleton pregnancy, has had live twins and a previous ectopic	3	1 + 1
Is not pregnant, has had a twin pregnancy resulting in two live births	1	1 + 0

1–2 weeks after the date calculated. Use a gestation wheel calculator or computer to calculate the expected date of delivery (Fig. 10.33).

Legal age of viability

The legal age of viability of the fetus in the UK is currently 24 weeks but occasionally a baby may be born alive before this time. The World Health Organization (WHO) recommends that a fetus should be considered viable after 22 weeks or if it weighs more than 500 g.

Miscarriage

The expulsion of the fetus before it reaches viability may be spontaneous or induced (termination of pregnancy). The term 'abortion' is rarely used in clinical practice but is in lay use to describe termination of pregnancy.

Live birth

A live birth refers to a baby that shows signs of life after delivery, irrespective of the length of gestation. These signs include beating of the heart, pulsation of the umbilical cord or definite movements of the voluntary muscles.

Stillbirth

This term is used to describe a baby delivered after 24 weeks that does not breathe or show any other sign of life.

Gestation

Gestation refers to the duration of pregnancy from the last menstrual period, expressed in weeks plus days: for example, 7(+6) weeks.

Gravidity

Gravidity is the total number of present and previous pregnancies.

Parity

Parity is the number of pregnancies resulting in a live birth (at whatever gestation), together with all stillbirths plus the number of miscarriages, terminations and ectopic pregnancies. A multiple pregnancy is counted as one. Parity is expressed as two numbers: for example, 2 + 1 (Box 10.21).

Neonatal death

A baby who dies before 28 completed days of life is deemed to be a neonatal death. Early neonatal death occurs before 7 days and late neonatal death from then until 28 days.

Perinatal mortality rate

The standard perinatal mortality rate is the number of stillbirths plus the number of early neonatal deaths per 1000 total births. The extended perinatal mortality rate is the number of stillbirths plus early and late neonatal deaths per 1000 total births. Factors affecting the perinatal mortality rate include maternal age, maternal health, antenatal care and the management of labour.

Maternal mortality

A woman who dies while pregnant, or within 42 days of delivery, miscarriage or termination, is classed as a maternal mortality. Death can be from any cause but must be related to or aggravated (directly or indirectly) by the pregnancy or its management. Deaths from accidents or incidental causes are not included. Late maternal deaths are those occurring between 42 days and 1 year.

10

10

Puerperium

The puerperium is the time from the end of the third stage of labour until involution of the uterus is complete: approximately 6 weeks.

Lie of the fetus

The lie is the relationship of the long axis of the fetus to the long axis of the uterus. It is normally longitudinal but may be oblique or transverse (Fig. 10.34).

Presentation of the fetus

The presentation describes the leading part of the fetus in the lower pole of the uterus. Normally this is cephalic, with the head presenting. It may be breech, with the bottom presenting, or shoulder, or compound when the head and a limb are present. The lie (the axis of the fetus in relation to the mother) is always longitudinal when the presentation is cephalic or breech. Transverse and oblique lies are associated with a shoulder presentation. These are more common in multiparous women when the abdominal wall musculature is lax. If the placenta is located in the lower segment of the uterus (placenta praevia), this may cause an oblique or transverse lie. The position of the presenting part is its relationship to the maternal pelvis. You may be given clues during the abdominal examination but the position is most important during labour, when it is defined by vaginal examination (Fig. 10.35).

Polyhydramnios

Polyhydramnios is an excess of amniotic fluid relative to the fetus, resulting in the uterus feeling tense and measuring large for dates.

Oligohydramnios

Oligohydramnios is a lack of amniotic fluid; the uterus may measure small for dates.

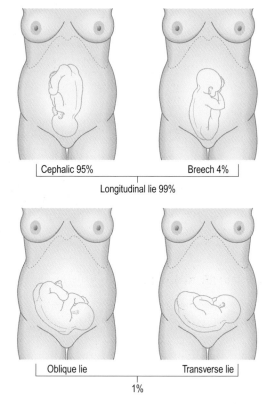

Cephalic 95%　　　　　　　　Breech 4%

Longitudinal lie 99%

Oblique lie　　　　　　　Transverse lie

1%

Fig. 10.34 The lie and presentation of the fetus.

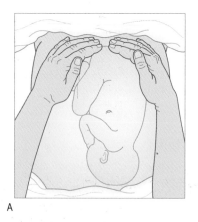

A

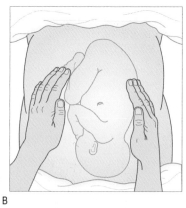

B

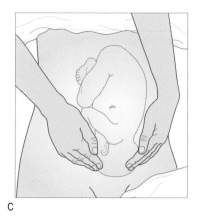

C

Fig. 10.35 Abdominal examination. (A) First manoeuvre — fundal palpation. Estimate the height of the fundus and palpate the fundal area gently to identify which pole of the fetus (breech or head) is occupying the fundus. **(B)** Second manoeuvre — lateral palpation. Slip your hands gently and quickly down the sides of the uterus to try to identify on which side the firm back and knobbly limbs of the fetus are positioned. **(C)** Pelvic manoeuvre. Turn to face the patient's feet and slide your hands gently on the lower part of the uterus, pressing down on each side to determine the presenting part. If it is the fetal head, it feels hard and may be ballotted between your fingers.

10

THE HISTORY

Presenting complaint

A pregnant patient often has no presenting complaint and is seen routinely to monitor the progress of her pregnancy. She may, however, complain of symptoms caused by pregnancy, such as nausea and vomiting, constipation, haemorrhoids, urinary frequency, backache, symphysial pain, breathlessness, ankle swelling, varicose veins and pruritus. Any disease may also occur that is unrelated to the pregnancy. Think of the latter from two points of view:

- the effect of the disease on the pregnancy
- the effect of pregnancy on the disease.

Address the patient's FIFE (p. 10). Establish her age and parity, and the gestational age of the pregnancy. Ask about her menstrual history and previous use of contraception. Find out her past obstetric history, noting all of her previous pregnancies, including miscarriages, terminations and ectopic pregnancy. Include the gestation at delivery, method of delivery and any complications she or her babies experienced.

Past medical history

Include operations and psychiatric illnesses. Identify women with diabetes, epilepsy or other chronic conditions so that you can give them appropriate advice about their medication and risks, and refer them early to a specialist in the relevant disease so that shared care can be arranged.

Drug history

Ask about any prescribed medication, over-the-counter drugs and natural remedies, illegal drugs, alcohol intake and smoking habits. Advise the patient to stop smoking and to abstain from alcohol. Check that she is taking 400µg of folic acid until 12 weeks' gestation to reduce the incidence of neural tube defects, including spina bifida.

Family history

A good family history is important, because a patient may have unwarranted anxiety about her baby; taking a proper history allows you to identify those women with a high risk of having a baby with a genetic disorder (Box 10.22).

Patients can be offered the opportunity of early diagnosis by chorion villus biopsy or amniocentesis. Chromosomal abnormality is more common in older women. This relates to the increased risk of trisomies, trisomy 21 (Down's syndrome) being the most common (Box 10.23).

Social history

Lower socioeconomic status is linked with increased perinatal and maternal mortality. Ask the patient who her partner is and how stable the relationship; if she is not in a relationship, find out who will give her support during and after her pregnancy. Was the pregnancy planned or not? If unplanned, find out how the woman feels about it. Ask what her job entails and whether she plans to return to it. Use this opportunity to give her advice. Encourage her to exercise regularly and to avoid certain foods such as tuna (high mercury content), soft cheeses (risk of *Listeria*) and calves' liver (high vitamin A content) (Box 10.24).

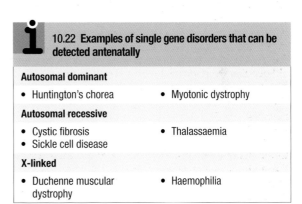

10.22 Examples of single gene disorders that can be detected antenatally

Autosomal dominant

- Huntington's chorea
- Myotonic dystrophy

Autosomal recessive

- Cystic fibrosis
- Sickle cell disease
- Thalassaemia

X-linked

- Duchenne muscular dystrophy
- Haemophilia

10.23 Age-related risk of Down's syndrome (trisomy 21)

Maternal age	Risk
20	1 in 1500
30	1 in 900
35	1 in 400
40	1 in 100
45	1 in 30

10.24 Checklist for the obstetric history

- Age
- Parity
- Menstrual history, last menstrual period, gestation, expected date of delivery
- Presenting complaint
- Past obstetric history
- Past medical and surgical history
- Drug history
- Family history
- Social history

10

THE PHYSICAL EXAMINATION
Abdominal examination

▶ Examination sequence
Obstetric examination of the abdomen

▶ Gain an impression of how your patient's pregnancy is proceeding by noting her demeanour from the moment you see her. Is she happy or does she appear exhausted and anxious? Is she pale or breathless? Does she get up with difficulty, and if so, why? Offer her the chance to empty her bladder before you examine her and ask her to collect a specimen of urine for testing.

▶ Measure her height and weight. Women <152 cm (5 feet) are more likely to have obstructed labour and small babies. Patients over 100 kg may develop gestational diabetes and have large (macrosomic) babies. Work out the body mass index (BMI) (kg/h^2; p. 59). Women are at higher risk in pregnancy if the BMI is <20 or >35. Serial weight measurements throughout pregnancy do not reliably predict problems such as pre-eclampsia or intrauterine growth restriction.

▶ Measure the patient's blood pressure and check a urine sample using dipstix for glycosuria and proteinuria.

▶ Ask her to lie down on a firm but comfortable couch, with her back resting at an angle of 30°. Ask her to uncover her abdomen from the lower chest to below her hips and place a sheet over any exposed underwear.

Inspection

▶ Look for the abdominal distension caused by the pregnant uterus rising from the pelvis. After 24 weeks you may see fetal movements, which confirm the baby's viability. Increased pigmentation, caused by increased melanocyte activity related to changes in sex hormones, commonly produces a dark line (linea nigra) stretching from the pubic symphysis upwards in the midline, and nipple pigmentation. Striae gravidarum are the red stretch marks of this pregnancy. Striae albicantes are white stretch marks from a previous pregnancy. Note any scars and check the umbilicus, which becomes flattened as pregnancy advances and everted in polyhydramnios (excess amniotic fluid) or multiple pregnancy.

Palpation

▶ Use your left hand to feel the uterus abdominally and estimate the height of the uterus above the symphysis pubis (Fig. 10.36).

▶ Note any fetal movements. Facing towards the woman's head, use both hands on either side of the fundus to gain an impression of which fetal part is lying there. Use your right hand on the woman's left side. Bring your hands down to palpate the sides of the uterus and identify which side is fuller; fullness suggests that the back is on that side. Now turn to face the patient's feet, so that your left hand is on the woman's left side. Feel the lower part of the uterus to determine the presenting part. Ballot the head by pushing it gently from one side to the other and feel its hardness against your fingers (Fig. 10.35).

▶ After 20 weeks measure the fundal height in centimetres. With a tape measure, fix the end at the highest point on the fundus and measure to the symphysis pubis. The highest point is not always in the midline. To avoid bias, do this with the blank side of the tape facing you, so that you only see the measurement on lifting

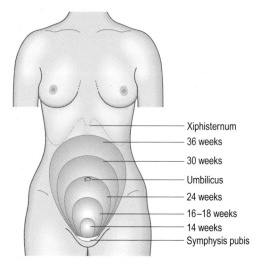

- Xiphisternum
- 36 weeks
- 30 weeks
- Umbilicus
- 24 weeks
- 16–18 weeks
- 14 weeks
- Symphysis pubis

Fig. 10.36 Approximate fundal height with changing gestation.

the tape. The measurement equals the gestation in weeks ±3 cm and is an indicator of growth problems in the fetus. In a tall or thin patient, the fundal height may be less than expected; in an obese patient, it may be greater.

▶ You may be able to determine the position of the presenting part. When the presentation is cephalic, the vertex or top of the fetal head engages in the occipitolateral position.

▶ If the presentation is cephalic, assess how far into the true pelvis the head has descended by estimating how much of the head you can feel above the pelvic brim. The head is divided into fifths. The head is said to be fixed when it is three-fifths palpable and engaged when it is two-fifths or one-fifth palpable (Fig. 10.37)

Percussion

▶ Percussion is unhelpful unless you suspect polyhydramnios. Confirm this by eliciting a fluid thrill but no shifting dullness (p. 204).

Auscultation

▶ Use an electronic hand-held Doppler fetal heart rate monitor as early as 14 weeks (Fig. 10.38A).

▶ A Pinard stethoscope is not useful until after 28 weeks. Place the widest part over the anterior shoulder of the fetus (Fig. 10.38B). Facing the mother's feet, put your left ear against the smaller end and press against the mother's abdomen gently to keep the stethoscope in place. Take your hands away from the stethoscope so that it is kept in place by the pressure of your head. Listen for the fetal heart. This sounds like a distant ticking noise. Imagine you are listening for a clock ticking through a pillow.

Vaginal examination

In early pregnancy

Perform a bimanual pelvic examination only if ultrasound is not available to establish gestation. Ultrasound

Completely above	Sinciput +++ occiput ++	Sinciput ++ occiput +	Sinciput + occiput just felt	Sinciput + occiput not felt	None of head palpable
5/5	4/5	3/5	2/5	1/5	0/5
Free, above the brim	'Fixing'	Fixed, not engaged	Just engaged	Engaged	Deeply engaged

Level of pelvic brim

Fig. 10.37 Descent of the fetal head.

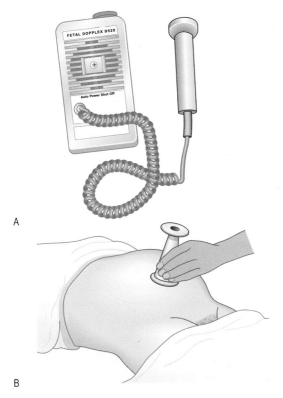

A

B

Fig. 10.38 Auscultation of the fetal heart. (A) Doppler fetal heart rate monitor. **(B)** Pinard fetal stethoscope. The fetal rate varies between 110 and 160/minute and should be regular.

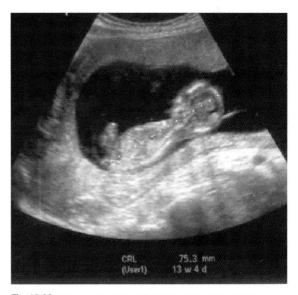

CRL 75.3 mm
(User1) 13 w 4 d

Fig. 10.39 Ultrasound scan showing fetal crown–rump measurement.

The pregnant uterus is equivalent to the size of:
- an apple at 6 weeks
- an orange at 8–10 weeks
- a grapefruit at 12–14 weeks.

Take a cervical smear only if this is clinically indicated; otherwise, defer it until the postnatal check.

In late pregnancy

Assess cervical status by vaginal examination before induction of labour. Feel the dilatation and length of the cervix, its consistency and position, and the station (level) of the head above or below the ischial spines (− or + respectively in cm). The cervix is most commonly located towards the posterior fornix behind the fetal head (Fig. 10.41).

establishes gestational age, confirms viability, excludes adnexal pathology and reveals multiple pregnancy (Figs 10.39 and 10.40). In a vaginal examination, the size of the uterus can be seen to reflect the gestation.

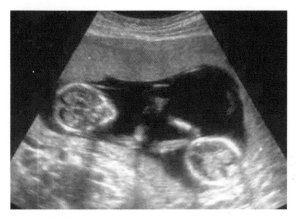

Fig. 10.40 Ultrasound scan taken at 12 weeks, showing a twin pregnancy.

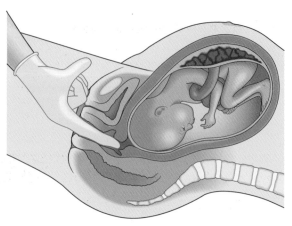

Fig. 10.41 Vaginal examination in late pregnancy to assess cervical status.

INVESTIGATIONS

10.25 Antenatal investigations

Investigation	Indication/Comment
Urinary glucose	Every visit: if persists, carry out glucose tolerance test
Urinary protein	Every visit Trace or +, check MSSU specimen: + + or more, consider pre-eclampsia
Full blood count	Booking, 28 weeks, 36 weeks: treat if haemoglobin level falls <100 g/l
Haemoglobin electrophoresis	Booking: sickle cell and thalassaemias. Routine for patients of mixed ethnicity
Blood grouping and antibody screen	Booking and as advised by laboratory Rhesus and Kell most common cause of isoimmunization
Rubella	Booking
Hepatitis B and C	Booking: if hepatitis B antigen-positive, baby will require vaccination soon after birth. Breastfeeding is best avoided. Hepatitis C tested if hepatitis B positive
HIV status	Booking (unless patient opts out): treating HIV-positive mother reduces risk of vertical transmission to baby. Deliver by caesarean section and avoid breastfeeding
Syphilis testing	Booking: if positive, treatment with penicillin will prevent congenital syphilis in neonate
Plasma glucose	28 weeks
Urine specimen for culture	As required
Cervical smear	If required
Serum screening for trisomy 21 and spina bifida	16 weeks: detects 60% of pregnancies affected by trisomy 21
Combined biochemical screening and nuchal translucency measurement for trisomy 21	11–14 weeks: detects 80–90% of pregnancies affected by trisomy 21
First trimester ultrasound scan	6–13 weeks: confirms viability, gestational age within 1 week, multiple pregnancy, adnexal mass
Detailed ultrasound scan	18–22 weeks: detects 90% of major congenital abnormalities. Confirms gestation within 10 days
Ultrasound scan for placental site	Antepartum haemorrhage after 24 weeks: more reliable as gestation advances when lower segment forms. 1 in 4 patients have a low placenta at 20 weeks
Ultrasound scan for growth	Clinical suspicion of poor growth, usually after 24 weeks
Amniocentesis	15 weeks for fetal karyotype: full karyotype takes 2–3 weeks. New methods for specific chromosomal abnormalities take 2–4 days. 0.5–1% risk of miscarriage
Chorion villus biopsy	10 weeks onwards for fetal karyotype, single gene disorders Short-term result in 2–5 days; long-term 2–3 weeks. 1–2% risk of miscarriage

> **10.26 Key points: obstetric examination**
>
> - Always establish maternal age, parity and gestation.
> - Do not routinely carry out a vaginal examination in early pregnancy.
> - A first-trimester scan accurately determines gestational age to within 1 week.
> - Fetal abnormality is best detected by an ultrasound scan at 18–22 weeks.
> - If the presentation is cephalic, the lie is always longitudinal.
> - In antepartum haemorrhage, exclude a low-lying placenta by ultrasound before carrying out a vaginal examination.

10

THE MALE GENITAL EXAMINATION

Anatomy

The male genitalia include the testes, epididymes and seminal vesicles, penis, scrotum and prostate gland (Fig. 10.42).

The testes

The testes develop intra-abdominally near the kidneys and migrate through the inguinal canal into the scrotum by birth, bringing their blood, lymphatic and nerve supply with them. This is why testicular problems may cause abdominal pain and enlargement of the para-aortic lymph nodes.

Each testis lies in the scrotum and separated from the other by a muscular septum; the left testis usually lies lower than the right. They are oval and 3.5–4 cm long. A fibrous layer, the tunica albuginea, covers them, and forms the posterior wall of the tunica vaginalis. This is a prolongation of the peritoneal tube that follows the testis down into the scrotum; if it persists, as the processus vaginalis, it may cause an indirect inguinal hernial sac or a congenital hydrocoele. Along the posterior border of each testis the epididymis is formed by efferent tubules draining the seminiferous tubules. Multiple veins in the pampiniform plexus form one vein at the deep inguinal ring. Varicosity of the plexus is called a varicocoele (Fig. 10.43).

The testes produce sperm and hormones, predominantly testosterone. Sperm are produced from the germinal epithelium, mature in the epididymis, and pass down the vas deferens to the seminal vesicles, where they are stored. They are ejaculated from the urethra, together with prostatic fluid, at orgasm. Testosterone is produced from the Leydig cells. Sperm and testosterone production starts at puberty, between 10 and 15 years old (Fig. 15.27, p. 425).

The penis

The penis is composed of two cylinders of endothelial-lined spaces surrounded by smooth muscle, known as the corpora cavernosa (Fig. 10.44). They are bound with the bulbospongiosus, which surrounds the urethra and expands into the glans penis. The skin covering the penis is reflected over the glans, forming the prepuce (foreskin). The penis is a conduit for urine and semen. Sexual arousal causes a parasympathetically mediated, increased blood flow into the corpora cavernosa with erection to enable vaginal penetration. Continued stimulation causes sympathetic mediated contraction of the seminal vesicles and prostate, closure of the bladder neck and ejaculation. Following orgasm, reduction in blood flow allows detumescence.

The scrotum

The scrotum is a pouch containing the testes, which sits posterior to the penis. It has thin pigmented, ridged or wrinkled skin and is lined by the dartos muscle (Fig. 10.45). Sperm production takes place most efficiently at a temperature lower than the body; hence the testes are held in the scrotum. The dartos muscle is highly contractile and helps regulate the temperature of the scrotal contents.

The prostate and seminal vesicles

The prostate produces a fructose-rich fluid as an energy substrate for sperm. After the age of 40 the prostate develops a 'trilobar' structure from benign hyperplasia, with a pair of lateral lobes and a variable median lobe, which protrudes into the bladder and may cause urethral and bladder outflow obstruction. Cancer of the prostate develops in the peripheral tissue in the lateral lobes and can then often be detected by digital rectal examination. Only the posterior aspect of the lateral lobes of the prostate is felt on rectal examination (p. 207).

SYMPTOMS AND DEFINITIONS

Testis and scrotal abnormalities

Hydrocoeles

These are due to fluid in the tunica vaginalis. They are usually idiopathic but may be secondary to inflammatory conditions or tumours. If you cannot

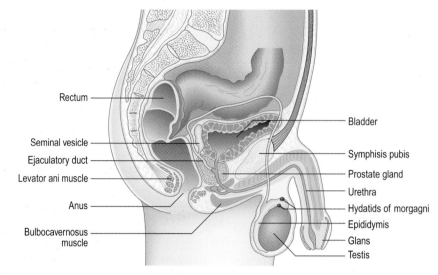

Fig. 10.42 Anatomy of the male genitalia. The male genitalia include the external organs, seminal vesicles and the prostate gland.

Labels: Rectum, Seminal vesicle, Ejaculatory duct, Levator ani muscle, Anus, Bulbocavernosus muscle, Bladder, Symphisis pubis, Prostate gland, Urethra, Hydatids of morgagni, Epididymis, Glans, Testis

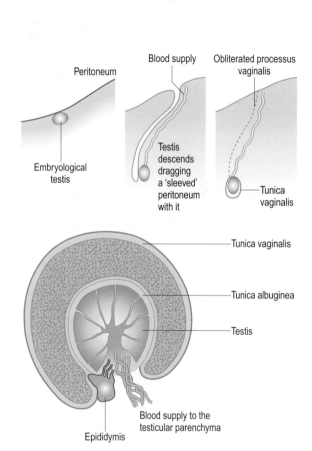

Labels: Peritoneum, Blood supply, Obliterated processus vaginalis, Embryological testis, Testis descends dragging a 'sleeved' peritoneum with it, Tunica vaginalis, Tunica vaginalis, Tunica albuginea, Testis, Blood supply to the testicular parenchyma, Epididymis

Fig. 10.43 Embryological development of the testis. The tunica vaginalis is the remnant of the peritoneum left behind after testicular descent. The tunica albuginea is the tough outer coating of the testis.

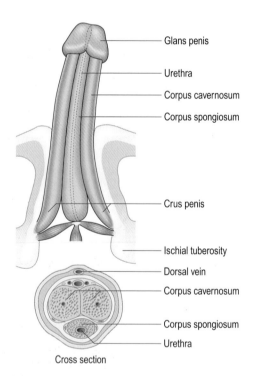

Labels: Glans penis, Urethra, Corpus cavernosum, Corpus spongiosum, Crus penis, Ischial tuberosity, Dorsal vein, Corpus cavernosum, Corpus spongiosum, Urethra, Cross section

Fig. 10.44 Anatomy of the penis. The shaft and glans penis are formed from the corpus spongiosum and the corpus cavernosum.

palpate the testis because of a hydrocoele, organize an ultrasound scan.

Epididymal cysts

These are swellings of the epididymis, which are completely separate from the body of the testis. Isolated

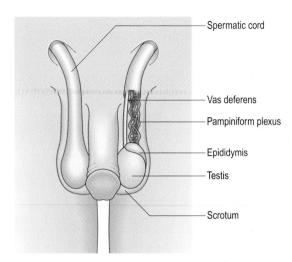

Fig. 10.45 The scrotum and its contents.

- Spermatic cord
- Vas deferens
- Pampiniform plexus
- Epididymis
- Testis
- Scrotum

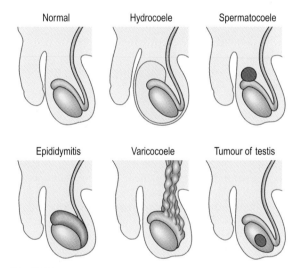

Fig. 10.46 **Swellings of the scrotum.** Some common abnormalities of the scrotal contents.

Normal | Hydrocoele | Spermatocoele
Epididymitis | Varicocoele | Tumour of testis

OSCEs 10.27 Examine this patient with an acutely swollen scrotum

1. 28% of torsions present with abdominal pain only, so examine the genitals of any boy presenting with this.
2. Look for scrotal bruising, redness and swelling. Examine the abdomen to exclude intra-abdominal causes of scrotal pain.
3. Try to palpate the cord structures, the body of the testis and the epididymis separately and note where the pain localizes. If the cord is short and thickened, and the testis retracted and swollen, then torsion is most likely. This requires immediate surgical referral.
4. If the testis is swollen, the cord is not shortened and the boy had facial swelling 10 days earlier, mumps orchitis is likely.
5. If the epididymis is palpable separately from the body of the testis and is tender and swollen, then epididymitis is possible, although it is rare in adolescents. In young men assume epididymitis is due to an STI, treat and refer to a specialist clinic. In the over-fifties and when urinalysis is abnormal, investigate and treat as urinary tract infection.
6. If there is an isolated tender swelling at the top of the testis, assume that it is probably torsion of a hydatid of Morgagni.
7. If in doubt, organize an urgent ultrasound s und is unavailable, then refer for immediate s avoid infarction of the testis.
8. Always explain the need for a possible testis is necrotic and for fixation of the prior to surgery, and obtain informed c
9. Carry out urinalysis.

swellings adherent to the epididymis alone are virtually never malignant. Painful swellings at the superior pole of the testis or adjacent to the head of the epididymis are usually due to torsion of a hydatid of Morgagni.

Epididymitis

Epididymitis is painful epididymal swelling; it is due to sexually transmitted infections (STIs) in young men or *E. coli* in the elderly.

Varicocoeles

These are varicosities of the spermatic vein, often described on palpation as feeling like a 'bag of worms' in the scrotum.

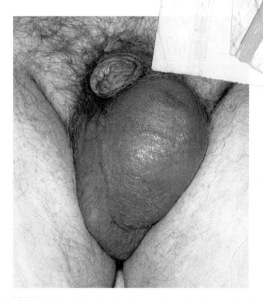

Fig. 10.47 **Left testicular torsion.** There is shortening of the cord with retraction of the testis and global swelling of the scrotal contents. The patient should be referred urgently to a surgeon for scrotal exploration.

Testicular tumours

Testicular tumours usually cause painless hard swellings of the body of the testis. Around 15% of tumours occur close to the head of the epididymis and may cause local discomfort.

A single testis

A single testis may be caused by incomplete testicular descent in the inguinal canal or an ectopic testis in the groin. Ask about previous surgery for a testicular tumour or ectopic testis.

Unilateral testicular atrophy

This may result from mumps infection, torsion of the testis or vascular compromise after inguinal hernia repair, or from a late orchidopexy for an undescended testis.

Bilateral testicular atrophy

This suggests primary or secondary hypogonadism or primary testicular failure. Check development of the secondary sexual characteristics (Fig. 15.27, p. 424), and look for hormonal abnormalities or signs of anabolic steroid usage.

Penile and urethral abnormalities

Urethritis

Urethritis is inflammation of the urethra, which may cause dysuria (pain on micturition) or a urethral discharge. The most common causes are non-specific urethritis and gonococcal infection.

Phimosis

Phimosis is narrowing of the preputial orifice, preventing retraction of the foreskin. This may cause recurrent infection of the glans penis (balanitis) or of the prepuce (posthitis) or both (balanoposthitis).

Paraphimosis

Paraphimosis is the inability to pull the foreskin forward after retraction due to the presence of a constriction ring in the prepuce (Fig. 10.48).

Peyronie's disease

This is a fibrotic condition of the shaft of the penis of unknown aetiology, producing curvature of the erect penis.

Genital ulcer

Genital ulcer refers to a break in the mucosa or skin anywhere on the genitals. Painful ulcers are usually caused by herpes simplex; if they are painless, consider reactive arthritis (p. 366), lichen simplex and (rarely) syphilis.

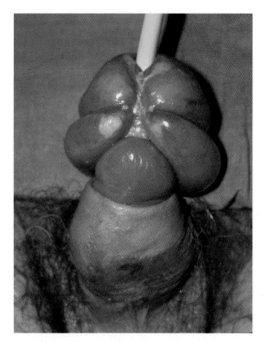

Fig. 10.48 Paraphimosis. Oedema of the foreskin behind an encircling constriction ring due to the foreskin not being replaced — in this case, after catheterization.

Sexual dysfunction

This may mean a change in libido, inability to achieve or maintain an erection, premature ejaculation, delayed ejaculation, failure to ejaculate or problems in attaining orgasm. Clarify what the exact problem is and consider possible causes, including psychological issues, alcohol, systemic disease (diabetes mellitus), peripheral vascular disease and drugs.

Prostate abnormalities

Prostatitis

Prostatitis is inflammation of the prostate gland; it is usually caused by STI in younger men and by *E. coli* in older men. It causes tender bogginess of the prostate.

Benign hypertrophy

This is common in patients >60 years and is associated with urinary symptoms (Box 9.3, p. 221). The median sulcus is preserved and the prostate may feel rubbery.

Prostate cancer

Prostate cancer is stony hard and often causes the lateral lobes to feel nodular. However, these changes are only 60% sensitive and should be investigated by biopsy.

◼◼▶ Examination sequence

Male genitals

◼◼▶ Explain to the patient what you are going to do and offer a chaperone. Record the chaperone's name; if the offer is refused, record the fact. Allow the patient privacy to undress.

◼◼▶ Ensure privacy and have a warm, well-lit room with a movable light source. Put on gloves. Ask the patent to stand and expose the area from his lower abdomen to the top of his thighs if you are examining the inguino-scrotal area; ask him to lie on his back to examine the penis or prostate.

◼◼▶ Look at the whole area for redness, swelling or ulcers. Note the hair distribution: in particular, alopecia or infestation. Shaving the pubic hair may cause dermatitis (inflammation of the dermis) or folliculitis (infection around the base of the hairs, leading to an irritating red rash). Check the groin, perineum and scrotal skin for rashes, intertrigo (infected eczema) in the skin creases, and lymphadenopathy.

The penis

◼◼▶ Enlarged sebaceous follicles may mimic warts. Numerous uniform pearly penile papules around the corona of the glans are normal. Look at the shaft of the penis and check the position of the urethral opening to exclude a hypospadias (the urethra opening part-way along the shaft of the penis (p. 408)).

◼◼▶ Retract the prepuce to check for phimosis, adhesions, inflammation, or swellings on the foreskin or glans. Always draw the foreskin forward after examination to avoid a paraphimosis.

◼◼▶ Examine the glans for red patches or vesicles.

◼◼▶ Examine the shaft for sebaceous cysts or hardness (usually on the dorsum) consistent with a plaque of Peyronie's disease.

◼◼▶ Take a urethral swab if your patient has a discharge or is having sexual health screening.

The scrotum

◼◼▶ Look at the scrotum for redness, swelling or ulcers; sebaceous cysts are common. Inspect the posterior surface. Note the position of the testes and any paratesticular swelling.

◼◼▶ Ask the patient whether he is experiencing any genital pain before examining the scrotal contents.

◼◼▶ If the patient is cold or apprehensive, the dartos muscle will contract and you will not be able to palpate the scrotal contents properly.

◼◼▶ Palpate the scrotum gently, using both hands. Check that both testes are present in the scrotum; if they are not, examine the inguinal canal and perineum.

◼◼▶ Place the fingers of both your hands behind the left testis to immobilize it and use your index finger and thumb to palpate the body of the testis methodically. Feel the anterior surface and medial border with your thumb and the lateral border with your index finger. Repeat on both sides (Fig. 10.49).

◼◼▶ Check the size and consistency of the testis and note any nodules or irregularities. Encourage all younger men to examine their testes regularly and to present any abnormal swellings to their doctor. This helps to detect testicular tumours early.

◼◼▶ You should barely be able to feel the normal epididymis, except for its head (Fig. 10.50).

◼◼▶ Palpate the spermatic cord with your right hand. Gently pull the right testis downward and place your fingers behind the neck

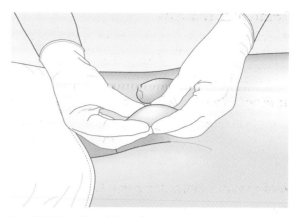

Fig. 10.49 Palpation of the testis.

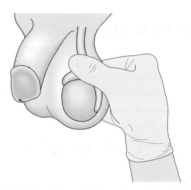

Fig. 10.50 Palpation of the epididymis. The epididymis is readily felt only at the top of the testis.

of the scrotum. You will be able to feel the spermatic cord and the vas deferens within it, like a thick piece of string. Feeling a 'bag of worms' in the cord suggests a varicocoele. This should disappear when the patient lies down; if it does not, then consider a retroperitoneal mass distending the testicular veins.

◼◼▶ Decide whether a swelling arises in the scrotum or from the inguinal canal. Use your fingers to see whether you can feel above the swelling; if so, it is a true scrotal swelling. If not, it may be a varicocoele or inguinal hernia, which has descended into the scrotum.

◼◼▶ If there is a bulky or painful mass in the scrotum and you cannot palpate the testis, request an ultrasound scan to clarify the anatomy of the intrascrotal structures (Fig. 10.51).

The prostate

◼◼▶ Carry out a rectal examination (p. 207).

◼◼▶ Feel the prostate anteriorly through the rectal wall and assess its size. The normal prostate is a smooth, non-tender structure in the anterior rectal wall.

◼◼▶ You may feel an indentation or sulcus between the two lateral lobes and sometimes the seminal vesicles above the prostate.

◼◼▶ Note any tenderness.

◼◼▶ Assess the consistency.

◼◼▶ Feel for any nodules.

◼◼▶ Withdraw your finger. Offer the patient tissues to clean himself up and privacy to get dressed.

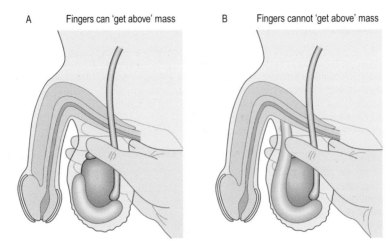

A   Fingers can 'get above' mass   B   Fingers cannot 'get above' mass

Fig. 10.51 Testing for scrotal swellings. (A) It is possible to 'get above' a true scrotal swelling. **(B)** This is not possible if the swelling is caused by an inguinal hernia that has descended into the scrotum.

INVESTIGATIONS

10.28 Investigations in male genital disease

Investigation	Indication/comment
Urinalysis	Protein and blood + + in urinary tract infection and epididymitis
Serum PSA	Raised in prostate cancer but increases with age, prostatic volume, following prostatic trauma and in seminal or urinary tract infection
Serum β-HCG, α-fetoprotein and leucocyte alkaline phosphatase	Raised in some types of testicular cancer and in bony metastases
Serum FSH and LH	In azoospermia FSH and LH levels may be low in pituitary causes. FSH may be normal in obstructive causes or maturation arrest and elevated in primary testicular failure
Serum prolactin	Raised prolactin suggests a pituitary tumour when libido is reduced
Serum testosterone and sex hormone-binding globulin (SHBG)	Low in lack of virilization or sometimes erectile dysfunction
MSU	Urinary tract infection, testicular pain, epididymitis
Urinary chlamydial PCR	STI, urethral discharge or epididymitis
Urethral swab	Suspected STI
Semen analysis/culture	In infertility or haemospermia to assess volume, number and quality of sperm in the ejaculate. Analyses two separate samples. Culture semen if pus cells are found or haemospermia persists
Genital ultrasound examination	Hydrocoele, acute scrotal pain or penile mass
Colour Doppler imaging	To assess blood flow in suspected testicular torsion, priapism and erectile dysfunction
Transrectal ultrasound examination	Increases the sensitivity and specificity of digital rectal examination in suspected prostate cancer. Defines the anatomy of the prostate and the seminal vesicles in infertility or haemospermia
CT scanning	To find the site of an undescended testis and to stage testicular cancer
MR scanning	To stage prostate cancer and delineate the seminal vesicles

10.29 Key points: the male genital examination

- Do not avoid examination of the male genitalia simply because the patient says everything is normal.
- Offer the patient a chaperone and record that person's name; document if the patient declines.
- Examine the scrotum and groin with the patient standing up initially. Examine the penis or prostate with the man lying on his back.
- Retract the foreskin to examine the glans fully; draw it forward when you have finished to avoid causing a paraphimosis.
- When you cannot feel the testis because of a large hydrocoele, organize an ultrasound scan to exclude an underlying cancer.
- Swellings of the epididymis are virtually never due to serious pathology.
- If you cannot palpate an abnormality in the scrotum, then there is no point in carrying out an ultrasound examination since it will be normal.
- A normal-feeling prostate gland does not exclude malignancy; if you suspect cancer, investigate by transrectal ultrasound scan-guided biopsy.

10

The nervous system

Brian Pentland
Richard Davenport
Richard Cowie

11

NERVOUS SYSTEM EXAMINATION

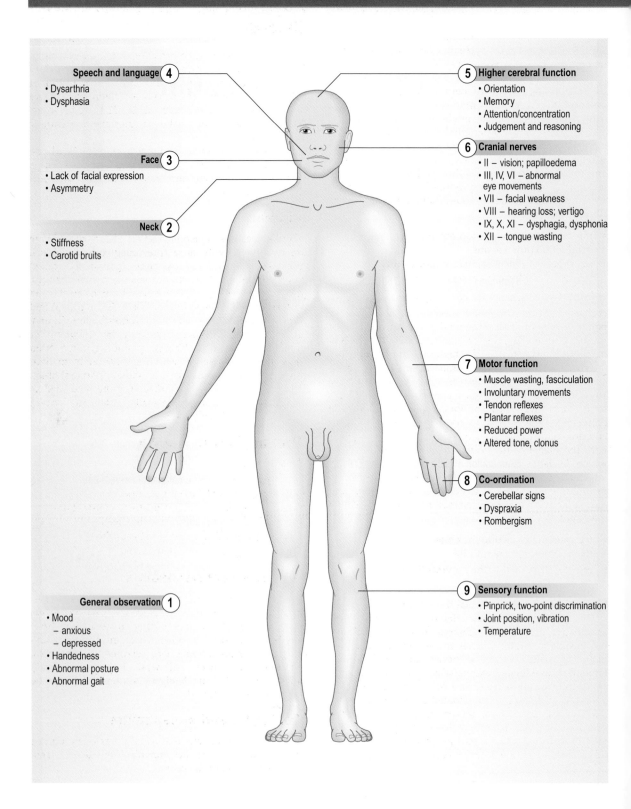

Speech and language ④
- Dysarthria
- Dysphasia

Face ③
- Lack of facial expression
- Asymmetry

Neck ②
- Stiffness
- Carotid bruits

General observation ①
- Mood
  - anxious
  - depressed
- Handedness
- Abnormal posture
- Abnormal gait

⑤ Higher cerebral function
- Orientation
- Memory
- Attention/concentration
- Judgement and reasoning

⑥ Cranial nerves
- II – vision; papilloedema
- III, IV, VI – abnormal eye movements
- VII – facial weakness
- VIII – hearing loss; vertigo
- IX, X, XI – dysphagia, dysphonia
- XII – tongue wasting

⑦ Motor function
- Muscle wasting, fasciculation
- Involuntary movements
- Tendon reflexes
- Plantar reflexes
- Reduced power
- Altered tone, clonus

⑧ Co-ordination
- Cerebellar signs
- Dyspraxia
- Rombergism

⑨ Sensory function
- Pinprick, two-point discrimination
- Joint position, vibration
- Temperature

ANATOMY

The nervous system consists of the brain and spinal cord (central nervous system, CNS) and peripheral nerves (peripheral nervous system, PNS). The neurone has a cell body and axon terminating at a synapse and is the functioning unit of the nervous system. Astrocytes provide the structural framework for the neurones, control their biochemical environment and form the 'blood–brain barrier'. Microglial cells are blood-derived mononuclear macrophages and have an immune and scavenging role. In the CNS, oligodendrocytes create and maintain a myelin sheath round the axons, while in the PNS the myelin is produced by Schwann cells. The functioning of the nervous system depends on two physiological processes:

- the generation of an action potential with its conduction down axons
- the synaptic transmission of impulses between neurones and/or muscle cells.

The brain consists of two cerebral hemispheres, each with four functionally specialized lobes (frontal, parietal, temporal and occipital), the brainstem and the cerebellum. The cerebral cortex over the cerebral hemispheres constitutes the highest level of function; the anterior half deals with executive ('doing') functions and the posterior half constructs a perception of the environment ('receiving and perceiving'). The brainstem, consisting of the midbrain, pons and medulla oblongata, contains all the sensory and motor pathways entering and leaving the cerebral hemispheres, together with the nuclei of the cranial nerves. The cerebellum, which lies below the cerebral hemispheres and posterior to the brainstem, is responsible for co-ordination, including gait and posture. Between the soft brain and the skull are three types of membranous covering called meninges:

- the dura mater next to the bone
- the arachnoid in the middle
- the pia mater next to the nervous tissue.

The subarachnoid space between the arachnoid and pia is filled with cerebrospinal fluid (CSF).

The spinal cord contains afferent and efferent fibres arranged in functionally discrete bundles which are responsible for motor reflexes and sensory information, including pain. Peripheral nerves are made up of large, fast, myelinated axons (which carry information about joint position sense and commands to muscles) and smaller, slower, unmyelinated axons (which carry information about pain, temperature and autonomic function). The sensory cell bodies of peripheral nerves are situated in the dorsal root ganglia, while the motor cell bodies are in the anterior horns of the spinal cord (Fig. 11.1).

SYMPTOMS AND DEFINITIONS

Headache

Headache is the most common neurological symptom. Headaches are either primary, e.g. migraine or secondary to other pathology, e.g. side-effects of medication or subarachnoid haemorrhage, and are common in many non-neurological conditions (Box 11.1). The most common causes of headache are migraine and chronic daily headache syndrome.

Use SOCRATES to define the nature of the headache (Box 2.10, p. 15). Ask what the patient does, or is prevented from doing, during an attack and how he or she feels between attacks.

Migraine

Migraine causes episodic, severe headache. There are two types: with aura (previously called classical migraine; ~20%) and without (previously called common migraine). Auras are usually visual changes, lasting from a few minutes up to an hour, often starting with scotoma (an area of diminished vision; p. 313) and then evolving positive symptoms (often flashing lights). Headache then follows. This may be unilateral or bilateral, is usually throbbing or pounding, and is often associated with nausea, vomiting, sensitivity to light (photophobia) or sensitivity to sound (phonophobia). Patients often lie in a darkened room and dislike movement. The headache usually lasts less than 24 hours, but occasionally longer.

Chronic daily headache

Causes include:
- cervicogenic (from cervical spondylosis)
- chronic (or transformed) migraine
- tension headache (usually bilateral, constant and described as a 'pressure' over the head)
- analgesic medication overuse headache
- a physical symptom of depression.

Sudden-onset headaches

Headaches that are maximal at onset suggest a sinister underlying cause, e.g. subarachnoid haemorrhage, SAH, and always require further investigation. SAH may be accompanied by other symptoms, including loss of consciousness (often brief), seizures, photophobia, vomiting and neck stiffness, but is clinically indistinguishable from benign 'thunderclap' headache where no cause is found.

Meningitis and encephalitis

These cause a headache that usually has a less abrupt onset, and may be accompanied by fever, rash, photophobia and neck stiffness.

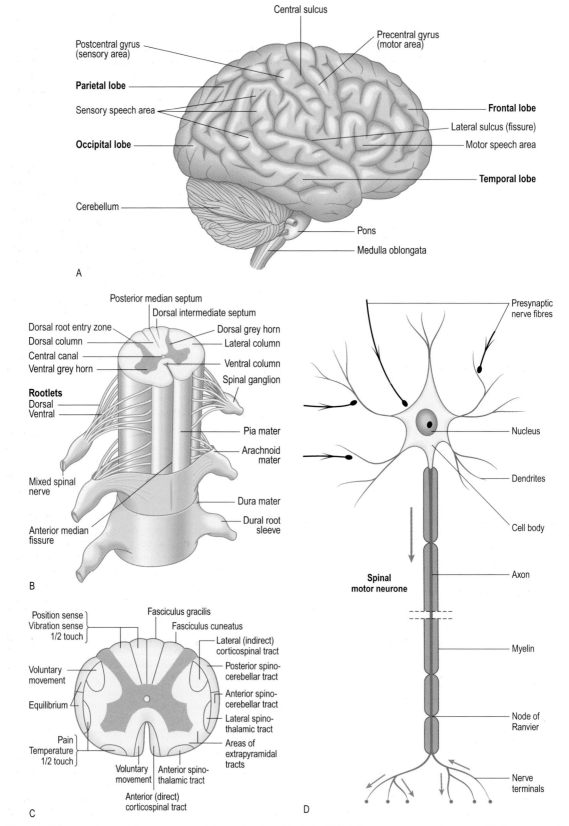

Fig. 11.1 Anatomy of the central nervous system. (A) Lateral surface of the brain. **(B)** Spinal cord, nerve roots and meninges. **(C)** Cross-section of the spinal cord. **(D)** Spinal motor neurone. The terminals of presynaptic neurones form synapses with the cell body and dendrites of the motor neurones.

11.1 Onset and course of headache

Acute single episode

- Subarachnoid haemorrhage
- Acute meningitis
- Vasodilator drugs
- Angle-closure glaucoma

Acute recurrent

- Migraine
- Cluster headache
- Neuralgias, e.g. trigeminal and post-herpetic
- Angle-closure glaucoma
- Sinusitis

Subacute single episode

- Infections, e.g. tuberculous meningitis, cerebral abscess
- Raised intracranial pressure, e.g. tumour, hydrocephalus
- Idiopathic intracranial hypertension
- Temporal arteritis

Chronic

- Chronic daily headache syndrome
- Depression
- Cervical spondylosis
- Drugs, e.g. nitrates, overuse of analgesics

Raised intracranial pressure

Raised intracranial pressure, e.g. due to an expanding intracranial tumour, causes a poorly localized headache, worse on waking in the morning and aggravated by activities such as stooping, coughing or straining at stool.

Neuralgias

These usually cause focal, knife-like or burning pain, affecting single nerves over the head. Paroxysms last seconds and are recurrent. In trigeminal and glossopharyngeal neuralgias, pain may be precipitated by activities such as talking, brushing the teeth, shaving or eating.

Temporal arteritis

This can cause new-onset headache in patients >55 years. There is often tenderness over the temporal arteries, but jaw or tongue claudication is rare.

Disturbances of consciousness

Take a history from the patient and witnesses wherever possible in episodic loss or alteration of consciousness. Patients often have difficulty describing these symptoms and may use terms such as 'blackout', 'faint', 'dizzy spells' and 'funny turns'. Establish where the attacks have taken place, possible triggers, any warning signs, how long the attacks last, how frequently they occur, how quickly the patient recovers, and how long the attacks have been happening. Allow both the patient and the witness to describe the entire episode from start to finish. Ask witnesses to act out any abnormal movements they have seen and enquire about skin colour change, breathing patterns and the recovery period. The history is vital, as examination and investigations rarely distinguish syncope from epileptic seizures.

Syncope

Syncope means loss of consciousness due to inadequate cerebral perfusion. Vasovagal syncope (fainting) is most common and is usually precipitated by stimulation of the parasympathetic nervous system: e.g., by pain, emotional upset, unpleasant sights or thoughts causing bradycardia and hypotension. There is often a pre-syncopal phase, when the patient is light-headed, has tinnitus and nausea, feels the vision 'greying out' and literally 'feels faint'. Fainting occurs with the patient upright — that is, head above heart — often in a warm environment. The patient is pale and slumps to the floor. Provided that he or she is kept lying flat, recovery is usually rapid but associated with nausea.

Syncope occurring during exercise suggests a cardiac cause, either left ventricular outflow obstruction, e.g. aortic stenosis or hypertrophic cardiomyopathy, or an arrhythmia, e.g. complete heart block.

Epileptic seizures

The most common type of generalized seizure is tonic-clonic. A generalized epileptic seizure or fit occurs due to sudden paroxysmal electrical discharges from the brain. These may involve the whole (generalized seizures) or part of the brain (focal seizures). Generalized seizures always involve disturbance (usually loss) of consciousness (Box 11.2). However, not all seizures cause loss of consciousness or convulsions.

Focal seizures arising from an abnormal electrical discharge in a localized area of cerebral cortex are simple or complex. Simple focal seizures arise from the frontal (motor) cortex and may be associated with jerking movements over a part of the body. Complex focal seizures usually arise from the temporal lobe and may cause unpleasant sensations (Box 11.3). Focal seizures can evolve into a secondary generalized seizure, and the patient may describe brief stereotyped warning symptoms suggestive of epilepsy, i.e. different to pre-syncope (Box 11.4).

Dizziness and vertigo

Dizziness has many meanings, so it is vital to establish what the patient is describing. Vertigo is the illusion of movement, due to mismatch of visual, proprioceptive and vestibular information reaching the brain. Vertigo can only be caused by peripheral (vestibular) or central (brain) lesions, whereas light-headedness rarely localizes and typically is a global symptom. Peripheral causes of vertigo are far more common than central ones (Box 11.5).

11

11.2 The typical pattern of a generalized seizure

Prodromal phase

- Change of mood or 'odd' feeling (aura)

Tonic phase

- Loss of consciousness
- Spasm of all muscles
- Cyanosis
- Fall

Clonic phase

- Jerking of limbs and trunk
- Tongue biting

Post-ictal phase

- Flaccidity
- Confusion
- Headache
- Amnesia

11.3 Features of focal seizures arising from temporal lobes

- Dream-like states
- Hallucinations of smell or taste; auditory hallucinations
- Disturbances of memory (déjà-vu, jamais vu)
- Emotional disturbance
- Abnormal behaviour

11.4 Features which suggest epileptic seizure rather than syncope

- Little or no warning or warning suggestive of focal onset
- Onset whilst lying flat, e.g. in bed
- Neat, synchronized rhythmical jerking of limbs
- Cyanosis (rather than pallor)
- Tongue biting (usually the side of the tongue)
- Confused and amnesic following event

Recurrent 'dizzy spells' affect at least 30% of people >65 years. These may be due to:

- Postural hypotension: light-headedness or even loss of consciousness on standing from a sitting or lying position is often caused by drugs, e.g. diuretics or antihypertensive medications
- Cerebrovascular disease/vertebrobasilar insufficiency
- Arrhythmia
- Hyperventilation: dizziness is associated with acute anxiety or panic.

Falls

Around 30% of people >65 years fall each year. The four main causes are:

- simple trip or accident
- acute illness
- loss of consciousness
- multiple risk factors

11.5 Common causes of vertigo

Central

- Migraine
- Brainstem ischaemia or infarction
- Multiple sclerosis

Peripheral

- Ménière's disease
- Benign paroxysmal positional vertigo
- Vestibular neuronitis
- Trauma
- Drugs, e.g. gentamicin, anticonvulsants

Risk factors for falls are:

- Disease, e.g. cerebrovascular, Alzheimer's and Parkinson's diseases
- Disability, e.g. impaired balance, vision, gait, cognition
- Drugs (either a side-effect of a particular drug or due to polypharmacy).

THE HISTORY

Nature and location of symptoms

Neurological symptoms may be difficult for patients to describe in words, so it is vital to clarify what the patient is telling you. Words such as 'blackouts', 'dizziness', 'weakness' and 'numbness' may indicate a different symptom from what you first imagined, so ensure you understand exactly what the patient is describing.

Witness evidence

If patients are unaware of their symptoms, e.g. disturbances of consciousness or cognition, obtain a witness account. This is more valuable than an unfocused neurological examination.

Time relationships

The onset, duration and pattern of symptoms over time often provide vital clues to the underlying pathological process.

- When did the symptoms start (or when was the patient last well)?
- Are they constant or intermittent?
  If intermittent, how long do they last?
  If constant, are they getting better or worse, or staying the same?
- Did they come on suddenly or gradually?

Precipitating, exacerbating or relieving factors

- What was the patient doing when the symptoms occurred?

- Does anything make the symptoms better or worse, e.g. time of day, menstrual cycle, position?

Associated symptoms

Associated symptoms might aid diagnosis. For example, headache may be associated with other symptoms suggestive of migraine, such as nausea, vomiting, photophobia or phonophobia.

Past history

Previous neurological symptoms forgotten by patients may be important and may be documented in their medical records. Birth history and childhood development may be important in some situations, e.g. epilepsy. Be prepared to contact parents or family doctors to seek important information. If considering a vascular cause for neurological symptoms, ask about important risk factors, e.g. other vascular disease, hypertension, family history and smoking.

Drug history

Always consider a drug-related cause for symptoms. Make a complete list of recent and current medications, including prescribed, over-the-counter and complementary therapies. Many neurological symptoms are caused by drugs taken for other conditions (Box 11.6). Adverse reactions may be idiosyncratic, dose-related or caused by chronic use.

Family history

Many neurological disorders are genetic, and are either caused by single gene defects, e.g. cerebellar ataxias or Huntington's disease, or having an important polygenic influence, e.g. migraine, or multiple sclerosis (Box 11.7). Many conditions have a mixture of modes of inheritance, e.g. the hereditary motor and sensory neuropathies. Consider the possibility of an uncommon genetic condition in every neurological diagnosis.

Social history

Occupational factors are relevant to several neurological disorders, e.g. toxic peripheral neuropathies. Alcohol is the most common toxin, damaging both the CNS (ataxia, seizures, cognitive symptoms) and the PNS (neuropathy). Poor diet with vitamin deficiency compounds these problems. Other recreational drugs, e.g. cocaine, ecstasy, cause seizures or strokes, and smoking contributes to both vascular and malignant disease.

Ask about sexual habits, particularly exposure to high-risk sexual practices, as both HIV infection and syphilis cause neurological disorders.

Social circumstances are highly relevant. How are patients coping with their symptoms? Do they drive? If so, should they? What are the emotional and support circumstances? Always ask patients what they think or fear might be wrong with them, as neurological symptoms cause much anxiety.

11.6 Neurological symptoms/syndromes due to drugs

Ataxia

- Phenytoin
- Carbamazepine
- Benzodiazepines
- Ciclosporin
- Fluorouracil

Dizziness/vertigo

- Aspirin
- Enalapril
- Antihistamines
- Flecainide

Epilepsy

- Tricyclic antidepressants
- Phenothiazines
- Fentanyl
- Aminophylline

Headaches

- Glyceryl trinitrate
- Statins
- Sildenafil

Memory impairment

- Benzodiazepines
- Corticosteroids
- Chlorpromazine
- Isoniazid

Myopathy

- Statins
- Corticosteroids
- Bretylium tosilate
- Guanethidine

Parkinsonism

- Neuroleptics
- Prochlorperazine

Peripheral neuropathy

- Isoniazid
- Metronidazole
- Amiodarone
- Procainamide
- Cimetidine
- Statins

Tremor

- Salbutamol
- Terbutaline
- Tricyclic antidepressants
- Amphetamines

Syncope

- Antihypertensives
- Anti-arrhythmic agents
- Levodopa

11.7 Examples of inherited neurological disorders

Autosomal dominant

- Myotonic dystrophy
- Neurofibromatosis types I and II
- Tuberous sclerosis
- Huntington's disease

Autosomal recessive

- Wilson's disease
- Friedreich's ataxia
- Tay–Sachs disease

X-linked recessive

- Duchenne muscular dystrophy
- Becker muscular dystrophy
- Fragile X syndrome

THE PHYSICAL EXAMINATION

Neurological assessment begins with your first contact with the patient and continues during history taking. Note facial expression, general demeanour, dress, posture, gait and speech to help assess the individual's mood and cognitive and physical state. Detailed mental state examination (p. 25) and general examination (p. 47) are integral parts of a neurological examination. Vascular disease is the most common cause of neurological disorders in later life, so measure the blood pressure and examine the cardiovascular system. Listen for cranial bruits or arteriovenous malformations by placing the stethoscope bell gently over the supraclavicular fossa, carotid bifurcation, closed eye and cranium (Fig. 11.2).

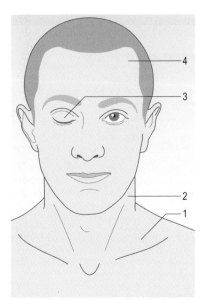

Fig. 11.2 Auscultation for cranial and cervical bruits. (1) Supraclavicular fossa. **(2)** Carotid bifurcation. **(3)** Over the closed eye. **(4)** Over the cranium.

Assessment of conscious level

Consciousness describes how awake a person is, and has two main components: state and content.

- The state of consciousness is largely dependent on integrity of the ascending reticular activating system, which extends in the brainstem from the lower pons to the thalamus
- The content of consciousness refers to how aware the person is and depends on the cerebral cortex, the thalamus and their connections.

In the early stages of deterioration of consciousness, subtle changes of mental function, such as disorientation, short-term memory impairment and slow cerebration, may occur, which can be assessed with the Abbreviated Mental Test (Box 2.50, p. 31).

Avoid ill-defined terms such as stuporose, obtunded or semiconscious. Use the Glasgow Coma Scale (Box 17.13, p. 446), a reliable and reproducible tool, to record conscious level.

Meningeal irritation

Inflammation or irritation of the meninges (meningism) can lead to increased resistance to passive flexion of the neck (neck stiffness) or the extended leg (Kernig's sign). Absence of meningism never excludes meningitis or subarachnoid haemorrhage. Meningism should always raise the possibility of infection, blood or tumour within the subarachnoid space, but it can also occur with non-neurological infections, e.g. urinary tract infection.

◼▶ Examination sequence
Meningeal irritation

- Position the patient supine with no pillow.
- Expose and fully extend both legs.

Neck stiffness

- Support the patient's head with the fingers of your hands placed at the occiput and the ulnar border of your hands against the paraspinal muscles of the patient's neck (Fig. 11.3A).
- Flex the patient's head gently until the chin touches the chest.
- Ask the patient to hold that position for 10 seconds. If neck stiffness is present, the neck cannot be passively flexed and you may feel spasm in the neck muscles.

Kernig's sign

- Flex one of the patient's legs at the hip and knee, with your left hand placed over the medial hamstrings.
- Use your right hand to extend the knee while the hip is maintained in flexion. Look at the other leg for any reflex flexion (Fig. 11.3B). Kernig's sign is positive when extension is resisted by spasm in the hamstrings, and the other limb may flex at the hip and knee. Kernig's sign is not present in local causes of neck stiffness, e.g. cervical spine disease or raised intracranial pressure.

Disorders of movement

Lesions in various parts of the motor system produce distinctive patterns of motor deficit. The principal motor pathway consists of the corticospinal (pyramidal) tract and the anterior horn cell (Fig. 11.8).

- Lower motor neurone lesions. The group of muscle fibres innervated by a single anterior horn cell (lower motor neurone) form a 'motor unit'. Loss of function of a lower motor neurone results in weakness and wasting in these muscle fibres, reduced tone (flaccidity), and reduced or absent reflexes

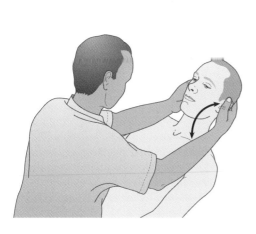
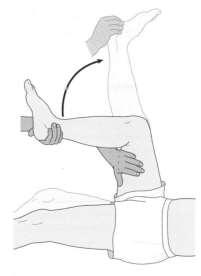

A   B

Fig. 11.3 **Testing for meningeal irritation. (A)** Neck rigidity. **(B)** Kernig's sign.

• Upper motor neurone lesions. If the connection between the spinal cord and the modulating influences of the cerebral cortex are interrupted (as occurs with a stroke), the anterior motor neurones are under the uninhibited influence of the spinal reflex. The motor units then have an exaggerated response to stretch with increased tone (spasticity) and brisk reflexes. Weakness is present but wasting is not seen in acute upper motor neurone lesions, although atrophy may develop with longstanding lesions. Primitive reflexes, such as plantar extensor response, recur.

Stance and gait

Stance and gait depend upon intact visual, sensory, corticospinal, extrapyramidal and cerebellar pathways, together with functioning lower motor neurones and spinal reflexes. Non-neurological gait disorders are discussed in Chapter 14.

Abnormal findings

• Unsteadiness on standing with the eyes open is common in cerebellar disorders, particularly those involving the vermis
• Instability which only occurs, or is markedly worse, on eye closure is indicative of proprioceptive sensory loss, referred to as sensory ataxia or Rombergism
• Hemiplegic gait, due to a unilateral upper motor neurone lesion, is characterized by leg extension at the knee and ankle and circumduction at the hip, such that the plantar flexed foot describes a semicircle as the patient walks
• Bilateral upper motor neurone damage causes a scissor-like gait due to spasticity
• Cerebellar dysfunction leads to a broad-based, unsteady (ataxic) gait, which usually makes tandem

walking (walking heel to toe in a straight line) impossible
• In Parkinsonism, initiation of walking may be delayed, while the steps are short and shuffling with loss/reduction of arm swing. The stooped posture and impairment of postural reflexes can result in a rapid short-stepped hurrying (festinant) gait. As a doorway or other obstacle approaches, the person may freeze. Turning involves many short steps, with the risk of unsteadiness and falls
• Proximal muscle weakness may lead to a waddling gait with bilateral Trendelenburg signs (p. 388)
• Bizarre gaits with no other neurological signs may be associated with Huntington's disease but are usually due to non-organic disorders.

Examination sequence

Stance and gait

Stance

▪▪ Ask the patient to stand up straight, with the feet close together (preferably bare) and eyes open.
▪▪ Swaying or lurching with the eyes open suggests a cerebellar ataxia.
▪▪ Ask the patient to close his eyes (Romberg's test). Repeatedly falling is a positive result, and indicates sensory ataxia due to a proprioceptive deficit.

Gait

▪▪ Ask the patient to walk a measured 10 metres, with a walking aid if needed, then to turn through 180° and return.
▪▪ Record the time taken to complete the first 10 metres and note stride length, arm swing, steadiness (including during turning), limping or other difficulties.
▪▪ Ask the patient to walk heel to toe in a straight line (tandem gait). This emphasizes any gait instability (gait ataxia).

Speech

Disturbance of articulation is dysarthria. Impairment of voice or sound production from the larynx is dysphonia. In both cases language function is intact, but patients' intelligibility may be a problem. They understand what is being said and the grammatical construction of their speech is normal. When language areas in the dominant hemisphere are damaged, there is disturbance of understanding and/or expression of words. This is dysphasia.

Dysarthria and dysphonia

Abnormal findings

Dysarthria

Disturbed articulation may result from local lesions of the tongue, lips or mouth, ill-fitting dentures or any disruption of the neuromuscular pathways. Lesions differ in the patterns of speech disturbance they cause and vary in their associated features.

- Bilateral upper motor neurone lesions of the corticobulbar tract cause a pseudobulbar (or spastic) dysarthria. This is characterized by a contracted, spastic tongue and difficulty pronouncing consonants, and may be accompanied by a brisk jaw jerk and emotional lability
- Bulbar palsy is the result of lower motor neurone lesions affecting the same group of cranial nerves. The nature of the speech disturbance is determined by the specific nerves and muscles involved. Weakness of the tongue results in difficulty with lingual sounds, while palatal weakness gives a nasal quality to the speech
- Extrapyramidal dysarthria causes the monotonous speech of Parkinsonism, while cerebellar dysarthria may be slow and slurred similar to the speech of a drunken person
- Myasthenia gravis is the most common cause of fatiguing speech.

Dysphonia

This usually results from either vocal cord pathology, as in laryngitis, or damage to the vagal (X) nerve supply to the vocal cords (recurrent laryngeal nerve). Inability to abduct the vocal cords leads to a 'bovine' (and ineffective) cough (p. 156).

◼▶ Examination sequence

Dysarthria and dysphonia

- Listen to the patient's spontaneous speech, noting volume, rhythm and clarity.
- Ask the patient to repeat phrases such as 'yellow lorry' (to test tongue (lingual) sounds) and 'baby hippopotamus' (for lip (labial) sounds), then a tongue twister, e.g. 'the Leith Police dismisseth us'.
- Ask the patient to count steadily to 30 to assess muscle fatigue.
- Ask the patient to cough and to say 'Aaah'.

Dysphasias

Anatomy

The language areas are located in the dominant cerebral hemisphere, which is the left in the vast majority of right-handed and most left-handed people. About 30% of left-handers have language areas on the right or bilaterally.

- Broca's area (inferior frontal region) is concerned with word production and language expression
- Wernicke's area (superior posterior temporal lobe) is the principal area for comprehension of spoken language. Adjacent regions of the parietal lobe are involved in the understanding of written language and numbers.

The arcuate fasciculus contains the main connections between Broca's and Wernicke's areas (Fig. 11.4).

Abnormal findings

- Expressive (motor) dysphasia results from damage to Broca's area and is characterized by a reduction in the number of words used and by non-fluent speech with errors of grammar and syntax. It has been described as 'telegraphic' in nature. Comprehension is, however, intact
- Receptive (sensory) dysphasia occurs with dysfunction in Wernicke's area. There is poor comprehension, and although speech may be fluent, it may be meaningless and contain paraphasias (incorrect words) and neologisms (nonsense or meaningless new words)
- Conduction dysphasia is due to damage to the arcuate fasciculus and, while comprehension and

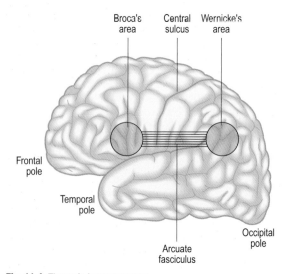

Fig. 11.4 The main language areas.

understanding may be intact, the patient is unable to repeat words or phrases spoken by the examiner

- Global dysphasia refers to a combination of expressive and receptive difficulties due to damage to both Broca's and Wernicke's areas, resulting in poor comprehension and lack of fluency
- Dominant parietal lobe lesions affecting the supramarginal gyrus may cause difficulty comprehending written language (dyslexia), problems with simple addition and subtraction (dyscalculia), and impairment of writing (dysgraphia).

▶ Examination sequence:

Dysphasias

▸ During spontaneous speech, listen to the fluency and appropriateness of the content, particularly for paraphasias and neologisms.

▸ Show the patient a common object, e.g. coin or pen, and ask its name.

▸ Give a simple three-stage command, e.g. pick up this piece of paper, fold it in half and place it under the book. Avoid visual clues by giving instruction from behind the patient's head.

▸ Ask the patient to repeat a simple sentence, e.g. 'Today is Tuesday'.

▸ Ask the patient to read a passage from a newspaper.

▸ Ask the patient to write a sentence; examine his or her handwriting.

Cortical function

Thinking, emotions, language, behaviour, planning and initiating movements, and perceiving sensory information are functions of the cerebral cortex and are central to awareness of and interaction with the environment. Certain cortical areas are associated with specific functions, so that particular patterns of dysfunction can help localize the site of intracranial pathology (Fig. 11.5). Our understanding of the relationships between structure and function in the cerebral cortex is incomplete but improving rapidly due to advances in neuroradiology.

Frontal lobe

Anatomy

The posterior part of the frontal lobe is the motor strip (precentral gyrus) which controls voluntary movement. It is organized with the lower limbs represented superiorly and the head inferiorly. Unless a cortical lesion is very large, it results in upper motor neurone signs in one limb or one side of the face. Lesions deeper within the cerebral hemisphere cause weakness on one side of the body (hemiplegia) and facial weakness.

The area anterior to the precentral gyrus is concerned with personality, social behaviour, emotions, cognition and expressive language, and contains the frontal eye fields and cortical centre for micturition.

Abnormal findings

The range of findings in frontal lobe damage includes:

- changes of personality and behaviour, e.g. apathy or disinhibition
- loss of emotional responsiveness or emotional lability
- cognitive impairments (particularly memory, attention and concentration)
- expressive dysphasia (dominant lobe)
- conjugate gaze deviation to the side of the lesion
- urinary incontinence
- primitive reflexes, e.g. grasp.

Temporal lobe

Anatomy

Both temporal lobes are important for memory and the perception of smell, and damage to either may result in a form of epilepsy with complex focal seizures characterized by hallucinations and memory disturbances. The lower fibres of the optic radiation are located in this lobe and it is the area of auditory perception.

Abnormal findings

Dysfunctions of the temporal lobe may manifest with:

- memory impairment
- complex focal seizures
- contralateral upper quadrantanopia
- receptive dysphasia (dominant lobe).

Parietal lobe

Anatomy

The postcentral gyrus (sensory strip) is the most anterior part of the parietal lobe and is the principal destination of conscious sensations. The upper fibres of the optic radiation pass through it. The dominant hemisphere contains aspects of language function and the non-dominant lobe is concerned with spatial awareness.

Abnormal findings

Damage to the parietal lobes is often associated with re-emergence of primitive reflexes. Signs of parietal lobe dysfunction include:

- cortical sensory impairments
- contralateral lower quadrantanopia
- dyslexia, dyscalculia, dysgraphia
- apraxia
- primitive reflexes, e.g. grasp.

Occipital lobe

Anatomy

The occipital lobe blends with the temporal and parietal lobes, and forms the posterior part of the cerebral

11

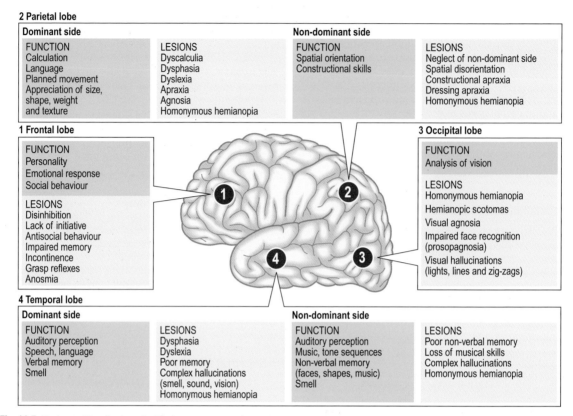

2 Parietal lobe

Dominant side		Non-dominant side	
FUNCTION Calculation Language Planned movement Appreciation of size, shape, weight and texture	**LESIONS** Dyscalculia Dysphasia Dyslexia Apraxia Agnosia Homonymous hemianopia	**FUNCTION** Spatial orientation Constructional skills	**LESIONS** Neglect of non-dominant side Spatial disorientation Constructional apraxia Dressing apraxia Homonymous hemianopia

1 Frontal lobe

FUNCTION
Personality
Emotional response
Social behaviour

LESIONS
Disinhibition
Lack of initiative
Antisocial behaviour
Impaired memory
Incontinence
Grasp reflexes
Anosmia

3 Occipital lobe

FUNCTION
Analysis of vision

LESIONS
Homonymous hemianopia
Hemianopic scotomas
Visual agnosia
Impaired face recognition
(prosopagnosia)
Visual hallucinations
(lights, lines and zig-zags)

4 Temporal lobe

Dominant side		Non-dominant side	
FUNCTION Auditory perception Speech, language Verbal memory Smell	**LESIONS** Dysphasia Dyslexia Poor memory Complex hallucinations (smell, sound, vision) Homonymous hemianopia	**FUNCTION** Auditory perception Music, tone sequences Non-verbal memory (faces, shapes, music) Smell	**LESIONS** Poor non-verbal memory Loss of musical skills Complex hallucinations Homonymous hemianopia

Fig. 11.5 Features of localized cerebral lesions.

cortex. The main function of the occipital lobe is the analysis of visual information.

Abnormal findings

Visual field defects with loss of part of a visual field (hemianopia) or a blind spot (scotoma) may occur. Other abnormalities are the inability to recognize visual stimuli (visual agnosia) and distorted perceptions of visual images. Examples of the latter are seeing things larger (macropsia) or smaller (micropsia) than in real life. Visual hallucinations also occur. Occipital damage may be associated with:

- visual field defects
- visual agnosia
- disturbances of visual perception
- visual hallucinations.

Frontal lobe damage is common in severe head injury, other forms of severe acquired brain injury, e.g. subarachnoid haemorrhage, anoxia, hypoglycaemia and dementias. The temporal and occipital lobes may also be affected in severe traumatic brain injury. Localization of damage to a particular lobe or lobes can be helpful in situations where a space-occupying lesion, e.g. tumour or abscess, is present or a particular arterial territory is involved in a vascular incident.

EXAMINATION OF THE CRANIAL NERVES

There are 12 cranial nerves arising from the brainstem (Fig. 11.6). Cranial nerves II, III, IV and VI relate to the eye (pp. 308–310) and cranial nerve VIII is involved in hearing and balance (p. 340).

The olfactory (I) nerve

The olfactory nerve conveys the sense of smell.

Anatomy

Bipolar cells in the olfactory bulb form olfactory filaments with small receptors projecting through the cribriform plate high in the nasal cavity. These cells synapse with second order neurones, which project centrally via the olfactory tract to the medial temporal lobe and ipsilateral amygdaloid body.

Abnormal findings

If the patient does not have nasal congestion or disease, loss of the sense of smell (anosmia) may result from damage to the olfactory filaments after head injury,

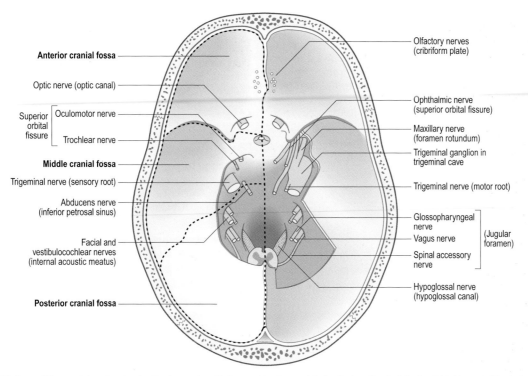

Fig. 11.6 Base of the cranial cavity: showing the dura mater, with the cranial nerves and their exits from the skull. On the right side, part of the tentorium cerebelli and the roof of the trigeminal cave have been removed.

local compression or invasion by skull base tumours. Patients usually complain of altered ability to taste when they have lost the sense of smell. Anosmia may also occur in Parkinson's and Huntington's diseases.

When pleasant odours are perceived as unpleasant, this is called parosmia. It is uncommon but may occur after head trauma, with sinus infection or as a side-effect of drugs. Olfactory hallucinations may occur in Alzheimer's disease and focal epilepsies.

Although bedside testing is usually sufficient in clinical practice, there are more objective smell tests available: for example, the University of Pennsylvania Smell Identification Test (UPSIT).

Examination sequence

Olfactory nerve

- Check that the nasal passages are clear.
- Ask the patient to close his eyes and shut one nostril with a finger.
- Present commonly available odours, e.g. coffee, chocolate, soap or orange peel, and ask the patient to sniff and identify them.

The optic (II), oculomotor (III), trochlear (IV) and abducens (VI) nerves

These are discussed in Chapter 12.

The trigeminal (V) nerve

The V nerve provides sensation to the face, mouth and part of the dura, and motor supply to the muscles of the jaw involved in chewing.

Anatomy

The cell bodies of the sensory fibres are located in the trigeminal (Gasserian) ganglion, which lies in a cavity (Meckel's cave) in the petrous temporal dura (Fig. 11.6). The peripheral processes of these cells give rise to the three major branches of the nerve:

- ophthalmic (V_1)
- maxillary (V_2)
- mandibular (V_3).

The ophthalmic branch leaves the ganglion and passes forward to the superior orbital fissure via the wall of the cavernous sinus. In addition to the skin of the upper nose, upper eyelid, forehead and scalp, V_1 supplies sensation to the eye (cornea and conjunctiva) and the mucous membranes of the sphenoidal and ethmoid sinuses and upper nasal cavity.

The maxillary branch (V_2) passes from the ganglion to leave the skull by the foramen rotundum. It contains sensory fibres from the mucous membranes of the upper mouth, roof of pharynx, gums, teeth and palate of the upper jaw and the maxillary, sphenoidal and ethmoid sinuses.

11

The mandibular branch (V$_3$) exits the skull via the foramen ovale and supplies the floor of the mouth, common sensation, i.e. not taste, to the anterior two-thirds of the tongue, the gums and teeth of the lower jaw, mucosa of the cheek and the temporomandibular joint in addition to the skin of the lower lips and jaw area, but not the angle of the jaw (Fig. 11.7).

From the trigeminal ganglion, the V nerve passes to the pons. The central sensory connections are three nuclei:

- the principal sensory nucleus (touch, joint position sense)
- the mesencephalic nucleus (unconscious proprioception)
- the spinal trigeminal tract and nucleus (pain and temperature).

The latter descends from the pons to the C2 segment of the spinal cord.

The motor fibres of V run in the mandibular branch (V$_3$) and innervate the temporalis, masseter, medial and lateral pterygoids (muscles of mastication), and some smaller muscles not examined clinically.

Abnormal findings

Unilateral loss of sensation in one or more branches of the V nerve may result from direct injury in association with facial fractures (particularly V$_2$) or local invasion by cancer.

Lesions within the cavernous sinuses, e.g. cancer, often result in loss of the corneal reflex and V$_1$ cutaneous sensory loss. Dysfunction of cranial nerves III, IV and VI may accompany such lesions.

Herpes zoster — re-activation of latent herpes varicella zoster (chickenpox) — can affect any dorsal root ganglion of sensory nerves. Although thoracic dermatomes are often involved, the ophthalmic division of the trigeminal (V) nerve is commonly affected (Fig. 11.8A). A brisk jaw jerk occurs with bilateral upper motor neurone lesions above the level of the pons.

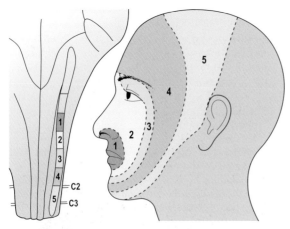

Fig. 11.7 Trigeminal nerve. Areas 1–5 indicate distribution of pain fibres in the spinal tract of V, with 1 being the pons and 5 being the upper cervical cord.

Examination sequence

Trigeminal nerve

There are four functions of the V nerve: sensory, motor and two reflexes.

Sensory

- Ask the patient to close his eyes and say 'yes' each time he feels you lightly touch them using the edge of a tissue. Do this in the areas of V$_1$, V$_2$ and V$_3$.
- Repeat, using a fresh neurological pin, e.g. Neurotip® to test superficial pain.
- Use an orange stick to test touch on the anterior two-thirds of the tongue. Ask the patient to close his eyes and indicate when they feel you touch the tongue.

Motor

- Inspect for wasting of the muscles of mastication.
- Ask the patient to clench his teeth; feel the masseters, estimating their bulk.
- Ask the patient to open his jaw against your hand, which is providing resistance, and note any deviation.

Corneal reflex

- Explain to the patient what you are going to do.
- Ask the patient to look upwards to the ceiling and gently depress the lower eyelid.
- Very lightly touch the lateral edge of the cornea with a wisp of damp cotton wool (Fig. 11.9).
- Look for both direct and consensual blinking.

Jaw jerk

- Ask the patient to let his mouth hang loosely open.
- Place your forefinger in the midline between lower lip and chin.
- Percuss your finger gently with the tendon hammer (Fig. 11.10), noting any reflex shutting of the jaw. The normal response is absent or just present.

The facial (VII) nerve

The facial nerve sends motor fibres to the muscles of facial expression, and parasympathetic secretomotor fibres to the lacrimal, submandibular and sublingual salivary glands (via nervus intermedius). It receives taste sensation from the anterior two-thirds of the tongue (via the chorda tympani branch), and also provides the efferent supply to several reflexes.

Anatomy

From its motor nucleus in the lower pons, fibres of the VII nerve pass back to loop around the VI nucleus before emerging from the lateral pontomedullary junction in close association with the VIII nerve; together they enter the internal acoustic meatus (Fig. 11.6). At the lateral end of the meatus the VII nerve continues in the facial canal within the temporal bone, exiting the skull via the stylomastoid foramen. Passing through the parotid gland, it gives off its

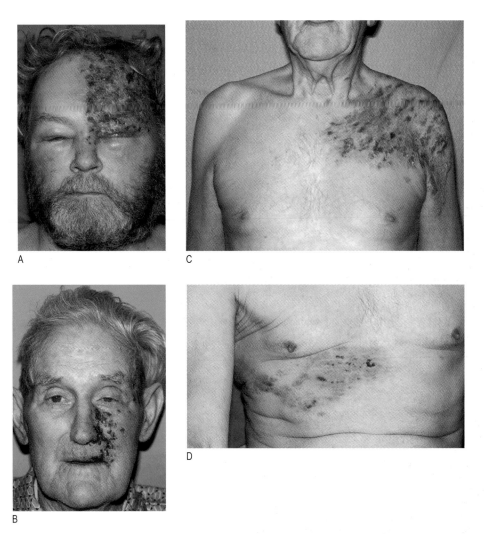

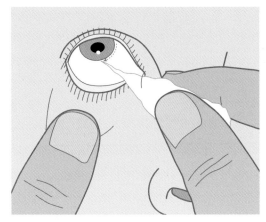

Fig. 11.8 Herpes zoster. (A) The ophthalmic division of the left trigeminal (V) nerve is involved. **(B)** The maxillary division of the left V nerve. **(C)** Cervical spinal root left C5. **(D)** Thoracic spinal root right T8.

Fig. 11.9 Testing the corneal reflex.

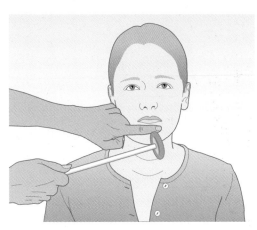

Fig. 11.10 Eliciting the jaw jerk.

terminal branches. In its course in the facial canal it gives off branches to the stapedius muscle and its parasympathetic fibres, as well as being joined by the taste fibres of the chordae tympani (Figs 11.11 and 11.12).

Abnormal findings

In a unilateral lower motor neurone VII nerve lesion, there is weakness of both upper and lower facial muscles. Bell's palsy is an idiopathic condition presenting with acute lower motor neurone VII nerve paralysis, often preceded by pain. It may be associated with impairment or loss of taste (hypogeusia, ageusia) and high-pitched sounds appearing unpleasantly louder than normal (hyperacusis). Bell's phenomenon occurs when the patient is unable to close the eye. As he or she tries, the eyeball rolls upwards, exposing the conjunctiva below the cornea (Fig. 11.13B).

In unilateral VII nerve upper motor neurone lesions, weakness (facial paresis) is marked in the lower facial muscles with relative sparing of the upper face. This is because there is bilateral cortical innervation of the upper facial muscles. While the nasolabial fold may be flattened and the corner of the mouth drooping, eye closure is usually well preserved. Involuntary emotional movements, e.g. smiling, employ different neural pathways and may be preserved in the presence of paresis.

In lesions distal to the stylomastoid foramen, taste and lacrimation are preserved. Hypogeusia or ageusia is most commonly due to oral conditions, but may accompany damage to the VII nerve in the facial canal

or proximally. Damage involving the nerve to stapedius can result in hyperacusis.

Bilateral facial palsy is less common than unilateral lesions, but both upper and lower motor neurone disorders occasionally occur. Extrapyramidal disorders, particularly Parkinson's disease, can result in a loss of spontaneous facial movements, but involuntary facial movements often complicate advanced Parkinson's

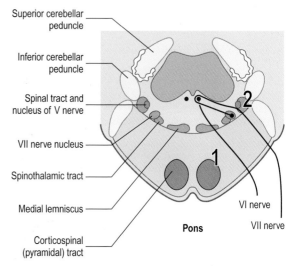

Fig. 11.12 Lesions of the pons. Lesions at (1) may result in ipsilateral VI and VII nerve palsies and contralateral hemiplegia; at (2) ipsilateral cerebellar signs and impaired sensation on the ipsilateral side of the face and on the contralateral side of the body may occur.

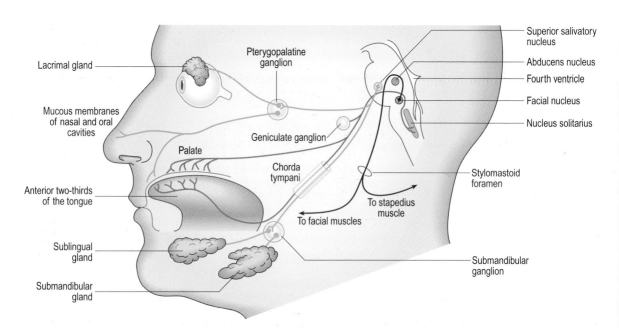

Fig. 11.11 Component fibres of the facial nerve and their peripheral distribution. Red shows motor fibres; green, sensory; and blue, parasympathetic.

disease. These movements (dyskinesias) commonly involve the mouth and tongue (orolingual), or mouth and face (orofacial), or may take the form of facial grimacing.

Ramsay Hunt syndrome occurs in herpes zoster infection of the geniculate (facial) ganglion. This produces a severe lower motor neurone facial palsy, ipsilateral loss of taste and buccal ulceration, and a painful vesicular eruption within the external auditory meatus.

▶ Examination sequence

Facial nerve

Clinical examination is usually confined to motor function and taste.

Motor function

▶ Carefully inspect the whole face for any asymmetry or for differences in blinking or eye closure on one side.

▶ Watch for spontaneous or involuntary movement. Minor asymmetry of the face is common and rarely pathological; ask the patient's partner if they have noticed a difference.

▶ Ask the patient to wrinkle the forehead or look up above his head (which has the same effect).

▶ Ask the patient to bare the teeth. Demonstrate this yourself; asking the patient to mimic you is helpful. Look for asymmetry (Figs 11.14A and B).

▶ Test power by saying 'Screw your eyes tightly shut and stop me from opening them,' then 'Blow out your cheeks with your mouth closed' (Figs 11.14C and D).

Taste

▶ Instruct the patient not to speak during the test.

▶ Ask the patient to put out his tongue.

▶ Use cotton buds dipped in sugar (sweet), salt, vinegar (sour) and quinine (bitter) solutions. Apply them one at a time to the anterior two-thirds of the tongue.

▶ Ask the patient to point to sweet, salt, sour and bitter on a card to indicate his response.

▶ The patient should rinse out his mouth with water between each test.

The vestibulocochlear (VIII) nerve

This is discussed in Chapter 13, page 340.

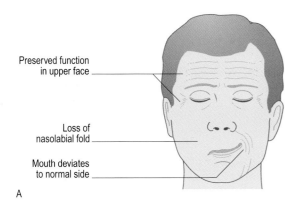

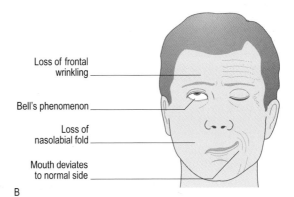

Preserved function in upper face

Loss of nasolabial fold

Mouth deviates to normal side

A

Loss of frontal wrinkling

Bell's phenomenon

Loss of nasolabial fold

Mouth deviates to normal side

B

Fig. 11.13 Types of facial weakness. (A) Weakness is caused by a lesion of the precentral area of the pyramidal tract (upper motor neurone). **(B)** The cause is a lesion of the facial nerve or nucleus (lower motor neurone); Bell's phenomenon is also shown.

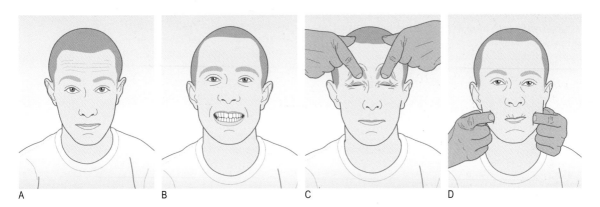

A B C D

Fig. 11.14 Testing the motor function of the facial nerves. (A) Ask the patient to raise the eyebrows. **(B)** Then ask him to show the teeth. **(C)** Next close the eyes against resistance. **(D)** Then blow out the cheeks.

11

The glossopharyngeal (IX) and vagus (X) nerves

The IX and X nerves have an intimate anatomical relationship. Both contain sensory, motor and autonomic components. The glossopharyngeal (IX) nerve mainly carries sensation from the pharynx and tonsils, and sensation and taste from the posterior third of the tongue. The vagus (X) nerve carries important sensory information but also innervates upper pharyngeal and laryngeal muscles.

Anatomy

Both nerves arise as several roots from the lateral medulla and leave the skull together via the jugular foramen (Fig. 11.6). The IX nerve passes down and forward to supply the stylopharyngeus muscle, the mucosa of the pharynx, the tonsillar area and the posterior third of the tongue, and sends parasympathetic fibres to the parotid gland. The X nerve courses down in the carotid sheath and into the thorax, giving off several branches, including pharyngeal and recurrent laryngeal branches, which provide motor supply to the pharyngeal, soft palate and laryngeal muscles. The main nuclei of these nerves in the medulla are the nucleus ambiguus (motor), the dorsal motor vagal nucleus (parasympathetic) and the solitary nucleus (visceral sensation) (Fig. 11.15).

Abnormal findings

Isolated unilateral IX nerve lesions are rare. Damage to the X nerve on one side leads to deviation of the uvula when the soft palate is elevated saying 'Aaah'. Damage to the recurrent laryngeal branch of the X nerve due to lung cancer, thyroid surgery, mediastinal tumours and aortic arch aneurysm causes dysphonia and a 'bovine' cough (p. 156). Bilateral X nerve lesions cause both bulbar and pseudobulbar palsies. They are associated with dysphagia, dysarthria and either lower or upper motor neurone lesions of the hypoglossal (XII) nerve. Less severe cases can result in nasal regurgitation of fluids and nasal air escape when the cheeks are puffed out. The gag reflex produces elevation of the palate and the pharynx, very similar to the motions seen at the beginning of vomiting.

Some clinical conditions causing IX and X nerve lesions are shown in Box 11.8.

Examination sequence

Glossopharyngeal and vagus nerves

Assess the patient's speech for dysarthria or dysphonia.

Ask him or her to say 'Aaah'; look at the movements of the palate and uvula using a torch.

Ask the patient to puff out the cheeks with the lips tightly closed. Look and feel for air escaping from the nose. Normally, both sides of the palate elevate symmetrically and the uvula remains in the midline. In order for the cheeks to puff out, the palate must elevate

and occlude the nasopharynx. If palatal movement is weak, air will escape audibly through the nose.

Ask the patient to cough; assess the strength of the cough.

Testing pharyngeal sensation and the gag reflex is unpleasant for the patient. Use the more reliable water swallow test instead, in fully conscious patients only. Administer 3 teaspoons of water and observe for absent swallow, cough or delayed cough, or change in voice quality after each teaspoon. If there are no problems, watch for the same reactions as above while the patient swallows a glass of water.

The accessory (XI) nerve

The accessory nerve has two components:
- a cranial part closely related to the vagus
- a spinal part which provides fibres to the upper trapezius and the sternocleidomastoid muscles.

The spinal component is discussed here.

Anatomy

The spinal nuclei arise from the anterior horn cells of C1–5. Fibres emerge from the spinal cord, ascend through the foramen magnum, and exit via the jugular foramen (Fig. 11.6), passing posteriorly.

Abnormal findings

Isolated XI nerve lesions are uncommon but the nerve may be damaged during surgery in the posterior triangle of the neck, penetrating injuries or local invasion by tumour. Wasting of the upper fibres of

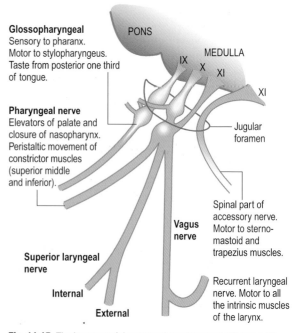

Glossopharyngeal Sensory to pharanx. Motor to stylopharyngeus. Taste from posterior one third of tongue.

Pharyngeal nerve Elevators of palate and closure of nasopharynx. Peristaltic movement of constrictor muscles (superior middle and inferior).

Superior laryngeal nerve

Internal

External

PONS

MEDULLA

IX X XI

XI

Jugular foramen

Spinal part of accessory nerve. Motor to sterno-mastoid and trapezius muscles.

Vagus nerve

Recurrent laryngeal nerve. Motor to all the intrinsic muscles of the larynx.

Fig. 11.15 The lower cranial nerves: glossopharyngeal (IX), vagus (X) and accessory (XI).

11.8 Common causes of IX and X nerve lesions

Unilateral of IX and X

- Skull base tumours (including meningioma)
- Skull base fracture

- Lateral medullary syndrome

Recurrent laryngeal

- Lung cancer
- Mediastinal lymphoma

- Aortic arch aneurysm
- Post-thyroid surgery

Bilateral X

- Progressive bulbar palsy (motor neurone disease)

- Bilateral supranuclear lesions (pseudobulbar palsy):
  Cerebrovascular disease
  Multiple sclerosis

trapezius may be associated with displacement of the upper vertebral border of the scapula away from the spine, while the lower border is displaced towards it. Wasting and weakness of the sternocleidomastoids is characteristic of dystrophia myotonica, and head drop may be seen in myasthenia, motor neurone disease and some myopathies.

Examination sequence

Accessory nerve

- Face the patient and inspect the sternocleidomastoid muscles for wasting or hypertrophy; palpate them to assess their bulk.
- Stand behind the patient to inspect the trapezius muscle for wasting or asymmetry.
- Ask the patient to shrug the shoulders while you apply downward pressure with your hands to assess their power (Fig. 11.16A).
- Test power in the left sternocleidomastoid by asking the patient to turn the head to the right while you provide resistance with your hand placed on the right side of the patient's chin (Fig. 11.16B). Reverse the procedure to check the right sternocleidomastoid.

The hypoglossal (XII) nerve

The XII nerve innervates the muscles of the tongue; the nucleus lies in the dorsal medulla beneath the floor of the fourth ventricle.

Anatomy

The nerve emerges anteriorly and exits the skull in the hypoglossal canal, passing to the root of the tongue (Fig. 11.6).

Abnormal findings

Unilateral lower motor XII nerve lesions lead to wasting of the tongue on the affected side and deviation to that side on protrusion (Fig. 11.17). Bilateral lower motor

neurone damage results in global wasting — the tongue lies thin and shrunken like an autumn leaf and involuntary twitching (fasciculation) may be evident. When associated with lesions of IX, X and XI nerves, typically in motor neurone disease, these features are called bulbar palsy.

Upper motor XII nerve lesions on one side are uncommon, while bilateral lesions lead to a tongue

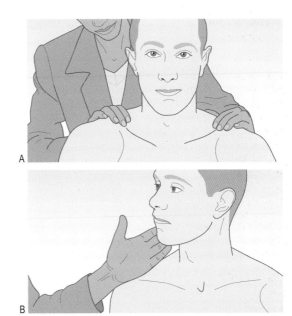

Fig. 11.16 Testing the trapezius and left sternocleidomastoid muscles. **(A)** Trapezius. **(B)** Left sternocleidomastoid.

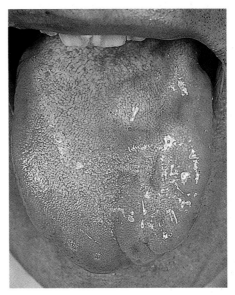

Fig. 11.17 Left hypoglossal nerve lesion.

11.9 Comparison of bulbar and pseudobulbar palsy		
	Bulbar palsy	**Pseudobulbar palsy**
Motor lesion	Lower motor neurone	Upper motor neurone
Speech	Dysarthria	Dysarthria and dysphonia
Swallowing	Dysphagia	Dysphagia
Tongue	Weakness, wasting and fasciculation	Conical, spastic
Jaw jerk	Absent	Brisk
Emotional lability	Absent	Present

with increased tone (spastic), which appears bunched-up, almost conical or acorn-like. Bilateral upper motor lesions of IX–XII nerves usually also affect the V and VII, and are called pseudobulbar palsy. They usually result from vascular disease, motor neurone disease or occasionally multiple sclerosis (Box 11.9). Tremor of the resting or protruded tongue is common in Parkinson's disease. Other involuntary movements of the mouth and tongue (orolingual dyskinesias) are often drug-induced: for example, by levodopa or neuroleptics.

Examination sequence

Hypoglossal nerve

- Ask the patient to open the mouth. Look at the tongue at rest for wasting, fasciculation or involuntary movement.
- Ask the patient to put out the tongue. Look for deviation or involuntary movement.
- Ask the patient to move the tongue from side to side.
- Test power by asking the patient to press the tongue against the inside of each cheek in turn while you press from the outside with your finger.
- Assess speech by asking the patient to say 'yellow lorry'.
- Assess swallowing with a water swallow test.

In a full neurological examination all 12 cranial nerves should be examined in sequence as summarized in Box 11.10.

EXAMINATION OF THE MOTOR SYSTEM

The motor system is assessed under the following headings:

- inspection and palpation of muscles
- assessment of tone
- examination of reflexes
- testing movement and power
- testing co-ordination.

Inspection and palpation of the muscles

Anatomy

Motor fibres, together with input from other systems involved in the control of movement, including extrapyramidal, cerebellar, vestibular and proprioceptive afferents, all converge on the cell bodies of lower motor neurones in the anterior horn of the grey matter in the spinal cord (Fig. 11.18).

Abnormal findings

Muscle bulk

Lower motor neurone lesions may cause muscle wasting. Wasting is not seen in acute upper motor neurone lesions but atrophy may develop with longstanding lesions. A motor neurone lesion in childhood impairs growth or produces a deformity of the limb. Muscle disorders usually result in proximal wasting (the notable exception is dystrophia myotonica, in which it is distal). Certain occupations and sports lead to muscle hypertrophy. This can also occur in muscular dystrophy but this gives a 'doughy' feeling on palpation which differs from healthy hypertrophic muscles.

Fasciculation

Fasciculation looks like irregular ripples or twitches under the skin overlying muscles at rest. This occurs in lower motor neurone disease, usually in wasted muscles. Flick the skin over wasted muscle to try to elicit fasciculation. Non-pathological fasciculation is common in healthy people and not associated with weakness or wasting.

Myoclonic jerks

These are sudden shock-like contractions of one or more muscles which may be focal or diffuse and occur singly or repetitively. Healthy individuals commonly experience these when falling asleep. They may also occur in association with epilepsy, diffuse brain damage and dementias.

Tremor

Tremor is an oscillatory movement about a joint or a group of joints resulting from alternating contraction and relaxation of muscles. Tremors are described according to their speed (fast or slow), amplitude (fine or coarse) and whether they are maximal at rest, on maintaining a posture or on carrying out an active movement.

- Physiological tremor is a fine, fast postural tremor seen with anxiety. A similar tremor occurs in hyperthyroidism and with excess alcohol or caffeine intake, and is a side-effect of β-agonist bronchodilators used in asthma and chronic obstructive pulmonary disease (COPD)
- Essential tremor is the most common cause of an action tremor, typically affecting the upper limbs and sometimes the head, with a postural and action component. It may be reduced by alcohol, and often

11.10 Summary of all 12 cranial nerves

Nerve	Examination	Abnormalities/Symptoms
I	Sense of smell, each nostril	Anosmia/parosmia
II	Visual acuity	Partial sight/blindness
	Visual fields	Scotoma; hemianopia
	Pupil size and shape	Anisocoria
	Pupil light reflex	Impaired or lost
	Fundoscopy	Optic disc and retinal changes
III	Accommodation reflex	Impaired or lost
III, IV and VI	Eye position and movements	Strabismus, diplopia, nystagmus
V	Facial sensation	Impaired, distorted or lost
	Corneal reflex	Impaired or lost
	Muscles of mastication	Weakness of chewing movements
	Jaw jerk	Increased in upper motor neurone lesions
VII	Muscles of facial expression	Facial weakness
VIII	Taste over anterior {2/3} tongue	Ageusia
	Whisper and tuning fork tests	Impaired hearing/deafness
	Vestibular tests	Nystagmus and vertigo
IX	Pharyngeal sensation	Not routinely tested
X	Palate movements	Impaired unilaterally or bilaterally
XI	Trapezius and sternomastoid	Weakness of neck movement
XII	Tongue appearance and movement	Dysarthria and chewing/swallowing problems

demonstrates an autosomal dominant pattern of inheritance
- Action tremors, which are coarse and even violent, are associated with lesions of the red nucleus (rubral tremor) and subthalamic nucleus. They are most often caused by cerebrovascular disease or multiple sclerosis
- Parkinson's disease demonstrates a slow, coarse tremor, which is worst at rest but reduced by voluntary movement. It is more common in the upper limbs and usually asymmetrical
- Intention tremor is absent at rest but maximal on movement, and is usually due to cerebellar damage. It can be assessed with the finger–nose test (p. 294).

Other involuntary movements (dyskinesias)

These are classified according to their appearance:
- Dystonia is caused by sustained muscle contractions, leading to twisting, repetitive movements and sometimes tremor
- Chorea and athetosis are both writhing movements. The former tends to be irregular, jerky and brief; the latter is slower and more sustained. They are often combined, when they are called choreoathetosis.
- Ballism refers to violent flinging movements caused by contractions of proximal limb muscles, sometimes affecting only one side of the body (hemiballismus)

- Tics are repetitive, stereotyped movements which can be briefly suppressed by the patient.

Examination sequence

Inspection and palpation of muscles

▶▎ Proper inspection of the muscles requires complete exposure in keeping with the patient's comfort and dignity.

▶▎ Look for asymmetry, inspecting both proximally and distally. Note any deformities, such as clawing of the hands or pes cavus. Examine specifically for wasting or hypertrophy, fasciculation and involuntary movement.

▶▎ Palpate muscles to assess their bulk. Wasted muscles feel 'flabby'; inflamed muscles (myositis) may be tender; and some forms of acute muscle necrosis (rhabdomyolysis) produce a firm 'woody' feel.

Tone

Tone is the resistance felt by the examiner when moving a joint passively through its range of movement.

Abnormal findings

Muscle tone may be decreased (hypotonia) or increased (hypertonia). There are two principal types of hypertonia: spasticity and rigidity.

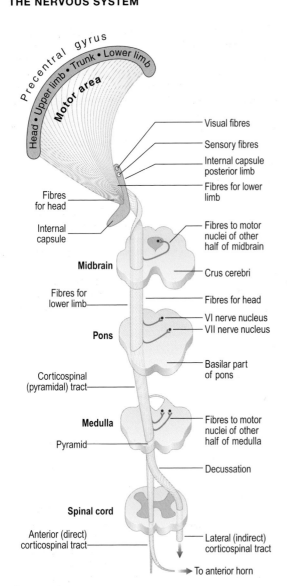

Fig. 11.18 Principal motor pathways.

Flaccidity or Hypotonia

This may occur in lower motor neurone lesions and is usually associated with muscle wasting, weakness and hyporeflexia. It may be a feature of cerebellar disease and occur in the early phases of cerebral or spinal shock, when the paralysed limbs are atonic prior to developing spasticity.

Spasticity

Spasticity is velocity-dependent resistance to passive movement: that is, it is detected with quick movements and is a feature of an upper motor neurone lesion. It is usually accompanied by weakness, hyper-reflexia, an extensor plantar response and sometimes clonus. In mild forms it is detected as a 'catch' at the beginning or end of passive movement. In severe cases it limits the range of movement possible and may be associated with contracture. In the upper limbs it may be more obvious on attempted extension; in the legs it is more evident on flexion.

Rigidity

Rigidity is a sustained resistance throughout the range of movement and is most easily detected when the limb is moved slowly. In Parkinson's disease this is classically described as 'lead-pipe rigidity'. In the presence of a Parkinsonian tremor there may be a regular interruption to the movement, giving it a jerky feel ('cog-wheel' rigidity). Other extrapyramidal conditions may also be associated with rigidity.

Clonus

This is a rhythmic series of contractions evoked by sudden stretch of the muscles. Unsustained clonus can occur in healthy individuals. When sustained, it indicates upper motor neurone damage and is accompanied by spasticity.

◼▶ Examination sequence

Tone

▪◢ The examination room should be warm.

▪◢ Ask the patient to lie supine on the examination couch, and to relax and 'go floppy'.

▪◢ Passively move each joint through as full a range as possible, both slowly and quickly.

Upper limb

▪◢ Hold the patient's hand as if shaking hands, using your other hand to support his elbow. Then rotate the forearm, and flex and extend the wrist, elbow and shoulder, varying the speed and direction of movement.

Lower limb

▪◢ Begin by rolling or rotating the leg from side to side, then briskly lift the knee into a flexed position (Figs 11.19A and B).

Knee clonus

▪◢ With the patient relaxed and the knee extended, sharply push with your thumb and forefinger above the patella towards the foot, sustaining the pressure for a few seconds.

Ankle clonus

▪◢ Support the patient's leg, with both the knee and ankle resting in 90° flexion. Briskly dorsiflex and partially evert the foot, sustaining the pressure (Fig. 11.19C).

Deep tendon reflexes

Anatomy

A tendon reflex is the involuntary contraction of a muscle in response to stretch. It is mediated by a reflex arc consisting of an afferent (sensory) and an efferent (motor) neurone with one synapse between: that is, a monosynaptic reflex. Muscle stretch activates the muscle spindles, which send a burst of afferent signals

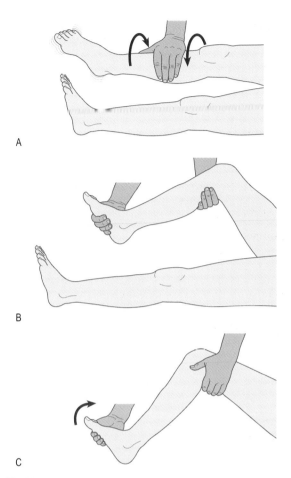

A

B

C

Fig. 11.19 Testing for tone. (A) Rock the leg to and fro. **(B)** Check the full range of movement at the knee. **(C)** Test for ankle clonus.

that in turn lead to direct efferent impulses, causing muscle contraction. These stretch reflex arcs are served by a particular spinal cord segment which is modified by the influence of descending upper motor neurones.

Abnormal findings

Abnormally brisk reflexes (hyper-reflexia) are generally a sign of upper motor neurone damage. Diminished or absent jerks are most commonly due to lower motor neurone lesions. In healthy elderly people the ankle jerks may be reduced or lost, and in the Holmes–Adie syndrome myotonic pupils (p. 324) are associated with loss of some deep tendon reflexes. Isolated loss of a reflex suggests a mononeuropathy or radiculopathy, e.g. loss of ankle jerk with lumbosacral (S1) disc prolapse. A normal reflex contraction with delayed relaxation may occur in hypothyroidism.

Positive Hoffmann's reflex (excess thumb flexion) and finger jerks suggest hypertonia, but can occur in healthy individuals.

In cerebellar damage the reflexes may be pendular, and muscle contraction and relaxation tend to be slow.

Inverted reflexes are caused by combined spinal cord and root pathology. For example, in an inverted biceps reflex, when the biceps tendon is tapped, there may be no biceps jerk but finger flexion occurs. This suggests a lesion at the C5/6 level, affecting not only the efferent arc of the biceps jerk (C5 nerve root), but also the spinal cord, causing reflexes below this level (including the finger jerks) to be increased. It is most commonly seen in cervical spondylotic myeloradiculopathies.

Examination sequence

Deep tendon reflexes

The patient should be as relaxed and comfortable as possible, as anxiety and pain can cause an increased response. For similar reasons reflexes should be performed after testing tone and before testing power and co-ordination in the motor examination sequence.

Flex your wrist and allow the weight of the tendon hammer head to determine the strength of the blow. Strike the tendon, not the muscle. Deciding whether a tendon reflex is normal or not requires practice.

Record the response as:

increased or hyperactive (+ + +)

normal (+ +)

diminished (+)

absent (−)

only present when using reinforcement (±).

Principal reflexes

Ask the patient to lie supine on the examination couch in a comfortable, relaxed position with the limbs exposed.

Comparing each reflex with that of the other side, check for symmetry of response and ensure that both the limbs are positioned identically (Figs 11.20 and 11.21).

Use reinforcement whenever a reflex appears to be absent. For knee and ankle reflexes, ask the patient to interlock the fingers and pull one hand against the other on your command immediately before you strike the tendon (Jendrassik's manœuvre; Fig. 11.22). To reinforce upper limb reflexes, ask the patient to clench the teeth or to make a fist with the contralateral hand. If you use reinforcement, the patient must relax between repeated attempts.

Hoffmann's reflex (Fig. 11.23A)

Place your right index finger under the distal interphalangeal joint of the patient's middle finger .

Using your right thumb, flick the patient's finger downwards.

Look for any reflex flexion of the patient's thumb.

Finger jerk (Fig. 11.23B)

Place your middle and index fingers across the palmar surface of the patient's proximal phalanges.

Tap your own fingers with the hammer.

Observe for flexion of the patient's fingers.

Superficial reflexes

This group of reflexes is polysynaptic and elicited by cutaneous stimulation.

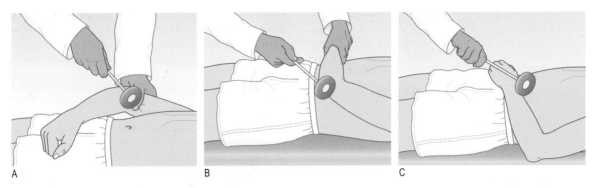

Fig. 11.20 **Testing the deep tendon reflexes of the upper limb. (A)** Eliciting the biceps jerk, C5 (C6). **(B)** Triceps jerk, C6, C7. **(C)** Supinator jerk (C5), C6.

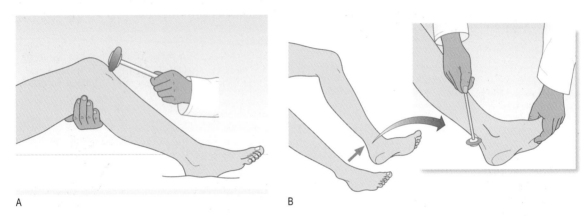

Fig. 11.21 **Testing the deep tendon reflexes of the lower limb. (A)** Eliciting the knee jerk (note that the legs must not be in contact with each other), L3, L4. **(B)** Ankle jerk of recumbent patient, S1.

Abnormal findings

An abnormal plantar response (S1–2) is extension of the large toe (extensor plantar response), often accompanied by flexion and abduction of the other toes (Babinski response). This is an unequivocal sign of upper motor neurone damage and is usually associated with spasticity, clonus and hyper-reflexia.

Superficial abdominal reflexes (T8–12) are lost in upper motor lesions but will also be affected by lower motor neurone damage affecting T8–12. They may be difficult to elicit in the obese, the elderly or those who have had abdominal surgery.

The cremasteric reflex (L1 and L2) is used to assist in identifying the level of spinal cord lesions, particularly after injury.

▶️ Examination sequence

Superficial reflexes

Plantar response (S1–2)

▶️ Run a blunt object (orange stick) along the lateral border of the sole of the foot towards the little toe (Fig. 11.24).

▶️ The normal response is flexion of the great toe and flexion of the other toes too.

Abdominal reflexes (T8–12)

▶️ The patient should be supine and relaxed.

▶️ Use an orange stick and stroke briskly but lightly in a medial direction across the upper and lower quadrants of the abdomen (Fig. 11.25).

▶️ The normal response is contraction of the underlying muscle, with the umbilicus moving laterally and up or down depending upon the quadrant tested.

Cremasteric reflex (L1–2): males only

▶️ Explain what you are going to do and why it is necessary.

▶️ Abduct and externally rotate the patient's thigh.

▶️ Use an orange stick to stroke the upper medial aspect of the thigh.

▶️ Normally the testis on the side stimulated will rise briskly.

Primitive reflexes

The primitive reflexes (snout, grasp, palmomental and glabellar tap) have little localizing value and when present singly are of limited significance, but in combination they suggest diffuse or frontal cerebral damage (Box 11.11). These reflexes are present in normal neonates and young infants — indeed, their absence in the 4 months after birth may indicate pathology — but they disappear as the nervous system matures. People with congenital or hereditary cerebral lesions and a few healthy individuals retain these reflexes, but their return after early childhood is usually associated with brain damage or degeneration.

In adults these reflexes are often present in severe acquired brain damage from trauma, anoxia, diffuse vascular or malignant disease, and in encephalopathy and dementia. Unilateral grasp and palmomental reflexes are strongly suggestive of contralateral frontal lobe pathology. The glabellar tap is positive in Parkinson's disease.

Power

Strength varies with age and occupation and according to whether the patient exercises regularly. Pain, particularly joint pain, may impair the ability to test muscle strength. Grade muscle power according to the Medical Research Council scale (Box 11.12). In practice, most cases of weakness are grade 4 and using + or − signs, e.g. 4+ or 4−, is helpful.

Use the following list of joint movements. Record what the patient can actually do in terms of daily

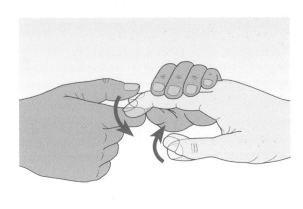

Fig. 11.22 Reinforcement while eliciting the knee jerk.

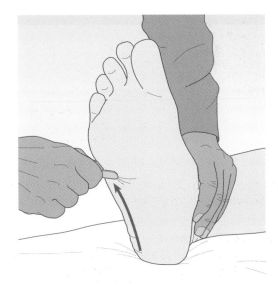

Fig. 11.24 Eliciting the plantar reflex.

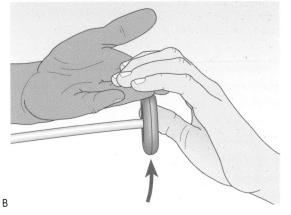

A   B

Fig. 11.23 Testing the deep tendon reflexes of the hand. **(A)** Hoffmann's sign. **(B)** Eliciting a finger jerk.

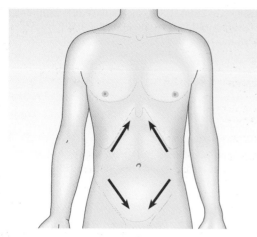

Fig. 11.25 Abdominal reflexes. Sites and direction of stimuli to elicit the reflexes.

activities that require some muscle strength (Boxes 11.13–11.15): for example, whether he or she can stand, walk, raise both arms above the head, and so on.

Always test both proximal and distal muscle groups in each limb, e.g. shoulder and finger abduction in the upper limb, even if the patient has not complained of weakness. For more specific complaints, and particularly in trauma, carefully assess individual muscles if necessary.

Upper limbs

- Shoulder: abduction, adduction, flexion and extension
- Elbow: flexion and extension
- Wrist: flexion and extension
- Finger: abduction, adduction, flexion and extension
- Thumb: extension and opposition.

Lower limbs

- Hip: abduction, adduction, flexion and extension
- Knee: flexion and extension
- Ankle: dorsiflexion, plantarflexion, inversion and eversion of the foot
- Large toe: extension, i.e. dorsiflexion.

Abnormal findings

Upper motor neurone lesions result in weakness of a relatively large group of muscles, e.g. a limb or more than one limb. In contrast, lower motor neurone damage can cause paresis of an individual and specific muscle (Box 11.16). In these circumstances, more detailed examination of individual muscles is required, as described in Chapter 14. Myopathies tend to cause proximal weakness, whereas neuropathies cause distal weakness.

11.11 Primitive reflexes

Snout reflex

- Lightly tap the lips. An abnormal response is lip pouting

Grasp reflex

- Firmly stroke the palm from the radial side. In an abnormal response, your finger is gripped by the patient's hand

Palmomental reflex

- Apply firm pressure to the palm next to the thenar eminence with a tongue depressor. An abnormal response is ipsilateral puckering of the chin

Glabellar tap

- Stand behind the patient and tap repeatedly between his eyebrows with the tip of your index finger. Normally the blink response stops after 3 or 4 taps

11.12 Medical Research Council scale for muscle power

0	No muscle contraction visible
1	Flicker of contraction but no movement
2	Joint movement when effect of gravity eliminated
3	Movement against gravity but not against examiner's resistance
4	Movement against resistance but weaker than normal
5	Normal power

11.13 Definitions of paralysis

Term	Definition
Paresis	Partial paralysis
Plegia	Complete paralysis
Monoplegia	Involvement of a single limb
Hemiplegia	Involvement of one-half of the body
Paraplegia	Paralysis of the legs
Tetraplegia	Paralysis of all four limbs

11.14 Patterns of motor dysfunction

- Paralysis or weakness
- Impairment of co-ordination
- Involuntary movements (dyskinesia)
- Changes in the rate at which movements are performed (hypokinesis and bradykinesis)
- Loss of learned movement patterns (dyspraxia)

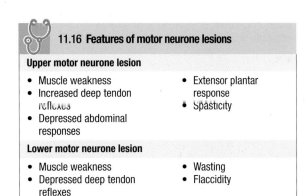

11.15 Causes of muscle weakness

Anatomical aetiology	Associated features	Common causes
Lower motor neurone	Muscle atrophy (wasting) Fasciculation Reflexes absent or diminished Hypotonia	Peripheral neuropathies Radiculopathies Anterior horn cell damage, e.g. poliomyelitis or motor neurone disease
Upper motor neurone	'Patterned' weakness Little or no muscle wasting Hyper-reflexia Hypertonia Hypokinesia of movement	Cerebrovascular disease, e.g. hemiplegia Spinal injury or disease, e.g. paraplegia Multiple sclerosis
Myopathies	Muscle wasting (usually proximal) Hypotonia Tenderness (myositis)	Hereditary conditions, e.g. muscular dystrophy Alcohol and other toxins
Non-organic	Inconsistent weakness No associated features	Stress Anxiety Compensation claims

11.16 Features of motor neurone lesions

Upper motor neurone lesion

- Muscle weakness
- Increased deep tendon reflexes
- Depressed abdominal responses
- Extensor plantar response
- Spasticity

Lower motor neurone lesion

- Muscle weakness
- Depressed deep tendon reflexes
- Fasciculation
- Wasting
- Flaccidity

Examination sequence

Power

- Test the power of individual muscle groups in both limbs alternately to compare.
- Ask the patient to contract a group of muscles to maintain a position and resist your attempt to displace the limb (isometric testing).
- Ask the patient to put the joint through a movement while you try to oppose the action (isotonic testing).

Co-ordination

Performing complex movements smoothly and efficiently depends upon intact sensory, as well as motor, function. Tests of co-ordination may therefore be influenced by muscle weakness, proprioceptive loss or extrapyramidal dysfunction.

Anatomy

The cerebellum lies in the posterior fossa and consists of two hemispheres with a central vermis. It is attached to the brainstem by three pairs of cerebellar peduncles. Afferent and efferent pathways convey information to and from the cerebral motor cortex, basal ganglia, thalamus, vestibular and other brainstem nuclei and the spinal cord. In general, midline structures, e.g. vermis, influence body equilibrium, while each hemisphere controls co-ordination on the same (ipsilateral) side.

Abnormal findings

In cerebellar disorders, the displaced outstretched arm may fly up past the original position (the rebound phenomenon), while the normal response is to return to the original position.

The finger–nose test may reveal a tendency to fall short or overshoot the examiner's finger (past-pointing or dysmetria). In more severe cases there may be a tremor of the finger as it approaches the target finger and the patient's own nose (intention tremor). The movement may be slow and generally disjointed and clumsy (dyssynergia).

The heel–shin test is the equivalent test for the lower limbs. It is abnormal if the heel wavers away from the line of the shin.

Impairment of rapid alternating movements is dysdiadochokinesis, which is evident as slowness, disorganization and irregularity of movement. Dysdiadochokinesis is typical of cerebellar disorders.

In disorders which predominantly affect midline cerebellar structures, e.g. tumours of the vermis and alcoholic cerebellar damage, the finger–nose test, heel–shin test and tests of dysdiadochokinesis may be normal. Check the stance and gait, as truncal ataxia may be the only abnormal finding.

Cerebellar dysfunction occurs in many conditions, and the differential diagnosis varies with age. Common causes of acute signs are potential toxins, e.g. phenytoin or alcohol, vascular lesions, trauma and demyelination (multiple sclerosis).

Examination sequence

Co-ordination

In addition to the following tests of limb co-ordination, examination of cerebellar function includes tests for dysarthria (p. 276), nystagmus (p. 323), stance and gait (p. 370). Dysfunction may also be accompanied by hypotonia and pendular tendon reflexes.

Rebound phenomenon

▪ Ask the patient to stretch his arms out in front and maintain this position.
▪ Push the patient's wrist quickly downward and observe the returning movement.

Finger–nose test (Fig. 11.26)

▪ Ask the patient to touch the nose with the tip of the forefinger and then reach out to touch your finger tip, held just within the patient's arm's reach.
▪ Ask the patient to repeat the movement between nose and target finger as quickly as possible.
▪ Make the test more sensitive by changing the position of your target finger. Timing is crucial — move your finger just as the patient's finger is about to leave his nose.

Heel–shin test (Fig. 11.27)

▪ Ask the patient to lie supine on the examination couch.
▪ Ask the patient to raise one leg and place the heel on the opposite knee, and then slide the heel up and down the shin between knee and ankle.

Rapid alternating movements

▪ Demonstrate the act of repeatedly patting the palm of one hand with the palm and back of your opposite hand as quickly and regularly as possible.
▪ Ask the patient to copy your actions.
▪ Repeat with the opposite hand.

Apraxia

Dyspraxia or apraxia is difficulty or inability to perform a motor action, despite the patient understanding the task and in the absence of motor weakness and cerebellar, extrapyramidal or sensory impairment.

Abnormal findings

- In ideational apraxia, the patient may understand the nature of the task but cannot initiate it
- In ideomotor apraxia, the patient may perform it in an odd or bizarre fashion. Both types are associated with either frontal or parietal lesions
- Constructional apraxia (difficulty drawing a figure) is a feature of parietal disturbance
- Dressing apraxia, which is often associated with spatial disorientation and neglect, is usually due to non-dominant hemisphere parietal lesions.

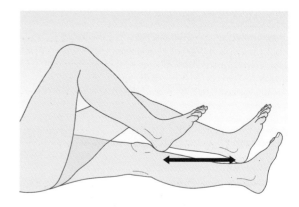

Fig. 11.27 Performing the heel–shin test with the right leg.

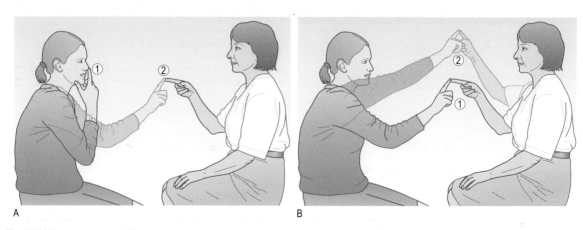

A   B

Fig. 11.26 Finger–nose test. **(A)** Ask the patient to touch the tip of her nose and then your finger. **(B)** Move your finger from one position to another, towards and away from the patient, as well as from side to side.

Examination sequence

Apraxia

▶ Ask the patient to perform an imaginary act, e.g. drinking a cup of tea, combing the hair, folding a letter and placing it in an envelope.

▶ Ask the patient to draw a geometrical figure and to write a sentence.

▶ Ask the patient to put on a pyjama top or dressing gown, one sleeve of which has been pulled inside out (Boxes 11.17 and 11.18).

EXAMINATION OF THE SENSORY SYSTEM

Detailed examination of sensation is time-consuming and unnecessary, unless the patient volunteers sensory symptoms or you suspect a specific pathology, e.g. spinal cord compression, syringomyelia, a peripheral nerve disorder or a parietal lesion.

Anatomy

Conscious joint position sense (proprioception) and vibration are conveyed in large, fast-conducting fibres in the posterior (dorsal) columns. Pain and temperature sensation are carried by small, slow-conducting fibres of the spinothalamic tract. The posterior column remains ipsilateral from the point of entry up to the medulla, but most pain and temperature fibres cross within one or two segments of entry to the contralateral spinothalamic tract. All sensory fibres relay in the thalamus before sending information to the sensory cortex in the parietal lobe (Fig. 11.28).

Abnormal findings

Sensory symptoms include pain, spontaneous abnormal sensations usually of 'tingling' or 'pins and needles' (paraesthesia), and loss of sensation or numbness. Neurogenic pain is often particularly unpleasant, is difficult to describe and may not conform to a dermatomal or peripheral nerve distribution (dysaesthesia). Clarify that by 'numbness' the patient means lack of sensation rather than weakness or clumsiness. Reduced ability to feel pain (hypoalgesia or hypoaesthesia) or temperature (thermoanaesthesia) on testing may be accompanied by scars from injuries or burns which have gone unnoticed. Touch or other simple sensory stimuli may be perceived by the patient as heightened (hyperalgesia or hyperaesthesia), or as unpleasant or painful (hyperpathia or allodynia).

The sensory modalities

In addition to the modalities conveyed in the principal ascending pathways (touch, pain, temperature, vibration and joint position sense), sensory examination includes tests of discriminative aspects of sensation which may be impaired by lesions of the sensory cortex. Only assess these cortical sensory functions if the main pathway sensations are intact. This is usually only required in cases where a parietal lesion is suspected. In general, it is better to ask patients to look away rather than close the eyes. The exceptions are tests of joint position and cortical sensation and where you suspect functional disturbance. When mapping out an area of altered sensation, move from reduced to higher sensibility: that is, from hypoaesthesia to normal, or normal to hyperaesthesia.

Abnormal findings

Abnormalities on sensory testing are best considered according to whether the lesion(s) is in the peripheral

---

OSCEs 11.17 Examine this patient with sudden-onset headache

1. Assess and record level of consciousness (intracranial lesions).
2. Measure pulse, blood pressure and temperature.
3. Look for signs of meningeal irritation: photophobia, neck stiffness and Kernig's sign (bacterial or viral meningitis, subarachnoid haemorrhage).
4. Examine the optic fundi for papilloedema (a late sign of raised intracranial pressure; absence of papilloedema does not exclude raised intracranial pressure).
5. Examine for focal neurological signs (cerebral haemorrhage, other structural lesions).
6. Examine for a purpuric rash (meningococcal meningitis).
7. In those >55 years feel for palpable temporal arteries and scalp tenderness (temporal arteritis).

OSCEs 11.18 Examine this patient with progressive clumsiness of the arm and leg, slurred speech and morning headache

1. Examine optic fundi for papilloedema (raised intracranial pressure).
2. Assess the motor and sensory systems of the limbs; exclude impaired joint position sense.
3. Examine eye movement — nystagmus.
4. Assess the lower cranial nerves — bulbar palsy.
5. Test co-ordination of the limbs using finger–nose and heel–shin tests, and for rebound phenomenon. Assess ability to undertake rapid alternating movements — cerebellar ataxia.
6. Check the stance and gait, and ability to sit without support (truncal ataxia).

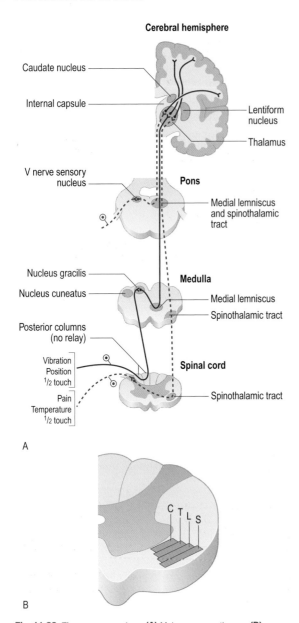

Fig. 11.28 The sensory system. (A) Main sensory pathways. **(B)** Spinothalamic tract: layering of the spinothalamic tract in the cervical region. C represents fibres from cervical segments which lie centrally; fibres from thoracic, lumbar and sacral segments (labelled T, L and S respectively) lie progressively more laterally.

11.19 Tests of sensation	
Modality	**Pathway**
Light touch	Large fast-conducting axons
Proprioception	Dorsal columns
Vibration	Medial lemniscus
Two-point discrimination	
Pinprick (superficial pain)	Smaller slower-conducting axons
Deep pain	Spinothalamic tracts
Temperature	
Stereognosis	Parietal cortex (only valid if peripheral sensory function intact)
Graphaesthesia	
Two-point discrimination	

the lower limbs first and more prominently. In many cases, touch and pinprick sensation are lost in a 'stocking and glove' distribution (Fig. 11.29A).

In some large fibre peripheral neuropathies, vibration and joint position sense are disproportionately affected. Patients may report staggering when they close their eyes during hair washing (Rombergism, p. 275). Occasionally when such patients are asked to close their eyes and hold their hands outstretched, their fingers will make involuntary slow wandering movements (pseudoathetosis).

Injuries and other damage to individual nerves lead to loss of all modalities in that nerve's territory. Sensory root damage leads to dermatomal sensory loss (Fig. 11.30).

Polyneuropathies may be classified by:
- mode of onset (acute, subacute or chronic)
- pathology (axonal or demyelinating)
- principal function disturbed (motor, sensory, autonomic or mixed)
- cause (Box 11.20).

Spinal cord

Traumatic and compressive lesions of the spinal cord cause loss or impairment of sensation in a dermatomal distribution below the level of the lesion. A zone of hyperaesthesia may be found immediately above the level of sensory loss.

Anterior spinal artery syndrome usually results in loss of spinothalamic sensation and motor function, with sparing of dorsal column sensation. A similar pattern of pain and temperature loss and sparing of dorsal column sensation (dissociated loss) occurs in syringomyelia.

When one half of the spinal cord is damaged, the Brown–Séquard syndrome may occur. This is characterized by ipsilateral motor weakness and loss of vibration and joint position sense, with contralateral loss of pain and temperature (Fig. 11.29B).

nerve(s), dorsal root(s) or spinal cord, or is intracranial (Box 11.19).

Peripheral nerve and dorsal root

A large number of pathological processes affect peripheral nerves, generally resulting in peripheral neuropathies or polyneuropathies. Peripheral neuropathies tend to affect

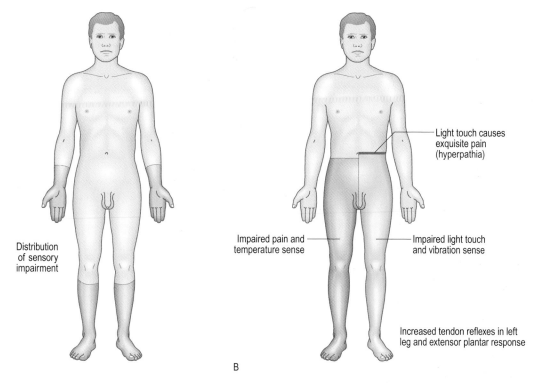

Light touch causes
exquisite pain
(hyperpathia)

Distribution
of sensory
impairment

Impaired pain and
temperature sense

Impaired light touch
and vibration sense

Increased tendon reflexes in left
leg and extensor plantar response

A   B

Fig. 11.29 **Patterns of sensory loss. (A)** In peripheral neuropathy. **(B)** Brown–Séquard syndrome. Note the distribution of corticospinal, posterior column and lateral spinothalamic tract signs. The cord lesion is in the left half of the cord.

Intracranial

Brainstem lesions are often vascular in origin, and determining the site of the lesion relies on understanding the relevant anatomy (Fig. 11.33). Alternating analgesia is a term for the loss of pain and temperature sensation on one side of the face (V nerve nucleus damage) and the opposite side of the body (spinothalamic tract damage); it occurs in lower brainstem lesions.

Thalamic lesions may cause a patchy sensory impairment on the opposite side with a very unpleasant, poorly localized pain, often of a burning quality (dysaesthesiae).

Cortical lesions in the parietal lobe lead to impairment of some of the principal presenting pathway sensations, particularly joint position sense, but are more likely to result in the abnormalities described above. The parietal lobe is involved in two-point discrimination, tactile recognition (stereognosis) and localization of a point touched by the doctor.

■▪◢ Examination sequence

Sensory modalities

Light touch

▪◢ While the patient looks away or closes his eyes, use a wisp of cotton wool (or lightly apply your finger) and ask the patient to respond to each touch.

▪◢ Time the stimuli irregularly and make a dabbing rather than a stroking or tickling stimulus.

▪◢ Compare each side for symmetry.

Superficial pain

▪◢ Use a fresh neurological pin, e.g. Neurotip®. Do not use a hypodermic needle. Dispose of the pin after each patient to avoid transmitting infection.

▪◢ Explain and demonstrate that the ability to feel a sharp pinprick is being tested.

▪◢ Follow the testing points in Figure 11.30, comparing for symmetry.

▪◢ Map out the boundaries of any area of reduced, absent or increased sensation.

Deep pain

▪◢ Explain the test and ask the patient to report it as soon as he feels discomfort.

▪◢ Squeeze the muscle bellies, e.g. calf, biceps, or apply pressure to fingernail or toenail beds. Do not apply pressure with an instrument, e.g. pen.

Temperature

▪◢ Touch the patient with a cold metallic object, e.g. tuning fork, and ask if it feels cold. More sensitive assessment requires tubes of hot and cold water at controlled temperatures but this is seldom performed.

Vibration

▪◢ Place a vibrating 128 Hz tuning fork over the sternum. Ask the patient, 'Do you feel it buzzing?'

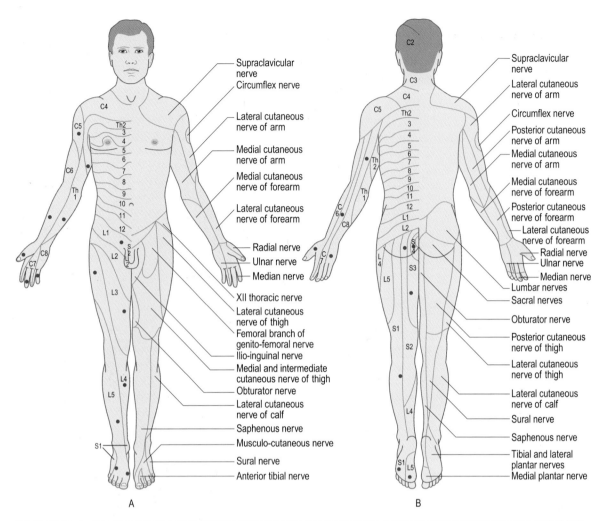

Fig. 11.30 Segmental and peripheral nerve innervation. Points for testing cutaneous sensation of limbs. By applying stimuli at the points marked, both the dermatomal and main peripheral nerve distributions are tested simultaneously.

Next place it on the tip of the great toe (Fig. 11.31). If sensation is impaired, place the fork on the interphalangeal joint and progress proximally — the medial malleolus, tibial tuberosity and anterior iliac spine — depending upon the response.

Repeat the process in the upper limb. Start at the distal interphalangeal joint of the forefinger, and if sensation is impaired, proceed proximally — radial styloid, olecranon, acromion.

If in doubt as to the accuracy of the response, ask the patient to close his eyes and to report when you stop the fork vibrating with your fingers.

Joint position sense

With the patient's eyes open, demonstrate the procedure. Hold the distal phalanx of the patient's great toe at the sides to avoid giving information from pressure (or middle finger) and move it up and down (Fig. 11.32).

Ask the patient to respond with 'up' or 'down' as you make these movements, without him or her assisting or resisting.

Now ask the patient to close his or her eyes and to identify the directions in a random sequence of small movements, e.g. up, down, down, up.

Test both great toes (or middle fingers). If impaired, move to more proximal joints in each limb.

Two-point discrimination

Use a two-point discriminator (an instrument like a pair of blunt-tipped school compasses) or an opened-out paper clip.

Ask the patient to look away or close the eyes.

Apply either one or two points to the pulp of the patient's forefinger and ask whether one or two stimuli were felt.

Adjust the distance between the two points to determine the minimum separation at which they are felt separately.

Test both fingers and thumbs.

11.20 Causes of polyneuropathies

Genetic

- Hereditary motor and sensory neuropathies (Charcot–Marie–Tooth disease)
- Refsum's disease
- Hereditary sensory and autonomic neuropathies

Drugs and toxins

- Alcohol
- Statins, isoniazid, metronidazole, amiodarone, perhexiline, phenytoin
- Lead, arsenic, mercury
- Solvents, carbon disulphide, herbicides, pesticides

Vitamin deficiencies

- Vitamins B_1, B_6, B_{12}
- Vitamin E

Infections

- Leprosy
- HIV
- Diphtheria

Inflammatory

- Acute inflammatory or idiopathic (Guillain–Barré syndrome)
- Chronic idiopathic demyelinating polyneuropathy (CIDP)
- Connective tissue disorders (rheumatoid arthritis, systemic lupus erythematosus, polyarteritis nodosa, systemic sclerosis)

Systemic medical conditions

- Diabetes mellitus
- Renal failure
- Hypothyroidism
- Acromegaly
- Critical illness neuropathy
- Sarcoidosis

Malignant disease

- Cancer (paraneoplastic)
- Lymphoproliferative disorders

Others

- Amyloidosis
- Paraproteinaemias

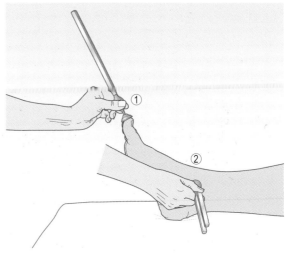

Fig. 11.31 Testing vibration sensation. At the big toe (1) and the ankle (2).

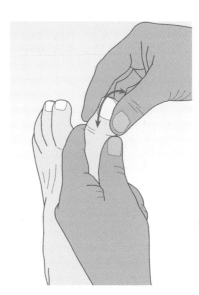

Fig. 11.32 Testing for position sense in the big toe.

Point localization

▶ With the patient's eyes closed, lightly touch various body parts, e.g. hand, finger, shoulder; and ask which part has been touched and whether on the right or left side.

▶ Repeat, touching individual fingers and asking the patient to identify which is touched. (Ensure that the patient knows the names of the fingers first.) Inability to do so is finger agnosia.

Stereognosis and graphaesthesia

▶ Ask the patient to close the eyes.

▶ Place familiar small objects, e.g. coin, key, matchstick, in the patient's hand and ask him or her to identify what they are after feeling them (stereognosis).

▶ Use the blunt end of a pencil or orange stick and trace letters or digits on the patient's palm. Ask the patient to identify the figure (graphaesthesia).

Sensory inattention

▶ Ask the patient to close the eyes. Touch the back of each of the patient's hands in turn and ask which has been touched.

▶ Next touch both hands simultaneously and ask whether the left, right or both sides were touched.

EXAMINATION OF THE PERIPHERAL NERVES

A peripheral nerve may be damaged generally (peripheral neuropathy) or specifically. Certain peripheral

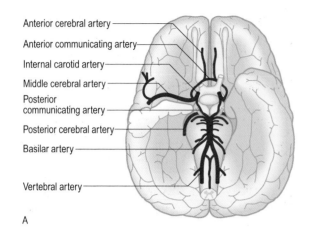

A

B

Midbrain

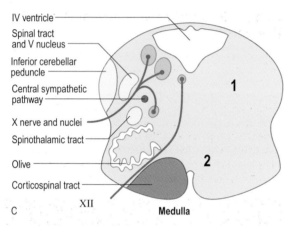

C   XII   **Medulla**

Fig. 11.33 Anatomy of brainstem lesions. (A) Arteries at the base of the brain. **(B)** Lesions of the midbrain, according to lesion site: (1) ipsilateral III nerve palsy, contralateral cerebellar signs and rubral tremors; (2) ipsilateral III nerve palsy and contralateral hemiplegia; (3) quadriparesis. **(C)** Lesions of the medulla: (1) ipsilateral cerebellar signs, jerking nystagmus on turning the eyes to the side of the lesion, impaired sensation on the ipsilateral face and contralateral body, Horner's syndrome, dysphonia and dysphagia; (2) crossed paralysis with ipsilateral wasting and weakness of tongue and contralateral hemiplegia.

nerves are especially prone to trauma or compression (compression or entrapment neuropathies); these include the radial, ulnar and median nerves in the upper limb, and the lateral cutaneous nerve of thigh and the common peroneal nerve in the leg.

Median nerve

This may be compressed as it passes between the flexor retinaculum and the carpal bones at the wrist (carpal tunnel syndrome); it is the most common entrapment neuropathy. The diagnosis is principally made from the history (Boxes 11.21 and 11.22).

Examination sequence

- Test for weakness of thumb opposition and abduction.
- Test opposition by asking the patient to touch the thumb and ring finger together while you attempt to pull them apart (opponens pollicis).
- Test for abduction with the patient's hand held palm up on a flat surface. Ask the patient to move the thumb vertically against your resistance (abductor pollicis brevis).

- Look for altered sensation over the dorsum of the hand involving the thumb, first and second fingers and the lateral half of the ring finger (Fig. 11.34A and Fig. 14.31, p. 379).

Radial nerve

This may be compressed as it runs through the axilla, or injured in fractures of the humerus.

Examination sequence

- Test for weakness of arm extensors (especially the wrist and fingers).
- Look for sensory loss over the dorsum of the hand (Fig. 11.34B) and loss of triceps tendon jerk.

Ulnar nerve

This is most often affected at the elbow by external compression or injury, e.g. dislocation.

Examination sequence

- Test for weakness of abduction and adduction of the fingers.
- With the patient's fingers on a flat surface, test abduction by asking the patient to spread the fingers against resistance.

• Test adduction by placing a card between the patient's fingers and pulling it out against resistance.
• Look for wasting of small muscles of the hand (can result in claw or 'benediction' hand) and sensory loss on the ulnar side of the hand (Fig. 11.34C).

Common peroneal nerve

This is most commonly damaged in fractures of the head of the fibula, but can also be compressed by tight bandages, by plaster of Paris or as a result of repetitive kneeling or squatting. This damage may result in foot drop.

11.21 Common features of carpal tunnel syndrome

• More common in women
• Paraesthesiae and/or pain in the hand (usually spares the little finger)
• May radiate up the arm to the elbow
• Weakness in the hand
• Symptoms commonly occur at night, and may wake the patient from sleep
• The patient may hang the hand and arm out of the bed for relief
• Thenar muscle wasting (in longstanding cases)

11.22 Causes of carpal tunnel syndrome

• Idiopathic
• Pregnancy, oral contraceptive pill and premenstrual
• Rheumatoid arthritis
• Distal radial fractures, e.g. Colles' fracture
• Hypothyroidism
• Acromegaly
• Amyloidosis
• Nephrotic syndrome

Examination sequence

• Test for weakness of dorsiflexion and eversion of the foot and sensory loss over the dorsum of the foot (Fig. 11.34D).

Lateral cutaneous nerve of thigh

The lateral branch of this purely sensory nerve may be trapped or kinked as it passes through the inguinal ligament, producing paraesthesiae in the lateral thigh (Fig. 11.34E). This condition (meralgia paraesthetica) is most common in obesity or pregnancy.

Examination sequence

• Test for loss of or heightened sensation over the lateral aspect of the thigh.

Subacute combined degeneration of the cord

This is an uncommon disorder due to vitamin B_{12} deficiency. It is a subacute myelopathy with damage to the posterior column and corticospinal tract, associated with peripheral nerve degeneration. Sensory impairment, particularly of joint position and vibration, is common but pain and temperature sensation may be defective in a glove and stocking distribution. Similarly, spasticity and extensor plantar responses may be associated with loss of ankle and knee reflexes. It is important because it is readily treatable.

PUTTING IT ALL TOGETHER

The first stage in neurological diagnosis is to decide whether a lesion has occurred within the nervous system. Then you need to determine the site(s) of damage

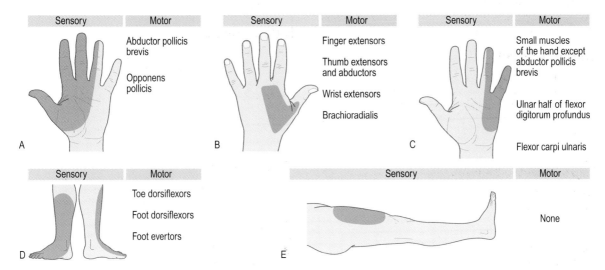

Fig. 11.34 Sensory and motor deficits in nerve lesions. (A) Median. **(B)** Radial. **(C)** Ulnar. **(D)** Common peroneal. **(E)** Lateral cutaneous of the thigh.

and the underlying pathology (where and what is the lesion?). This process is not necessarily straightforward, and interpretation of history and examination findings is an exercise in pattern recognition.

Neurological symptoms are common and do not always indicate underlying pathology. Non-organic symptoms — that is, those with no evidence of underlying disease — are also common. Always exclude organic disease before considering a non-organic diagnosis. Differentiating organic disease and non-organic symptoms is difficult, even for experts (p. 32).

The history provides the best clues to the pathology of any lesion and guides subsequent examination. Deciding whether there is a single lesion, multiple sites of damage or diffuse disorder in the nervous system is useful. For instance, tumours and strokes may lead to damage at a specific site; multiple sclerosis is characterized by lesions scattered in site and time; and chronic alcohol misuse can lead to widespread cerebral, brainstem, spinal cord and peripheral nerve disturbances.

OSCEs 11.23 Examine this patient with slowly progressive weakness and numbness of the legs

1. Carry out general examination to exclude heart failure, anaemia and hypothyroidism.
2. Examine the lymph nodes, liver and spleen (metastatic tumours, lymphoma and other reticuloses, immunodeficiency).
3. Examine the neurological system to determine the pattern and location of the lesion:
   Truncal sensory level with hyper-reflexia, weakness and spasticity below level — cord lesion.
   Loss of limb reflexes, wasting of limb muscles, and glove and stocking sensory deficit — peripheral neuropathy.
4. Examine the spine for deformity and local tenderness.

INVESTIGATIONS

Lumbar puncture

Lumbar puncture is the key investigation in suspected meningitis and is used selectively in a number of other conditions. The procedure may be hazardous in the presence of raised intracranial pressure. The CSF pressure is measured and the appearance of the fluid, normally crystal-clear, is noted. CSF specimens are routinely examined for cells, protein content, and glucose levels in comparison to simultaneously taken blood levels; they are also stained and cultured for bacteria. Other specific tests may be carried out, e.g. oligoclonal bands, meningococcal and pneumococcal antigens, malignant cells and haemoglobin breakdown products in subarachnoid haemorrhage. Box 11.25 summarizes findings in health and some common disorders.

Neurophysiological tests

- Electroencephalography (EEG) records the spontaneous electrical activity of the brain, using electrodes placed on the scalp. It is used in the investigation of epilepsy, encephalitis or dementia. Modifications to the standard EEG improve sensitivity, including sleep-deprived studies and prolonged video telemetry
- Electromyography (EMG) is used to investigate disorders affecting muscles, using a concentric needle electrode inserted into the muscle. Electrical activity is displayed on an oscilloscope and an audio monitor, allowing the neurophysiologist to see and hear the pattern of activity
- Nerve conduction studies involve applying electrical stimuli to nerves and measuring the speed of impulse conduction. They are used for both motor and sensory nerves, and are helpful in diagnosing peripheral nerve disorders such as nerve compressions or polyneuropathies.

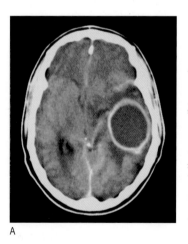
A

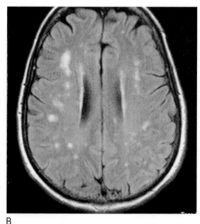
B

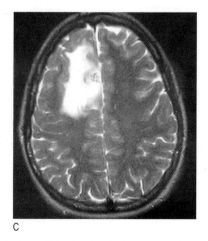
C

Fig. 11.35 Scanning of the head. (A) CT scan showing a cerebral abscess. **(B)** MR scan of the head showing multiple sclerosis with white demyelinating plaques. **(C)** MR scan showing a glioma involving the right cerebral hemisphere.

11.24 Investigations in nervous system disease

Investigation	Indication/Comment	Investigation	Indication/Comment
Urine tests		DNA (nuclear and mitochondrial) analysis	Huntington's disease Hereditary ataxias and neuropathies Mitochondrial disorders
Glucose	Diabetic peripheral neuropathy		
Ketones	Diabetic coma (ketoacidosis)	Edrophonium (Tensilon) test	Myasthenia gravis
Bence Jones protein	Myeloma	**Neurophysiology**	
Porphobilinogen	Porphyria	EEG	Epilepsy Encephalopathy/encephalitis Sleep disorders
Blood tests			
Haemoglobin	Syncope, seizures, stroke		
MCV	Vitamin B_{12} deficiency	EMG	Myopathy Muscular dystrophy Motor neurone disease
White cell count	Infection, e.g. meningitis		
Blood culture	Meningitis, endocarditis, stroke		
ESR/C-reactive protein	Cranial arteritis	Single-fibre EMG	Myasthenia gravis
Vitamin B_{12} and folic acid	Peripheral neuropathy, dementia	Nerve conduction studies	Entrapment neuropathy Peripheral neuropathy
Clotting/thrombophilia screen	Stroke		
VDRL–TPHA	Neurosyphilis	Visual evoked potentials	Multiple sclerosis
HIV	Central nervous system involvement	Brainstem auditory evoked potentials	Acoustic neuroma
Antinuclear factor and dsDNA	Stroke		
Rheumatoid factor	Peripheral neuropathy	Somatosensory evoked potentials	Brachial plexus lesions
Antiphospholipid antibody	Stroke		
Acetylcholine receptor and muscle-specific kinase (MuSK) antibodies	Myasthenia gravis	ECG	Epilepsy/syncope Stroke Muscular dystrophy
Serum immunoglobulins	Myeloma	**Radiology (Figs 11.35 and 11.36)**	
Thyroid function test	Tremor Carpal tunnel syndrome	Chest X-ray	Source of cerebral metastases Tuberculosis Sarcoidosis
GH, ACTH, FSH/LH, prolactin, TSH	Pituitary tumour	Skull X-ray	Fracture Bone erosion, e.g. tumour Calcification, e.g. tumour, Sturge–Weber syndrome
Liver function tests	Ataxia Peripheral neuropathy		
Urea/creatinine	Encephalopathy Peripheral neuropathy	CT brain scan	Trauma: fractures, intracranial haematoma Stroke and subarachnoid haemorrhage Tumours, tuberculoma Cerebral atrophy
Electrolytes	Diabetes insipidus/SIADH Periodic paralysis		
Glucose	Coma Stroke Neuropathies		
		CT angiography	Suspected subarachnoid haemorrhage
Serum lipids and cholesterol	Stroke	MR brain scan	Multiple sclerosis Infection Metastases Infiltrative malignancy Pontine myelinolysis
Calcium	Epilepsy Tetany		
Drug/toxin screen	Coma Epilepsy Peripheral neuropathy		
		MR spine	Tumours Prolapsed intervertebral disc Syringomyelia Vascular malformations
Caeruloplasmin/serum copper	Wilson's disease		
Creatine phosphokinase	Muscular dystrophy, myopathy		
Lactate	Myophosphorylase deficiency (McArdle's syndrome)	SPECT scan	Dementia Malignancy

(*Continued*)

11.24 (Continued)

Investigation	Indication/Comment	Investigation	Indication/Comment
PET scan	Parkinson's disease	Brain biopsy	Mass lesions of uncertain cause (most commonly tumours)
Ultrasound of extracranial arteries	Atherosclerotic stenosis	Needle aspiration of brain	Cerebral abscess
Transcranial ultrasound	Hydrocephalus (in infants)	Needle aspiration of spine	Tuberculosis
Echocardiogram	Stroke: source of embolism	Rectal biopsy	Amyloidosis
Angiography	Atheroma of extracranial vessels Aneurysms Arteriovenous malformations	Bone marrow aspiration	Vitamin B$_{12}$ deficiency Myeloproliferative disorders
Invasive		Lumbar puncture	Meningitis, encephalitis Multiple sclerosis Malignant infiltration
Nerve biopsy	Peripheral neuropathies		
Muscle biopsy	Muscular dystrophies or myopathies	Intracranial pressure monitoring	Trauma Normal pressure hydrocephalus

ACTH, adrenocorticotrophic hormone; EEG, electroencephalography; EMG, electromyography; FSH/LH, follicle-stimulating hormone/luteinizing hormone; GH, growth hormone; MCV, mean corpuscular volume; PET, positron emission tomography; SIADH, syndrome of inappropriate antidiuretic hormone; SPECT, single photon emission computerized tomography; TSH, thyroid-stimulating hormone; VDRL–TPHA, Venereal Disease Research Laboratory–*Treponema pallidum* haemagglutination assay.

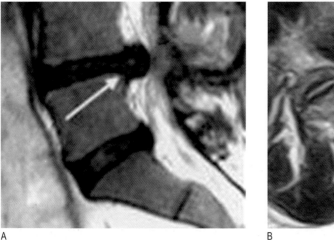
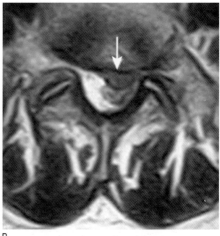

A   B

Fig. 11.36 T2 MR images showing a large left paracentral L4/5 disc protrusion (arrowed). **(A)** Sagittal section. **(B)** Axial section.

OSCEs 11.25 Examine this patient with right leg pain paraesthesiae and numbness in the foot

1. Assess the distribution of pain and sensory loss. Do they fit a dermatomal pattern consistent with compression of one nerve root?
2. Examine the power of the lower limb muscles, particularly the flexors (L5 nerve root) and extensors (S1 nerve root) of the ankle and toes.
3. Examine the reflexes of the leg. Is the ankle reflex present? Which nerve root is responsible for the ankle reflex?
4. Assess nerve compression using the sciatic and femoral nerve stretch tests.
5. Examine the circulation of the leg for arterial and venous insufficiency (peripheral vascular disease, deep venous thrombosis).
6. Examine the hip joint for evidence of degenerative osteoarthritis.

11.26 Cerebrospinal fluid (CSF) findings in some common disorders

Condition	Pressure	Appearance	Cells/μl	Protein (g/l)	Glucose	Microbiology
Normal	15–180 mm	Crystal clear	<5 lymphocytes	0.1–0.4	>60% of blood glucose	Sterile
Acute bacterial meningitis	Usually increased/normal	Cloudy/turbid	100–50 000 polymorphs (lymphocytes in early stages)	Increased	Reduced	Gram stain of organism + culture
Tuberculous meningitis	Usually increased/normal	Clear/cloudy	25–500 lymphocytes (polymorphs in early stages)	Increased	Reduced	Auramine/Ziehl–Neelsen stain + culture
Viral meningitis	Usually normal/slight increase	Crystal clear	5–200 lymphocytes (occasional polymorphs in early stages)	Normal/slightly increased	Normal/occasionally reduced	Sterile
Tumour	Normal/increased	Crystal clear/occasionally cloudy	0–500 lymphocytes + malignant cells	Increased	Normal/reduced	Sterile
Subarachnoid haemorrhage	Increased	Bloodstained or xanthochromic supernatant	Red cells + normal/slightly raised white cells	Increased	Normal	Sterile
Multiple sclerosis	Normal/increased	Crystal clear	0–50 lymphocytes	Normal/increased oligoclonal bands	Normal	Sterile

11.27 Key points: the nervous system

- Most neurological diagnoses are made on the history, not the examination.
- Most headaches presenting to doctors are either migraine or chronic daily headache.
- If a patient cannot talk properly, consider the five Ds: **d**eafness, **d**ementia, **d**ysphasia, **d**ysarthria and **d**ysphonia.
- Dysphasia is often mistaken for confusion.
- Additional witness history is invaluable when assessing symptoms such as loss of consciousness or cognitive disturbance.
- A witness description is always more valuable than an unfocussed neurological examination.
- Most cases of loss of smell (anosmia) and deafness are due to local disorders of the nose and ear and not neurological disease.
- Sensory loss in trigeminal (V) nerve lesions does not extend on to the pinna or beyond the angle of the mandible.
- Vertigo rarely has a central cause.
- Solitary lesions of IX and X nerves are uncommon.
- Severe muscle wasting is usually due to a lower motor neurone lesion.

11

John Olson
Richard Cowie

The visual system

12

12

ANATOMY

Eyelids, conjunctiva and lacrimal system

The eyelids protect the eye from injury and excessive light, and help distribute tears. Secretions from three types of gland within the eyelids moisten the eye:

- mucin from goblet cells
- aqueous humour from accessory lacrimal glands
- oil from Meibomian glands.

The conjunctiva is a thin mucous membrane lining the eyelids and reflected at the superior and inferior fornices on to the surface of the eye. Most tears come from multiple, small, accessory lacrimal glands in the eyelids. The lacrimal gland secretes tears to wash away foreign bodies and to express emotion in crying. Lying anterolaterally in the roof of the orbit, its ducts drain into the superior fornix. Tears that do not evaporate drain through the lacrimal canaliculi at the medial edge of each eyelid into the lacrimal sac in the anterior part of the medial wall of the orbit, and from there into the nasolacrimal duct which opens into the nasal inferior meatus.

The eye

The eye focuses an image on to the neurosensory retina. The eyeball is made up of the anterior chamber, the lens and vitreous body.

- The anterior chamber is filled with aqueous humour and lies behind the cornea and in front of the iris. Aqueous is produced by the ciliary body in the

posterior chamber, and passes through the pupil to leave through the trabecular meshwork of the angle of the anterior chamber

- The lens is a transparent, biconvex structure behind the iris and in front of the vitreous. It is suspended by the suspensory ligaments of the ciliary body. It becomes less elastic with age, causing increasing difficulty with accommodation (presbyopia)
- The vitreous is a transparent gel behind the lens. Posteriorly, it is firmly attached to the margins of the optic disc, and anteriorly, to the retina at the ora serrata.

The outer aspect of the eyeball has three layers:

- an outer fibrous layer, five-sixths of which is the opaque sclera and one-fifth the transparent cornea
- a middle vascular pigmented layer, the uveal tract, which posteriorly forms the choroid and anteriorly forms the iris/ciliary body complex
- an inner neurosensory layer, the retina (Fig. 12.1).

Sensation from the cornea, conjunctiva and intraocular structures is conveyed by the ophthalmic branch (V_1) of the trigeminal nerve (p. 279).

The optic (II) cranial nerve

The visual pathway consists of the retina, the optic chiasm, the optic tracts, the lateral geniculate bodies, the optic radiations and the visual cortex. The retina consists of an outer pigmented layer, and an inner neurosensory layer which is continuous with the optic nerve. The retinal pigment epithelium lies adjacent to the highly vascular choroid. Around 90% of the blood supply to the eye passes through the choroid, supplying the posterior

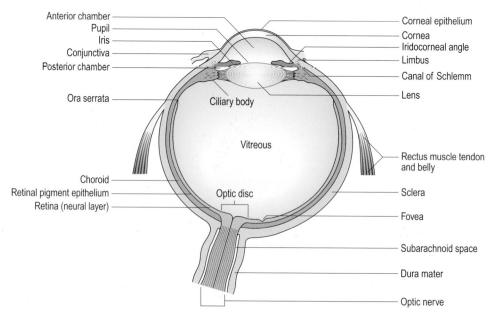

Fig. 12.1 Schematic diagram of the human eye in horizontal section.

two-thirds of the retina, the optic nerve and the fovea. The retinal blood supplies the relatively inert layers of the inner retina. The neurosensory retina consists of photoreceptors, ganglion cells and interconnecting bipolar cells.

- Rod photoreceptors are responsible for night vision and detection of peripheral movement

- Cone photoreceptors are responsible for colour and central vision
- Photoreceptors synapse with the vertically oriented bipolar cells of the retina, which in turn synapse with the ganglion cells of the optic nerve (Fig. 12.2).

The optic nerve is purely sensory and, similar to 'white matter' rather than peripheral nerve, is unable to regenerate. Initially unmyelinated, the fibres of the optic nerve myelinate on leaving the eye through the optic disc. The optic nerve enters the cranium through the optic canal. The two optic nerves join at the optic chiasm, where the nasal fibres, responsible for the temporal visual field, decussate. Leaving the chiasm, the visual pathway is confusingly renamed the optic tract. The optic tracts terminate in the lateral geniculate bodies of the thalamus. However, some fibres leave the tract before the lateral geniculate nucleus to form the afferent limb of the pupillary reflex.

Optic radiations

These pass through the cerebral hemisphere in the posterior part of the internal capsule and the parietal and temporal lobes to terminate in the occipital cortex (Fig. 12.3).

Occipital lobe

The occipital lobe analyses visual information, and damage to the primary visual cortex produces a homonymous

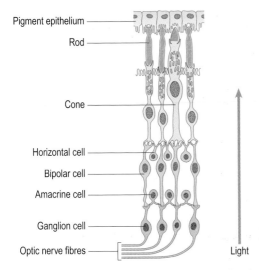

Fig. 12.2 Schematic drawing showing the cellular organization of the retina.

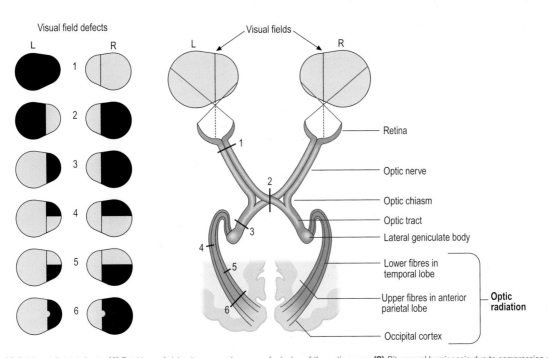

Fig. 12.3 Visual field defects. (1) Total loss of vision in one eye because of a lesion of the optic nerve. **(2)** Bitemporal hemianopia due to compression of the optic chiasm. **(3)** Right homonymous hemianopia from a lesion of the optic tract. **(4)** Upper right quadrantanopia from a lesion of the lower fibres of the optic radiation in the temporal lobe. **(5)** Lower quadrantanopia from a lesion of the upper fibres of the optic radiation in the anterior part of the parietal lobe. **(6)** Right homonymous hemianopia with sparing of the macula due to lesion of the optic radiation in the posterior part of the parietal lobe.

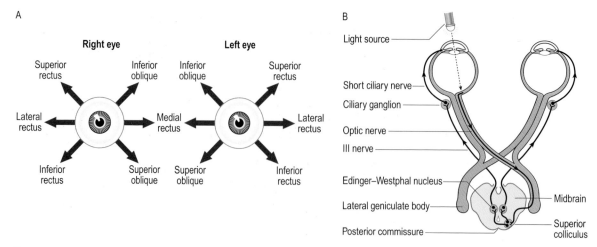

Fig. 12.4 Control of eye movement and pupil size. **(A)** Fields of action of pairs of extraocular muscles. This diagram will help you to work out which eye muscle is paretic. For example, a patient whose diplopia is maximum on looking down and to the right has either an impaired right inferior rectus or a weak left superior oblique. **(B)** Pathway of pupillary constriction and the light reflex (parasympathetic).

hemianopia or scotoma. Loss of function of the secondary visual areas causes inability to recognize visual stimuli (visual agnosia) and distorted perceptions of visual images, such as seeing things larger (macropsia) or smaller (micropsia) than reality. Visual hallucinations may occur.

The oculomotor (III), trochlear (IV) and abducens (VI) cranial nerves

The oculomotor (III), trochlear (IV) and abducens (VI) nerves innervate the six external ocular muscles controlling eye movement and, through parasympathetic nerves, also affect pupillary size (Fig. 12.4). They are examined together because of their close functional inter-relationships.

The oculomotor (III) nerve passes just below the free edge of the tentorium in relation to the posterior communicating artery and enters the dura surrounding the cavernous sinus. It enters the orbit through the superior oblique fissure, and subdivides into its terminal branches. The nerve innervates the superior, medial and inferior recti, the inferior oblique and levator palpebrae superioris muscles. These muscles open the upper lid (levator palpebrae superioris) and move the globe upwards (superior rectus, inferior oblique), downwards (inferior rectus) and medially (medial rectus). Through the parasympathetic fibres arising from the Edinger–Westphal nerves, the nerve indirectly supplies the sphincter muscles of the iris, causing constriction of the pupil, and the ciliary muscle which focuses the lens for near vision (accommodation).

The trochlear (IV) nerve fibres decussate before leaving the midbrain posteriorly (the left nucleus innervates the right trochlear nerve and vice versa). The nerve enters the orbit in the superior orbital fissure, supplying the superior oblique muscle which causes downward movement of the globe when the eye is adducted.

The abducens (VI) nerve has a long course around the brainstem before it pierces the dura to enter the cavernous sinus. The nerve is in direct relation to the internal carotid artery before it passes through the superior orbital fissure to the lateral rectus muscle. Lateral rectus abducts the eye (Fig. 12.5).

The pupils are round, regular, equal in size and symmetrical in their responses. The autonomic nervous system and integrity of the iris determine the size of the resting pupil. The afferent limb of the pupillary reflex involves the optic nerve, chiasm (where some fibres decussate) and the optic tract, bypassing the lateral geniculate nucleus to terminate in the III nerve (Edinger–Westphal) nucleus. The efferent limb involves the inferior division of the III nerve, passing through the ciliary ganglion in the orbit to the constrictor muscle of the iris. Sympathetic stimulation causes pupillary dilatation and upper and lower eyelid retraction. With parasympathetic stimulation (the fibres travel with the III nerve), the opposite occurs.

SYMPTOMS AND DEFINITIONS

Ocular pain

Pain in the eyes is common and ranges from irritating to the excruciating pain of scleritis. You must note if the affected eye is red or not to make the diagnosis.

Ocular pain with a 'white eye'

If the patient feels something in the eye, the problem involves the surface of the eye. The most common cause is a dry eye secondary to inflammation of the skin of the eyelids, chronic blepharitis, from disruption of eyelid glandular secretions. Paradoxically, patients

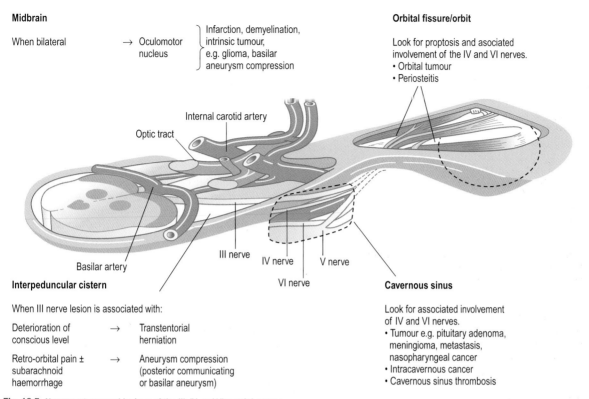

Midbrain

When bilateral → Oculomotor nucleus ⎱ Infarction, demyelination, intrinsic tumour, e.g. glioma, basilar aneurysm compression

Internal carotid artery

Optic tract

Orbital fissure/orbit

Look for proptosis and asociated involvement of the IV and VI nerves.
• Orbital tumour
• Periosteitis

III nerve   IV nerve   V nerve

VI nerve

Basilar artery

Interpeduncular cistern

When III nerve lesion is associated with:

Deterioration of conscious level → Transtentorial herniation

Retro-orbital pain ± subarachnoid haemorrhage → Aneurysm compression (posterior communicating or basilar aneurysm)

Cavernous sinus

Look for associated involvement of IV and VI nerves.
• Tumour e.g. pituitary adenoma, meningioma, metastasis, nasopharyngeal cancer
• Intracavernous cancer
• Cavernous sinus thrombosis

Fig. 12.5 Neuroanatomy and lesions of the III, IV and VI cranial nerves.

often complain of watery eyes due to overproduction of tears from the lacrimal gland. Blepharitis occurs in low-grade infection or inflammation of the eyelids or systemic skin conditions, such as atopic eczema, acne rosacea or seborrhoeic dermatitis. Dry eyes are a feature of Sjögren's syndrome.

Preceding visual disturbance associated with headache or eye pain suggests migraine. Although patients may describe flashing lights in a zigzag pattern, many just notice blurring of vision. Cluster headaches may present as ocular pain. In subacute episodes of angle-closure glaucoma (raised intraocular pressure) patients describe seeing haloes around lights.

Pain on eye movement usually indicates either optic neuritis or scleritis. The eye in optic neuritis is white; in scleritis it is red.

Ocular pain with a 'red eye'

Redness around the white of the eye adjacent to the limbus (circumciliary injection) reflects involvement of the anterior ciliary arteries supplying the cornea, iris and ciliary body. Diffuse redness suggests scleritis or conjunctivitis.

An inverted eyelid (entropion) leads to painful corneal erosion and an everted eyelid (ectropion) causes dryness in the exposed eye (Fig. 12.6). Rarely, watery

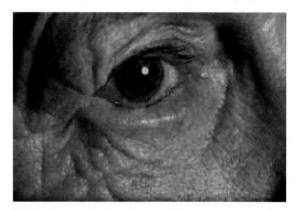

Fig. 12.6 Senile entropion of the lower lid.

eyes may result from a blocked drainage system. This is aggravated when the lacrimal gland is stimulated.

Foreign bodies on the surface of the eye are associated with a clear history of an at-risk activity, e.g. grinding metal without eye protection.

Severe unilateral pain with a cloudy cornea and an oval non-reactive pupil indicates acute angle-closure glaucoma. Long-sighted people with a relatively shallow anterior chamber, and the elderly in whom thickening of the lens makes the anterior chamber shallower, are at risk. Acute angle-closure glaucoma is precipitated by pupillary dilatation, which becomes fixed by ischaemia, inducing high intraocular pressure and circumciliary injection. The cornea is cloudy and the underlying iris cannot be clearly seen. The pain is severe and may be associated with systemic symptoms. Both eyes require treatment to prevent recurrence.

Acute iritis leads to a small, irregularly shaped pupil (Fig. 12.7) and redness around the limbus. The inflamed iris becomes stuck to the underlying lens. The pain is not as severe as in angle-closure glaucoma and photophobia may be prominent. Recurrence is common and the patient may have the human leucocyte antigen,

HLA B27, with an associated condition, e.g. ankylosing spondylitis, inflammatory bowel disease or psoriasis. Rarely, iritis presents bilaterally.

Corneal ulceration may be due to herpes simplex virus (Box 12.1), but in contact lens wearers, dry eyes or debilitated patients raises suspicion of bacterial infection. Depending on severity, redness may vary from circumciliary injection to the diffuse redness associated with spontaneous lacrimation.

Pain on moving a red eye indicates scleritis (Fig. 12.8) and may be the first manifestation of systemic vasculitis. The redness is frequently bilateral and involves the whole sclera or a sector of the sclera, unlike the circumciliary injection of iritis or angle-closure glaucoma. Episcleritis is uncomfortable rather than painful and appears less dramatic than scleritis. A drop of topical phenylephrine makes the redness of episcleritis disappear, but not that of scleritis.

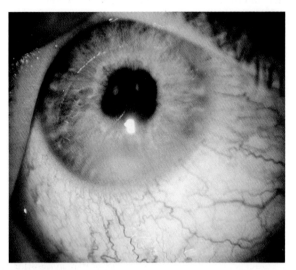

Fig. 12.7 Acute iritis. Irregular pupil and circumciliary injection.

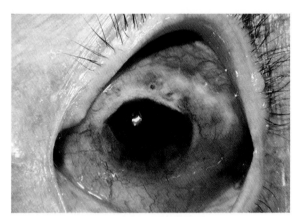

Fig. 12.8 Necrotizing scleritis. Areas of pallor within diffuse areas of redness, indicating ischaemia.

12.1 Causes of corneal ulceration

Cause	History	Examination
Bacterial	Previous corneal disease Dry eyes, contact lenses	Ulcer affecting central cornea
Herpes simplex	Previous episode, general	Dendritic pattern most common manifestation
Herpes zoster	Ophthalmic shingles affecting external nose	Crusting vesicles affecting ophthalmic division of trigeminal nerve
Acanthamoeba	Contact lens users washing lens with tap water	Severe ocular pain and photophobia
Fungal	Ocular trauma with vegetable matter or immunocompromised patient	Feathery indistinct white lesion or non-responding 'bacterial ulcer'
Neurotrophic	Previous brainstem stroke	Absent or reduced corneal sensation
Alkali burn	Injury with chemicals	Loss of adjacent conjunctival vessels indicates poor prognosis
Corneal abrasion	Trauma	A linear scratch indicates a foreign body under eyelid
Marginal keratitis	Blepharitis	Ulcer affecting peripheral cornea

Conjunctivitis is an inflammation of the conjunctivae and feels uncomfortable. There is always an associated discharge. Unlike in scleritis or episcleritis, the inner eyelid is inflamed and red (Fig. 12.9). Conjunctivitis due to bacterial infection is associated with a yellow/green discharge, while chlamydial and viral infection causes a clear discharge and pre-auricular lymphadenopathy. Persistent watery discharge with itchy eyes and no lymphadenopathy suggests an allergic cause.

Visual disturbance

Double vision (diplopia)

This may be uniocular or binocular. Binocular diplopia is caused by imbalance of eye movements, whereas uniocular is due to intraocular disease.

Blurred vision

Distinguish true blurring of the whole visual field from a discrete defect (scotoma). Blurring of the whole visual field is due to an ocular problem, such as an uncorrected refractive error, e.g. myopia, hypermetropia or presbyopia, or opacities in the cornea, lens, aqueous chamber or vitreous gel. A patient with a central scotoma, common with age-related macular degeneration, will not be able to see a face clearly but the rest of the visual field is unaffected.

Sudden-onset visual loss

Sudden-onset visual loss may be temporary or permanent, and may affect one or both eyes. Patients may not notice gradual visual loss in one eye but complain of sudden visual loss when they close their unaffected eye.

Transient visual loss or disturbance is caused by the aura of migraine or unilateral transient retinal ischaemia (amaurosis fugax). Absence of headache does not exclude migraine. The aura of classical migraine usually takes the form of coloured lines, often scintillating, and is always homonymous (present in both visual fields), even if the patient mistakenly attributes it to one eye. Unlike amaurosis fugax, it is still seen with the eyes shut. In contrast, retinal migraine causes unilateral visual loss and may be difficult to differentiate from amaurosis fugax.

Amaurosis fugax produces a negative unilateral visual phenomenon which is black or grey. Classically, this is a short-lasting visual disturbance (minutes) appearing like a shutter coming down, up or from the side, and resolves in a similar fashion. It may be confused with the aura of migraine or the homonymous hemianopia of transient occipital lobe ischaemia.

Visual impairment following exercise or a hot bath is characteristic of demyelinating optic neuritis (Uthoff's phenomenon).

Permanent, sudden visual loss is usually due to vascular occlusion. Establish whether the symptoms are uniocular or homonymous (Box 12.2).

Retinal artery occlusion is usually embolic. It resembles amaurosis fugax but is permanent. Always consider giant cell arteritis in anterior ischaemic optic neuropathy. The diagnosis is more likely in the presence of a swollen and white optic nerve head and evidence of inflammation (raised erythrocyte sedimentation rate (ESR), C-reactive protein (CRP) or platelet count).

Homonymous visual loss, in the absence of hemiparesis or dysphasia, usually indicates occipital lobe infarction.

Gradual-onset visual loss

Gradual onset of visual loss is commonly caused by cataract or atrophic age-related macular degeneration. Both cause glare from bright lights. Slowly progressive visual loss, accompanied by optic atrophy, occurs when the optic nerve or chiasm is compressed by tumours of the skull base, e.g. meningioma or pituitary adenoma.

Distortion of vision

Distortion is caused by disruption of the photoreceptors at the macula, most commonly macular degeneration in the elderly. Untreated, central visual loss is rapid and irreversible. In those <65 years, it may be caused by fluid (oedema) or blood under the central retina. Scarring of the outer surface of the vitreous (epiretinal membrane) may distort the normally smooth surface of the macula. This may occur following any insult to the vitreous, such as haemorrhage, inflammation or trauma.

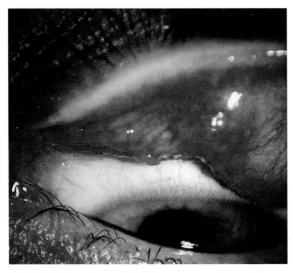

Fig. 12.9 Giant papillary conjunctivitis seen on everting upper lid. A form of allergic conjunctivitis induced by contact lens wear.

12.2 Causes of uniocular permanent sudden-onset visual loss

- Retinal artery occlusion
- Anterior ischaemic optic neuropathy
- Retinal vein occlusion
- Traumatic optic neuropathy

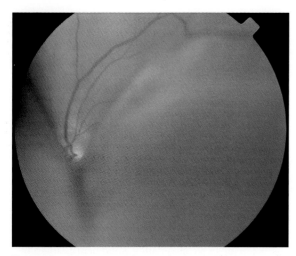

Fig. 12.10 Retinal detachment. Elevation of the retina around the 'attached' optic disc. The retina may be so elevated that it is visible on viewing the red reflex.

Flashes and floaters

Flashes and floaters are common in those >65 years and in short sight (myopia); they are caused by vitreous degeneration. As the vitreous degenerates, the gel liquefies and fluid escapes through perforations in the outer surface of the vitreous overlying the macula. The fluid peels the vitreous off the retina and the remaining contents swirl about on eye movement. The patient can see something floating within the eye. If the vitreous has an abnormal attachment to the retina then, as it detaches, the retina may tear and the patient sees flashes of light. Retinal tears allow fluid from the vitreous cavity to enter the space between the retina and the retinal pigment epithelium, causing retinal detachment (Fig. 12.10). The patient notices visual loss starting peripherally and moving centrally.

Haloes

Haloes are coloured lights seen around bright lights due to fluid in the cornea (corneal oedema) which acts as a prism. They occur with angle-closure glaucoma.

Oscillopsia

Oscillopsia, when objects appear to oscillate, causes mild blurring to rapid and periodic jumping, and is common in nystagmus affecting primary gaze.

THE HISTORY

Although many ocular diagnoses can be made on examination alone, the history is crucial to diagnose visual disorders. For example, vascular symptoms are often sudden in onset, whereas a slow, inexorable progression of symptoms suggests compression of the optic pathway by a tumour. Symptoms which come on

12.3 Past history and the eye

History	Implication
Diabetes mellitus	Diabetic retinopathy, diabetic macular oedema, ocular ischaemia, III or VI nerve palsy, retinal vein occlusion
Thyroid disease	Exophthalmos (proptosis in autoimmune thyroid eye disease), ophthalmoplegia
Hypertension	Retinal vein occlusion, arteriosclerosis, hypertensive retinopathy (accelerated), non-arteritic anterior ischaemic optic neuropathy
Cerebrovascular or ischaemic heart disease, peripheral vascular disease	Retinal vein occlusion, retinal artery occlusion, non-arteritic anterior ischaemic optic neuropathy, ocular ischaemia, occipital lobe infarction
Atrial fibrillation	Embolic retinal artery occlusion, occipital lobe infarction
Tuberculosis	Uveitis
Multiple sclerosis	Optic neuritis, VI nerve palsy, bilateral internuclear paresis
Hayfever, asthma, eczema	Allergic eye disease
Myeloma, hyperviscosity syndrome, leukaemia	Retinal vein occlusion
Inflammatory bowel disease, rheumatoid arthritis	Episcleritis, scleritis
Ankylosing spondylitis	Recurrent anterior uveitis
Persistent ear, nose and throat symptoms	Wegener's granulomatosis
Glaucoma	Retinal vein occlusion
Cataract surgery	Retinal detachment

over about 2 weeks, last 2–3 weeks and then resolve suggest demyelination. Always clarify terms used by patients to describe the symptoms; for example, diplopia and blurring are easily confused.

Past history

Information about previous visual and non-visual illnesses can help diagnosis (Box 12.3).

Drug history

List the patient's current medications (Box 12.4).

Family history

Always ask about the family history, especially in children. There is an increased incidence of multiple sclerosis in those with a family history, and many patients with

12.4 Drugs and the eye

Visual condition	Drug
Keratopathy	Amiodarone
Cataract	Corticosteroid
Anterior uveitis	Rifabutin
Angle closure glaucoma	Anticholinergics
Retinal toxicity	Chloroquine, chlorpromazine, phenothiazine, tamoxifen, interferon
Optic neuropathy	Amiodarone, sildenafil, amiodarone, ethambutol, isoniazid
Demyelination	Infliximab
Nystagmus	Anticonvulsants

12.5 Causes of acute anterior uveitis (iritis)

- Idiopathic
- HLA B27 association
- Sarcoidosis
- Herpes simplex keratitis
- Post-cataract surgery
- Tuberculosis
- Neurosyphilis
- Trauma

12.6 Causes of proptosis

- Thyroid eye disease (exophthalmos)*
- Carotico-cavernous fistula
- Orbital cellulitis
- Orbital haematoma
- Wegener's granulomatosis
- Orbital metastasis or meningioma
- Pseudoproptosis (pathological myopia, shallow orbits, contralateral enophthalmos)

* Most common cause.

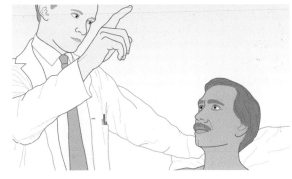

Fig. 12.11 Testing for lid lag.

thyroid eye disease have a family history of autoimmune thyroid disease. A family history of tuberculosis increases the likelihood of uveitis, representing re-activation of previous subclinical disease.

Social history

Cigarette smoking is the most important cause of vascular disease affecting the eye. A history of hayfever or allergies to animals suggests an allergic eye disorder. Recreational drug use may be associated with visual loss, particularly cocaine-induced vascular occlusions. Uveitis may be the first manifestation of HIV infection or neurosyphilis, so a sexual history is important in all patients with ocular inflammation or unexplained neuro-ophthalmic symptoms (Box 12.5).

Occupational history

Ultraviolet keratitis may be experienced by arc welders who do not use appropriate eye protection, but also occurs with unprotected recreational use of tanning beds or exposure to bright sunlight without sunglasses, e.g. snow blindness.

EXAMINATION OF VISION

Examination of vision requires assessment of cranial nerves II, III, IV and VI and their central connections:
- inspection
- visual acuity

- visual fields
- ocular alignment
- pupillary examination
- colour vision
- ophthalmoscopy.

Inspection

Examination sequence

Inspection of vision

Carefully and systematically look at:

- Head position.
- Position of eyelids when looking straight ahead and on eye movement.
- Proptosis (forward bulging of the eyeball) (Box 12.6).
- Lid lag. With the patient sitting, position yourself on his right side. Watch how the upper eyelid moves with the downward movement of the eye as the patient follows your finger, moving from a point approximately 45° above the horizontal to a point below this plane. Normally, there is perfect co-ordination as the upper lid follows the downward movement of the eye. In lid lag, as occurs in thyroid eye disease, sclera can be seen above the iris (Fig. 12.11).
- Periorbital appearance (Box 12.7).
- Lacrimal apparatus.
- Eyelid margin.

12.7 Causes of periorbital oedema

- Allergic eye disease
- Thyroid eye disease
- Orbital cellulitis
- Nephrotic syndrome
- Heart failure
- Angio-oedema

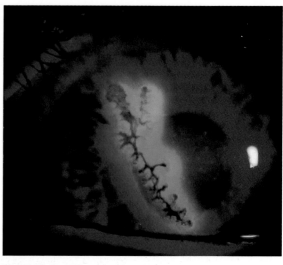

Fig. 12.13 Dendritic conjunctival ulcer. Fluorescein staining showing branching dendritic ulcer.

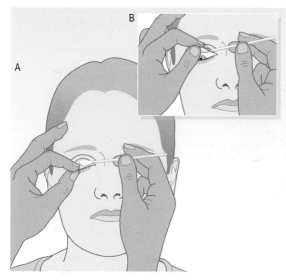

Fig. 12.12 Everting the upper eyelid to look at the conjunctiva.

12.8 Causes of ptosis

Mechanical	
• Chronic orbital inflammation • Degenerative • Eyelid tumour	• Intraocular surgery • Long-term use of contact lenses • Trauma

Myogenic	
• Chronic progressive external ophthalmoplegia • Congenital myogenic ptosis secondary to levator dysgenesis	• Myotonic dystrophy • Oculopharyngeal dystrophy

Neuromuscular junction	
• Myasthenia gravis	

Neurogenic: congenital	
• Congenital Horner's syndrome	• Congenital III nerve palsy

Neurogenic: acquired	
• Acquired Horner's syndrome • III cranial nerve palsy	• Synkinetic neurogenic ptosis, e.g. Marcus Gunn

▶ Conjunctiva. Ask the patient to look down, hold the eyelashes of the upper lid, press gently on the upper border of the tarsal plate with a cotton bud and gently pull the eyelashes up. Look for the giant papillae of allergic eye disease or a hidden foreign body (Fig. 12.12).
▶ Sclera.
▶ Cornea. Carry out fluorescein testing for corneal ulceration. Ask the patient to look down and gently touch a fluorescein strip on to the sclera, where it will leave a yellow mark. Ask the patient to blink to distribute the dye on the cornea. This yellow dye reveals epithelial defects which are sometimes obvious to the naked eye. Use your ophthalmoscope with a +10 lens to visualize the cornea more accurately. A light with a cobalt blue filter will make any defects more obvious but is not essential (Fig. 12.13).
▶ Resting appearance of pupils.

Abnormal findings

Congenital and longstanding paralytic squint often causes an abnormal head posture with the head turned or tilted to minimize the diplopia.

Narrowing of the palpebral fissure (the gap between upper and lower eyelids) suggests ptosis (drooping eyelid) (Box 12.8) or blepharospasm (tonic spasm in the orbicularis oris muscle). If the sclera is visible above the cornea, suspect eyelid retraction or proptosis; below, consider ectropion.

Causes of ptosis include:
- III nerve palsy: causes unilateral ptosis that is often complete. The pupil is large because of loss of parasympathetic innervation of the iris. The unopposed action of the IV and VI cranial nerves results in the eye looking inferolaterally. Acute III nerve palsy may herald the onset of a posterior communicating artery aneurysm and requires urgent investigation

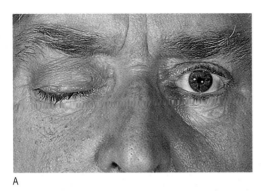
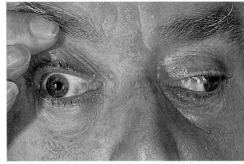

A   B

12

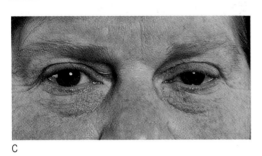
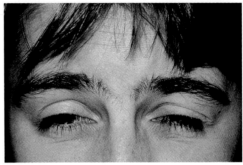

C   D

Fig. 12.14 Ptosis. (A) Complete right ptosis in third nerve palsy. **(B)** The same patient looking down and to the left; the right eye has rotated medially, demonstrating that the trochlear (IV) nerve is intact. **(C)** Left Horner's syndrome. **(D)** Myasthenia gravis. The patient is attempting to open his eyelids. Raised forehead browlines (frontalis overactivity) reflect the effort of attempting to open the eyelids.

- Horner's syndrome (damage to the cervical sympathetic nerves): gives a partial ptosis and involves both upper and lower lids, leading to a pseudo-enophthalmos (small eye). The pupil is small due to lack of sympathetic innervation to the iris (miosis)
- Myasthenia gravis: causes bilateral ptosis due to fatiguability of the muscle, levator palpebrae superioris. The patient may be unable to 'bury the eyelashes', which strongly suggests either a neuromuscular junction disorder, a myopathy or a meningeal disorder, as it is not possible for a single lesion to affect both III and VII ipsilateral cranial nerves (Fig. 12.14).

Periorbital oedema may be associated with oedema of the conjunctiva (chemosis).

The lacrimal gland may become swollen through:

- inflammation (sarcoidosis)
- infection (dacroadenitis or mumps)
- malignancy (lymphoma, cancer).

Nasolacrimal duct blockage produces watering and sticky discharge, and may cause acute inflammation of the lacrimal sac (dacrocystitis). It is common in neonates and usually resolves spontaneously.

Blepharitis (inflammation of the eyelid margin) is a common cause of dry eyes. Although often isolated, it may be associated with systemic skin involvement. Look for features of more widespread skin disease:

- 'ace of clubs' appearance of rosacea (erythema on forehead, cheeks and chin)
- flexural dermatitis of atopic eczema
- dandruff or seborrhoeic dermatitis.

Common lumps on the eyelids include:

- stye (eyelash microabscess)
- chalazion (pea-like swellings of the tarsal glands)
- basal cell skin cancer.

If the sclera is thin, it becomes transparent and the blue-green choroid is seen. This occurs in scleromalacia, osteogenesis imperfecta and Ehlers–Danlos syndrome. A yellow tinge to the sclera is found in the early stages of jaundice (Fig. 8.10, p. 195).

Scleritis causes a dark-red colour, tenderness and pain on eye movement. White patches within red areas suggest impending necrosis and the presence of systemic vasculitis.

The epithelium of the cornea may be affected if the cornea is dry, traumatized or infected. Peripheral corneal deposition is seen with hyperlipidaemia (corneal arcus; Fig. 6.7, p. 115) due to lipid deposition. In Wilson's disease, copper is deposited round the cornea, causing Kayser–Fleischer rings (Fig. 12.15). Calcium may also be deposited in chronic ocular inflammation and chronic hypercalcaemia.

12

Visual acuity

A clear focused image requires adaptation of the focal length of the optic lens by alteration of its curvature to suit the varying distance of the entering rays. There are several common refractive errors:

- Hypermetropia (long-sightedness) is the most common refractive error. Rays of light from a distant object are brought to focus behind the retina. It is common in infants and can be compensated for by contraction of the ciliary muscle, which increases the refractive power of the lens (Fig. 12.16)
- Myopia (or short-sightedness) is when rays from a distant object are focused in front of the retina. Simple myopia usually starts in childhood and worsens during the growing years (Fig. 12.17)
- Presbyopia occurs as the lens ages and becomes less able to change its curvature. It is very common in those >45 years
- Astigmatism is when the cornea is irregularly curved and requires correction with cylindrical lenses.

■▶ Examination sequence

Visual acuity

■▶ Ask patients to put their glasses on, if they use them. Only use reading glasses when testing near vision.

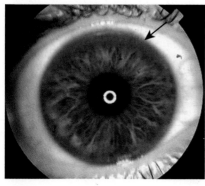

Fig. 12.15 Kayser–Fleischer ring (arrowed).

■▶ Ensure good ambient lighting.

■▶ Use a Snellen or LogMar chart 6 metres from the patient (Fig. 12.18). Ask the patient to cover one eye with a card and read from the top down until he can no longer distinguish the letters.

■▶ Switch over and repeat with the other eye.

■▶ If the patient cannot read down to line 6 (6/6 vision), place a pinhole directly in front of his glasses to correct refractive errors. This allows only central rays of light to enter the eye and can correct for about 4 dioptres of refractive error (Fig. 12.19).

■▶ If patients cannot see the top line of the chart at 6 metres, bring them forward till they can and record that vision, e.g. 1/60 — can see top letter at 1 metre.

■▶ If patients still cannot see the top letter at 1 metre, check whether they can count fingers, see hand movements or just see light.

■▶ For children, use different-sized objects instead of letters.

■▶ For patients complaining of central blurred vision, record the near vision in each eye using reading glasses and standard charts.

■▶ Repeat the process above for near vision. Use a test card, held at a comfortable reading distance, to assess near vision. N5 is the smallest size that an unimpaired eye can see (N8 is the size of normal newsprint). A Snellen visual acuity of 6/60 (LogMar = 1.0) indicates that at 6 metres patients can only see letters they should be able to read 60 metres away. Normal vision is said to be 6/6 (LogMar = 0.0). In UK visual acuity of 6/10 or better is required for a driving licence.

Macular function

■▶ Use an Amsler grid (Fig. 12.20) to record visual defects, including central scotomas, quadrantanopias and hemianopias, and distortion of the central 10° of vision.

■▶ Ask the patient to hold the grid at a comfortable reading distance.

■▶ They fix on the central black spot with the eye being tested.

■▶ Tell them to keep their eye still and look at the grid using the 'sides of their vision'.

■▶ Ask them to outline the areas where the lines are broken, distorted or missing.

Visual fields

The normal visual field extends 160° horizontally and 130° vertically. The blind spot is located 15° to the temporal side of the point of visual fixation and represents the optic nerve head. At the bedside, test visual fields by confrontation; the exact method depends on the patient's

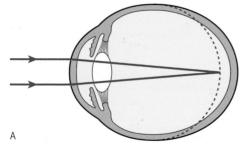

A

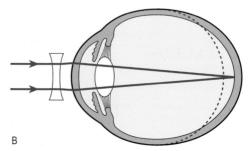

B

Fig. 12.16 The myopic (short-sighted) eye. (A) The eye is too long and the image on the retina is not in focus. **(B)** The use of a concave (minus) lens brings the image on the retina into focus.

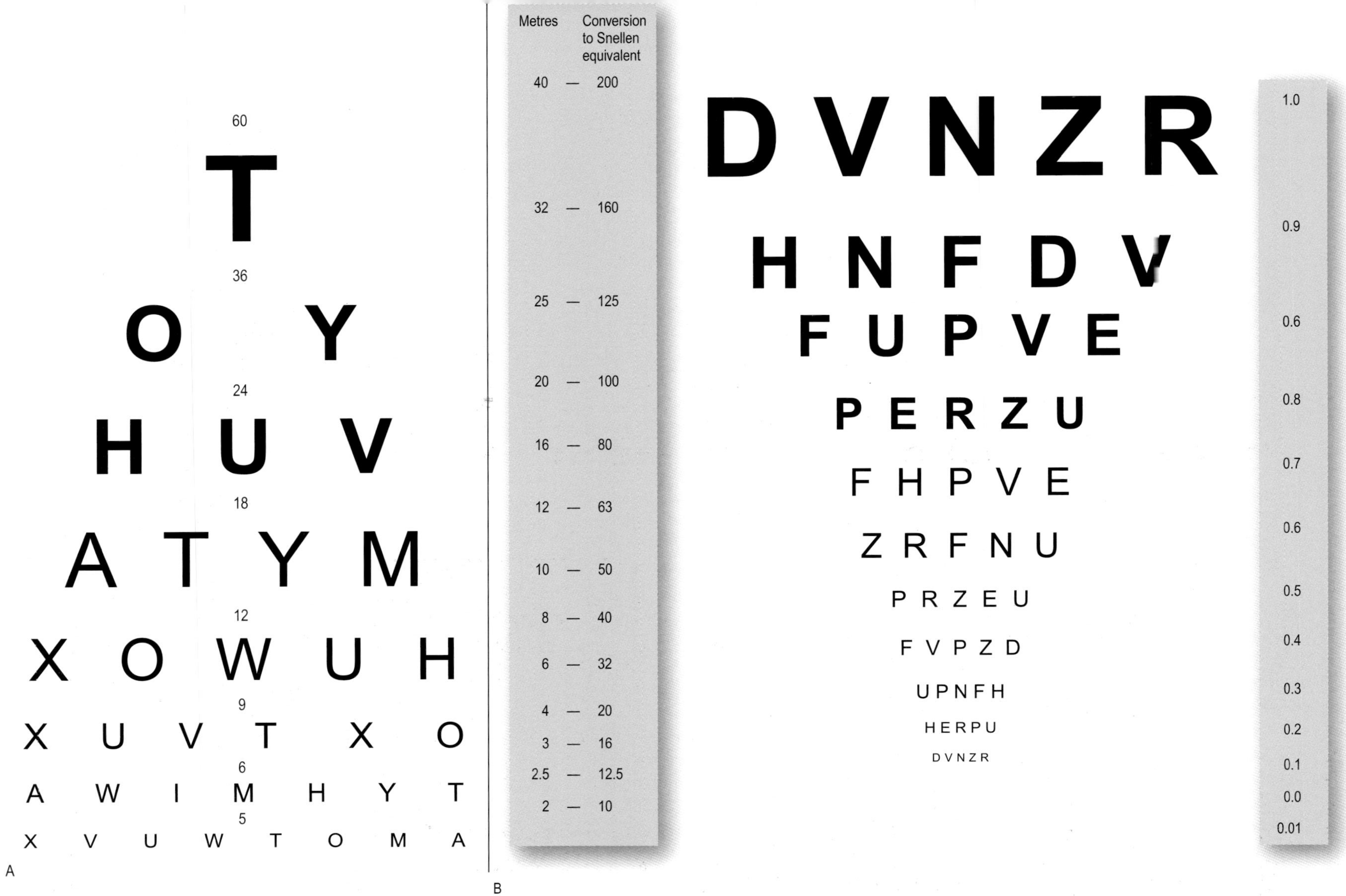

Fig. 12.17 Visual acuity charts. (A) Snellen visual acuity chart; this is increasingly replaced by the LogMar visual acuity chart. **(B)** LogMar chart; this is usually illuminated.

A

(Snellen size)	Letters
60	T
36	O Y
24	H U V
18	A T Y M
12	X O W U H
9	X U V T X O
6	A W I M H Y T
5	X V U W T O M A

B

LogMar	Letters	Metres	Conversion to Snellen equivalent
1.0	DVNZR	40	200
0.9	HNFDV	32	160
0.6	FUPVE	25	125
0.8	PERZU	20	100
0.7	FHPVE	16	80
0.6	ZRFNU	12	63
0.5	PRZEU	10	50
0.4	FVPZD	8	40
0.3	UPNFH	6	32
0.2	HERPU	4	20
0.1	DVNZR	3	16
0.0		2.5	12.5
0.01		2	10

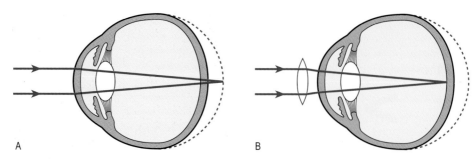

Fig. 12.18 The hypermetropic (long-sighted) eye. (A) The eye is too short and the image on the retina is not in focus. **(B)** The use of a convex (plus) lens brings the image on the retina into focus.

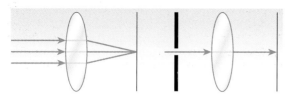

Fig. 12.19 Pinhole. Normally, the lens focuses rays of light on to a discrete point on the retina. The pinhole partially negates the role of the lens by only allowing rays from directly in front to pass through.

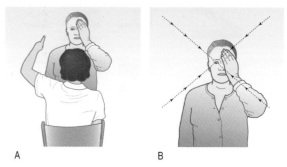

Fig. 12.21 Testing the visual fields.

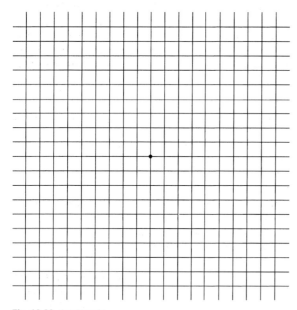

Fig. 12.20 Amsler grid.

ability to cooperate. For more accurate assessment use an automated visual field analyser.

Examination sequence

Visual fields

- Sit directly facing the patient, about 1 metre away.
- Ask the patient to keep looking at your eyes.

Homonymous defects

- Keep your eyes open and ask the patient to do the same (Fig. 12.21).
- Hold your hands out to their full extent. Wiggle your finger tip and ask the patient to point to it as soon as he sees it move. Do this at 10 and 2 o'clock, and then 8 and 4 o'clock (each of the four outer quadrants of the patient's visual field — superotemporal, superonasal, inferotemporal, inferonasal).

Sensory inattention

- Both you and the patient should keep your eyes open.
- Test both left and right fields at the same time. Note whether the patient reports seeing only one side move and which quadrant or side is affected.

Peripheral visual fields

- Test each eye separately.
- Ask the patient to cover one eye and look directly into your opposite eye.
- Shut the eye that is opposite the patient's covered eye.
- Test each quadrant separately. Start with your finger in the periphery and wiggle the tip, bring your wiggling finger along the diagonal towards the centre of vision till the patient sees it move.
- Repeat for the other quadrants.
- Compare your visual field with the patient's.

Central visual field

- Use a red hatpin to test one eye qualitatively at a time.
- Ask the patient to cover one eye and look directly at you.
- Shut your eye that is opposite the patient's covered eye.

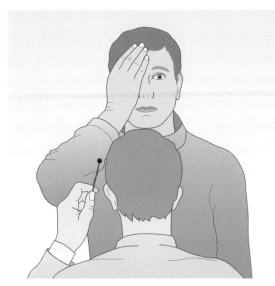

Fig. 12.22 Testing visual fields by confrontation.

▪▶ Hold the hatpin in the centre of the visual field, as close to fixation as possible.
▪▶ Ask the patient what colour the hatpin is. If it is pale or pink, this implies colour desaturation, usually affecting the optic nerve.
▪▶ Compare the four quadrants of the visual field centrally; each time ask about colour desaturation (Fig. 12.22). Note that the visual field for red may be smaller than for white.

Blind spot

This is a physiological scotoma corresponding to absence of photoreceptors where the optic nerve leaves the eye.

▪▶ Ask the patient to cover one eye and look directly at you.
▪▶ Shut the eye that is opposite the patient's covered eye.
▪▶ Hold the hatpin at the fixation point; you and the patient focus on each other's eye.
▪▶ Move the hatpin temporally and horizontally until it disappears from your visual field. Maintaining the same temporal horizontal position, move it anteriorly or posteriorly until it also disappears from the patient's visual field.
▪▶ Compare the size of the patient's blind spot to yours.

Abnormal findings

Reduced visual acuity indicates a central visual field defect. The most common cause is cataract. There are three retinal forms of central visual field defect:

• Macular lesions cause central scotomas, which may be incomplete and associated with distortion, allowing the patient to see partially through them
• Peripheral retinal lesions spare central vision, causing ring scotomas
• Optic disc lesions cause horizontal or arcuate scotomas.

Lesions of the optic nerve within the orbit cause different central scotomas from those of macular origin because red desaturation (red colours appear orange or pink) occurs early and there is no visual distortion.

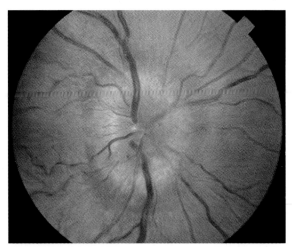

Fig. 12.23 Swollen optic disc. Papilloedema is suggested if visual acuity is unaffected, colour vision is normal and there is an enlarged blind spot.

• Unilateral optic nerve lesions cause a relative afferent pupillary defect, even with normal vision; in macular lesions this is a late finding
• Distension of the nerve sheath around the optic nerve, e.g. papilloedema (Fig. 12.23), causes an enlarged blind spot. Optic atrophy occurs later.

Lesions at the optic chiasm cause bilateral temporal visual field defects (bitemporal hemianopia; Fig. 12.3). As the optic chiasm is a continuation of the optic nerve, central red desaturation is the first sign of involvement, not peripheral visual field loss.

Optic tract lesions are uncommon; they are usually suprasellar lesions, such as pituitary tumours, and produce asymmetrical (incongruous) homonymous visual field defects.

The visual radiations are more commonly affected and produce:

• symmetrical (congruous) visual field defects (homonymous hemianopia)
• lack of awareness of visual field loss, suggesting parietal lobe involvement
• visual field defects affecting only central vision because of the dual blood supply of the occipital cortex.

Functional visual loss is common, particularly bilateral visual field constriction that does not expand on testing further away. This tubular constriction differentiates it from the funnel constriction of bilateral retinal disorders, such as retinitis pigmentosa (Fig. 12.24) or bilateral homonymous hemianopia (cortical visual impairment).

In normal funnel vision, the visual field, no matter how small, doubles when the patient is tested in front of a tangent screen and is moved back from a 1 metre distance to 2 metres. Patients with tunnel vision will claim that their visual field is unchanged or sometimes even smaller (Fig. 12.25).

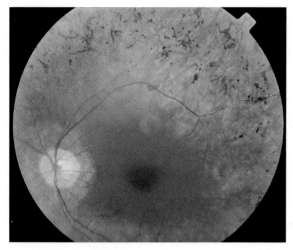

Fig. 12.24 Retinitis pigmentosa. A triad of optic atrophy, attenuated retinal vessels and pigmentary changes. Pigmentary changes typically start peripherally in association with a ring scotoma and symptoms of night blindness.

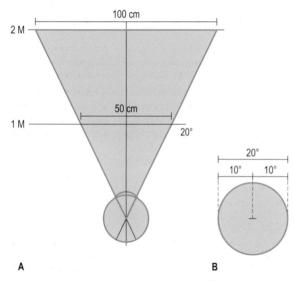

Fig. 12.25 Tangent screen.

Ocular alignment

The eyes are normally parallel in all positions of gaze, except convergence. If not, a squint is present. Squints are associated with:

- paresis of one of the extraocular muscles (paralytic or incomitant squint)
- defective binocular vision (non-paralytic or concomitant squint).

Acquired paralytic squints cause diplopia (double vision); the images are maximally separated and squint is greatest in the direction of action of the paretic muscle. Concomitant squints are the same in all positions of gaze. They usually become manifest in childhood when they are not associated with diplopia (Fig. 12.26). In

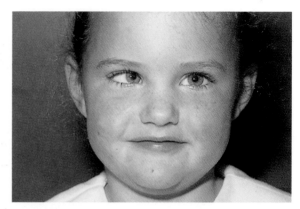

Fig. 12.26 Concomitant right convergent squint in a child.

children, the visual acuity of the squinting eye falls, causing a 'lazy eye' (amblyopia).

Examination sequence

Ocular alignment

The examination sequence depends on whether the patient complains of double vision (diplopia) or squint.

Diplopia

- Look for head turns or tilts in the direction of underacting muscles.
- Sit directly facing the patient, about 1 metre away.
- Hold a pen-torch and ask the patient to look at the light; observe the position of the pen-torch's reflection on the cornea. The fixating (non-paretic) eye has the pen-torch's reflection in the centre; the eye with weak muscles (paretic) has an off centre reflection. If the paretic eye has better vision than the non-paretic eye the patient fixates with it, producing confusing eye movements.
- Hold your finger vertically, at least 50 cm away, and ask the patient to follow it.
- Look for the direction of gaze where diplopia is maximal.
- Ask whether the diplopia is horizontal, vertical, tilted or a mixture of both.
- Cover one of the patient's eyes to see if diplopia is monocular or binocular.
- If diplopia is binocular, ask which image disappears; the outer image corresponds to the affected eye. Note the direction of gaze in which diplopia is worst and work out which muscle is affected (Fig. 12.4A).
- On horizontal movement, in the absence of proptosis, no ipsilateral sclera should be seen on extreme gaze ('burying the white'). Its presence suggests ipsilateral muscle weakness.
- On down-gaze hold the eyelids open.
- For each eye, look for nystagmus while examining eye movements. Note the direction of any fast component and whether it changes direction with the direction of gaze.

Squint (cover test)

- Sit directly facing the patient, about 1 metre away.
- Examine visual acuity and the visual fields as above.
- Cover one eye and ask the patient to look at the light of your pen-torch.

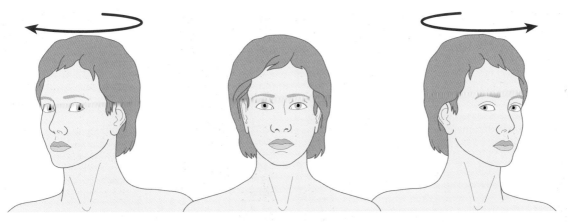

Fig. 12.27 Performing the doll's head manœuvre in the horizontal plane. Note the eyes move in the opposite direction to head movement.

Closely observe the uncovered eye for any movements.

If it moves to take up fixation, that eye was squinting.

Repeat the sequence for the other eye.

Oculocephalic (doll's eye) reflex

With the patient supine, hold his head in both hands with your thumbs holding the eyes open; if the patient is conscious, ask him to focus on your eyes.

Rock the head gently from side to side, noting the movement of the eyes as they hold their gaze.

An impaired reflex indicates an impaired brainstem (Fig. 12.27).

Abnormal findings

Monocular diplopia is created by 'ghosting' from structural abnormality anywhere between the cornea and fovea.

Pure horizontal diplopia usually results from involvement of the VI cranial nerve. The symptoms are worse looking to the affected side.

- Orbital trauma may trap a medial rectus muscle
- In demyelination the lesion is often in the pons and may be associated with ipsilateral lower motor neurone nerve palsy
- Disruption of the neuronal connection between the medial rectus and the contralateral VI nerve (median longitudinal fasciculus) — for example, in multiple sclerosis — causes under-action of the medial rectus and an internuclear ophthalmoplegia. Unlike VI nerve palsy, diplopia is worse on looking to the contralateral side. There is often a vertical component to the diplopia, skewing the image
- VI nerve palsy occurs with raised intracranial pressure when the nerve is stretched as it passes upward to the cavernous sinus.

Other causes of impaired horizontal movement include:

- pontine gaze palsies (nuclear VI nerve palsy)
- convergence spasm (impaired uniocular lateral gaze associated with small pupils bilaterally) — miosis.

Impaired vertical gaze can occur in:

- Brainstem stroke, demyelination and children with hydrocephalus (when the inferior segment of the cornea lies below the lower lid — the 'sun setting' sign)

- IV nerve palsies, which cause vertical diplopia, particularly noticeable on down-gaze. The IV cranial nerve is particularly susceptible to a blow to the back of the head, as it is the only nerve to emerge from the posterior brainstem and damage is often bilateral
- Thyroid eye disease, a common cause of vertical diplopia. The patient often also complains about the appearance of lid retraction or proptosis, or both.

If the patient's complaint is of 'squint' rather than double vision, this suggests non-paralytic squint resulting from defective binocular vision. An amblyopic eye often diverges while monocular eye movements will be intact. The cover test is useful in children.

The oculocephalic test differentiates supranuclear lesions from cranial nerve lesions. An impaired response in an unconscious patient may indicate brainstem stroke, metabolic dysfunction or drug intoxication.

Nystagmus

Nystagmus is an involuntary oscillation of the eyes that is often rhythmical, with both eyes moving synchronously. It may be vertical, horizontal, rotatory or multidirectional. The most common form is biphasic or jerk nystagmus, in which there is a slow drift in one direction, followed by a fast correction in the opposite direction.

The convention is to describe nystagmus in the direction of the fast phase or jerk. Oscillations occurring at the same speed and over the same range about a central point are pendular nystagmus.

Examination sequence

Nystagmus

Ask the patient to look straight ahead at your finger, held an arm length away.

Move your finger to each side and up and down.

If nystagmus is present, note:
- the position in which it occurs
- the direction in which it is most marked
- whether it is horizontal, vertical, rotatory or multidirectional

323

– whether there are fast and slow phases (jerk) or equal oscillations about a central point (pendular)

▶ At extremes of lateral gaze, normal subjects may show a few nystagmoid jerks.

The most common cause of jerk nystagmus is vestibular.

- Peripheral vestibular nystagmus often has horizontal, vertical and rotatory components, and is usually associated with vertigo. The amplitude of the oscillation increases with gaze towards the direction of the fast phase and is markedly suppressed by visual fixation using Frenzel lenses. Common peripheral causes are vestibular neuronitis and Ménière's disease.

- Central vestibular nystagmus, in contrast, is usually unidirectional, does not alter with direction of gaze or with visual fixation, and is less likely to be accompanied by vertigo. Central causes include multiple sclerosis and cerebrovascular disease.

Vertical nystagmus is relatively rare and indicates brainstem damage. Upbeat nystagmus, with the fast phase on looking upwards, occurs with upper brainstem lesions in multiple sclerosis, infarction and Wernicke's encephalopathy. Lesions around the craniocervical junction, such as Arnold–Chiari malformation or demyelination, can result in downbeat nystagmus, which is also seen with phenytoin and lithium intoxication.

In gaze-evoked nystagmus there is no nystagmus in the primary position but only on eccentric gaze. This is of limited localizing value. Periodic alternating nystagmus is present in the primary position but changes direction in a crescendo-decrescendo manner, often every 90 seconds with a null period of up to 10 seconds. This may be congenital, due to lesions at the craniocervical junction, or a feature of drug intoxication. Demyelination of the medial longitudinal bundle within the brainstem can cause ataxic nystagmus, where the oscillations are more marked in the abducting eye than in the adducting one. This is often associated with an internuclear ophthalmoplegia with reduced adduction.

Congenital nystagmus is usually a horizontal jerk nystagmus but can be pendular. Acquired pendular nystagmus results from cerebellar or brainstem disease,

most commonly multiple sclerosis, but is also found in spinocerebellar degenerations and brainstem ischaemia.

When a person looks out of a train window at the passing scenery, a physiological opticokinetic nystagmus occurs. This can be tested using a vertically striped drum that is spun in front of the subject, the fast phase being in the opposite direction to the spin. It can be impaired in people with visual field defects and the test can be useful in cases of hysterical blindness.

Pupillary examination

▶ Examination sequence

Pupils

▶ Examine the pupils for shape and symmetry, taking account of ambient lighting.

▶ Ask the patient to fix the eyes on a distant point straight ahead.

▶ Bring a bright torchlight from the side to shine on the pupil. Look for constriction of that pupil (direct light reflex) and for constriction of the opposite pupil (consensual light reflex).

▶ With the patient's vision fixed on a distant point, present an object about 15 cm in front of the eyes and ask the patient to focus on it (convergence). Look for pupil constriction (accommodation reflex).

Abnormal findings

Old family photographs can help you to assess the onset of pupillary abnormalities.

Essential anisocoria, in which one pupil is bigger than the other but otherwise both behave normally, is a common normal variant.

In diabetes mellitus, autonomic neuropathy may lead to small pupils that respond poorly to pharmacological dilatation. They may mimic the Argyll Robertson pupils of syphilis (pin-point, irregular pupils that constrict only on convergence).

An Adie pupil is usually mid-dilated and responds poorly to convergence. It is a result of ciliary ganglion malfunction within the orbit. With time it may shrink in size and be confused with an Argyll Robertson pupil. It is frequently bilateral, and when associated with

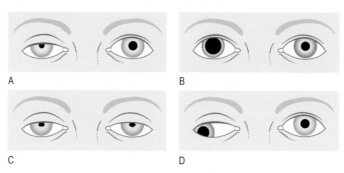

A   B

C   D

Fig. 12.28 Pupillary defects. (A) Right Horner's syndrome (ptosis and miosis). **(B)** Right Holmes–Adie pupil. **(C)** Argyll Robertson pupils with bilateral ptosis and small irregular pupils. **(D)** Right III nerve palsy (looking down and out, ptosis and a dilated pupil).

absent neurological reflexes, it is termed the Holmes–Adie syndrome.

Optic nerve damage results in an afferent pupillary defect (Marcus Gunn pupil). Both pupils are dually innervated at the level of the midbrain. Normally, both pupils constrict to light, regardless of which eye is illuminated. If one optic nerve is damaged, whatever lighting the dominant optic nerve is exposed to determines the size of both pupils (Fig. 12.28).

A unilateral dilated pupil in a patient with deteriorating conscious level secondary to intracranial mass lesions, e.g. tumour or enlarging haematoma, occurs when brain herniation compresses the III nerve.

Colour vision

Red desaturation, the impaired ability to identify red objects, is an early indicator of optic nerve pathology.

▶ Examination sequence

Colour vision

▶ Red-green colour vision can be assessed using Ishihara test plates (Fig. 12.29). These are coloured spots forming numbers which the patient reads out.

▶ The first plate is a test plate; if the patient cannot see the number, they have poor visual acuity or functional visual loss.

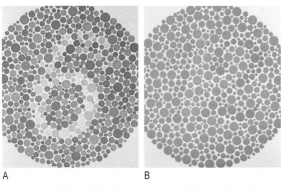

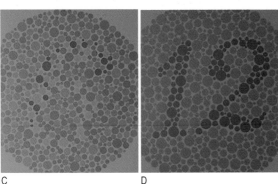

A   B

C   D

Fig. 12.29 Plates from the Ishihara series. (A and **B)** Normal colour vision. **(C** and **D)** The plates as they appear to someone with colour blindness. The person is unable to read '6' in plate A, and can just read '12' in plate B.

Abnormal findings

Congenital red-green blindness is an X-linked recessive condition and affects 7% of the male population. Optic nerve damage anywhere from the photoreceptors to the lateral geniculate nucleus of the thalamus impairs red-green colour vision before loss of visual acuity.

Ophthalmoscopy

Examine the eye undilated first to see the pupils and iris; then, ideally, examine the eye dilated using tropicamide drops, to visualize the lens, vitreous and retina. Only the optic nerve can be reliably assessed without pupillary dilatation. If patients have particularly thick lenses, examine their eyes with their glasses in place; however, this will reduce the examiner's field of vision. Patients should not drive or use machinery until the effect of the mydriatic has completely worn off, which may take several hours.

▶ Examination sequence

Ophthalmoscopy

▶ Examine the patient's right eye, holding the ophthalmoscope in your right hand and vice versa (Fig. 12.30).

▶ Find '0' and then rotate the 'lenses' clockwise until the number 10 is obtained (plus '10'). This should be the same colour as the '1' clockwise to '0'. If not, you have gone too far.

▶ Place your other hand on the patient's forehead and ask the patient to look down. Catch the lowered upper eyelid and gently retract it against the orbital rim. Holding the eyelid against the brow enables you to approach the patient's head as closely as possible without bumping into it, and prevents the upper eyelid from obscuring your view.

▶ Ask the patient to fixate on a distant object straight ahead.

▶ From a distance of about 10 cm bring the red reflex into focus. Any opacity will appear black. In this way the cornea, iris and lens can be visualized.

▶ Now come close to the patient's head such that you are touching the hand you are resting on the patient's forehead.

▶ As you do so, rotate the lenses anticlockwise, progressively increasing the focal length.

▶ Observe for black opacities in the vitreous until the retina comes into focus.

Fundal examination

▶ Find the optic disc, which comes into view if you approach at a slight angle above the horizontal from the temporal side.

▶ Normally, the disc is pink with a pigmented temporal margin (Fig. 12.31). Pallor can be difficult to judge, but if unilateral, should always be accompanied by a relative afferent pupillary defect (Fig. 12.32). Change the focus if you cannot see the disc clearly. Assess its shape, colour and vessels.

▶ Follow the blood vessels as they extend from the optic disc in four directions: superotemporally, inferotemporally, superonasally and inferonasally.

▶ Ask the patient to look superiorly (examine horizontally), temporally (examine vertically), inferiorly (examine horizontally) and nasally (examine vertically).

▶ Ask the patient to look directly at the light to locate the centre of the macula. Ask him to keep the eye still while you look around the macula.

12

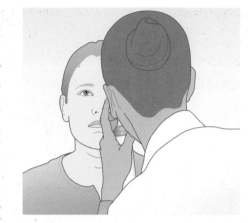

Fig. 12.30 Ophthalmoscopy: correct method. The patient's gaze is fixed on a distant point.

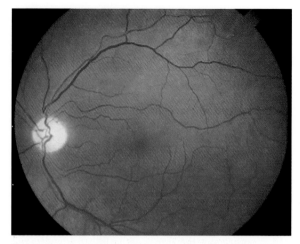

Fig. 12.32 Left optic atrophy. Note the lack of a pink neuroretinal rim.

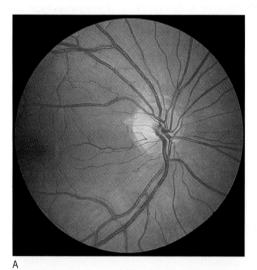

A

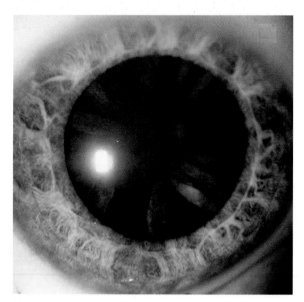

Fig. 12.33 Cortical cataract.

Abnormal findings

Cornea

Asymptomatic corneal scars from foreign bodies, often accompanied by remnants of rust, and previous ulceration are common.

Lens

There are three common forms of cataract:

- Peripheral cortical cataract is common in diabetes mellitus (Fig. 12.33). It appears as incomplete black spokes radiating from the periphery of the lens
- Posterior subcapsular cataract, the typical 'steroid cataract', appears as a black opacity coming from the centre of the lens

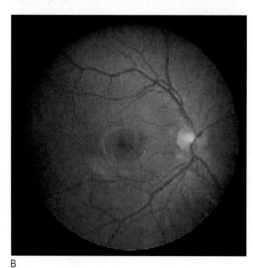

B

Fig. 12.31 Normal fundi. (A) Caucasian. **(B)** Asian.

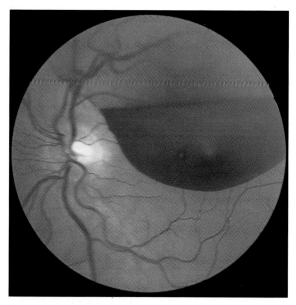

Fig. 12.34 Pre-retinal haemorrhage.

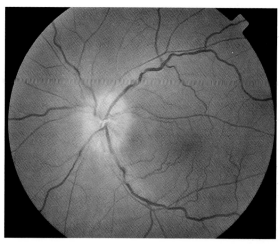

Fig. 12.35 Pale white swollen disc. This is highly suggestive of giant cell arteritis, particularly if associated with visual loss.

- Nuclear sclerosis ('ageing cataract') is the normally transparent lens yellowing before it becomes brown, then black. It cannot usually be detected in the red reflex, but symptoms and an inability to focus clearly on the retina confirm its presence.

Vitreous

Vitreous haemorrhage appears to the patient as black blobs that move with eye movement (intra-gel vitreous haemorrhage). Abnormal vitreous adhesion to normal retinal vessels may cause vitreous haemorrhage, and 'flashes of light' indicate that the retina may have torn. Haemorrhage in the space between the retina and the posterior surface of the vitreous causes a subhyaloid (pre-retinal) vitreous haemorrhage (Fig. 12.34).

Optic disc

A swollen white optic disc (Fig. 12.35) suggests arteritic anterior ischaemic optic neuropathy (giant cell arteritis and polyarteritis nodosa). Pseudophakic patients with artificial intraocular lenses following cataract extraction often have falsely pale discs. Increased cup-to-disc ratio (cupped disc) is seen with chronic open-angle glaucoma (a group of diseases of the optic nerve involving loss of retinal ganglion cells, associated with raised intraocular pressure and visual field loss). Typically, the vertical margins are affected first.

12.9 Common causes of arteriolar occlusion

- Accelerated hypertension
- Diabetic retinopathy
- HIV retinopathy
- Retinal vein occlusion
- Systemic lupus erythematosus
- Systemic vasculitis

The optic disc is a common site for new vessel formation. In the presence of an enlarged blind spot, blurring of the optic disc indicates distension of the optic nerve sheath. Reduced colour vision and a relative afferent pupillary response suggest an intrinsic optic nerve lesion.

Horizontal nerve fibre layer

The nerve fibre layer runs horizontally and over the retinal blood vessels. Lesions within this are therefore flat and striated, and obscure retinal blood vessels.

Arteriolar occlusion (Box 12.9) causes 'cotton wool' spot formation (Fig. 12.36A) and flame haemorrhages (Fig. 12.36B).

Roth's spots are flame-shaped haemorrhages with a central cotton wool spot. They are caused by immune complex deposition, and are seen in subacute bacterial endocarditis and serum sickness (Fig. 6.10, p. 116).

Retinitis due to infection with the herpes viruses causes a large, rapidly progressive area of 'cotton wool' spot formation. Differentiation can be difficult from the cotton wool spots caused by arterial occlusion and the two may co-exist in HIV infection. Cotton wool spots, however, do not enlarge over time, whereas areas of retinitis do (Box 12.10).

Retinal artery occlusion or embolism causes corresponding retinal pallor because of anterior retinal layer infarction. The optic nerve head, the fovea and the posterior retina, including the photoreceptors, are unaffected by retinal artery occlusion, as their blood supply is from the short posterior ciliary arteries of the ophthalmic artery. This explains the cherry red spot sign of central retinal artery occlusion, where the healthy fovea is surrounded by an oedematous retina (Fig. 12.37). Retinal emboli may be seen at vessel bifurcations. As only the luminal contents of the vessel are normally apparent and not the wall, the embolus

12.10 Causes of retinitis

- Cytomegalovirus
- Herpes simplex
- Herpes zoster
- Varicella zoster

may appear to be paradoxically wider than the vessel it is lodged in.

Vertical bipolar layer

The retinal capillaries are found in this layer. The most common causes of capillary disease are diabetes mellitus and retinal vein occlusion (Fig. 12.38). Capillary occlusion is also seen with HIV and radiation retinopathies. When a capillary occludes, microaneurysm formation may occur

at the site. Capillaries are too small to visualize with the naked eye. On ophthalmoscopy microaneurysms appear as round dots separate from blood vessels; they can haemorrhage and leak, leading to:

- dot haemorrhages: thin, vertical haemorrhages that may be difficult to differentiate from microaneurysms
- blot haemorrhages: larger, full-thickness bipolar layer haemorrhages that represent larger areas of capillary occlusion (Fig. 12.39).

Intra-retinal microvascular anomalies are perfused, dilated stumps of capillaries within areas of widespread capillary occlusion.

Venous beading is associated with adjacent capillary bed destruction.

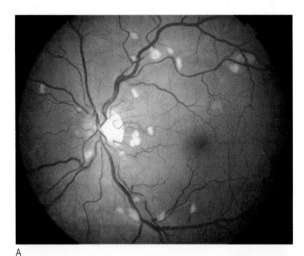

A

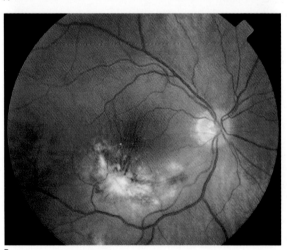

B

Fig. 12.36 Arteriolar occlusion of the horizontal nerve fibre layer. **(A)** Multiple cotton wool spots in HIV retinopathy. **(B)** Cytomegalovirus retinitis. Note the large superficial retinal infiltrate associated with flame haemorrhage.

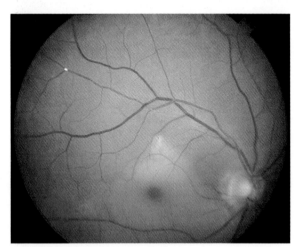

Fig. 12.37 Central retinal artery occlusion. Note the milky-white pale infarcted retina surrounding healthy pink fovea ('cherry red spot').

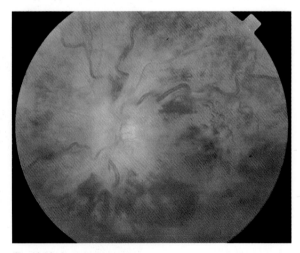

Fig. 12.38 Central retinal vein occlusion. Note the widespread retinal haemorrhages and swollen optic disc.

Microaneurysms, dot and blot haemorrhages, intra-retinal microvascular anomalies and venous beading are all surrogate markers for capillary occlusion. If sufficient capillaries occlude, then new vessels, originating from postcapillary venules, will form. These new vessels grow in the potential space between the retina and the posterior vitreous surface. They can be differentiated from normal retinal vessels because, instead of branching into smaller and finer vessels that eventually terminate, they form returning loops that distally are often more dilated than their proximal origins. New vessels grow intimately into the posterior surface of the vitreous and are found, unlike intra-retinal microvascular abnormalities, at the border of perfused and non-perfused retina (Fig. 12.40).

The vitreous is most strongly attached to the optic disc, and new vessels at this site are more likely to haemorrhage than elsewhere. New vessel formation is also commonly seen along the arcades, where the vitreous is less strongly adherent, and temporal to the macula.

Retinal veins and arteries share a common tunica adventitia where their branches cross over. Arteriosclerosis, commonly seen with hypertension, produces arteriovenous nipping, where the thickened artery, trapped by its tunica adventitia, twists and compresses the underlying vein. Arteriosclerosis is the most common cause of retinal vein occlusion. Raised intracapillary pressure subsequent to retinal vein occlusion results in capillary rupture and retinal haemorrhage. In central retinal vein occlusion, new

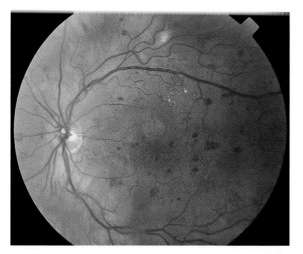

Fig. 12.39 Diabetic retinopathy. Note the presence of multiple dot and blot haemorrhages, indicating widespread capillary occlusion — a precursor of new vessel formation.

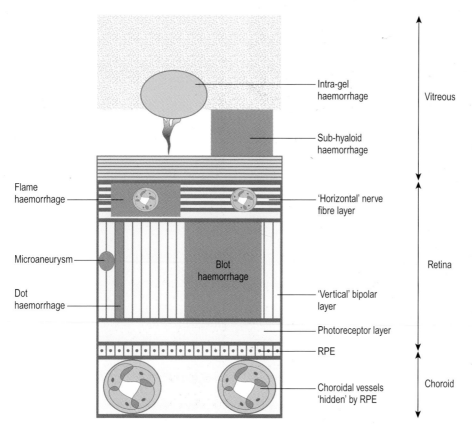

Fig. 12.40 Types of optic fundal haemorrhage, according to the retinal level. RPE, retinal pigment epithelium.

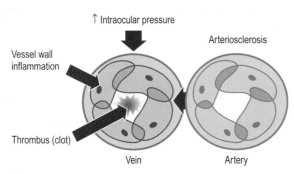

Fig. 12.41 Causes of retinal vein occlusion.

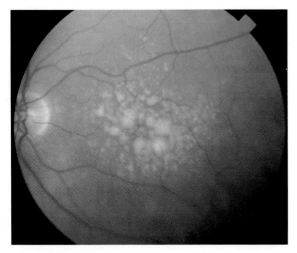

Fig. 12.42 Numerous large retinal drusen affecting the central retina (drusen maculopathy).

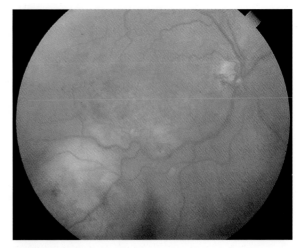

Fig. 12.43 Melanoma. Large and more significantly raised pigmented lesion deep to the retinal vessels, indicating its choroid origin.

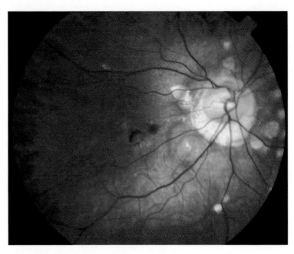

Fig. 12.44 Choroiditis. Multiple white lesions (multifocus choroiditis) with additional greenish choroidal neovascular membrane and adjacent retinal haemorrhage.

vessel formation may occur on the iris (rubeosis iridis). Subsequent scarring of the drainage angle leads to rubeotic glaucoma, which is blinding and extremely painful. Eyes at risk often have a relative afferent pupillary defect and profound visual loss (Fig. 12.41).

Arteriosclerotic retinal vein compression usually occurs in elderly patients or those with arteriosclerotic risk factors, such as smoking, hypertension, hyperlipidaemia or diabetes mellitus. Raised intraocular pressure from chronic open-angle glaucoma is also a common cause. In younger patients, strongly consider idiopathic retinal vasculitis or thrombophilia.

Retinal pigment epithelium and photoreceptors

Around 90% of the blood supply to the eye goes, via the short posterior ciliary arteries, to fenestrated choroidal blood vessels that supply the retinal pigment epithelium and the posterior retina by diffusion. Disease of the retinal pigmented cells often leads to death of the overlying photoreceptors. This is seen as

areas of depigmentation revealing the normally hidden choroidal vessels with adjacent clumps of precipitated pigment.

The most common disorder of the retinal pigment epithelium is age-related macular degeneration. It is preceded by drusen formation: amorphous depositions under the retinal pigment epithelium (Fig. 12.42). Drusen are differentiated from hard exudates, in people with diabetes mellitus, by the absence of adjacent microaneurysms. Atrophic age-related macular degeneration results in areas of pigment atrophy leading to gradual loss of central vision. Neovascular

OSCEs 12.11 Examine this patient with sudden loss of vision in one eye

1. Look at the hands for signs of smoking.
2. Examine the pulse for arrhythmia (atrial fibrillation).
3. Measure the blood pressure (hypertension).
4. Listen for cardiac murmurs and carotid bruits (valvular heart disease, carotid artery stenosis).
5. Measure the visual acuity in both eyes.
6. Check colour vision (optic nerve disease).
7. Assess both peripheral visual fields for homonymous hemianopia (cerebrovascular accident) and the affected eye's visual field for an altitudinal or arcuate field defect (optic nerve disease).
8. Examine for a relative afferent pupillary defect (optic nerve disease).
9. Assess pain on eye movement (optic neuritis).
10. Perform ophthalmoscopy. The optic nerve is:
    White and swollen in arteritic anterior ischaemic optic neuropathy (giant cell arteritis)
    Pink and swollen in non-arteritic anterior ischaemic optic neuropathy.
11. Look at the optic fundus:
    Numerous retinal haemorrhages indicate venous occlusion
    Pallor indicates arterial occlusion
    Retinal embolism is seen at arterial bifurcations (thromboembolic disease).

12

OSCEs 12.12 Examine this patient with acute redness and pain in one eye

1. Assess the distribution of the redness:
    Diffuse redness suggests conjunctivitis, episcleritis, scleritis
    Redness of the lower inner eyelid suggests conjunctivitis
    Circumciliary injection suggests keratitis, iritis or angle-closure glaucoma
    Redness resolving with phenylephrine drops suggests episcleritis.
2. Look for evidence of ocular discharge (conjunctivitis).
3. Examine the clarity of the iris — a hazy iris suggests corneal oedema (acute angle-closure glaucoma) or aqueous chamber inflammatory cells (acute iritis).
4. Look for the small, irregularly shaped pupil of acute iritis, or an oval, mid-dilated, poorly reactive pupil (acute-angle closure glaucoma).
5. Ask the patient to move the eye — pain indicates scleritis.
6. Examine the red reflex with direct ophthalmoscopy: corneal ulceration appears black — confirm with fluorescein dye.
7. Examine the urine for microscopic haematuria or proteinuria (systemic vasculitis).
8. Assess visual acuity.

age-related macular degeneration is more severe and is associated with rapid-onset visual distortion and central visual loss. Visual loss results from choroidal new vessels growing under the photoreceptors.

Hyperpigmentation of the retinal pigment epithelium (choroidal naevi) is a common asymptomatic finding. In contrast, malignant melanomas (Fig. 12.43) are usually symptomatic and elevated, progress in size and may be associated with retinal detachment and vitreous haemorrhage.

Choroiditis (inflammation of the choroid) appears as white spots (Fig. 12.44). When active, they have a white, poorly defined, fluffy edge with an overlying hazy vitreous, causing blurring of vision. When inactive, they have a well-defined pigmented edge. As the nerve fibre layer is not involved, the overlying retinal blood vessels are unaffected, and are clearly visible as they cross the choroiditis. Choroiditis is associated with toxoplasmosis, sarcoidosis and tuberculosis.

INVESTIGATIONS

Visual symptoms and signs often result from systemic disorders. Specialized tests include:

- lumbar puncture to examine the cerebrospinal fluid
- electrical recordings of brain, muscle, nerve, etc. (neurophysiology)
- radiological procedures (neuroradiology)
- automated visual field analysis
- fundal photography
- specific genetic tests (neurogenetics) (Boxes 12.13 and 12.14).

12.13 Investigations in eye disease

Investigation	Indication/Comment
Bedside tests	
Refraction	Short and long sight, lens disorders, cataract, corneal disorders
Corneal staining	Corneal epithelial disease
Schirmer's tear test	Dry eyes
Intraocular pressure	Glaucoma
Urinalysis	Vasculitis, renal disease and diabetes mellitus
Mantoux skin test	Tuberculosis
Blood tests	
Renal function, ESR, CRP	Systemic disease, including vasculitis
Autoantibodies	Autoimmune disease
ACE activity	Sarcoidosis
HIV and syphilis serology	Atypical uveitis or neurological signs
Prolactin	Optic neuropathy, pituitary macroadenoma
Neurophysiology	
Electrophysiology	Optic nerve and retinal disorders
Radiology	
Chest X-ray	Sarcoidosis, tuberculosis
Orbital ultrasound	Inadequate fundal view because of cataract
Digital photography	Documentation of fundal findings
Optical coherence tomography	Macular disorders
Fundus fluorescein angiography	Retinal disorders
CT brain	Intracranial tumours, compressive lesions
MRI brain	Pituitary lesion, demyelination
Invasive tests	
Lumbar puncture	Multiple sclerosis, inflammatory optic neuropathies
Temporal artery biopsy	Giant cell arteritis

12.14 Key points: the visual system

- Blepharitis is a common cause of dry eyes and ocular discomfort.
- Pain on moving one eye suggests optic neuritis or scleritis.
- Circumciliary injection indicates iris root/ciliary body inflammation, e.g. iritis, keratitis, angle-closure glaucoma.
- Patients describe the deficit of amaurosis fugax as black or grey.
- The aura of migraine is a positive visual phenomenon that may be white, coloured or scintillating.
- Sudden-onset permanent visual loss is usually caused by vascular occlusion.
- A white, swollen optic disc with visual loss suggests giant cell arteritis.
- Distortion of vision suggests disruption of the macular photoreceptors by blood, fluid, scar or traction.
- Flashes and floaters are forerunners of retinal detachment.
- Haloes are associated with angle-closure glaucoma.
- Pain on eye movement is common in optic neuritis; review the diagnosis if it is not present.
- Unilateral optic nerve lesions cause a relative afferent pupillary defect, even with apparently normal vision; with macular lesions this is a late finding.
- In oculomotor (III) nerve palsy in a comatose patient the pupillary reflex is preserved when coma is metabolic, but is lost with a structural brain lesion.

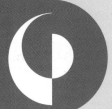

Fiona Nicol
Robert Mills

The ear, nose and throat

13

13

THE EAR

ANATOMY

The ear is divided into external, middle and inner ear and is concerned with hearing and balance.

External ear

This consists of the pinna, the external auditory canal (meatus) and the lateral surface of the tympanic membrane (Fig. 13.1). The skin of the outer third of the external auditory meatus contains hair, and sebaceous and ceruminous glands. Squamous debris from the outer part of the drum migrates to the outside, mixing with cerumen and sebum to become wax.

Middle ear

The middle ear is the medial surface of the tympanic membrane, the tympanic cavity and the Eustachian tube. Three bones — the malleus, incus and stapes (the ossicles) — transmit sound from the external ear to the inner ear. The Eustachian tube communicates with the pharynx. The tympanic membrane (eardrum) lies obliquely across the external auditory meatus. It is normally grey and semitranslucent; the lower part, the pars tensa, has a fibrous middle layer which the upper pars flaccida lacks. The handle of the malleus attaches on to the fibrous layer of the pars tensa. Both this and the short process of the malleus can be seen using an otoscope (Fig. 13.2).

The chorda tympani, a branch of the facial (VIII) nerve, passes horizontally medial to the malleus and lateral to the incus. It carries taste fibres from the anterior two-thirds of the tongue and may be damaged by severe trauma to the middle ear.

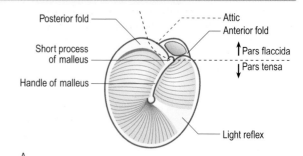

A

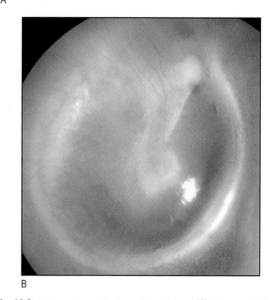

B

Fig. 13.2 Auriscopic examination of the right ear. (A) Diagram showing the main structures. **(B)** A normal tympanic membrane.

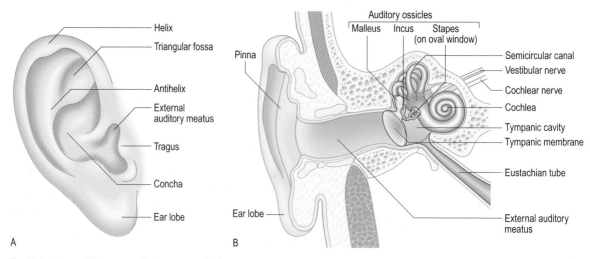

A   B

Fig. 13.1 The ear. (A) The pinna. **(B)** Cross-section of the outer, middle and inner ears.

Inner ear

The inner ear or labyrinth comprises the cochlea (hearing) and the vestibular portion (balance). The hair cells in the cochlea convert the mechanical energy from sound into electrical impulses, which are transmitted in the cochlear division of cranial nerve VIII.

The vestibular part of the inner ear contains the lateral, superior and posterior semicircular canals, arranged at right angles to each other and opening into the vestibule which contains the utricle and the saccule. They contain a fluid called endolymph. Head movement causes movement of the endolymph to stimulate hair processes embedded in the membrane lining, and these movements are converted into nerve impulses in the vestibular division of the vestibulocochlear (VIII) nerve. The vestibulo-ocular reflex maintains gaze during head movement and generates conjugate eye movement to preserve macular fixation.

SYMPTOMS AND DEFINITIONS

Pain and itching

These are common. Earache may be referred from the throat (Boxes 13.1 and 13.2).

Otorrhoea

A chronic offensive scanty discharge may be a sign of a cholesteatoma (a mass of keratin which grows in a pocket formed by retraction of part of the tympanic membrane, usually in the attic). Bleeding is most often due to the formation of granulation tissue in the ear. In chronic discharge, pain suggests otitis externa, not malignant change or cholesteatoma. A new traumatic perforation in the tympanic membrane has a ragged edge; chronic perforations have smooth margins.

Hearing loss

Hearing loss can be mild, moderate, severe or profound, and is commonly progressive. People who develop hearing loss before they acquire speech have unusual speech that is vowel-based and lacks clear articulation of specific consonants (Box 13.3).

Tinnitus

This subjective sensation of sound with no auditory stimulus can be caused by almost any pathology in the auditory apparatus. Objective tinnitus is a sound heard by both the patient and the doctor, and may be due to a variety of causes, e.g. palatal myoclonus. Tinnitus is often, but not always, accompanied by hearing loss.

13.2 Causes of earache (otalgia)

Otological

- Acute otitis externa
- Acute otitis media
- Perichondritis
- Trauma
- Herpes zoster (Ramsay Hunt syndrome)
- Tumour

Non-otological

- Tonsillitis and pharyngitis
- Temporomandibular joint dysfunction
- Dental disease
- Cervical spine disease
- Cancer of the pharynx or larynx

13.1 Symptoms and definitions in ear disease

Symptom	Definition	Common cause
Otalgia	Pain	Otitis media or externa, referred from pharyngitis, trauma or rarely cancer
Pruritus	Itching	Otitis externa
Otorrhoea	Discharge	
	Purulent	Eardrum perforation with infection Otitis externa
	Mucoid	Eardrum peroration, severe trauma causing leak of cerebrospinal fluid (CSF)
	Bloodstained	Granulation tissue from infection, trauma
Hearing loss	Deafness	Box 13.3
Tinnitus	Noise in the absence of an objective source	Presbyacusis, noise damage
Vertigo	Hallucination of movement	Inner ear disease
Unsteadiness		Vestibular or central disease

13.3 Causes of hearing loss

Conductive[1]

- Wax
- Otitis externa
- Middle ear effusion
- Trauma to the tympanic membrane/ossicles
- Otosclerosis
- Chronic middle ear infection
- Tumours of the middle ear

Sensorineural[2]

- Genetic, e.g. Alport's syndrome, Jervell–Lange–Nielsen syndrome
- Prenatal infection, e.g. rubella
- Birth injury
- Infection:
  - Meningitis
  - Measles
  - Mumps
- Trauma
- Ménière's disease
- Degenerative (presbyacusis)
- Occupation- or other noise-induced
- Acoustic neuroma
- Idiopathic

[1] Disruption to the mechanical transfer of sound in outer ear, eardrum or ossicles.
[2] Cochlear or central damage.

Vertigo

Patients feel that they or their surroundings are moving, most commonly rotating. Vertigo is usually peripheral and due to disease of one or both inner ears, but may rarely be central and due to disturbance of the vestibular nerve nuclei, brainstem or cerebellum (Box 13.4).

The following help make the diagnosis:

- the duration of the episodes
- the presence or absence of hearing loss, particularly unilateral or asymmetrical hearing loss
- a history of fluctuations in hearing level
- the presence or absence of tinnitus
- the presence or absence of aural fullness, particularly with the episodes
- precipitating factors
- a past history of significant head injury
- headaches with the episodes (Boxes 13.5 and 13.6).

Vestibular neuronitis is acute vestibular failure of unknown cause. It causes acute vertigo and vomiting, worsened by any head movements, along with malaise and ataxia. It lasts days or weeks and resolves completely.

13.4 Causes of vertigo

Peripheral vertigo

- Vestibular neuronitis
- Benign positional vertigo
- Drugs e.g. gentamicin, anticonvulsants
- Ménière's disease
- Trauma

Central vertigo

- Brainstem ischaemia or infarction
- Migraine
- Multiple sclerosis (MS)

13.6 Drugs that cause ototoxicity

Type	Examples
Antibiotics	Gentamicin
Cytotoxics	Cisplatin
Diuretics	Furosemide given IV after aminoglycosides
Analgesics	Aspirin
Others	Quinine

13.5 Diagnosing vertigo

	Acute labyrinthitis (vestibular neuronitis)	Benign paroxysmal positional vertigo	Ménière's disease	Central vertigo
Duration	Days	Seconds or minutes	Hours	Hours — migraine Days and weeks — MS Long term — cerebrovascular accident (CVA)
Hearing loss	–	–	++	–
Tinnitus	–	–	++	–
Aural fullness	–	–	++	–
Episodes	Rarely	Yes	Recurrent vertigo; persistent tinnitus and progressive sensorineural deafness	Migraine — recurs CNS damage — usually some recovery but often persistent
Triggers	May have upper respiratory symptoms	Lying on affected ear	None	Drugs Cardiovascular disease

Benign paroxysmal positional vertigo (BPPV) causes attacks of vertigo particularly marked when lying on one side. It may be due to debris in the posterior semicircular canals. Ménière's disease is thought to be due to increased pressure within the endolymph.

Unsteadiness

Unsteadiness is a feeling of instability and is different from vertigo, although patients may experience both. Unsteadiness and a feeling of light-headedness are vague, common symptoms and often unrelated to vertigo. It can be very difficult to understand exactly what patients are complaining of when they use these terms or say they are 'giddy' or 'dizzy', so clarify exactly what they mean and how their symptoms affect them. Light-headedness is not a vestibular symptom but unsteadiness may be. Patients with ataxia may complain of being unsteady. The only life-threatening causes of vertigo and unsteadiness are central, i.e. from brainstem or cerebellar changes, and uncommon, but it is important to differentiate them.

Nystagmus

Nystagmus is an involuntary rhythmical oscillation of the eyes. It may be vertical, horizontal, rotatory or multidirectional. The most common form is biphasic or jerk nystagmus with a slow (pathological) drift in one direction followed by a fast correction in the opposite direction. The direction of the fast phase or jerk is used to describe the direction of the nystagmus. Pendular nystagmus (oscillations equal in rate and amplitude about a central point) occurs with central defects of vision.

THE HISTORY

Past history

A past history of previous ear problems (notably discharge), particularly in childhood, indicates that the hearing problem is the result of previous chronic otitis media. Past medical history may identify a systemic disease associated with hearing loss, e.g. Wegener's granulomatosis.

Family history

Family history is important, since some types of sensorineural deafness are inherited. Otosclerosis, a cause of conductive deafness in which the stapes footplate becomes fixed, is also inherited in some cases.

Drug history

This may identify the previous administration of ototoxic medication. Ototoxicity may primarily affect hearing, e.g. cisplatinum, or balance, e.g. gentamicin.

Social history

A history of previous noise exposure, either at work or during leisure activities, is important, since prolonged exposure to loud noise can cause sensorineural hearing loss.

THE PHYSICAL EXAMINATION

Examination sequence

The ear

▶ Look at the pinna, noting its shape, size and any deformity. Gently pull on the pinna and ask if it is sore. Look at the size of the meatus. If it is very wide, this suggests previous mastoid surgery. Note any discharge or colour change in the skin.

▶ Use an auriscope with the largest speculum that will comfortably fit the external auditory meatus. Explain to the patient what you are going to do.

▶ Hold the auriscope comfortably and rest the ulnar border of your hand against the patient's cheek (Fig. 13.3). If the patient moves his head during your examination, your hand will move too and limit any trauma to the ear.

▶ Gently pull the pinna upwards and backwards to straighten the cartilaginous external auditory meatus. Introduce the speculum and inspect the skin of the external auditory meatus for infection, wax and foreign bodies. Look at the tympanic membrane. You should see a cone of light as the concave surface of the tympanic membrane reflects the light forwards — the light reflex. Note the pearly grey translucent appearance of the normal drum.

Abnormal findings

Congenital atresia of the ear canal is frequently associated with deformity (microtia) or even absence of the pinna. Trauma may produce a haematoma of the pinna. Basal cell and squamous cell cancers typically occur on the superior aspect of the pinna, which is

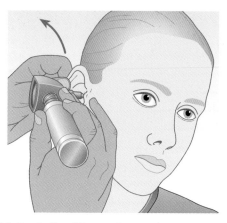

Fig. 13.3 Examination of the ear using an auriscope.

particularly vulnerable to sun damage (Fig. 13.4). Tenderness on palpation of the tragus suggests infection of the external auditory meatus or temporomandibular joint problems.

Discharge without a perforation or retraction pocket of the tympanic membrane indicates otitis externa (Fig. 13.5). In severe otitis externa or furunculosis where a boil is present, the external auditory meatus may be completely occluded, and any attempt at otoscopy will provoke severe pain. The lumen may be also be partially or completely occluded by exostoses (Fig. 13.6). A solitary bony swelling of the ear canal is likely to be an osteoma.

White patches on the tympanic membrane are tympanosclerosis, a form of scarring. Note the position of any perforations in relation to the handle of the malleus (Fig. 13.7). If the perforation includes most of the tympanic membrane, it is subtotal. Differentiate perforations from retraction pockets of the pars tensa

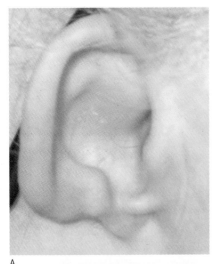

A

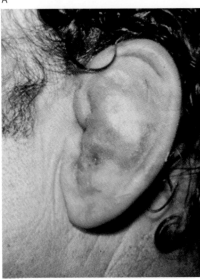

B

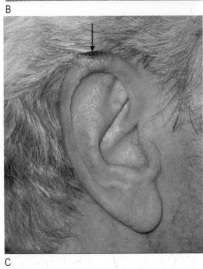

C

Fig. 13.4 The pinna. **(A)** Microtia. **(B)** Haematoma. **(C)** Squamous cancer (arrow).

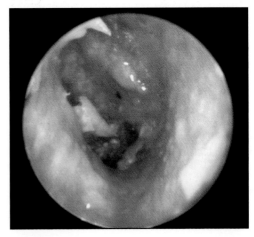

Fig. 13.5 Otitis externa.

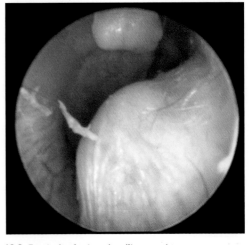

Fig. 13.6 Exostosis of external auditory meatus.

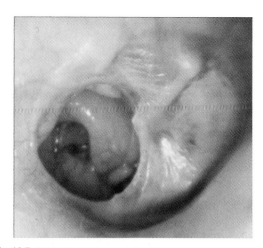

Fig. 13.7 Tympanic membrane perforation.

where the drum is intact, but thinned and collapsed on to the medial wall of the middle ear (Fig. 13.8). A retraction pocket containing a mass of keratin is a cholesteatoma (Fig. 13.9). It is most commonly found in the attic region, but may also involve the pars tensa. The presence of fluid behind the tympanic membrane indicates otitis media with effusion (OME; Fig. 13.10). Typically, the drum is dull and there are dilated blood vessels radiating across its surface. In adults the fluid is more likely to be serous and the drum yellow in colour. There may be a fluid level behind the drum (Fig. 13.11). Surgical treatment of OME usually involves insertion of a ventilation tube or grommet (Fig. 13.12). In acute suppurative otitis media the drum appearances are similar to those of OME in the early stages (Fig. 13.13). Subsequently the drum becomes red. With further progression the drum bulges and perforation with discharge may occur.

13

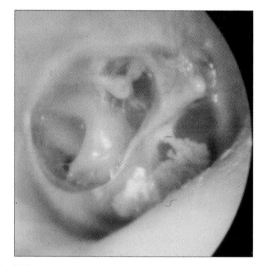

Fig. 13.8 Retraction pocket of the pars tensa.

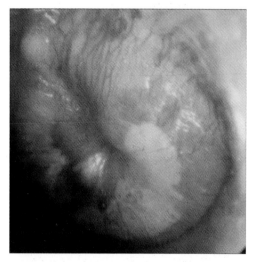

Fig. 13.10 Otitis media with effusion.

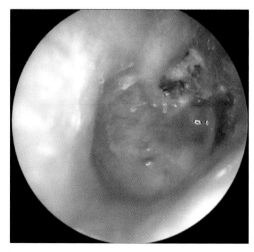

Fig. 13.9 Cholesteatoma.

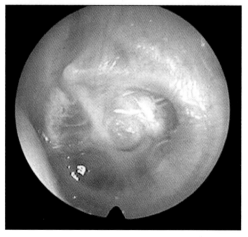

Fig. 13.11 Fluid level behind tympanic membrane in otitis media.

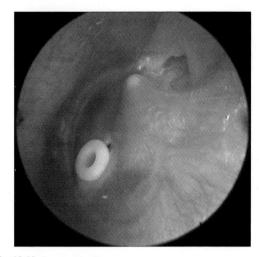

Fig. 13.12 Grommet in situ.

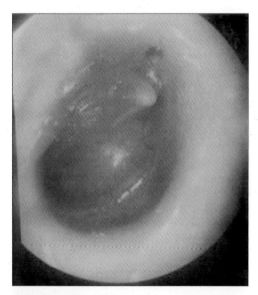

Fig. 13.13 Acute otitis media.

TESTING HEARING

Testing hearing and vestibular function assesses the vestibulocochlear (VIII) nerve. Hearing can only be properly assessed by audiometry, but an impression of the severity of the hearing loss may be gained by noting how the patient responds to normal speech. Adults complain of hearing loss but children usually do not. Parents may notice that children turn up the sound on the TV or report poor concentration and performance at school.

▶ Examination sequence

Whispered voice test

- ▶ Stand behind the patient.
- ▶ Start with your mouth about 15 cm from the ear you are testing.
- ▶ Mask hearing in the other ear by rubbing the tragus.
- ▶ Ask the patient to repeat your words. Use a combination of numbers and letters. Start at 15 cm with a normal speaking voice to confirm that the patient understands the test.
- ▶ Repeat, but this time at arm's length from the patient's ear. Typically, if a patient can hear a whispered voice at 60 cm, his hearing is better than 30 dB: that is, normal.

Tuning fork tests

Use a 512 Hz or 256 Hz tuning fork to help differentiate conductive or sensorineural hearing loss.

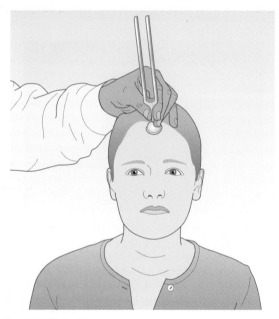

Fig. 13.14 Weber's test.

▶ Examination sequence

Weber's test (Fig. 13.14)

- ▶ Hit the prongs of the fork against a hard surface to make it vibrate.
- ▶ Place the base of the vibrating tuning fork on top of the patient's head or in the middle of the forehead.
- ▶ Ask the patient where he hears the sound; normally this is in the middle or equally in both ears.
- ▶ Note to which side Weber's test lateralizes.

Abnormal findings

In symmetrical hearing loss, the sound is also heard in the middle. It is heard loudest in the ear with conductive deafness, since there is no interference from extraneous noise. In unilateral sensorineural deafness the sound is loudest in the unaffected ear.

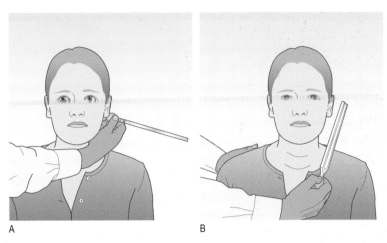

Fig. 13.15 **Rinne's tests. (A)** Testing bone conduction. **(B)** Testing air conduction.

◼▶ Examination sequence

Rinne's test (Fig. 13.15)

- Hit the prongs of the fork against a hard surface to make it vibrate.
- Place the vibrating prongs at the patient's external auditory meatus; ask if he can hear it.
- Place the still-vibrating base on the mastoid process and ask whether it is louder in front of or behind the ear.

Abnormal findings

If the sound is louder at the ear canal, the test is positive and air conduction is better than bone conduction. Record this as AC > BC; this is normal.

If the sound is louder on the mastoid process, the test is negative; bone conduction is better than air conduction. Record this as BC > AC.

Rinne's test is negative in conductive deafness. An exception is when one ear has no hearing at all. The test may be negative because sound is conducted through the skull bones to the 'good' ear — a false-negative Rinne's test. The Weber test is more sensitive than Rinne's test in unilateral conductive deafness, so a positive Rinne with a Weber referred to the deafer ear indicates a relatively mild conductive deafness.

Testing vestibular function

◼▶ Examination sequence

Testing for nystagmus

- With the patient seated, hold your finger an arm's length away, level with the patient's eyes.
- Ask the patient to look at and follow the tip of your finger as you slowly move it up and down and then side to side.
- Look at the patient's eyes for any oscillations and note:
  - whether they are horizontal, vertical or rotatory
  - which direction of gaze causes the most marked nystagmus

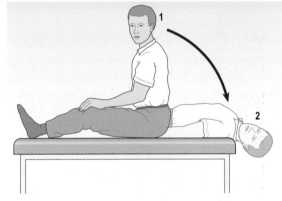

Fig. 13.16 Dix–Hallpike position test.

- in which direction the fast phase of jerk nystagmus occurs
- whether jerk nystagmus changes direction when the direction of gaze changes
- if nystagmus is more obvious in one eye than the other (ataxic or dysconjugate nystagmus).

- At extremes of lateral gaze normal subjects may show a few nystagmoid jerks (Box 13.7).

Dix–Hallpike positional test (Fig. 13.16)

- Ask the patient to sit upright, close to the edge of the couch.
- Turn the patient's head 45° to one side.
- Rapidly lower him, so that the head is now 30° below the horizontal. Ask patients to keep their eyes open.
- Watch their eyes carefully for nystagmus. Repeat the test, turning the head to the other side.

Abnormal findings

In benign paroxysmal positional vertigo there is a latent period of up to 20 seconds before the patient experiences vertigo, accompanied by rotatory nystagmus which

13

341

13.7 Characteristics of nystagmus

Nystagmus type	Clinical pathology	Characteristics	
		Fast phase	**Maximal on looking**
Pendular	Eyes, e.g. congenital blindness, albinism	No fast phase	Straight ahead
Jerk Peripheral	Semicircular canal, vestibular nerve	Unidirectional Dix–Hallpike fatigues on repetition	Away from affected side
Central	Brainstem, cerebellum	Bidirectional (changes with direction of gaze) Dix–Hallpike persists	To either side
Dysconjugate (ataxic)	Interconnections of III, IV and VI nerves (medial longitudinal bundle)	Typically affects the abducting eye	To either side

OSCEs 13.8 Examine this patient who complains of earache

1. Carry out a general examination, looking for evidence of systemic upset (acute otitis media).
2. Inspect and palpate the pinna and surrounding area (acute mastoiditis, acute otitis externa, trauma (haematoma), previous surgery).
3. Inspect both external auditory meati for signs of discharge, crusting and excoriation (acute otitis media, acute otitis externa).
4. Feel the tragus for tenderness (acute otitis externa).
5. Using the otoscope, examine the external auditory meati (lift the pinna upwards and backwards to straighten the canal).
6. Inspect the tympanic membrane for surface appearance and integrity. If the view is obscured with wax/debris, consider manual removal or microsuction.
7. Ask the patient to open and close the jaw while you palpate the temporomandibular joints, listening for a click (temporomandibular joint dysfunction).
8. Examine the throat (referred pain from the oropharynx).
9. Consider other investigations such as audiology (hearing test).

OSCEs 13.9 Examine this patient who complains of being dizzy and lightheaded

1. Is the patient pale (anaemia) or sweating (cardiac disease, anxiety, labyrinthitis)?
2. Check pulse, blood pressure lying and standing, and temperature (dysrhythmias, hypotension or viral infection).
3. Look for a facial palsy (cholesteatoma).
4. Examine the ears (cholesteatoma).
5. Examine for nystagmus.
6. Carry out the Dix–Hallpike test.
7. Perform Romberg's test (sensory ataxia).
8. Carry out Unterberger's test (labyrinthitis, vestibular disease).
9. Watch the patient walk: slow, fast and turn, heel to toe (cerebellar disease).

13.10 Investigations in ear disease

Investigation	Indication/Comment
Swab from external auditory meatus	Otitis media and externa
MRI scan	Acoustic neuroma
Audiometry	Hearing loss A single-frequency tone at different noise levels is presented to each ear in turn through headphones in a soundproof booth. The intensity is reduced in 10-decibel steps until patients can no longer hear it. The threshold is the quietest sound they can hear
Impedance audiometry (tympanometry)	Otitis media with effusion Eustachian tube dysfunction Ossicular discontinuity The compliance of the eardrum is measured during changes in the pressure in the ear canal. Compliance should be maximal at atmospheric pressure
Vestibular testing Caloric tests	Unilateral vestibular hypofunction Water at 30°C and then 44°C is irrigated into the external ear canal. Electronystagmography records nystagmus. The response is reduced in vestibular hypofunction
Posturography	Vestibular hypofunction Reveals whether patients rely on vision or proprioception more than usual

beats towards the lower ear. This response fatigues, so if you repeat the test immediately there will be a lesser response. This is adaptation. Central pathology produces immediate nystagmus, not necessarily with vertigo, and shows no adaptation.

Unterberger's test

Patients march on the spot with their eyes closed. They rotate to the side of the damaged labyrinth.

Fistula test

Repeatedly compress the tragus against the external auditory meatus to occlude the meatus. If this produces a sense of imbalance or vertigo with nystagmus, it suggests an abnormal communication between the middle ear and the vestibular apparatus, e.g. erosion due to cholesteatoma.

THE NOSE AND SINUSES

ANATOMY

The nose is formed from two nasal bones. The shape is dictated by the cartilages in the lower two-thirds of the nose. The septal cartilage divides the nose into two nasal cavities. The outer skin continues just inside these cavities and contains hair and sebaceous glands. The nasal cavities open to the exterior through the nostrils (anterior nares), and on their lateral wall the paired superior, inferior and middle turbinates are found (Fig. 13.17).

The paranasal sinuses — maxillary, frontal, ethmoid and sphenoid — are air-filled spaces in the bones of the skull which open through ostia into the nasal cavity. The nose warms and humidifies inspired air and detects smells.

SYMPTOMS AND DEFINITIONS

Nasal obstruction

Persistent unilateral obstruction is often due to a deviated nasal septum caused by trauma, but it may be congenital. Bilateral obstruction may be due to polyps from chronic rhinitis.

Nasal discharge

Discharge may be unilateral or bilateral. A watery discharge suggests allergic rhinitis but purulent discharge suggests bacterial infection and occurs in the later stages

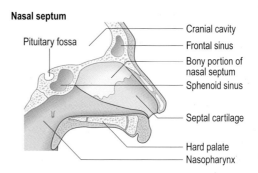

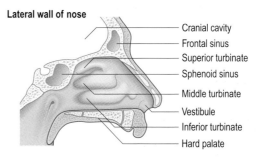

Fig. 13.17 The nose and paranasal sinuses.

of coryza, in sinus infection or when there is a foreign body in the nose.

Epistaxis

This is bleeding from inside the nose. There is a rich blood supply to an area of the anterior nasal septum (Little's area) that is easily traumatized and is a common site for bleeding, especially in children. Epistaxis may be life-threatening in the elderly.

Sneezing

This is the protective sudden expulsive effort which clears the nasal passages of irritants. It is common in viral upper respiratory infection and allergic rhinitis.

13.11 Symptoms and definitions in nasal disease

Symptom	Definition	Common cause
Nose blocked		Viral illness, deviated nasal septum, nasal polyp
Rhinorrhoea	Discharge	Watery — allergic rhinitis, CSF leak Purulent — infection, foreign body
Epistaxis	Nose bleed	Trauma, infection
Sneezing		Allergy, infection
Coughing		Postnasal drip
Anosmia	Absence of smell	Head injury, viral neuropathy
Hyposmia	Reduced smell	Nasal polyps, nasal blockage
Cacosmia	Unpleasant smell	Chronic anaerobic sepsis
Nasal deformity		Trauma, rhinophyma
Pain		Sinus infection, dental infection
Septum perforation		Nose-picking, granulomatous disease, e.g. Wegener's granulomatosis, cocaine use, inhalation of industrial dusts, e.g. nickel, chromium

Disturbance of smell

Anosmia (complete loss of olfaction) may follow head injury with damage to the olfactory epithelium/olfactory nerve or can occur after a viral upper respiratory tract infection. Mechanical obstruction of the nose by nasal polyps or severe mucosal oedema and swelling in allergic rhinitis usually causes hyposmia (reduced sense of smell). Cacosmia is an unpleasant smell due to chronic sepsis in the nose.

Nasal deformity

Swelling and bruising from trauma settle over 2 weeks but the nose may remain deformed if the nasal bones have been displaced. Skin affected by acne rosacea over the course of years causes rhinophyma (Fig. 13.18). Destruction of the nasal septum produces flattening of the bridge and a 'saddle' deformity. Causes include Wegener's granulomatosis, congenital syphilis and chronic abuse of cocaine. Widening of the nose is an early feature of acromegaly and a late feature of neglected nasal polyposis.

Nasal and facial pain

Nasal pain is extremely rare, except following trauma. Facial pain is common and caused by migraine, sinusitis, dental sepsis and trigeminal neuralgia and cluster headache, characteristically with unilateral nasal discharge and eye watering.

THE HISTORY

Past history

A past history of atopy, including allergic or perennial rhinitis, is related to nasal polyps and sinusitis. Recurrent upper respiratory tract infections may cause sinusitis. Prolonged bleeding is associated with, but not caused by, hypertension and bleeding diathesis. Trauma, both recent and old, to the face and nose may cause nasal blockage, deformity and anosmia.

Drug history

Anticoagulants and non-steroidal anti-inflammatory drugs (NSAIDs) may aggravate epistaxis. 'Snorting'

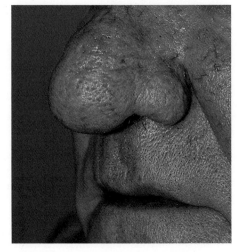

Fig. 13.18 Rhinophyma as a complication of rosacea.

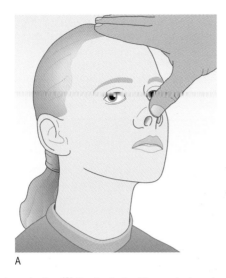
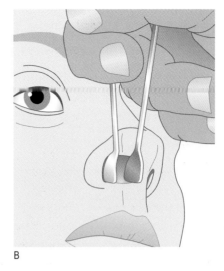

A

B

Fig. 13.19 Nasal examination. (A) Elevating the tip of the nose to give a clear view of the anterior nares. **(B)** Anterior rhinoscopy using a Thudicom's nasal speculum.

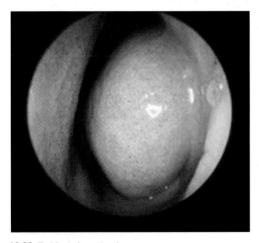

Fig. 13.20 Turbinate hypertrophy.

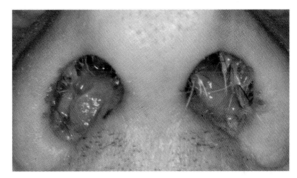

Fig. 13.21 Nasal polyps.

cocaine can cause perforation of the nasal septum. Alcohol worsens acne rosacea and rhinophyma.

Family history

Family history of atopy is relevant in hayfever and nasal polyposis.

Social history

Exposure to inhaled wood dust in certain occupations was associated with an increase of sinus cancer. Exposure to other dusts, particularly at work, may exacerbate allergic rhinitis.

OSCEs 13.12 Examine this patient who complains of a blocked nose

1. Inspect the external nasal pyramid for asymmetry or evidence of trauma.
2. Using your thumb, lift the nasal tip to inspect the nostrils, e.g. septal haematoma following a blow to the nose.
3. Ask the patient to sniff while gently occluding each nostril in turn. In children hold a mirror or metal spatula under their nostrils, looking for two patches of condensation from expired air — the 'mirror test'.
4. Examine the anterior nasal cavity, especially the position of the septum and size of the inferior turbinates, using a large speculum on an otoscope. Look for nasal polyps, foreign bodies (especially in children) or other soft tissue swellings.
5. Refer to visualize the postnasal space (nasopharynx): with endoscopy in adults and older children, or lateral soft tissue X-ray in young children/infants (adenoidal hypertrophy).
6. Consider further investigations, such as allergy testing (allergic rhinitis) and a CT scan of the paranasal sinuses (chronic rhinosinusitis).

13.13 Investigations in nasal disease

Investigation	Indication/Comment
Plain X-ray	Nasal bone fracture Not required for the diagnosis
Lateral X-ray nasopharynx	Adenoidal hypertrophy Young children
Nasal endoscopy	Sinus disease
CT scan	Sinus disease, trauma and cancer Radiation dose to the eyes is significant, so avoid repeat imaging

THE PHYSICAL EXAMINATION

▶ Examination sequence

The nose and sinuses

Inspection

▶ Look at the external surface and appearance of the nose. Note any skin disease or deformity.

▶ Stand behind the patient and ask him to look upwards.

▶ Look down the nose from above to detect any deviation.

▶ Press on the tip of the nose to elevate it and inspect the anterior nares (Fig. 13.19).

▶ In children, you may see the nasal vestibule, the anterior end of the septum and the anterior end of the inferior turbinates. In adults, use a nasal speculum or a large-bore speculum on an auriscope.

▶ Note if the septum is in the midline, any bleeding points, clots where bleeding has recently stopped, crusting and perforations.

▶ On the lateral wall, inspect the anterior end of the inferior turbinate.

Palpation

▶ Feel the nasal bones gently to distinguish bony from cartilaginous deformity.

▶ Feel any facial swelling for tenderness. Block each nostril in turn and ask the patient to breathe in so that you can assess nasal obstruction.

▶ Specialists can see the postnasal space by using a small mirror inserted through the mouth and passed beyond the soft palate or by passing a nasal endoscope to the back of the nose.

Abnormal findings

The nasal mucosa is pale, moist and hypertrophied in allergic rhinitis (Fig. 13.20). In chronic rhinitis, it is swollen and red. A pale grey, moist swelling blocking the nostril may be a polyp (Fig. 13.21). If you probe a polyp in the nasal cavity, it will feel soft, mobile and pain-free. This is difficult to do without using a head-light so that your hands are free. Facial swelling is unusual in sinusitis but occurs with a dental root abscess and with cancer of the maxillary antrum.

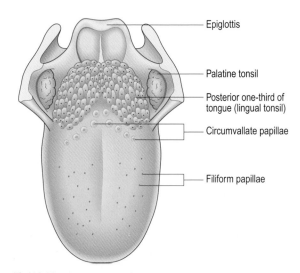

Fig. 13.23 Anatomy of the tongue.

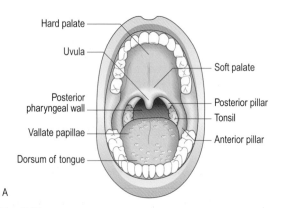

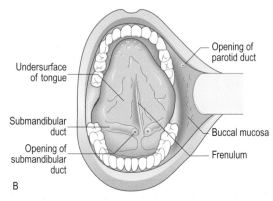

Fig. 13.22 Anatomy of the mouth and throat. (A) Examination with the mouth open. **(B)** With the tongue touching the roof of the mouth.

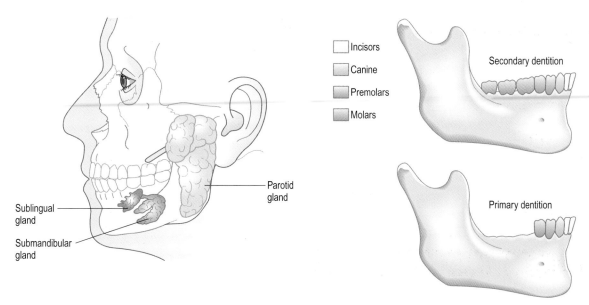

Sublingual gland

Submandibular gland

Parotid gland

Incisors

Canine

Premolars

Molars

Secondary dentition

Primary dentition

Fig. 13.24 The position of the major salivary glands.

Fig. 13.25 Primary and secondary dentition.

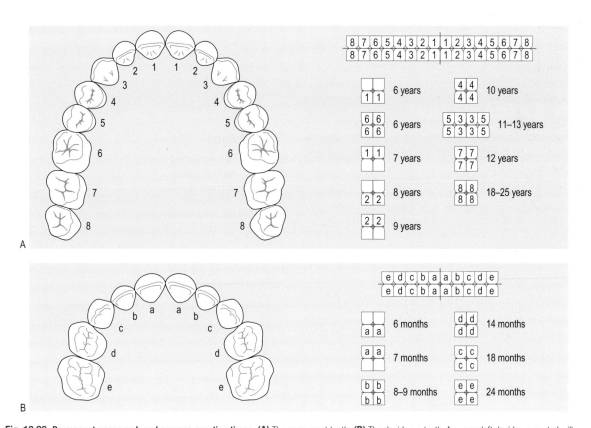

A

B

Fig. 13.26 Permanent upper arch and average eruption times. (A) The permanent teeth. **(B)** The deciduous teeth. An upper left deciduous central will be designated ⌐a; a lower right permanent lateral incisor 2 ⌐, a lower left permanent third molar ⌐ 8, etc.

13.14 Symptoms and definitions in mouth and throat disease

Symptom	Definition	Common cause
Pain		Dental caries, periodontal infection
Odynophagia	Pain on swallowing	Infection, cancer of oesophagus, larynx or pharynx
Stridor	Noise from upper airway on breathing	Upper airways obstruction, e.g. laryngeal cancer
Dysphonia	Change in the quality of the voice	Cysts, polyps, cancer, laryngitis
Dysphagia	Difficulty swallowing	Figure 13.28 and page 187
Lumps		Lymphadenopathy
Halitosis	Bad breath	Poor dental hygiene
Trismus	Inability to open mouth fully	Quinsy, tetanus
Xerostomia	Dry mouth	Anticholinergic drugs, Sjögren's syndrome

13.15 The gums in systemic conditions

Condition	Description
Phenytoin treatment	Firm and hypertrophied
Scurvy	Soft and haemorrhagic
Acute leukaemia	Hypertrophied and haemorrhagic
Cyanotic congenital heart disease	Spongy and haemorrhagic
Chronic lead poisoning	Punctate blue line

THE MOUTH AND THROAT

ANATOMY

The mouth extends from the lips anteriorly to the tonsils posteriorly. Within are the anterior two-thirds of the tongue, the lips, the hard palate, the teeth and the alveoli of the maxilla and mandible, and the gums (Fig. 13.22). The throat includes the pharynx and the larynx.

The mouth

The lips form a seal for the oral cavity. The tongue's normal appearance varies from pink through red to very dark brown. The surface has a velvety texture because of the filiform papillae containing taste buds (Fig. 13.23). Circumvallate papillae are groups of taste buds at the junction of the anterior two-thirds of the tongue and the posterior third. At the base of the tongue are the anterior and posterior tonsillar pillars laterally with the tonsils between them.

The parotid, submandibular and sublingual salivary glands secrete saliva into the oral cavity (Fig. 13.24).

The parotid gland sits in front of the ear and is traversed by the facial nerve (p. 280). It opens into the mouth on the buccal mucosa, opposite the second upper molar. The submandibular gland lies anterior and medial to the angle of the jaw, and its duct opens into the floor of the mouth next to the frenulum of the tongue.

The teeth

In children the primary dentition is complete by 3 years and consists of 20 'milk' teeth. Secondary dentition starts at around 6 years and is complete by the late teens. Adults have 32 permanent teeth (Figs 13.25 and 13.26).

The throat

The pharynx refers to the upper parts of the digestive and respiratory tract.

The larynx consists of muscles and cartilage. It produces the voice, and prevents food and saliva from entering the respiratory tract. Its sensory supply is via the superior and recurrent laryngeal branches of cranial nerve X (vagus). Its motor supply is mainly from the recurrent laryngeal nerve, which loops round the arch of the aorta on the left and the subclavian artery on the right before entering the larynx inferiorly.

SYMPTOMS AND DEFINITIONS

Pain

Sore mouth

Inflammation of the gums (gingivitis) may cause a narrow red line at the border of the gums (Box 13.15).

Aphthous ulcers are small painful superficial ulcers on the tongue, palate or buccal mucosa. The cause is

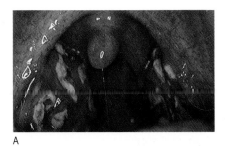

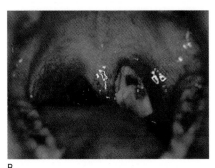

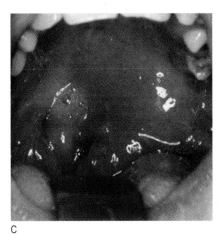

Fig. 13.27 Sore throat. (A) Acute tonsillitis. **(B)** Glandular fever. **(C)** A peritonsillar abscess.

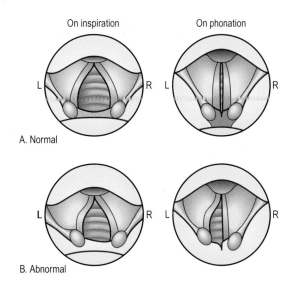

On inspiration   On phonation

A. Normal

B. Abnormal

Fig. 13.28 Laryngoscopic views of the vocal cords. (A) Normal movements. **(B)** Movements in the presence of recurrent laryngeal nerve paralysis, most commonly caused by lung cancer. Note that the paralysed left cord is in the cadaveric position (between inspiration and expiration).

13.16 Causes of dysphonia

Neonate

- Congenital abnormality
- Neurological disorder

Child

- Infection:
  Croup
  Laryngitis
- Voice abuse (screamer's nodes)

Adult

- Infection:
- Upper respiratory tract infection
- Laryngitis
- Trauma
- Lung cancer
- Vocal cord nodules (singer's nodes)
- Neurological
- Cancer of the larynx
- Functional

not known and they heal within a few days. Ulceration on the gums, tongue or buccal or lingual surfaces may also be due to trauma, vitamin or mineral deficiency (anaemia), cancer or lichen planus, or may be associated with Crohn's disease. Unilateral painful vesicles on the palate can be caused by herpes zoster.

Diffuse oral thrush may be secondary to the use of inhaled steroids or immunodeficiency, e.g. HIV infection or leukaemias.

Sore throat

Many viruses cause acute inflammation of the pharynx (pharyngitis). Acute tonsillitis may be viral or caused by *Streptococcus pyogenes* (Fig. 13.27A). There may be a pustular exudate on the tonsils and associated systemic features of fever, malaise, anorexia and cervical lymphadenopathy. It is not possible to distinguish viral from bacterial tonsillitis clinically. In glandular fever, palatal petechiae can be seen and the tonsil may be covered in a white pseudomembrane (Fig. 13.27B).

Diphtheria caused by *Corynebacterium diphtheriae* causes a true grey membrane over the tonsil but is rarely seen because of immunization.

A peritonsillar abscess causes extreme pain, so that the patient dribbles saliva out of the mouth (Fig. 13.27C). Trismus is present and the uvula is displaced to the opposite side. Any persistent mass or ulcer on the tonsil associated with pain may be a squamous cancer.

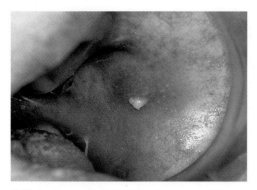

Fig. 13.29 Pus discharging from parotid duct.

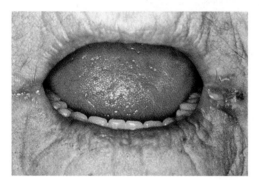

Fig. 13.30 Angular stomatitis.

Throat pain often radiates to the ear because of the dual innervation of the pharynx and external auditory meatus via the vagus nerve.

The feeling of a lump in the throat with normal examination (globus pharyngeus) is due to anxiety or acid reflux. Rarely, it is a sign of underlying malignancy. Warning signs are progressive symptoms and associated features, including dysphagia, hoarseness, odynophagia and weight loss.

Stridor

Inspiratory stridor (p. 164) indicates narrowing at the vocal cords, biphasic stridor suggests obstruction in the trachea, while noise on expiration (wheeze) indicates narrowing of the smaller, peripheral airways (Fig. 13.28).

Dysphonia

Any disturbance of vocal cord function may cause dysphonia (Box 13.16).

Refer all smokers with hoarseness for more than 4 weeks for direct laryngoscopy to exclude cancer.

Dysphonia associated with stridor needs urgent referral for specialist assessment. Recurrent laryngeal nerve damage or infiltration by tumour causes vocal cord palsy. The most common cause is lung cancer, but it may also be caused by oesophageal or thyroid cancers and aortic or subclavian aneurysm. If dysphonia varies over time and is associated with a normal cough, confirm good apposition of the vocal cords; it is unusual to find a physical cause.

Lymphadenopathy

Sudden unilateral salivary gland swelling is due to a stone obstructing the duct. Other causes of enlarged salivary glands include mumps, sarcoidosis and bacterial infection (suppurative parotitis; Fig. 13.29) or tumour.

Disorders of the lips

Hypoxia or cold causes central cyanosis or blue discoloration. Cold exposure causes desquamation and cracking of the lips; riboflavin deficiency causes red cracking of the lips. Inflamed painful cracking of the skin at the corners of the mouth may be due to excess saliva, poorly fitting dentures or iron deficiency (Fig. 13.30). Squamous and basal cell cancers occur on the lips and are associated with smoking and sun exposure.

Disorders of the mucosa

Abnormal buccal pigmentation is found in Addison's disease (Fig. 5.12B, p. 100), haemochromatosis or the Peutz–Jeghers syndrome (polyposis of the small intestine with pigmentation on the fingers and lips and in the mouth).

Assume any painless persistent mass is oral cancer and refer urgently to an oral surgeon. Even if the patient has only just noticed it, the lump may have been present for some time. Mucous retention cysts occur in younger people on the mucosa of the cheeks and lips as bluish domes less than 1 cm in diameter.

Disorders of the tongue and teeth

Areas of changing denuded smooth mucosa (geographic tongue) or of excessive furring are normal. Black discoloration occurs in heavy smokers, while a smooth red tongue due to diffuse atrophy of the papillae may indicate iron or vitamin B_{12} deficiency (Fig. 13.31A).

The tongue may be enlarged (macroglossia) in Down's syndrome, acromegaly (Fig. 3.17A, p. 55), hypothyroidism and amyloidosis. Wasting and fasciculation of the tongue are features of motor neurone disease. White patches due to thrush (*Candida* yeast infection; Fig. 13.31B) scrape off

13

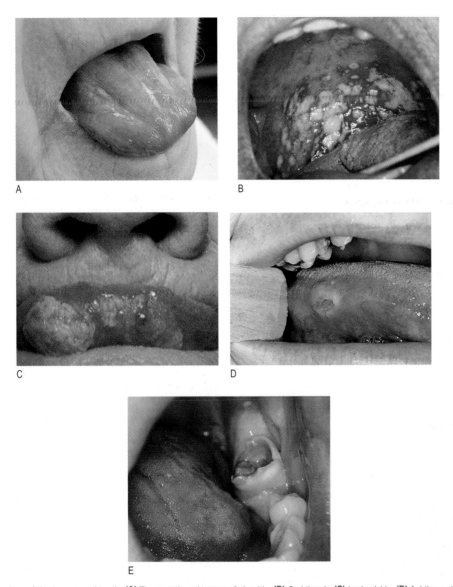

A

B

C

D

E

Fig. 13.31 Disorders of the tongue and teeth. (A) The smooth, red tongue of glossitis. **(B)** Oral thrush. **(C)** Leukoplakia. **(D)** Aphthous stomatitis causing a deep ulcer in a patient with inflammatory bowel disease. **(E)** Dental caries.

with a tongue depressor. Leukoplakia, a premalignant condition, cannot be scraped off and requires excision biopsy (Fig. 13.31C).

Aphthous ulcers (Fig. 13.31D) are small and painful, and occur on the inner sides of the lips, the edges of the tongue and the insides of the cheeks. They occur in crops and usually heal within a few days. Mouth ulcers may be the first presentation of inflammatory bowel disease, e.g. Crohn's disease or ulcerative colitis. Any mouth ulcers persisting for over 3 weeks require biopsy to exclude oral cancer.

Rotten teeth (dental caries) are common in patients with poor oral hygiene (Fig. 13.31E).

THE HISTORY

Past history

Ask about dental problems and systemic disease, particularly affecting the gastrointestinal tract; the mouth is part of this. Neurological conditions may affect ability to masticate and swallow, and drooling or dry mouth with superimposed infection may result. Note any recent or past facial trauma. Ask about any cosmetic operations.

Drug history

Many drugs, including tricyclic antidepressants and anticholinergics used in incontinence, cause a dry mouth. Recent and multiple courses of antibiotics increase the chance of oral thrush, as does any prolonged debilitating illness.

Social history

Piercings and sexually transmitted infection may affect the mouth. Oral cancer is more common in smokers, those who chew tobacco or betel nut, or those who have an excess alcohol intake or poor oral hygiene.

Timing of symptoms

Epiglottitis usually presents with rapidly progressive airway obstruction occurring within a few hours, sore throat, fever and drooling. The condition usually occurs in small children, although it is also seen in adults. Acute laryngotracheobronchitis (croup) in infants usually has a longer history (24–48 hours) and the airway obstruction is less severe. Do not try to examine the throat in a patient with stridor, as this may induce laryngospasm and total airway obstruction.

THE PHYSICAL EXAMINATION

Examination sequence

Mouth and throat

Have a good light source. A head mirror or head light leaves both your hands free to manipulate instruments.

Inspection

Look at the patient's lips, then ask him to open the mouth. Inspect the buccal mucosa, gums and teeth. Ask the patient to remove any dentures. Note dental hygiene and any gingivitis.

Use a tongue depressor to display the inner surface of the lips. Look for areas of discoloration, inflammation, ulceration or nodules.

Look at the hard palate. Note any cleft, abnormal arched palate or telangiectasia.

Look at the tongue inside the mouth; then ask the patient to put it out so that you can look at the lateral borders. This gives a better view of the posterior part of the tongue and allows you to assess the XII (hypoglossal) nerve function.

Ask the patient to touch the roof of the mouth with the tongue; inspect the floor of the mouth. Note the punctum of the submandibular glands.

Look at the posterior aspect of the oral cavity and the oropharynx. Ask the patient to say 'Aaah'. Some patients open wide enough to allow a good view of all the structures, but to obtain a clear view use a tongue depressor. These are usually made of wood or plastic and are disposable.

Place the depressor firmly on the patient's tongue, as far back as the posterior third.

Ask the patient to say 'Aaah' as you hold the tongue down. Some people are very sensitive to the tongue depressor and even a gentle examination stimulates their gag reflex.

Look at the uvula and see if it moves symmetrically.

Look at the soft palate for any cleft or structural abnormality. Note any telangiectasia.

Look at the tonsils and note their size, colour, any discharge or membrane, and whether they are symmetrical in shape and size. Tonsils are largest at age 8; they then involute and may be difficult to see in adults.

Use the tongue depressor to scrape off any white plaques gently.

Deliberately touch the posterior pharyngeal wall gently to stimulate the gag reflex. Check for symmetrical movement of the soft palate.

Ask the patient to put out the tongue and move it to the left; use the tongue depressor to see into the right posterolateral edge of the tongue.

Repeat this for the other side.

Palpation

If you have noted any lesion in the mouth, put on a pair of gloves and palpate it with one hand outside on the patient's cheek or jaw and a gloved finger inside the mouth.

Feel the lesion and identify its characteristics. Use a similar technique for the salivary glands if they are affected.

Palpate the cervical lymph nodes systematically (Figs 3.19A,B and C, p. 57).

Abnormal findings

Neurological disease, painful mouth and a tight frenulum may all limit protrusion of the tongue. White plaques of thrush come away easily when scraped but leukoplakia does not. Rarely a stone may be felt in the parotid or submandibular duct. The posterolateral edge of the tongue is a site for some cancers and is hidden from easy view.

The neck

Examine the neck in all patients with disease of the mouth and throat. A neck mass or rash may be the main presenting complaint.

The distribution of common neck swellings is shown diagrammatically in Fig. 13.32, while causes of neck lumps are listed in Box 13.18.

▶ Examination sequence

The neck

▶ With the patient sitting down, look at the neck from in front to identify any visible masses and observe pulsation of any visible swellings.

▶ From behind, palpate the neck.

▶ Work systematically around the neck, checking both the anterior and posterior triangles and feeling for midline swellings.

▶ Assess the mobility of any swellings found and record their size.

▶ Palpate swellings between your fingers to determine whether they are compressible, suggesting that they are cystic, or pulsatile, suggesting that they are vascular.

▶ If you find a midline swelling, ask the patient to swallow (offer a glass of water if needed), and note if it moves superiorly on swallowing (thyroid).

▶ Ask the patient to put out the tongue and note any movement superiorly (thyroglossal cyst; Fig. 13.33).

13.18 Causes of neck lumps

Midline structures

- Thyroid isthmus swelling — most common cause in adults
- Thyroglossal cyst (Fig. 13.33) — (lump moves when patient sticks out tongue)
- Laryngeal swellings
- Submental lymph nodes
- Dermoid cysts

Lateral structures

In the anterior triangle (bounded by the midline, the anterior border of sternocleidomastoid muscle and body of mandible) (Fig. 13.32):

- Thyroid lobe swellings
- Pharyngeal pouch
- Submandibular gland swelling
- Branchial cyst
- Lymph nodes:
  Malignant: lymphoma, metastatic cancer
  Infection: any bacterial infection of head/neck (including teeth), viral infection, e.g. infectious mononucleosis, HIV, tuberculosis
- Parotid gland swelling, e.g. mumps, parotitis, stones, autoimmune disease, benign and malignant tumours

In the posterior triangle (bounded by the posterior border of sternocleidomastoid muscle, the trapezius and the clavicle) (Fig. 13.32):

- Lymph nodes:
  Malignant: lymphoma, metastatic cancer
  Infection: any bacterial infection of head/neck (including teeth) viral infection, e.g. infectious mononucleosis, HIV tuberculosis
- Carotid artery aneurysm
- Carotid body tumour
- Cystic hygroma
- Cervical rib

13

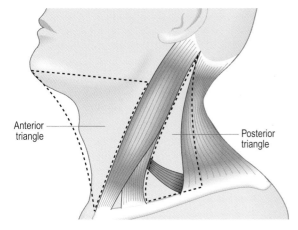

Fig. 13.32 Sites of swellings in the neck.

Anterior triangle

Posterior triangle

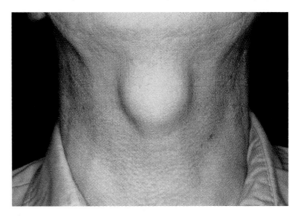

Fig. 13.33 Thyroglossal cyst.

13

INVESTIGATIONS

 13.19 Investigations in mouth and throat disease

Investigation	Indication/comment
Full blood count	Pharyngitis May show lymphopenia in acute viral infection or neutrophilia in bacterial infection
Monospot	Infectious mononucleosis
Throat swab	Acute tonsillitis and pharyngitis Patients may carry *Strep. pyogenes* and have a viral infection, so swab does not always help direct management
Endoscopy and biopsy	Cancer of larynx and pharynx, changes in vocal cords Under general anaesthetic
Ultrasound	Neck swellings
CT scan	Cancer and metastases Useful in staging

 13.20 **Key points: the ear, nose and throat**

- Pull the pinna upwards and backwards to straighten out the ear canal when performing otoscopy.
- Use the otoscope to visualize the anterior portion of the nasal cavity.
- Look for nasal deviation from above and behind the patient.
- A pearly grey mass obstructing a nostril, which is painless if probed, is a polyp.
- Many patients, particularly children, open their mouth wide enough for a good view without you using a tongue depressor.
- Palpate any masses in the mouth with your gloved finger inside the oral cavity.
- Vertigo is almost always caused by disease in the ear.
- Always examine the lateral borders of the tongue (using a tongue depressor if necessary) so that you do not miss hidden cancer.

The musculoskeletal system

14

Jim S. Huntley
Jane Gibson
A. Hamish R. W. Simpson

MUSCULOSKELETAL EXAMINATION

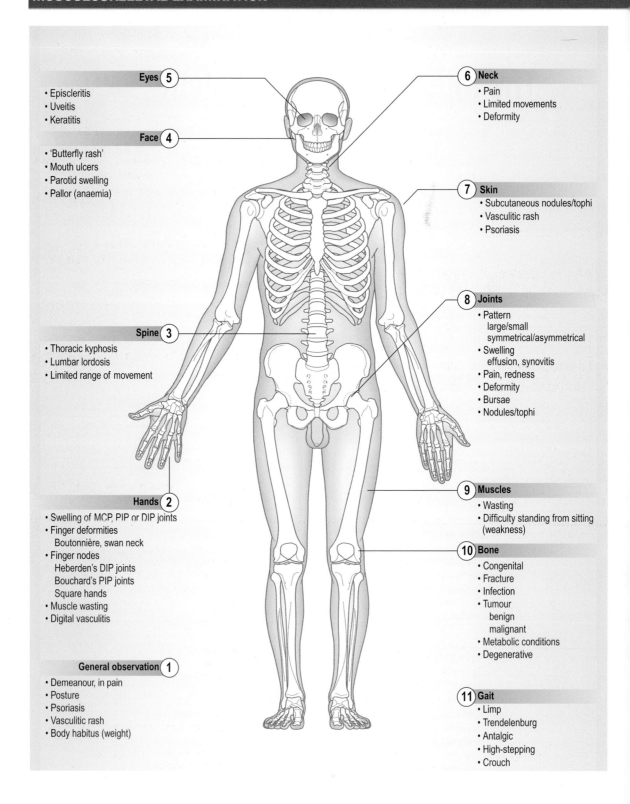

Eyes (5)
- Episcleritis
- Uveitis
- Keratitis

Face (4)
- 'Butterfly rash'
- Mouth ulcers
- Parotid swelling
- Pallor (anaemia)

Spine (3)
- Thoracic kyphosis
- Lumbar lordosis
- Limited range of movement

Hands (2)
- Swelling of MCP, PIP or DIP joints
- Finger deformities
  Boutonnière, swan neck
- Finger nodes
  Heberden's DIP joints
  Bouchard's PIP joints
  Square hands
- Muscle wasting
- Digital vasculitis

General observation (1)
- Demeanour, in pain
- Posture
- Psoriasis
- Vasculitic rash
- Body habitus (weight)

(6) Neck
- Pain
- Limited movements
- Deformity

(7) Skin
- Subcutaneous nodules/tophi
- Vasculitic rash
- Psoriasis

(8) Joints
- Pattern
  large/small
  symmetrical/asymmetrical
- Swelling
  effusion, synovitis
- Pain, redness
- Deformity
- Bursae
- Nodules/tophi

(9) Muscles
- Wasting
- Difficulty standing from sitting
  (weakness)

(10) Bone
- Congenital
- Fracture
- Infection
- Tumour
  benign
  malignant
- Metabolic conditions
- Degenerative

(11) Gait
- Limp
- Trendelenburg
- Antalgic
- High-stepping
- Crouch

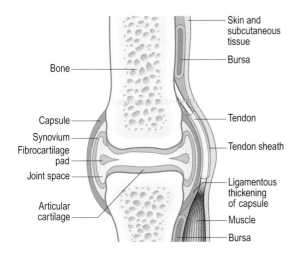

Fig. 14.1 Structure of a joint and surrounding tissues.

ANATOMY

Joint structure is shown in Fig. 14.1. Other aspects of anatomy are dealt with in the relevant section below.

SYMPTOMS AND DEFINITIONS

Several systemic disorders affect the musculoskeletal system, so be aware of clinical patterns. For example, psoriasis affects the skin, nails and sometimes the joints, and joint symptoms and erythema nodosum may occur in sarcoidosis. Follow a simple system to narrow down the diagnostic possibilities.

- Was the problem caused by, or is it related to, an injury? If so, follow Chapter 17
- If not, are the joints affected? (Box 14.1). If they are swollen, this may be a type of arthritis. Arthritis (joint inflammation) may be a misnomer: as in osteoarthritis, for example. Arthralgia means joint pain. Almost all adult patients with arthritis have arthralgia, but only a minority of patients with arthralgia have arthritis. If you suspect arthritis, establish whether it is 'inflammatory' or 'non-inflammatory'
- Inflammatory conditions produce pain at rest and on movement, and symptoms are often worse in the morning. Stiffness tends to ease with movement or after a warm bath or shower
- Non-inflammatory conditions tend to become more painful with activity and ease with rest. Non-inflammatory joint problems may be caused by a degenerative or, rarely, a neoplastic process. Some musculoskeletal cancers, especially if rapidly growing, may have an inflammatory type of presentation

- How many joints are involved? One joint implies a monoarthritis; 2–4 joints, oligoarthritis; and more than four, polyarthritis (Box 14.2)
- Are the joints affected symmetrically or asymmetrically? Are the small or large joints of the arms or legs affected? The different patterns of joint involvement help to establish a differential diagnosis (Fig. 14.8).

If joints are not involved, the problem may involve the surrounding tissues or be referred from another site. Surrounding structures include ligaments, tendons, tendon sheaths, bursae, muscle and bone (Fig. 14.1), and the process may be inflammatory (having an infective or non-infective cause) or non-inflammatory.

When examining the patient, distinguish between:

- focal pathology, e.g. lateral epicondylitis of the elbow — 'tennis elbow', medial meniscal tear of the knee, osteoarthritis at the hip
- systemic conditions with (one or more) local manifestations, e.g. rheumatoid arthritis, SLE, psoriasis
- referred pain from a different site, e.g. diaphragmatic irritation causing shoulder-tip pain

14

 14.1 Causes of joint pain (arthralgia)

Generalized

- Infective
  Viral, e.g. rubella, mumps, hepatitis B
  Bacterial, e.g. staphylococci, tuberculosis, *Borrelia*
  Fungal
- Post-infective
  Rheumatic fever, reactive arthritis
- Inflammatory
  Rheumatoid arthritis, systemic lupus erythematosus (SLE), ankylosing spondylitis, systemic sclerosis
- Degenerative
  Osteoarthritis
- Tumour
  Primary, e.g. osteosarcoma, chondrosarcoma
  Metastatic, e.g. from lung, breast, prostate
  Systemic tumour effects, e.g. hypertrophic pulmonary osteoarthropathy
- Crystal formation
  Gout, pseudogout
- Trauma, e.g. road traffic accidents
- Others
  Fibromyalgia syndrome
  Sjögren's syndrome
  Hypermobility syndromes

Localized

- Trauma, e.g. sports injuries
- Tendonitis, e.g. shoulder rotator cuff lesions, Achilles tendonitis
- Enthesopathies, e.g. tennis elbow, golfer's elbow
- Bursitis, e.g. trochanteric bursitis
- Nerve entrapment, e.g. carpal tunnel syndrome

14

14.2 Differential diagnosis of monoarthritis, oligoarthritis and polyarthritis

	Type	Examples
Monoarthritis (single joint involvement)	Infective	*Staphylococcus aureus*, *Staph. epidermidis*, *Salmonella*, tuberculosis, *Neisseria gonorrhoeae*, *Escherichia coli*, *Haemophilus*
	Traumatic	Haemarthrosis
	Bleeding diathesis	Haemarthrosis
	Post-traumatic	
	Degenerative	Acute exacerbation of underlying state, Charcot joint
	Metabolic	Crystal arthropathies: gout, pseudogout
	Polyarthritis presenting as monoarthritis	Rheumatoid arthritis
Oligoarthritis (involvement of 2–4 joints)	Degenerative	Osteoarthritis
	Inflammatory polyarthritis presenting as oligoarthritis	Seronegative conditions: Reactive arthritis, psoriatic arthropathy, ankylosing spondylitis Infective: Bacterial endocarditis, *N. gonorrhoeae*, *M. tuberculosis* Sarcoidosis
Polyarthritis (involvement of ≥5 joints)	Inflammatory	Rheumatoid arthritis, SLE
	Non-inflammatory	Infective: Bacterial: Lyme disease, subacute bacterial endocarditis Viral: rubella, mumps, glandular fever, chickenpox, hepatitis B and C, HIV Post-infective: Rheumatic fever Osteoarthritis: Nodal with Heberden's/Bouchard's nodes Metabolic: Haemochromatosis Other: Hypertrophic pulmonary osteoarthropathy

- radicular pain, e.g. pain felt down the back of the leg from an intervertebral disc protruding on to a nerve root.

Also assess the functional significance of any abnormality: e.g. the degree of ligamentous laxity at a joint.

Pain

Determine whether the pain originates from a joint (arthralgia), muscle (myalgia) or other soft tissue. The site may be well localized and suggest the diagnosis: e.g. the first metatarsophalangeal joint in gout (Fig. 14.2). It may be difficult to determine the source of referred pain (Boxes 14.3 and 14.4).

Is the pain is mechanical or non-mechanical, and present at rest or aggravated by movement? Pain caused by a mechanical problem is worse on movement and eases with rest. Pain at rest may be due to inflammation, infection or tumour, and is often aggravated by movement.

The onset and timing of pain give clues to the diagnosis; pain from traumatic injury is usually immediate but is also exacerbated by later movement or if bleeding occurs into the affected joint (haemarthrosis).

- Crystal arthritis (gout and pseudogout) causes acute, sometimes extreme, pain which develops quickly and is often associated with redness (erythema) over the affected joint
- Joint sepsis causes pain that develops over a day or two
- Flitting joint pain which starts in one joint and moves to affect others over a period of days is a feature of rheumatic fever and gonococcal arthritis.

Pain is subjective and difficult to describe. Chronic pain is commonly associated with anxiety and depression, worsening the patient's perception and response. Ask if pain disturbs patients' sleep by preventing them getting to sleep or by waking them.

- Bone pain is penetrating, deep or boring, and is characteristically worse at night. Localized pain suggests tumour, infection (osteomyelitis), avascular necrosis or osteoid osteoma (a benign bone tumour)
- Generalized bony conditions, such as osteomalacia, usually cause diffuse pain
- Muscle pain (Box 14.5) is usually described as stiffness and is poorly localized, deep, and aggravated by use of the muscle. It is associated with muscle weakness in some conditions, e.g. polymyositis, but not in polymyalgia rheumatica

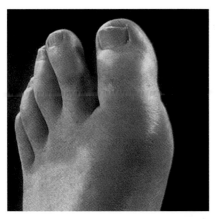

Fig. 14.2 Acute gout of the first metatarsophalangeal joint. This causes swelling, erythema, and extreme pain and tenderness (podagra).

14.3 Assessing musculoskeletal pain (*mnemonic SOCRATES*)

- **S**ite
- **O**nset
- **C**haracter
- **R**adiation
- **A**ssociated factors
- **T**iming (frequency, duration, periodicity)
- **E**xacerbating features (exercise, use, etc.)
- **S**everity

14.4 Common patterns of referred and radicular musculoskeletal pain

Site of pathology	Perceived at
Cervical spine	
C1/C2	Occiput
C3, 4	Interscapular region
C5	Tip of shoulder, upper outer aspect of arm
C6, 7	Interscapular region or the radial fingers and thumb
C8	Ulnar side of the forearm, ring and little fingers
Thoracic spine	Chest
Lumbar spine	Buttocks, knees, legs
Shoulder	Lateral aspect of upper arm
Elbow	Forearm
Hip	Anterior thigh, knee
Knee	Thigh, hip

- Partial muscle tears may be painful; complete rupture may be relatively pain-free
- Fracture pain is sharp and stabbing, aggravated by attempted movement or use, and relieved by rest and splintage
- 'Shooting' pain is often caused by mechanical trapping of a peripheral nerve: for example, buttock pain which 'shoots' down the back of the leg, caused by lumbar intervertebral disc protrusion
- Chronic joint pain in patients >40 years old with progression over years is commonly caused by osteoarthritis. Patients often say that their symptoms vary, with 'good' and 'bad' days
- 'Pain all over', which is unremitting with little diurnal variation and only 'dulled' by conventional analgesic or anti-inflammatory drugs, is a common feature of chronic pain syndromes (Fig. 2.2, p. 16)
- Neurological involvement in diabetes mellitus, leprosy, syringomyelia and syphilis (tabes dorsalis) may cause loss of pain from joints, or pain that is disproportionately less than you would expect from examination. Even grossly abnormal joints may be pain-free (Charcot joint)
- Chronic pain syndrome (fibromyalgia). Widespread joint pain (arthralgia) and muscle pain and tenderness (myalgia) is a common presentation of a chronic pain disorder. Chronic pain is defined as pain present for more than 3 months and is due to sensitization of the pain pathways. It is commonly associated with sleep disorders, psychological stress and depression. It should be differentiated from musculoskeletal disorders by a normal examination except for the presence of typical tender points (Fig. 14.3). Treatment should focus on coping mechanisms for pain, improvement in sleep and a graded exercise regimen
- Pain disproportionately greater than expected is seen in compartment syndrome (increased pressure in a fascial compartment, which compromises perfusion and viability of the compartmental structures) and complex regional pain syndrome

14.5 Causes of muscle pain (myalgia)

Infective

- Viral: Coxsackie, cytomegalovirus (CMV), echovirus
- Bacterial: *Strep. pneumoniae*, *Mycoplasma*
- Parasitic: schistosomiasis, toxoplasmosis
- Inflammatory: polymyalgia rheumatica, myositis, dermatomyositis

Traumatic

- Tears, haematoma, rhabdomyolysis

Drugs

- e.g. Alcohol, statins, zidovudine

Neuropathic

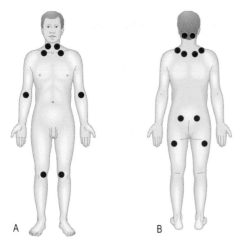

Fig. 14.3 Typical tender points in chronic pain syndrome (fibromyalgia).

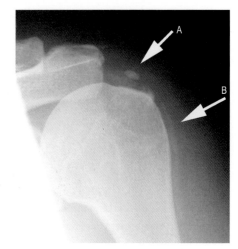

Fig. 14.4 Calcific deposits in supraspinatus (arrow A) and biceps tendons (arrow B). These deposits are a cause of arthralgia with a painful arc of movement.

(formerly reflex sympathetic dystrophy, or algodystrophy). This develops after injury or illness, or spontaneously, and is characterized by severe 'burning' pain, local tenderness, oedema, abnormal sweating and colour, temperature changes and localized osteoporosis.

Stiffness

Establish what the patient means by stiffness. Is it:
- a restricted range of movement?
- difficulty moving, but with a normal range?
- painful movement?
- localized to a particular joint or more generalized?

If stiffness predominates over pain, suspect a soft tissue contracture or spasticity (increasing muscle contraction in response to stretch) or tetany (involuntary sustained contraction), and examine for the increased tone of an upper motor neurone lesion (p. 288).

Stiffness may relate to the soft tissues rather than the joint itself. In polymyalgia rheumatica stiffness commonly affects the shoulder and pelvic areas. Other common soft tissue causes are:
- inflammation at tendon insertion sites (enthesopathies), e.g. at the medial and lateral epicondyles of the elbow ('golfer's' and 'tennis' elbow respectively)
- calcific tendonitis, e.g. supraspinatus tendonitis (Fig. 14.4)
- bursitis, e.g. trochanteric bursitis.

There are characteristic differences between inflammatory and non-inflammatory presentations of joint stiffness:
- Inflammatory arthritis presents with early morning stiffness that takes at least 1 hour to wear off with activity

- Non-inflammatory, mechanical arthritis tends to occur after resting, and stiffness lasts only a few minutes on movement. There may be pain on movement. This typically eases with rest, but may return later in the day.

Redness (erythema) and warmth

Erythema and warmth over a joint occur in acute inflammatory arthritis. Erythema is common in infective, traumatic and crystal-induced conditions, but unusual in rheumatoid arthritis or SLE. If present, it suggests co-existing joint infection.

Swelling

Establish the site, localization, extent and time course of any swelling. Swelling may be diffuse oedema or localized as a discrete fluid collection in a joint, bursa or tendon sheath (Fig. 14.5A). The time course is especially important when considering joint swelling caused by intra-articular fluid. Inflammatory arthritis from any cause results in swelling.

When vascular structures, such as bone and ligament, are injured, rapid tense swelling develops within minutes because of bleeding into the joint (Fig. 14.5B). This process is even more rapid and severe if the patient is taking anticoagulants or has an underlying bleeding disorder, e.g. haemophilia. If avascular structures, such as the menisci, are torn or articular cartilage is abraded, a reactive effusion takes hours or days to produce joint swelling.

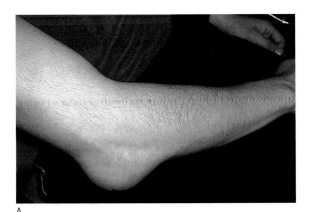

A

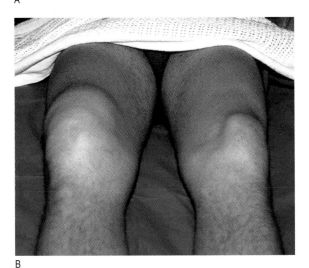

B

Fig. 14.5 Joint swelling. (A) Olecranon bursitis. **(B)** Right knee haemarthrosis.

<table>
</table>

14.6 **The muscular dystrophies**		
	Inheritance	**Gene product**
Duchenne	X-linked	Dystrophin
Becker	X-linked	Dystrophin
Dystrophia myotonica	Autosomal dominant	Myotonin
Facioscapulohumeral	Autosomal dominant	
Limb girdle	Autosomal recessive	

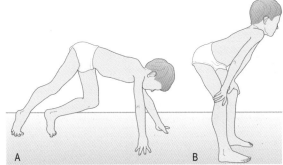

A   B

Fig. 14.6 Gower's sign. (A) Duchenne muscular dystrophy leads to great difficulty in getting up from a prone position. After rolling over, the affected individual walks the hands and feet towards each other. **(B)** He then uses the hands to climb up the legs, reaching an upright position by swinging the arms and trunk sideways and upwards.

Other primary muscle diseases include the heritable muscular dystrophies (Box 14.6 and Fig. 14.6).

Sudden onset of weakness, e.g. wrist or foot drop, may indicate a mononeuritis multiplex associated with rheumatoid arthritis, vasculitis or connective tissue disease, diabetes mellitus or HIV infection.

Weakness

Weakness suggests a joint disorder, peripheral nerve lesion, e.g. median nerve compression in carpal tunnel syndrome, or muscle disease. The problem may be secondary to pain, or focal or generalized.

Predominantly proximal weakness suggests a primary muscle disease, such as immune-mediated inflammatory muscle disease, e.g. dermatomyositis or polymyositis, or a non-inflammatory myopathy, e.g. secondary to chronic alcohol use, steroid therapy or thyrotoxicosis.

Distal weakness is more likely to be neurological: for example, the peripheral neuropathy of thiamine or vitamin B_{12} deficiency, connective tissue disorders or hereditary sensory motor neuropathy (Charcot–Marie–Tooth disease).

Intermittent weakness that worsens during activity suggests myasthenia gravis. Slowly progressive generalized weakness is a feature of motor neurone disease.

Locking and triggering

'Locking' is an incomplete range of movement at a joint because of an anatomical block. It may be associated with pain. Patients use 'locking' to describe a variety of problems, so establish precisely what they mean.

True locking is a block to the usual range of movement caused by a mechanical obstruction, e.g. a loose body or torn meniscus, within the joint. This prevents the joint from reaching the extremes of the normal range of movement. The patient is characteristically able to 'unlock' the joint by trick manœuvres.

Pseudo-locking is a loss of range of movement due to pain. For instance, some patients with patellofemoral pain (typically teenage girls) hold the knee in full extension and will not flex it.

Sometimes, when extending a finger from a flexed position, there is a block to extension, which then 'gives' suddenly. This is triggering. It results from nodular tendon thickening or a fibrous thickening of the flexor sheath. In adults it usually affects the ring or middle fingers. It can be congenital, usually affecting the thumb.

Deformity

Acute deformity may occur if there is a fracture, dislocation or swelling, e.g. haemarthrosis or intramuscular haematoma (Fig. 14.7). Malapposition of the joint surfaces may be partial (subluxation) or complete (dislocation). Establish if the joint deformity is fixed or mobile, and if mobile, whether it is passively correctable.

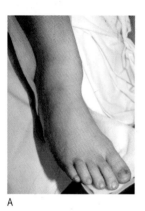
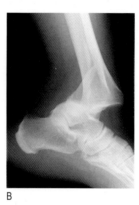

A B

Fig. 14.7 Ankle deformity. (A) Clinical appearance. **(B)** Lateral X-ray view showing tibiotalar fracture dislocation.

Extra-articular manifestations

Patients may present with symptoms of extra-articular disease, rather than musculoskeletal features. Weight loss, low-grade fever and malaise are associated with rheumatoid arthritis or SLE. High-spiking fevers in the evening with a rash occur in adult-onset Still's disease. Headache, jaw pain on chewing (claudication) and scalp tenderness are features of temporal arteritis. Although inflammatory arthritis is commonly associated with extra-articular features, patients may not connect them with musculoskeletal problems (Boxes 14.7 and 14.8). The pattern of the joint condition (a/symmetric, flitting) and extent (mono-, oligo- or polyarthritis) may suggest the diagnosis and direct the history relating to extra-articular features.

THE HISTORY

Presenting complaint

Record the nature and duration of pain (use SOCRATES, Box 14.3), stiffness, swelling, weakness and locking. The duration of swelling in inflammatory arthritis is especially important. Instability, deformity, sensory disturbance and loss of function may also be presenting complaints.

If the problem relates to an injury, obtain an exact account of the mechanism and subsequent events, e.g. development of swelling.

Establish the pattern of joints involved (Fig. 14.8). Predominant involvement of the small joints of the hands, feet or wrists suggests an inflammatory arthritis, e.g. rheumatoid arthritis or SLE. Medium or large joint swelling is more likely to be degenerative or a seronegative arthritis, e.g. psoriatic arthritis or ankylosing spondylitis (Box 14.9). Nodal osteoarthritis has a predilection for the distal interphalangeal joints and carpometacarpal joint of the thumb.

Ask about extra-articular features (Boxes 14.7 and 14.8).

Past history

Note features that might contribute to the complaint, such as pain and restricted movement in a joint that had been dislocated. Identify co-morbid factors, diabetes

---

 14.7 Arthritis and other manifestations outside the musculoskeletal system

Felty's syndrome

- Rheumatoid arthritis with splenomegaly, lymphadenopathy and neutropenia

Sjögren's syndrome

- Arthritis with 'dry eyes' (keratoconjunctivitis sicca), xerostomia (reduced or absent saliva production), salivary gland enlargement and Raynaud's phenomenon

Enteropathic arthritis

- Associated with inflammatory bowel disease — ulcerative colitis and Crohn's disease

Psoriatic arthritis

- With skin and nail features of psoriasis

Haemophilia

- Associated with (especially knee) arthropathy because of recurrent haemarthroses

Sickle cell disease

- Associated with osteonecrosis of the hip due to bone infarction

Still's disease

- Juvenile idiopathic arthritis

Reactive arthritis

- Urethritis, conjunctivitis and inflammatory oligoarthropathy about 1–3 weeks after sexually transmitted chlamydial infection or infective gastroenteritis

14.8 Association of arthropathy with extra-articular features

Type of arthropathy	Symmetry	Condition	Extra-articular features
Monoarthropathy		Septic arthritis	Fever, malaise, source of sepsis, e.g. skin, throat, gut
		Gout	Tophi, signs of renal failure (Fig. 9.5, p. 227)
		Osteoarthritis	
Oligoarthropathy	Asymmetrical	Reactive arthritis	Urethritis, mouth and/or genital ulcers, conjunctivitis, iritis, enthesopathy, e.g. Achilles tendinopathy/plantar fasciitis, rash (keratoderma blennorrhagica)
		Ankylosing spondylitis	Enthesopathy, iritis
		Psoriatic	Psoriasis, nail pitting
		Osteoarthritis	
Polyarthropathy	Symmetrical	Rheumatoid arthritis	Raynaud's phenomenon, subcutaneous rheumatoid nodules, episcleritis, dry eyes, pleurisy
		SLE	Raynaud's phenomenon, photosensitive rash, especially on face, alopecia, fever, episcleritis
		Osteoarthritis	

14

14.9 Nomenclature in inflammatory arthritis

Seropositive: indicates the presence of IgM rheumatoid factor (RF) in significant titre in the serum of patients with a polyarthritis
Seronegative: indicates the absence of RF in the serum of patients with inflammatory arthritis. If the disease is morphologically the same as rheumatoid arthritis, it is seronegative rheumatoid arthritis. Other inflammatory arthritides, such as psoriatic arthritis, reactive arthritis and ankylosing spondylitis, are also seronegative and are the seronegative arthritides. They are more likely to be associated with HLA B27, share extra-articular features and have an asymmetric pattern of joint involvement.

Highly specific anticyclic citrullinated peptides (ACPA) in the serum of patients with rheumatoid arthritis may change the definitions for rheumatoid arthritis in the future.

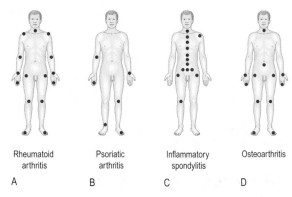

Rheumatoid arthritis   Psoriatic arthritis   Inflammatory spondylitis   Osteoarthritis

A   B   C   D

Fig. 14.8 Contrasting patterns of involvement in polyarthritis.
(A) Rheumatoid arthritis (symmetrical, small and large joints, upper and lower limbs). **(B)** Seronegative psoriatic arthritis (asymmetrical, large > small joints, associated periarticular inflammation, giving dactylitis). **(C)** Seronegative inflammatory spondylitis (axial involvement, large > small joints, asymmetrical). **(D)** Osteoarthritis (symmetrical, small and large joints).

mellitus, steroid therapy, ischaemic heart disease, stroke and obesity.

Drug history

Many drugs have side-effects that may either worsen or precipitate musculoskeletal conditions (Box 14.10).

Family history

A single gene defect (monogenic inheritance) is found in hereditary sensory motor neuropathy (Charcot–Marie–Tooth disease), osteogenesis imperfecta, Ehlers–Danlos syndrome, Marfan's syndrome and the muscular dystrophies. Osteoarthritis, osteoporosis and gout are heritable in a variable polygenic fashion. Seronegative spondyloarthritis is more common in patients with HLA B27 (Box 14.11). Rheumatoid arthritis is also associated with a familial tendency.

Environmental, occupational and social histories

Ask about current and previous occupations. Are patients working full- or part-time, on sick leave or receiving benefits? Have they had to take time off work because of their condition? If so, is their job at risk? Litigation may be pending in occupation-related complaints, such as repetitive strain disorder, hand vibration syndrome and fatigue fractures. Army recruits, athletes and dancers are at particular risk of fatigue fractures.

Identify functional difficulties, including ability to hold and use items such as pens, tools and cutlery. How does the condition affect activities of daily living (Box 14.12), such as washing, dressing and toileting? Can patients use stairs and do they need aids to walk?

14.10 Drugs associated with adverse musculoskeletal effects

Drug	Possible adverse musculoskeletal effects
Steroids	Osteoporosis, myopathy, avascular necrosis, infections
Statins	Myalgia, myositis, myopathy
Angiotensin-converting enzyme (ACE) inhibitors	Myalgia, arthralgia, positive antinuclear antibody
Antiepileptics	Osteomalacia, arthralgia
Immunosuppressants	Infections
Quinolones	Tendonopathy, tendon rupture

14.11 Conditions linked to human leucocyte antigen HLA B27 type

- Ankylosing spondylitis
- Reactive arthritis
- Psoriatic arthritis (some forms)
- Enteropathic arthritis — associated with ulcerative colitis and Crohn's disease

Ask about functional independence, especially cooking, housework and shopping.

Some conditions are seen in certain ethnic groups: for example, sickle cell disease may present with bone and joint pain in African patients; osteomalacia is more often seen in Asian patients; and bone and joint tuberculosis is more common in African and Asian patients.

Take a sexual history (p. 20) since sexually transmitted disease may be relevant, e.g. reactive arthritis, gonococcal arthritis and hepatitis B. Box 14.13 identifies other social factors.

THE PHYSICAL EXAMINATION

Dynamic tests are difficult to describe in pictures and text, so ask an experienced clinician to check your technique. Practise examining as many joints as possible to become familiar with normal appearances and ranges of movement.

General principles

- Observe the general appearance of the patient
- Do not cause the patient additional pain
- Compare one limb with the opposite side
- Assess active before passive movements

14.12 Joints involved in activities of daily living

Activity	Joint(s) involved	Function required
Pinch grip	Thumb, index finger	Opposition and flexion of thumb (note: sensation is also required for optimal function)
Key grip	Thumb, index finger	Adduction and opposition of thumb
Gripping taps, handles, bottle tops	Hand, wrist	Grasp
Eating, cleaning teeth and face	Hand, elbow	Grasp, elbow flexion
Dressing, washing, hair care	Hand, elbow, shoulder	Pinch, grasp, elbow flexion, shoulder abduction/rotation
Toileting, cleaning perineum	Hand, wrist, elbow, shoulder	Grasp, wrist/elbow flexion, forearm supination, internal shoulder rotation

14.13 Social factors and musculoskeletal conditions

Alcohol
- Trauma, myopathy, rhabdomyolysis, nerve palsies

Smoking
- Lung cancer with bony metastases, hypertrophic pulmonary osteoarthropathy

Drugs of misuse
- Trauma, hepatitis B, HIV

Diet
- Vitamin deficiencies, e.g. osteomalacia (vitamin D), scurvy (vitamin C)
- Anorexia nervosa, e.g. osteoporosis

- Use standard terminology to describe joint and limb positions and movement.

Movements are always described from the neutral position (Fig. 14.9). The commonly used terms are:
- flexion: bending at a joint from the neutral position
- extension: straightening a joint back to the neutral position
- hyperextension: movement beyond the normal neutral position because of a torn ligament or underlying ligamentous laxity, e.g. Ehlers–Danlos syndrome
- adduction: movement towards the midline of the body (finger adduction is movement towards the axis of the limb)
- abduction: movement away from the midline.

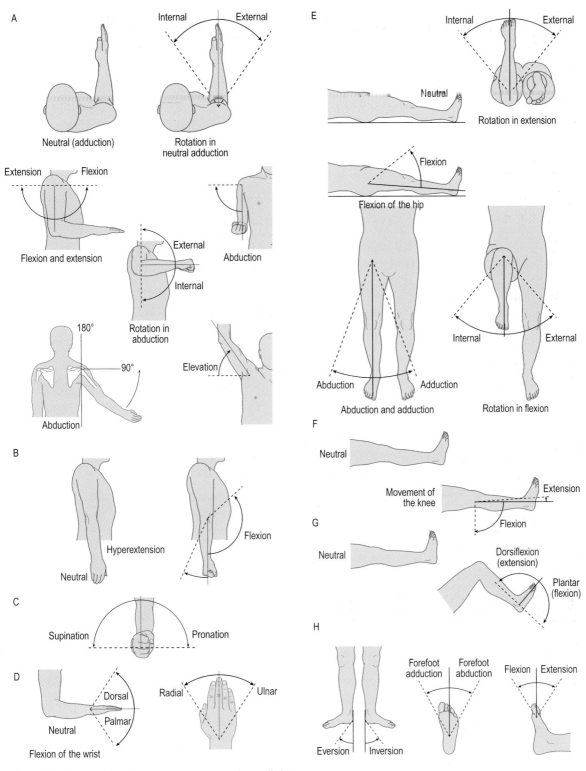

Fig. 14.9 Joint positions and movements of the upper and lower limbs.

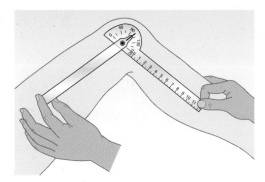

Fig. 14.10 Goniometer.

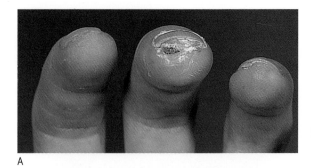

A

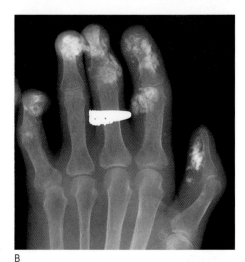

B

Fig. 14.11 Systemic sclerosis in the hand. (A) Calcium deposits ulcerating through the skin. (B) X-ray showing calcium deposits.

Two additional terms are used to describe the position of a limb because of deformity at an affected joint or bone:

- valgus: the distal part deviates away from the midline
- varus: the distal part deviates towards the midline.

Equipment

- Tape measure
- Tendon hammer
- Blocks for assessing leg-length discrepancy
- Goniometer (a protractor for measuring the range of joint movement) (Fig. 14.10).

Skin, nail and soft tissue features

The skin and related structures are the most common sites of associated lesions. Rashes, often aggravated by exposure to light, are common in vasculitis, e.g. SLE. The skin and nail appearances in psoriasis are usually obvious but may be hidden, e.g. the umbilicus, natal cleft, scalp (Fig. 3.16, p. 54, and Fig. 4.4, p. 75).

In systemic sclerosis the thickened, tight skin produces a characteristic appearance of the face (Fig. 3.10C, p. 51). In the hands, flexion contractures, calcium deposits in the finger pulps (Fig. 14.11) and tissue ischaemia leading to ulceration may occur. The telangiectasiae of systemic sclerosis are purplish, blanch with pressure and are most common on the hands and face.

Subcutaneous nodules in rheumatoid arthritis occur on the extensor surface of the forearm (Fig. 14.12). They are firm and non-tender, and may also be felt at sites of pressure or friction, e.g. the sacrum. Achilles tendons and toes are common sites for ulceration and infection. Rheumatoid nodules are strongly associated with a positive rheumatoid factor and can occur at other sites, such as the lungs.

Reactive arthritis (formerly Reiter's syndrome) has extra-articular features (Fig. 14.13A) and is associated with skin and nail changes similar to those of psoriasis,

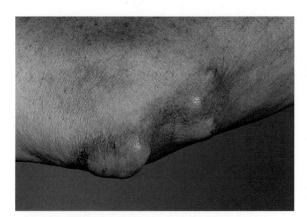

Fig. 14.12 Rheumatoid nodules and olecranon bursitis.

together with conjunctivitis, circinate balanitis (painless superficial ulcers on the prepuce and glans; Fig. 14.13B), urethritis and superficial mouth ulcers (Fig. 14.13C).

Bony nodules in osteoarthritis affect the hand, and are smaller and harder than rheumatoid nodules on the dorsal aspect of the interphalangeal (IP) joints.

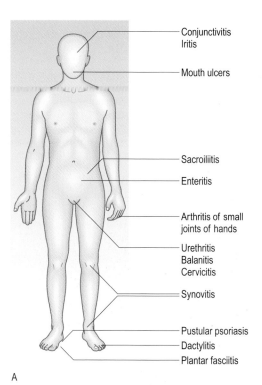

- Conjunctivitis
- Iritis
- Mouth ulcers
- Sacroiliitis
- Enteritis
- Arthritis of small joints of hands
- Urethritis
- Balanitis
- Cervicitis
- Synovitis
- Pustular psoriasis
- Dactylitis
- Plantar fasciitis

A

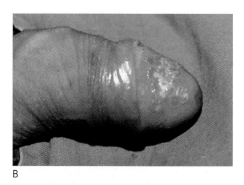

B

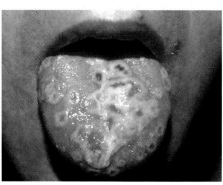

C

Fig. 14.13 Reactive arthritis. (A) Clinical features. **(B)** Lesions on the glans penis. **(C)** Ulcerated tongue.

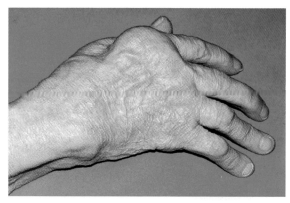

Fig. 14.14 Rheumatoid hand: showing ulnar deviation of the fingers, small muscle wasting and synovial swelling at carpus, metacarpophalangeal and proximal interphalangeal joints.

14

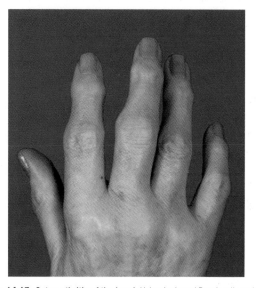

Fig. 14.15 Osteoarthritis of the hand. Heberden's and Bouchard's nodes.

At the distal interphalangeal (DIP) joints they are called Heberden's nodes, and at the proximal interphalangeal (PIP) joints, Bouchard's nodes (Fig. 14.15).

Gouty tophi are firm, white, irregular subcutaneous crystal collections (monosodium urate monohydrate). Common sites are the helix of the ear and extensor aspects of the fingers, hands and toes (Fig. 14.16). The overlying skin may ulcerate, discharging crystals, and become secondarily infected.

Small, dark red vasculitic spots due to small skin infarcts occur in many systemic inflammatory disorders, including rheumatoid arthritis, SLE (Fig. 3.16F, p. 54) and polyarteritis nodosa, and indicate active disease. Common sites for these lesions are the nail folds, finger and toe tips and other pressure areas.

Raynaud's phenomenon is episodic ischaemia of the fingers precipitated by stimuli such as cold, pain and stress. There is a typical progression of colour change. Blanching

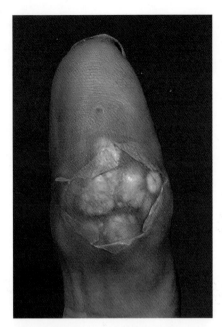

Fig. 14.16 Gouty tophus.

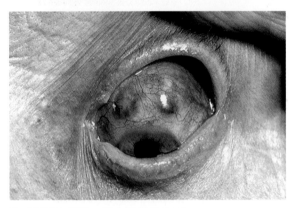

Fig. 14.17 Scleritis and scleromalacia.

(white) leads to cyanosis (blue), and is followed by reactive hyperaemia (red), associated with altered sensation (dysaesthesia) and pain. Raynaud's phenomenon is common in otherwise healthy individuals but is frequently present in systemic sclerosis and SLE.

Eye features

The eyes are affected in many inflammatory conditions.
- Conjunctivitis is a feature of reactive arthritis and ankylosing spondylitis
- Reduced tear production with 'dry eyes' (keratoconjunctivitis sicca) contributes to conjunctivitis and inflammation of the eyelids (blepharitis). This occurs in Sjögren's syndrome, rheumatoid arthritis and SLE
- Scleritis and episcleritis (Fig. 14.17) can be seen in rheumatoid arthritis and other vasculitic disorders

- Anterior uveitis (iritis) is seen in about 25% of patients with ankylosing spondylitis and reactive arthritis
- The sclerae are blue in certain types of osteogenesis imperfecta (Fig. 3.10A, p. 51).

▶ Examination sequence

▶ The Schirmer tear test is used to diagnose keratoconjunctivitis sicca.

▶ Hook a small strip of notched blotting paper about 40 mm long over the lower eyelid while the patient looks upwards. The notch is ~5 mm from one end of the strip and is the point at which the strip is bent over the eyelid.

▶ Ask patients to close their eye.

▶ Wait for exactly 5 minutes, then remove the strips.

▶ Measure the distance that tears travel down the strip with a millimetre rule; >15 mm is normal, 5–15 mm equivocal and <5 mm abnormal.

Extra-articular features of some musculoskeletal conditions are summarized in Figure 14.18.

Hypermobility

Some patients have a greater than normal range of joint movement. They may present with recurrent dislocations or sensations of instability if this is severe, but frequently do so just with arthralgia. Mild hypermobility is a normal variant but two inherited conditions affecting connective tissues — Marfan's syndrome and Ehlers–Danlos syndrome — cause hypermobility.

Hypermobility is assessed using the Beighton scoring system (Box 14.14).

14.14 The Beighton scoring system to assess hypermobility	
Ask the patient to:	**Score**
Bring the thumb to touch the forearm	1 point each side
Extend the little finger >90°	1 point each side
Extend the elbow >10°	1 point each side
Extend the knee >10°	1 point each side
Touch the floor with the palms of hands and the knees straight	1 point
A score of 4 or more indicates hypermobility.	

The GALS screen

The GALS (gait, arms, legs, spine) screen is a rapid screen for musculoskeletal and neurological deficits, and functional ability (Fig. 14.19).

Screening questions

- Do you have any pain or stiffness in your muscles, joints or back?

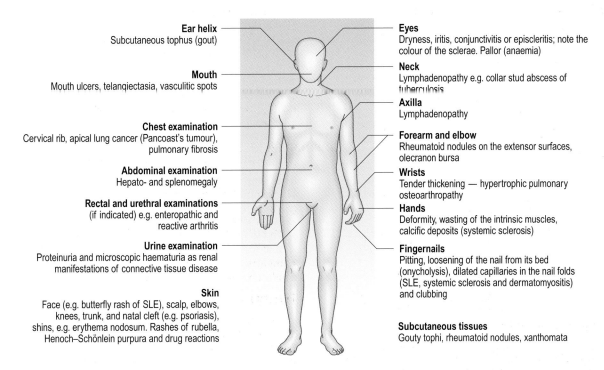

Ear helix
Subcutaneous tophus (gout)

Mouth
Mouth ulcers, telangiectasia, vasculitic spots

Chest examination
Cervical rib, apical lung cancer (Pancoast's tumour),
pulmonary fibrosis

Abdominal examination
Hepato- and splenomegaly

Rectal and urethral examinations
(if indicated) e.g. enteropathic and
reactive arthritis

Urine examination
Proteinuria and microscopic haematuria as renal
manifestations of connective tissue disease

Skin
Face (e.g. butterfly rash of SLE), scalp, elbows,
knees, trunk, and natal cleft (e.g. psoriasis),
shins, e.g. erythema nodosum. Rashes of rubella,
Henoch–Schönlein purpura and drug reactions

Eyes
Dryness, iritis, conjunctivitis or episcleritis; note the
colour of the sclerae. Pallor (anaemia)

Neck
Lymphadenopathy e.g. collar stud abscess of
tuberculosis

Axilla
Lymphadenopathy

Forearm and elbow
Rheumatoid nodules on the extensor surfaces,
olecranon bursa

Wrists
Tender thickening — hypertrophic pulmonary
osteoarthropathy

Hands
Deformity, wasting of the intrinsic muscles,
calcific deposits (systemic sclerosis)

Fingernails
Pitting, loosening of the nail from its bed
(onycholysis), dilated capillaries in the nail folds
(SLE, systemic sclerosis and dermatomyositis)
and clubbing

Subcutaneous tissues
Gouty tophi, rheumatoid nodules, xanthomata

Fig. 14.18 Extra-articular manifestations of musculoskeletal conditions.

14

- Do you have difficulty dressing yourself?
- Do you have difficulty walking up and down stairs?

If all three replies are negative, the patient is unlikely to have a significant musculoskeletal problem. If the patient answers positively, carry out a more detailed assessment.

▶ Examination sequence

GALS screen
▶ Ask the patient to undress to their underwear and stand in front of you. Demonstrate actions rather than only telling them what to do.

Gait
▶ Ask the patient to walk ahead in a straight line for several steps, then turn and walk back towards you. Look for smoothness and symmetry of the gait.

Arms
▶ Stand in front of the patient.
▶ Gently press the midpoint of each supraspinatus to detect hyperalgesia (Fig. 14.19A).
▶ Ask the patient to put his hands behind the head, with the elbows going back (Fig. 14.19B). This tests abduction and external rotation of the glenohumeral joint.
▶ Have the patient place the elbows by the side of the body and bend them 90°. Turn the palms up and down (Fig. 14.19C). This tests pronation and supination at the wrist and elbow.

▶ Ask the patient to bend the arms up to touch the shoulders. This tests elbow flexion.
▶ Show him how to make a 'prayer sign', bending the wrist back as far as possible. Put the backs of the hands together in a similar fashion. This tests wrist flexion and extension.
▶ Have the patient put his arms straight out in front of the body. This tests elbow extension.
▶ The patient next clenches the fists (Fig. 14.19D), and then opens the hands flat. This tests both wrists and hands. Inspect the dorsum of the hands and check for full finger extension at the metacarpophalangeal (MCP), PIP and DIP joints.
▶ Ask him to squeeze your index and middle fingers. This tests the strength of the power grip.
▶ Have him touch each finger tip with his thumb. This tests precision grip and problems in co-ordination or concentration.
▶ Gently squeeze the patient's metacarpal heads (Fig. 14.19E). Tenderness suggests inflammation, e.g. rheumatoid arthritis, involving the MCP and PIP joints.

Legs
▶ Ask the patient to lie supine (face up) on the couch.
▶ Carry out Thomas's test for fixed flexion deformity on both hips (p. 388) (if there is no contraindication).
▶ Flex each hip and knee with your hand on the patient's knee. Feel for crepitus in patellofemoral joint, knee and hip flexion (Fig. 14.19F).
▶ Flex the patient's knee and hip to 90°, and passively rotate each hip internally and externally, noting pain or limited movement. This tests hip rotation (internal and external).

▶ Palpate each knee for warmth and swelling. Check for patellar tap. These detect inflammation and effusions.

▶ Look at the feet for any abnormality. Examine the soles looking for calluses and ulcers, indicative of abnormal load bearing.

▶ Gently squeeze the metatarsal heads for tenderness (Fig. 14.19G).

Spine

▶ Stand behind the patient and assess the straightness of the spine, muscle bulk and symmetry in the legs and trunk. Look for any asymmetry at the level of the iliac crests (unilateral leg shortening), and swelling or other abnormality of the gluteal, hamstring, popliteal and calf muscles. Look at the Achilles tendons and hindfoot regions for swelling or deformity.

▶ Stand beside the patient and ask him to bend down and try to touch the toes (Fig. 14.19H). This highlights any abnormal spinal curvature or limited extension at the hips.

▶ Stand behind the patient, hold the pelvis, and ask him to turn from side to side without moving the feet. This tests mainly thoracolumbar rotation.

▶ Ask him to slide the hand down the leg towards the knee. This tests lateral lumbar flexion.

▶ Stand in front of the patient and ask him to put the ear on the shoulder (Fig. 14.19I) to test lateral cervical flexion.

▶ Ask him to look up at the ceiling and then down at the floor to test cervical flexion and extension.

▶ Have the patient let the jaw drop open and move it from side to side. This tests both temporomandibular joints.

The GALS screen provides a rapid, but limited, assessment. The following section describes the detailed examination required for full evaluation.

Gait

Gait is the cyclical pattern of musculoskeletal motion that carries the body forwards. Normal gait is smooth, symmetrical and ergonomically economical, with each leg 50% out of phase with the other.

For each leg, gait has two phases: stance and swing. The stance phase is from foot-strike to toe-off, when the foot is on the ground and load-bearing (Fig. 14.20). The swing phase is from toe-off to foot-strike, when the foot clears the ground. When both feet are on the ground this is double stance.

A limp is an abnormal gait due to pain, structural change e.g. lower limb length discrepancy, tone abnormality or weakness.

Pain

An antalgic gait is one which is altered to reduce pain. Pain in a lower limb is usually aggravated by weight-bearing, so the patient minimizes the time spent in the stance phase on that side. This results in a 'dot–dash' mode of walking.

If the source of pain is in the spine, then axial rotatory movements are minimized, resulting in a slow gait with small paces. Patients with hip pain may lean towards the affected side as this decreases the compression force on the hip joint.

Structural change

Patients with limb-length discrepancy may walk on tiptoe on the shorter side, and have compensatory hip and knee flexion on the longer side. There may be pelvic tilting on block testing (p. 387). Other structural changes producing an abnormal gait include deformities such as joint fusions, bone malunions and contractures.

Weakness

This may be due to nerve or muscle pathology or alteration in muscle tone.

In a normal gait the hip abductors of the stance leg raise the contralateral hemipelvis. In Trendelenburg gait, abductor function is poor when weight-bearing on the affected side, so the contralateral hemipelvis falls. This effect may be reduced by a truncal lurch over the affected hip (Duchenne sign; Fig. 14.46).

Common causes of a Trendelenburg gait are:

- weakness of the hip abductors, e.g. in polio or paresis of the superior gluteal nerve after total hip replacement
- structural hip joint problems, e.g. congenital dislocation of the hip
- painful hip joint problems, e.g. osteoarthritis.

Foot drop occurs in common peroneal nerve palsy. The gait is high-stepping to allow clearance of the weak foot.

Increased tone

This occurs following an upper motor neurone lesion, e.g. cerebrovascular accident (stroke) or cerebral palsy. The gait depends on the specific lesion, contractures and compensatory mechanisms. A common pattern in cerebral palsy is the energy-inefficient crouch gait, from gastrocnemius and soleus weakness in which the hips and knees are always flexed.

▶▶ **Examination sequence**

Gait

▶ Ask the patient to walk barefoot in a straight line; then repeat in shoes.

▶ Observe the patient from behind, in front and from the side.

▶ Evaluate what happens at each level (foot, ankle, knee, hip and pelvis, trunk and spine) during both stance and swing phases.

The procedure for examination of the joints is given in Box 14.15.

The spine

The spine is divided into the cervical, thoracic, lumbar and sacral segments. Most spinal diseases affect multiple segments and cause alteration in the posture or function of the whole spine. Spinal disease may occur without local symptoms and present with pain, neurological symptoms or signs in the trunk or limbs. The key

14

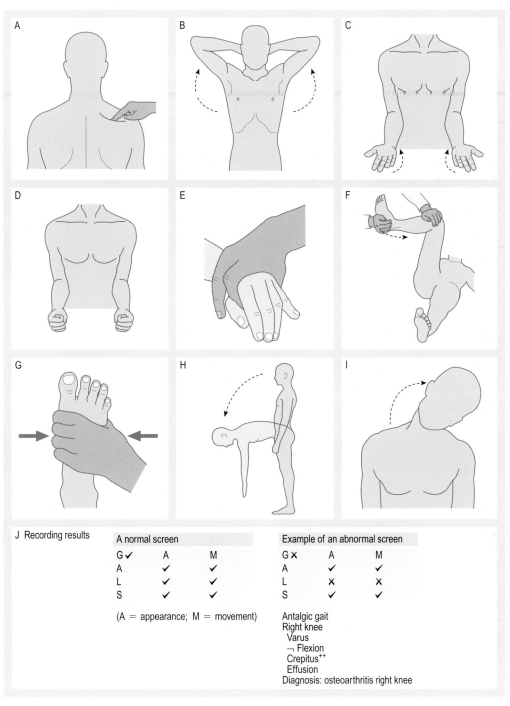

A

B

C

D

E

F

G

H

I

J Recording results

A normal screen		
G ✔	A	M
A	✔	✔
L	✔	✔
S	✔	✔

(A = appearance; M = movement)

Example of an abnormal screen		
G ✗	A	M
A	✔	✔
L	✗	✗
S	✔	✔

Antalgic gait
Right knee
 Varus
  ⌐ Flexion
 Crepitus++
 Effusion
Diagnosis: osteoarthritis right knee

Fig. 14.19 The GALS screen.

to accurate diagnosis depends on knowledge of the underlying bony and neurological anatomy (Fig. 14.21), a careful history, and eliciting signs and symptoms to differentiate between mechanical (non-inflammatory) and inflammatory causes (Box 14.16).

Nomenclature in spinal disease

- Scoliosis: lateral curvature of the spine (Fig. 14.22A)
- Kyphosis: curvature of the spine in the sagittal (anterior–posterior) plane, with the apex posterior

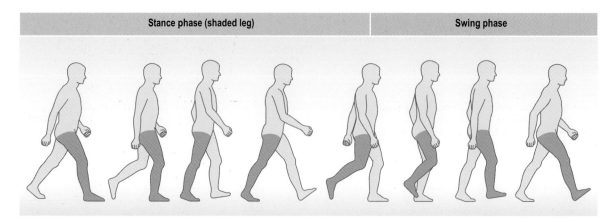

Stance phase (shaded leg)	Swing phase

Fig. 14.20 Phases of the normal gait cycle.

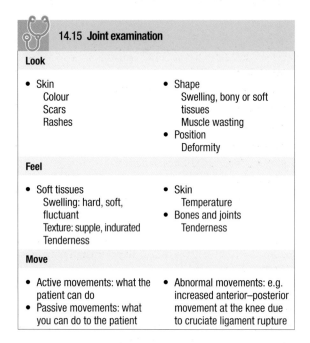

14.15 Joint examination

Look

- Skin
  Colour
  Scars
  Rashes
- Shape
  Swelling, bony or soft tissues
  Muscle wasting
- Position
  Deformity

Feel

- Soft tissues
  Swelling: hard, soft, fluctuant
  Texture: supple, indurated
  Tenderness
- Skin
  Temperature
- Bones and joints
  Tenderness

Move

- Active movements: what the patient can do
- Passive movements: what you can do to the patient
- Abnormal movements: e.g. increased anterior–posterior movement at the knee due to cruciate ligament rupture

(Fig. 14.22B). (The thoracic spine normally has a mild kyphosis)

- Lordosis: curvature of the spine in the sagittal (anterior–posterior) plane, with the apex anterior (Fig. 14.22C)
- Gibbus: spinal deformity caused by an anterior wedge deformity localized to a single vertebra producing an increase in forward flexion (Fig. 14.22D)
- Spondylosis: degenerative change in the spine.
- Spondylolisthesis: one vertebra slipping anteriorly on an inferior vertebra (Fig. 14.23A)
- Spondylolysis: defect in the pars interarticularis of a vertebral arch (Fig. 14.23B)
- Retrolisthesis: one vertebra slipping posteriorly on an inferior vertebra.

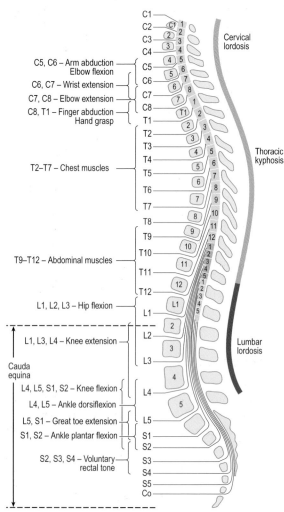

Fig. 14.21 The normal spinal curves and root innervations.

14.16 Common spinal problems

- Mechanical back pain
- Prolapsed intervertebral disc
- Spinal stenosis
- Ankylosing spondylitis
- Compensatory scoliosis from leg-length discrepancy
- Cervical myelopathy
- Pathological pain/deformity, e.g. osteomyelitis, tumour, myeloma
- Osteoporotic vertebral fracture resulting in kyphosis (or rarely lordosis), especially in the thoracic spine with loss of height
- Cervical rib
- Scoliosis
- Spinal instability, e.g. spondylolisthesis

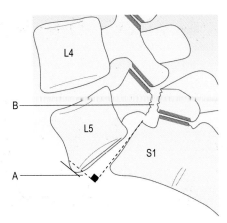

Fig. 14.23 Lumbosacral junction. (A) Anterior translation of L5 on S1 (spondylolisthesis). **(B)** Defect in pars interarticularis (spondylolysis).

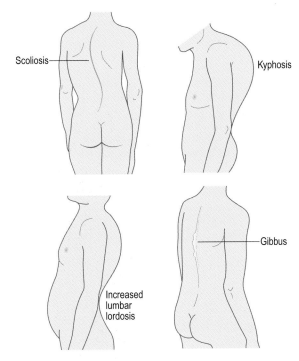

Fig. 14.22 Spinal deformities.

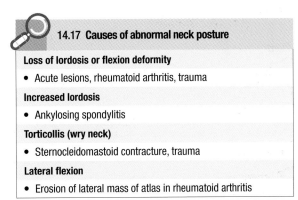

14.17 Causes of abnormal neck posture

Loss of lordosis or flexion deformity

- Acute lesions, rheumatoid arthritis, trauma

Increased lordosis

- Ankylosing spondylitis

Torticollis (wry neck)

- Sternocleidomastoid contracture, trauma

Lateral flexion

- Erosion of lateral mass of atlas in rheumatoid arthritis

Cervical spine

Anatomy

Head nodding occurs at the atlanto-occipital joints, and rotational neck movements mainly at the atlanto-axial joint. Flexion, extension and lateral flexion occur mainly at the midcervical level.

The neural canal contains the spinal cord and the emerging nerve roots, which pass through exit foramina bounded by the facet joints posteriorly and the intervertebral discs and neurocentral joints anteriorly. The nerve roots, particularly in the lower cervical spine, may be compressed or irritated by lateral disc protrusion or by osteophytes arising from the facet or neurocentral joints. A central disc protrusion may press directly on the cord.

The history

The most common symptoms are pain and difficulty turning the head and neck. Patients find difficulty driving, especially when attempting to reverse.

Neck pain is usually felt posteriorly but may be referred to the head, shoulder, arm or interscapular region. Cervical disc lesions cause radicular pain in one or other arm, roughly following the dermatomes of the nerve roots affected (Box 14.4).

If the spinal cord is compromised (cervical myelopathy), then lower limb weakness, difficulty walking, loss of sensation and sphincter disturbance may occur.

- Be particularly careful during examination of patients with rheumatoid arthritis, as atlanto-axial instability can lead to spinal cord damage when the neck is flexed
- In patients with a history of neck injury never elicit the range of movements. Splint the neck and check for abnormal posture. Check neurological function in the limbs and X-ray to assess bony injury.

◼◢ Examination sequence

Cervical spine

◼◢ Ask the patient to remove enough clothing for you to see the neck and upper thorax, then to sit on a chair.

Look

◼◢ Face the patient. Observe the posture of the head and neck and note any abnormality or deformity, such as loss of lordosis (usually due to muscle spasm) (Box 14.17).

Feel

◼◢ Feel the midline spinous processes from the occiput to T1 (the process of T1 is usually the most prominent).

◼◢ Feel the paraspinal soft tissues.

◼◢ Feel the supraclavicular fossae — for cervical ribs or enlarged cervical lymph nodes.

◼◢ Feel the anterior neck structures, including the thyroid.

◼◢ Note any tenderness in the spine, trapezius, interscapular and paraspinal muscles.

Move

◼◢ Assess active movements first (Fig. 14.24).

◼◢ Ask the patient to put his chin on to the chest so that you can assess forward flexion. The normal range is 0 (neutral) to 80°. Record a decreased range as the chin–chest distance.

◼◢ Ask the patient to look upwards at the ceiling as far back as possible, to assess extension. The normal range is 0 (neutral) to 50°. Thus the total flexion–extension arc is usually around 130°.

◼◢ Ask the patient to put his ear on to the shoulder, to assess lateral flexion. The normal range is 0 (neutral) to 45°.

◼◢ Ask the patient to look over his or her right/left shoulder. The normal range of lateral rotation is 0 (neutral) to 80°.

◼◢ Gently perform passive movements, if there are reduced active movements, and see if the end of the range has a sudden or a gradual resistance and whether it is pain or stiffness that restricts movement. Note any pain or paraesthesiae in the arm on passive neck movement, suggesting nerve root involvement.

◼◢ Perform a neurological assessment of the upper and lower limbs (Figs. 11.20 and 11.21, p. 290).

Thoracic spine

Anatomy

This segment of the spine is the least mobile and maintains a physiological kyphosis throughout life. Movement is mainly rotational with a very limited amount of flexion, extension and lateral flexion.

The history

The presenting symptoms in the thoracic spine are localized spinal pain (Box 14.18), pain radiating round the chest wall or, less frequently, symptoms of paraparesis, including sensory loss, leg weakness, and loss of bladder or bowel control. Disc lesions are rare but may be accompanied by pain radiating around the chest (girdle pain), mimicking cardiac or pleural disease. Patients with osteoporotic vertebral fractures may not complain of pain, but lose height and have deformity (increased kyphosis).

Pain from the thoracolumbar junction in ankylosing spondylitis may be confused with pulmonary, renal or cardiac problems. Patients with vertebral collapse due to malignancy may have associated spinal cord compression. Consider infection as a cause of acute pain, especially if systemic upset or fever is present. When thoracic pain is poorly localized, consider intrathoracic causes such as myocardial ischaemia or infarction, oesophageal or pleural pain, and aortic aneurysm.

◼◢ Examination sequence

Thoracic spine

◼◢ Ask the patient to undress to expose the neck, chest and back.

Look

◼◢ With the patient standing, inspect the posture from behind, the side and the front, noting any deformity, e.g. rib hump or abnormal curvature.

Feel

◼◢ The midline spinous processes from T1 to T12. Feel for increased prominence of one or more posterior spinal processes, implying anterior wedge-shaped collapse of the vertebral body — often related to osteoporosis.

◼◢ The paraspinal soft tissues for tenderness.

Move

◼◢ Ask the patient to sit with the arms crossed. Ask him to twist round both ways and look at you.

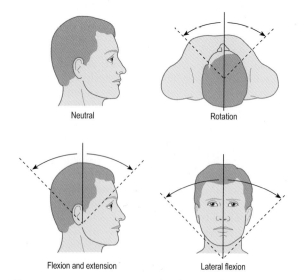

Neutral Rotation

Flexion and extension Lateral flexion

Fig. 14.24 Movements of the cervical spine.

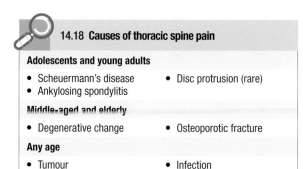

14.18 Causes of thoracic spine pain

Adolescents and young adults

- Scheuermann's disease
- Ankylosing spondylitis
- Disc protrusion (rare)

Middle-aged and elderly

- Degenerative change
- Osteoporotic fracture

Any age

- Tumour
- Infection

Lumbar spine

Anatomy

The surface markings are the spinous processes of L4/5, which are level with the pelvic brim, and the 'dimples of Venus', which overlie the sacroiliac joints. The normal lordosis may be lost in disorders such as ankylosing spondylitis and lumbar disc protrusion.

The principal movements are flexion, extension, lateral flexion and rotation. Most patients can bring the tips of their fingers at least to the level of the knees in forward and lateral flexion. Extension should be approximately 10–20°. In flexion, the upper segments move first, followed by the lower segments, to produce a smooth lumbar curve. However, even with a rigid lumbar spine, patients may be able to touch their toes if the hips are mobile.

In the adult, the spinal cord ends at L2. Below this, the spinal nerve roots may be injured or compressed by disc protrusion; above this level the spinal cord itself may be involved.

The history

Low back pain is extremely common. Most is 'mechanical', and due to degenerative disease. Radicular back pain due to nerve root compression radiates down the posterior aspect of the leg to the ankle (sciatica). Pain due to inflammation of the sacroiliac joints is commonly felt in the buttocks, but may be referred down both legs to the knees. Groin and thigh pain in the absence of hip abnormality suggests referred pain from L1, 2.

Red flag features suggest significant spinal pathology (Box 14.19). Consider abdominal and retroperitoneal pathology too, e.g. abdominal aortic aneurysm, pancreatitis, peptic ulcer and renal disorders.

Important spinal conditions are acute disc protrusion, spinal stenosis, ankylosing spondylitis (Fig. 14.25), osteoporotic fracture, infection and tumours. Infection and tumours are associated with weight loss or fever. In the majority of patients, however, backache reflects age-related degenerative change in discs and facet joints (spondylosis).

Mechanical low back pain is common after standing for too long or sitting in a poor position. Symptoms worsen as the day progresses and improve after resting or on rising in the morning.

Insidious onset of backache and stiffness in a young adult suggests inflammatory disease of the sacroiliac joints and lumbar spine. Symptoms are worse in the morning or after inactivity, and ease with movement. Morning stiffness is more marked than in osteoarthritis, lasting 30–60 minutes. There may be other clues to the diagnosis, such as peripheral joint involvement, extra articular features or a positive family history.

Acute onset of low back pain in a young adult, often associated with bending or lifting, is typical of acute disc protrusion (slipped disc). The acute episode may be superimposed on a background of preceding

14

14.19 'Red flag' features for acute low back pain

History

- Age <20 yrs or >55 yrs
- Recent significant trauma (fracture)
- Pain:
  - Thoracic (dissecting aneurysm)
  - Non-mechanical (infection/tumour/pathological fracture)
- Fever (infection)
- Difficulty in micturition
- Faecal incontinence
- Motor weakness
- Sensory changes in the perineum (saddle anaesthesia)
- Sexual dysfunction, e.g. erectile/ejaculatory failure
- Gait change (cauda equina syndrome)
- Bilateral 'sciatica'

Past medical history

- Cancer (metastases)
- Previous steroid use (osteoporotic collapse)

System review

- Weight loss/malaise without obvious cause, e.g. cancer

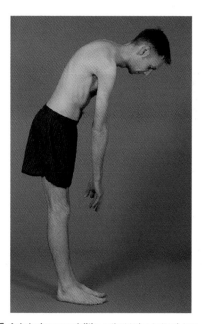

Fig. 14.25 Ankylosing spondylitis: patient trying to touch toes.

mild episodic backache due to disc degeneration. Activities such as coughing or straining to open the bowels exacerbate the pain. There may be symptoms of lumbar or sacral nerve root compression (cauda equina syndrome). If the sacral nerve roots are involved, there may be loss of sphincter control and perianal sensation.

Acute back pain in the middle-aged, elderly or those with preceding factors, e.g. steroid therapy, may be due to osteoporotic fracture. This is eased by lying, exacerbated by spinal flexion and not usually associated with neurological symptoms.

An acute onset of severe progressive pain, especially associated with malaise, weight loss or night sweats, may indicate pyogenic or tuberculous infection of the lumbar spine or sacroiliac joint. The patient may have a past history of diabetes mellitus or immunosuppression, e.g. steroid therapy or HIV infection, and complain of pain and great difficulty in moving. The infection may involve the intervertebral discs and adjacent vertebrae and may track into the psoas muscle sheath, presenting as a painful flexed hip or a groin swelling.

Consider malignant disease involving a vertebral body in patients with unremitting spinal pain of recent onset, disturbing sleep. Other clues are a previous history of cancer, and systemic symptoms or weight loss. Tumours rarely affect intervertebral discs.

Cauda equina syndrome and spinal cord compression are neurosurgical emergencies. If you suspect them, refer the patient immediately for assessment and possible surgical decompression.

Intermittent discomfort or pain in the lumbar spine occurring over a long period of time is typical of degenerative disc disease. There is stiffness in the morning or after immobility. Pain and stiffness are relieved by gentle activity but recur with, or after, excessive activity. Over years there is gradual loss of lumbar spine mobility, sometimes with spontaneous improvement in pain as the facet joints become increasingly stiff.

Diffuse pain in the buttocks or thighs brought on by standing too long or walking is the presenting symptom of lumbosacral spinal stenosis. This can be difficult to distinguish from intermittent claudication (p. 140). The pain may be accompanied by tingling and numbness and may be difficult for the patient to describe. Typically, it is relieved by rest or spinal flexion. Stooping or holding on to a supermarket trolley may increase exercise tolerance. Narrowing of the spinal canal or neural exit foraminae is caused by degenerative changes in the intervertebral discs and facet joints, and there is a long preceding history of discomfort typical of degenerative joint disease.

◼◥ Examination sequence

Lumbar spine
Look

◼◥ Examine the patient standing with the back fully exposed. Look for obvious deformity, such as decreased/increased lordosis, obvious scoliosis, soft tissue abnormalities like a hairy patch or lipoma that might overlie a congenital abnormality, e.g. spina bifida.

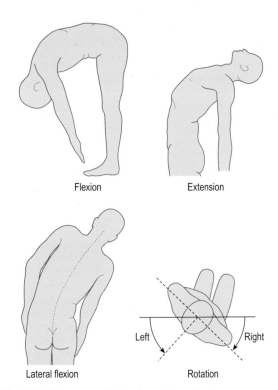

Flexion　　　　Extension

Lateral flexion　　　　Rotation

Left　　　Right

Fig. 14.26 Movements of the lumbar and dorsal spine.

Feel

◼◥ Palpate the spinous processes and paraspinal tissues. Note the overall alignment and focal tenderness (the L4/5 interspinous space is palpable at the level of the iliac crests). After warning the patient, lightly percuss the spine with your closed fist and note any tenderness.

Move (Fig. 14.26)

◼◥ Flexion: ask the patient to try to touch the toes with the legs straight. Record how far down the legs the patient can reach; a certain amount of such movement is dependent on hip flexion. Note any abnormality of this movement. Usually the upper segments should flex before the lower ones, and this progression should be smooth.

◼◥ Extension: ask the patient to straighten up and lean back as far as possible (normal 10–20° from neutral erect posture).

◼◥ Lateral flexion: ask the patient to reach down to each side, touching the outside of the leg as far down as possible while keeping the legs straight.

Special tests

◼◥ Examination sequence

Schober's test for forward flexion

◼◥ Mark the skin in the midline at the level of the dimples of Venus, which overlie the sacroiliac joints (Fig. 14.27; mark A).

◼◥ Using a tape measure, draw two more marks: one 10 cm above (mark B) and one 5 cm below this (mark C).

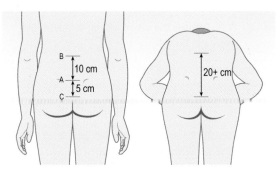

Fig. 14.27 Schober's test. Measuring forward flexion of the spine.

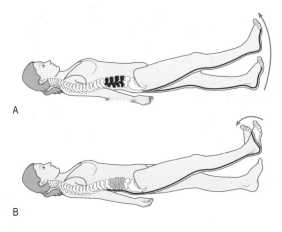

▪**➤** Place the end of the tape measure on the upper mark (B) and ask the patient to touch his toes. The distance from mark B to mark C should increase from 15 to more than 20 cm.

Root compression tests

Prolapse of an intervertebral disc causing pressure on a nerve root occurs most often in the lower lumbar region, leading to compression of the corresponding nerve roots.

The femoral nerve (L2, L3, L4) lies anterior to the pubic ramus, so straight leg-raising or other forms of hip flexion do not increase its root tension. Problems with the femoral nerve roots may cause quadriceps weakness and/or diminished knee jerk on that side.

The sciatic nerve (L4, L5; S1, S2, S3) runs behind the pelvis, so manœuvres designed to put tension on the lower nerve roots (L4 exiting the L4/5 foramen, L5 exiting the L5/S1 foramen) differ from those for the upper lumbar nerve roots (L2, L3).

■**➤ Examination sequence**

Straight leg raise

▪**➤** This tests L4, L5, S1 nerve root tension (L3/4, L4/5 and L5/S1 disc prolapse respectively).
▪**➤** With the patient lying supine, lift the foot to flex the hip passively, keeping the knee straight.
▪**➤** Measure the angle between the couch and the flexed leg to determine any limitation (normal 80–90° hip flexion) caused by thigh or leg pain.
▪**➤** If a limit is reached, raise the leg to just less than this level, and test for nerve root tension by dorsiflexing the foot (Fig. 14.28).

■**➤ Examination sequence**

Tibial nerve stretch

▪**➤** This tests L4, L5, S1, S2 and S3.
▪**➤** With the patient supine, flex the hip to 90°.
▪**➤** Extend the knee. In this position the tibial nerve 'bowstrings' across the popliteal fossa. Press over either of the hamstring tendons, and

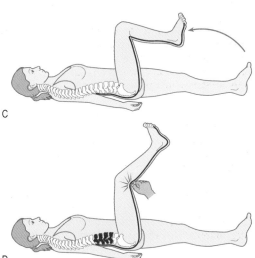

Fig. 14.28 Stretch tests: sciatic nerve. (A) Straight leg raising limited by tension of root over prolapsed disc. **(B)** Tension increased by dorsiflexion of foot (Bragard's test). **(C)** Root tension relieved by flexion at the knee. **(D)** Pressure over centre of popliteal fossa bears on posterior tibial nerve which is 'bowstringing' across the fossa, causing pain locally and radiation into the back.

then over the nerve in the middle of the fossa. The test is positive if pain occurs when the nerve is pressed, but not the hamstring tendons (Fig. 14.28D).

■**➤ Examination sequence**

Femoral nerve stretch test

▪**➤** This tests L2, L3 and L4.
▪**➤** With the patient lying on the front (prone) flex the knee and extend the hip (Fig. 14.29). This stretches the femoral nerve. A positive result is when pain is felt in the back or the front of the thigh.

14

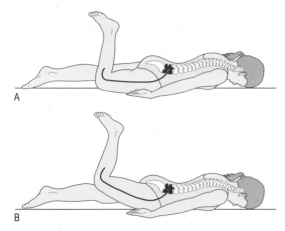

Fig. 14.29 Stretch test: femoral nerve. (A) Pain may be triggered by knee flexion alone. **(B)** Pain may be triggered by knee flexion in combination with hip extension.

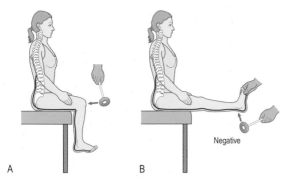

Fig. 14.30 Sciatic nerve. The 'flip' test. **(A)** Attention is diverted to the tendon reflexes. **(B)** The patient with actual nerve root compression cannot permit full extension of the leg.

▶ Examination sequence

Flip test (functional) overlay

- Ask the patient to sit on the end of the couch with the hips and knees flexed to 90° (Fig. 14.30A).
- Examine the knee reflexes.
- Extend the knee, as if to examine the ankle jerk. The patient with a prolapsed disc will lie back ('flip'; Fig. 14.30B).

▶ Examination sequence: the sacroiliac joints

- Tests for movement and pain in these joints are unreliable, but compressing the pelvis or pressing down on the sacrum with the 'heel' of your hand with the subject lying prone may produce pain if these joints are inflamed.

The upper limb

Distinguish between systemic and local conditions. Systemic conditions, e.g. rheumatoid arthritis, usually

---

OSCEs 14.20 Examine this patient with acute lumbar back pain

1. With the patient standing, look for spinal deformity, e.g. decreased lordosis, scoliosis, scars, and for skin abnormality, e.g. hairy patch found in spina bifida.
2. Feel the spinous processes and paraspinal tissues for any focal tenderness.
3. Gently percuss the vertebral column with your closed fist, noting any tenderness.
4. Ask the patient to try to touch his or her toes with the legs kept straight and record how far down the patient can reach.
5. Ask the patient to straighten up and lean back as far as possible and record the amount of movement.
6. Ask the patient to reach down to each side, touching the outside of the leg as far as possible, and record the amount of flexion.
7. Perform the straight leg-raising test.
8. Perform the femoral stretch test.
9. Check lower limb reflexes, power and sensation (including the perineum), and anal tone.

---

cause pathology at several sites. Local conditions must be distinguished from referred or radicular pain. Work out whether the condition is inflammatory or non-inflammatory on the basis of the pattern of diurnal stiffness and pain.

The prime function of the upper limb is to position the hand appropriately in space. This requires a range of movements at the shoulder, elbow and wrist. The hand may function in both precision and power modes. The intrinsic muscles of the hand allow both grip and fine manipulative movements, and the forearm muscles provide power and stability.

The patient should be seated, facing you, with the arms and shoulders exposed. Examine the hand and fingers first, and move proximally.

The hand and wrist

The wrist joint has metacarpocarpal, intercarpal, ulnocarpal and radiocarpal components. There is a wide range of possible movements, including flexion, extension, adduction (deviation towards the ulnar side), abduction (deviation towards the radial side) and circumduction (a composite movement where the hand can move in a conical fashion on the wrist).

The proximal and distal interphalangeal (PIP and DIP) joints are hinge joints and allow only flexion and extension. The metacarpophalangeal (MCP) joints allow flexion and extension, and abduction/adduction that is greatest when the MCP joints are extended.

When examining and documenting the fingers use their names, to avoid confusion (Fig. 14.31).

Motor innervation of the hand is shown in Box 14.21.

The patient will often localize complaints of pain, stiffness, loss of function, contractures, disfigurement and trauma. If symptoms are more vague or diffuse, then consider referred pain or a compressive neuropathy: for

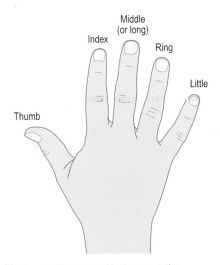

Fig. 14.31 Names of fingers used in documentation.

i	14.21 Motor innervation of the hand	
Nerve	**Muscles supplied**	
Median	Opponens and abductor muscles of the hand and most of the wrist and finger flexors	
Ulnar	Adductor of thumb, most of lumbricals and interossei	
Radial	Extensors of wrist and hand	

OSCEs 14.22 Examine the hands and forearms of this patient with joint pains in the hands, feet and wrists

1. Expose the arms to above the elbow.
2. Ask the patient if his hands are painful before moving or feeling them.
3. Look at the position of the fingers and note any deviation from the norm.
4. Look at the skin and nails for erythema, thinning, purpura, signs of psoriasis, nail-fold infarcts, scars and any other changes. Turn the hands over to see the palmar skin.
5. Note any small muscle wasting, swelling, nodules and deformity. Describe the deformities.
6. Feel each joint in turn for warmth and swelling. Note the character of any swelling and decide whether it is bony, soft tissue or a joint effusion. Are any deformities reducible?
7. Assess passive and active movements of each affected joint and note any limitation of movement.
8. Feel the ulnar border of the forearm for nodules (seropositive rheumatoid arthritis) and look for scaling (psoriasis).

example, compression of the median nerve as it traverses the carpal tunnel in the wrist, which leads to the symptoms and signs of carpal tunnel syndrome (Fig. 14.32). It can be idiopathic, but other causes are

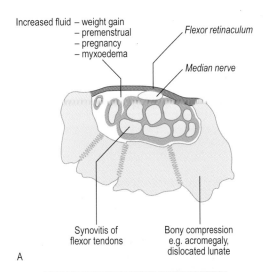

A

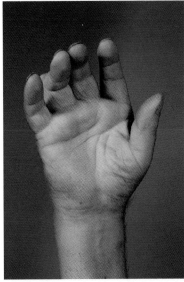

B

Fig. 14.32 Carpal tunnel syndrome. (A) Causes of median nerve compression. **(B)** Thenar muscle wasting.

inflammatory and degenerative arthritis, diabetes, hypothyroidism, acromegaly and pregnancy. Typical symptoms are pain, tingling and numbness in the thumb and fingers, and pain can extend proximally up the arm. Symptoms may wake the patient at night and can be alleviated by shaking the hand. Weakness can lead to a poor grip and a complaint of dropping things. Hands may feel swollen, particularly in the morning. Look for wasting of the thenar eminence (Fig. 14.32B). Examine for weakness of thumb abduction and opposition (Figs 14.38A and B). Percussion over the carpal tunnel elicits tingling in the affected fingers (Tinel's sign), and forced flexion of the wrist over 30 seconds will yield the same (Phalen's sign). There may be reduced sensation in the median nerve distribution.

Nerve conduction tests may support the diagnosis but can be normal.

◤ Examination sequence

The hand and wrist
Look

◢ Colour change: erythema suggests acute inflammation caused by soft tissue infection, septic arthritis, tendon sheath infection or crystal-induced disease (gout and pseudogout).

◢ Swelling: swelling at the MCP and/or IP joints suggests synovitis. Swelling of MCP joints produces loss of interdigital indentation on the dorsum of the hand, especially when the MCP and IP joints are fully flexed (loss of normal 'hill–valley–hill–valley' aspect; Fig. 14.33A). Swelling at the PIP joints produces a 'spindling' appearance, which is typically seen in rheumatoid arthritis and collateral ligament injuries.

◢ Deformity:

- The fingers are long in Marfan's syndrome (arachnodactyly; Fig. 3.27B, p. 63).
- Phalangeal fractures may produce rotational deformity. Detect by flexing the fingers together (Fig. 14.34) and then in turn.

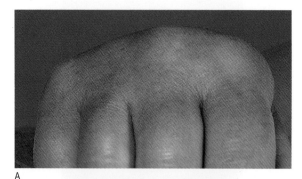

A

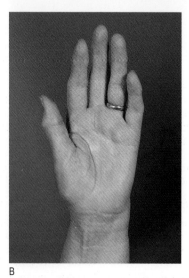

B

Fig. 14.33 Hand and wrist swelling. (A) Ask the patient to make a fist. Look at it straight on to detect any loss of 'hill and valley'. **(B)** Squaring of the wrist due to osteophytes at the carpometacarpal joint of the thumb.

Normally, with the MCP and IP joints flexed, the fingers should not cross, and should point to the scaphoid tubercle in the wrist.

- At the IP joints (Fig. 14.35), you may find 'mallet' finger, a flexion deformity at the DIP joint which is passively correctable. This is usually caused by minor trauma disrupting the terminal extensor expansion at the base of the distal phalanx, either with or without bony avulsion.
- Boutonnière (or button-hole) deformity is a flexion deformity at the PIP joint with hyperextension at the DIP joint (imagine the tip of the finger pressed firmly on to a button) and fixed flexion at the PIP joint (Fig. 14.35).
- 'Swan neck' deformity is hyperextension at the PIP joint with flexion at the DIP joint.
- There may be subluxation and ulnar deviation of the MCP joints.
- Dupuytren's contracture affects the palmar fascia, resulting in the MCP and PIP joints of the little and ring fingers becoming fixed in flexion (Fig. 3.12, p. 53).
- Anterior (or volar) displacement — partial dislocation — of the wrist may be seen in rheumatoid arthritis.

◢ Extra-articular signs (Box 14.23):

- Small muscle wasting, especially of the interossei in inflammatory arthritis (T1 nerve root lesion or ulnar nerve palsy)
- Vasculitis of the fingers, most commonly detected in the nail folds (Fig. 3.16E, p. 54).
- Palmar erythema.
- Nail changes, e.g. pitting (psoriasis) and loosening of the nail from its bed (onycholysis) in psoriatic arthritis (Fig. 3.16B, p. 54).

Feel

◢ Hard swellings suggest bony outgrowths (osteophytes) characteristic of osteoarthritis, mucous cysts or, rarely, tumours. Heberden's and Bouchard's nodes occur at the DIP and PIP joints respectively.

◢ Soft swellings suggest synovitis:

- Detect synovitis in the IP joints by gently squeezing with your thumb and index finger above and below the joint to detect sponginess.
- Test the MCP joints by examining for sponginess within the interphalangeal space by squeezing gently across the metacarpal joints.

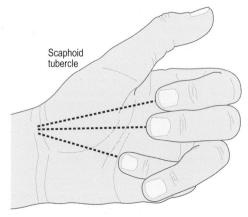

Scaphoid tubercle

Fig. 14.34 Flexion of the fingers showing rotational deformity of the ring finger.

14.23 Examples of visible abnormalities of the hands

Abnormality	Appearance and consistency	Typical site	Associated disease
Heberden's nodes	Small bony nodules	DIP joints	Osteoarthritis
Bouchard's nodes	Small bony nodules	PIP joints	Osteoarthritis
Rheumatoid nodules	Fleshy and firm	Extensor surface of knuckles	Rheumatoid arthritis
Tophi	White subcutaneous	Juxta-articular	Gout
Calcific deposits	White subcutaneous	Finger pulp	Systemic sclerosis, dermatomyositis
Dilated capillaries	(Use magnifying glass)	Nail folds	Systemic sclerosis, dermatomyositis, SLE

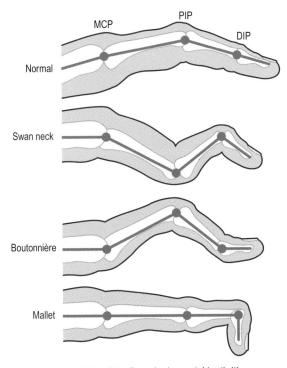

Fig. 14.35 Deformities of the finger in rheumatoid arthritis.

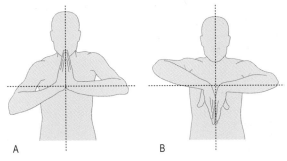

Fig. 14.36 Assessing the wrist. (A) Extension. (B) Flexion. Reduced range of movement at right wrist.

- Palpate the flexor tendon sheaths in the hand and fingers to detect local swellings or tenderness. If you detect any swelling (usually just proximal to the MCP joints) look for triggering or 'locking' during extension of the previously flexed finger.
- To detect crepitus, place your index finger across the patient's fully extended fingers and ask him to open and close the fingers. Swelling, tenderness and crepitus are found over the tendon sheaths of abductor pollicis longus and extensor pollicis brevis in De Quervain's tenosynovitis. Symptoms are aggravated by movements at the wrist and thumb. Crepitus at this site is often felt as a creaking sensation and may even be audible. Crepitus may also occur with movement of the radiocarpal joints in osteoarthritis, most commonly secondary to old scaphoid or distal radial fractures.

Move

▶ To assess active movements of the hand, ask the patient to make a fist, then extend his fingers fully. Lack of full extension of one or more fingers may indicate tendon rupture. To test grip, ask the patient to squeeze two of your fingers inserted from the thumb side into the palm of his or her hand.

- Assess flexor tendon sheath abnormalities by passive movements of the hand to look for triggering.

▶ To assess movements at the wrist, ask the patient to put the palms of the hands together and extend the wrists fully: 'prayer sign' (normal is 90° of extension) (Fig. 14.36A). To assess wrist flexion, ask the patient to put the backs of his hands together and flex the wrists fully: 'reverse prayer sign' (normal 90° of flexion) (Fig. 14.36B).

Examining the wrist and hand with a wound

Specifically test the tendons, nerves and circulation in a patient with wound(s) to the wrist or hand. The site of the wound and the position of the hand at the time of injury indicate the structure(s) possibly damaged. Normal movement may still be possible, even if 90% of a tendon has been divided. Careful surgical exploration is needed for correct diagnosis and treatment. Sensory aspects of nerve injury are covered on page 299.

14

14

▶ Examination sequence

Wrist and hand with a wound

Muscles and tendons

▶ Flexor digitorum profundus is the only flexor of the DIP joint. Ask the patient to flex the DIP joint while you hold the PIP joint in extension (Fig. 14.37A).

▶ Flexor digitorum superficialis flexes the PIP joint, but to test for flexor digitorum superficialis you have to eliminate the action of flexor digitorum profundus, as it can also flex the PIP joint. Do this by holding the other fingers fully extended and asking the patient to flex the PIP joint in question (Fig. 14.37B).

▶ To assess extensor digitorum, ask the patient to extend the fingers with the wrist in the neutral position (Fig. 14.37C).

▶ To assess flexor and extensor pollicis longus, hold the proximal phalanx of the patient's thumb firmly and ask him to flex and extend the IP joint (Fig. 14.37D).

▶ To assess extensor pollicis longus, ask the patient to place the hand palm down on a flat surface and to extend the thumb like a hitch-hiker (Fig. 14.37E). If the tendon is intact, the patient will be able to do this. Pain occurs in De Quervain's disease.

Nerves (motor function only)

▶ The median nerve supplies the thenar muscles, which abduct and oppose the thumb.
- Place the patient's hand flat, palm up, on a table. Ask the patient to abduct the thumb (a vertical movement up from the palm) and to hold it in that position against resistance (Fig. 14.38A).
- To test opposition, ask the patient to touch the tip of the little finger and keep it there against resistance (Fig. 14.38B).

▶ The ulnar nerve supplies the interossei and adductor pollicis muscles.
- To test the interossei, ask the patient to hold a sheet of card between the little and ring fingers (Fig. 14.38C). The fingers must be fully extended.

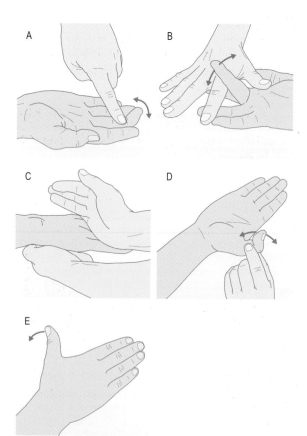

Fig. 14.37 Testing the flexors and extensors of the fingers and thumb. (A) Flexor digitorum profundus. **(B)** Flexor digitorum superficialis. **(C)** Extensor digitorum. **(D)** Flexor pollicis longus. **(E)** Extensor pollicis longus.

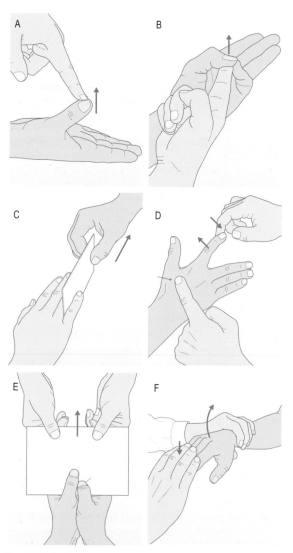

Fig. 14.38 Testing motor function of the median, ulnar and radial nerves. (A and B) The median nerve: **(A)** abducting the thumb; **(B)** testing opposition. **(C–E)** The ulnar nerve: **(C)** testing the interossei; **(D)** testing the first interosseus; **(E)** testing adductor pollicis. **(F)** The radial nerve: testing the extensors of the wrist and fingers.

- Test the first dorsal interosseus muscle by asking the patient to abduct the extended index finger against resistance (Fig. 14.38D).
- To test adductor pollicis, ask the patient to grip a piece of card between the palm and the adducted thumb. If the adductor is weak, the thumb cannot be held straight and will flex at the MCP and IP joints (Froment's sign) (Fig. 14.38E).

▪◢ The radial nerve supplies the extensors of the wrist and fingers.

- Ask the patient to flex the elbow to 90° and pronate the wrist. Support the wrist with your hand and ask the patient to extend the fingers and then the wrist (Fig. 14.38F). Watch the MCP joints, as extension of the IP joints can also be produced by the interossei and lumbrical muscles supplied by the median and ulnar nerves.
- For extensor pollicis longus, ask the patient to bend the thumb and extend it against resistance.

The elbow

The elbow joint has humero-ulnar, radio-capitellar and superior radio-ulnar articulations. The medial and lateral epicondyles are the flexor and extensor origins respectively for the forearm muscles. These two prominences and the tip of the olecranon are easily palpated. They normally form an equilateral triangle when the elbow is flexed to 90° and lie in a straight line when the elbow is fully extended. A subcutaneous bursa overlies the olecranon and may become inflamed or infected (bursitis). Pain at the elbow may be localized or referred from the neck. Rheumatoid arthritis and epicondylitis are common causes of pain at the elbow.

▪◢ Examination sequence

The elbow
Look

▪◢ At the overall alignment of the extended elbow. There is normally a valgus angle of 11–13° when the elbow is fully extended (the 'carrying angle').
▪◢ For swelling, bruising and scars.
▪◢ For evidence of synovitis between the lateral epicondyle and olecranon.
▪◢ For olecranon bursitis, tophi or nodules.
▪◢ For rheumatoid nodules on the proximal extensor surface of the forearm.

Feel

▪◢ The bony contours of the lateral and medial epicondyles and olecranon tip, defining an equilateral triangle with the elbow flexed at 90°.
▪◢ For sponginess on either side of the olecranon and ask about tenderness. Synovitis feels spongy or boggy when the elbow is fully extended.
▪◢ Focal tenderness, over the lateral or medial epicondyle. When isolated to one site, this may indicate 'tennis' (lateral) or 'golfer's' (medial) elbow.
▪◢ For bursae — fluid-filled sacs, usually soft, but if acutely inflamed or infected may be firm.
▪◢ For rheumatoid nodules on the proximal extensor surface of the forearm.

Move

▪◢ Assess the extension–flexion arc. Ask the patient to touch his shoulder on that side and then straighten the elbow as far as

possible. The normal range of movement is 0–145°; a range less than 30–110° will cause functional problems.

▪◢ To assess supination and pronation, ask the patient to put his elbows by the side of the body and flex them to 90°. Now ask the patient to turn the hands upwards to face the ceiling (supination: normal range 0–90°) and then downwards to face the floor (pronation: normal range 0–85°).

Special tests

▪◢ Examination sequence

Tennis elbow (lateral epicondylitis)

▪◢ Ask the patient to flex the elbow to 90°.
▪◢ Pronate and flex the hand/wrist fully.
▪◢ Support the patient's elbow. Ask him to extend the wrist against your resistance.
▪◢ Pain is produced at the lateral epicondyle and may be referred down the extensor aspect of the arm.

▪◢ Examination sequence

Golfer's elbow (medial epicondylitis)

▪◢ Ask the patient to flex the elbow to 90° and supinate the hand/wrist fully.
▪◢ Support the patient's elbow.
▪◢ Ask him to flex the wrist against your resistance. Pain is produced at the medial epicondyle and may be referred down the flexor aspect of the arm.

The shoulder

The shoulder joint consists of the glenohumeral joint and the acromioclavicular joint, but movement also occurs between the scapula and the posterior chest wall (Fig. 14.39).

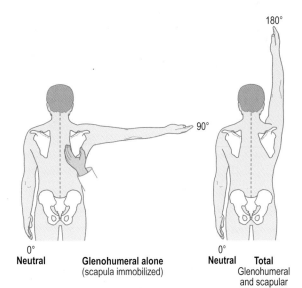

Fig. 14.39 Movements at the shoulder joint.

14.24 Causes of shoulder girdle pain

Rotator cuff

- Degeneration
- Tendon rupture
- Calcific tendonitis

Subacromial bursa

- Calcific bursitis
- Polyarthritis

Capsule

- Adhesive capsulitis

Head of humerus

- Tumour
- Osteonecrosis
- Fracture/dislocation

Joints

- Glenohumeral, sternoclavicular Synovitis, osteoarthritis, dislocation
- Acromioclavicular Osteoarthritis

14.25 Common conditions affecting the shoulder

Non-trauma

- Rotator cuff syndromes, e.g. supraspinatus, infraspinatus tendonitis
- Impingement syndromes (involving the rotator cuff and subacromial bursa)
- Adhesive capsulitis ('frozen shoulder')
- Calcific tendonitis
- Bicipital tendonitis
- Rheumatoid arthritis

Trauma

- Rotator cuff tear
- Glenohumeral dislocation
- Acromioclavicular dislocation
- Fracture of the clavicle
- Fracture of the head or neck of the humerus

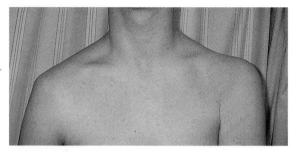

Fig. 14.40 Right anterior glenohumeral dislocation. Note loss of normal shoulder contour.

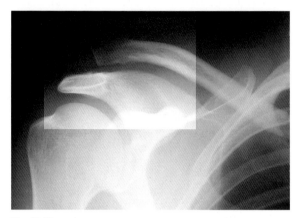

Fig. 14.41 X-ray of right acromioclavicular dislocation.

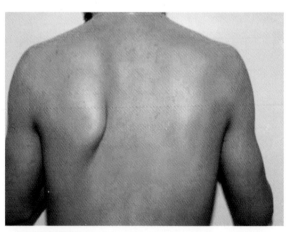

Fig. 14.42 'Winging' of the left scapula due to paralysis of the nerve to serratus anterior.

Movements of the shoulder girdle, especially abduction and rotation, also produce movement at the sternoclavicular joint.

Pain in the shoulder is common (Boxes 14.24 and 14.25) and frequently referred to the upper arm. Glenohumeral pain may occur over the anterolateral aspect of the upper arm. Pain felt at the shoulder may be referred from the cervical spine, radicular pain caused by central nerve root compression, or diaphragm and subdiaphragmatic peritoneum via the phrenic nerve. The most common cause of referred pain is cervical spondylosis, where disc space narrowing and osteophytes cause nerve root impingement and inflammation.

Stiffness and limitation of movement around the shoulder, caused by adhesive capsulitis of the glenohumeral joint, is common after immobilization or disuse following injury or stroke. This is sometimes termed 'frozen shoulder', but movement can still occur between the scapula and chest wall.

The rotator cuff muscles and their tendinous insertions help stability and movement (especially abduction; Fig. 14.9) at the glenohumeral joint. The rotator muscles are: supraspinatus, subscapularis, teres minor and infraspinatus. Some rotator cuff disorders, especially impingement syndromes and tears, present with a painful arc (Fig. 14.43).

Examination sequence

The shoulder
Look

- Examine the whole shoulder girdle front and back, including the axilla for:
- Deformity: the deformities of anterior glenohumeral and complete acromioclavicular joint dislocation are obvious (Figs 14.40 and 14.41), but the shoulder contour in posterior glenohumeral dislocation may only appear abnormal when you stand above the seated patient and look down on the shoulder.
- Swelling: in dislocations, proximal humeral fractures, haemarthrosis and inflammatory conditions.
- Muscle wasting: especially of the deltoid, supraspinatus and infraspinatus. Wasting of supraspinatus or infraspinatus indicates a chronic tear of their tendons.
- The size and position of the scapula, i.e. elevated, depressed or 'winged' (Fig. 14.42): a small elevated scapula occurs in the rare conditions of Sprengel's shoulder and Klippel–Feil syndrome.

Feel

- Start at the sternoclavicular joint and palpate along the clavicle to the acromioclavicular joint. Clavicular fractures and acromioclavicular joint injuries are accompanied by deformity and local tenderness.
- Palpate the acromion and coracoid (2 cm inferior and medial to the clavicle tip) processes, the scapula spine and the biceps tendon in the bicipital groove.
- Palpate the supraspinatus tendon by extending the shoulder to bring supraspinatus anterior to the acromion process. Tenderness is present with ligamentous tears and calcific tendonitis.

Move

- Screening tests for shoulder dysfunction: stand behind the patient. Ask the patient to put both hands behind the head, then to put the arms down and to reach behind the back to touch the shoulder blades. Fully examine the shoulder if he has pain, swelling or limitation of movement.
- Range of movement: determine the range of active and passive movement.
  - Ask the patient to flex and extend the shoulder as far as possible.
  - To test abduction, ask the patient to lift the arm away from the side of the body. Between 50 and 70% of abduction occurs at the glenohumeral joint (the rest occurs with movement of the scapula on the chest wall), but this increases if the arm is externally rotated. To determine how much movement occurs at the glenohumeral joint, palpate the inferior pole of the scapula between your thumb and index finger to detect scapular rotation. During abduction note the degree and smoothness of scapular movement. If the glenohumeral joint is excessively stiff, then movement of the scapula over the chest wall will predominate. If there is any limitation or pain (painful arc) associated with abduction, test the rotator cuff.
  - Measure internal and external rotation with the patient's arm by the side of the body and the elbow flexed at 90°. Document internal rotation as the highest spinous process that the patient can reach with the thumb.
  - Assess the ability of the deltoid to abduct against resistance; compare side with side.

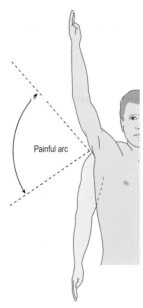

Fig. 14.43 Painful arc.

Special tests
Rotator cuff problems

Ask the patient to abduct the arm from the side of the body against resistance. If abduction cannot be initiated or is painful, this suggests a rotator cuff problem.

Examination sequence

Impingement

- Test for a painful arc by passively abducting the arm fully and asking the patient to lower (adduct) it slowly (Fig. 14.43). A painful arc occurs between 60° and 120° of abduction.
- If the patient cannot initiate abduction, passively abduct the patient's internally rotated arm to 30–45° while placing your hand over the scapula to confirm there is no scapular movement. Ask the patient to continue to abduct the arm. Pain on active movement, especially against resistance, suggests impingement.

Ligamentous tears and injuries

To test the component muscles of the rotator cuff, neutralize the effect of other muscles crossing the shoulder. Discrepancy between active and passive ranges suggests a tendinous tear — in particular with subscapularis, where there may be an excessive range of passive internal rotation.

- Subscapularis and pectoralis major produce powerful internal rotation of the shoulder. To isolate subscapularis, test internal rotation with the patient's hand behind the back. Loss of power suggests a tear, while pain on forced internal rotation suggests tendonitis.
- Supraspinatus. With the arm by the side, test abduction. Loss of power suggests a tear, while pain on forced abduction at 60° suggests tendonitis.

14

Infraspinatus and teres minor. Test external rotation with the arm in the neutral position, but with 30° flexion to reduce the contribution of deltoid. Loss of power suggests a tear, while pain on forced external rotation suggests tendonitis.

Bicipital tendonitis

Palpate the bicipital tendon in its groove, noting any tenderness.

Ask the patient to supinate the forearm, and then flex the arm against resistance. Pain is produced in bicipital tendonitis.

The lower limb

The hip

The hip is a ball and socket joint and allows movements of flexion, extension, abduction, adduction, internal/external rotation and the combined movement of circumduction. With age, the most common restrictions in movement are extension and internal rotation, followed by abduction.

Pain is usually felt in the groin, but can be referred to the anterior thigh, the knee or buttock. Hip pain is usually aggravated by activity, but avascular necrosis and tumours may be painful at rest and at night. Lateral hip or thigh pain, aggravated when lying on the side at night, suggests trochanteric bursitis.

Distinguish pain arising from the hip from:

- lumbar nerve root irritation (p. 375)
- spinal or arterial claudication (p. 140)
- abdominal causes, e.g. hernias (p. 205)
- knee pain referred to the hip.

Find out how the pain restricts patients' activities. In particular, ask about walking in terms of the time and distance they manage outside the house and up and down stairs, whether they do their own shopping and which walking aids they use.

Fracture of the neck of femur is common following relatively minor trauma in postmenopausal women and those aged over 70 years. The fracture may be minimally displaced or impacted and need not have the classical appearance of a shortened, externally rotated leg (Fig. 14.57A). The patient may even be able to weight-bear.

■◣ Examination sequence

The hip

Patients should undress to their underwear and remove socks and shoes. You should be able to see the iliac crests.

Look

Gait: assess as described above.

General inspection: ask the patient to stand. From the front, observe whether:

- Stance is straight.
- The shoulders are parallel to the ground and placed symmetrically over the pelvis.

- There is a pelvic tilt (which may mask a hip deformity or true shortening of one leg).
- There are deformities of hip, knee, ankle or foot.
- There is muscle wasting (from polio or disuse secondary to arthritis).

From the side, assess whether there is a stoop or increased lumbar lordosis (both may result from a flexion contracture).

From behind, assess whether:

- The spine is straight or curved laterally (scoliosis); if there is scoliosis, note the relative positions of the shoulders and pelvis, and measure leg lengths.
- There is any gluteal atrophy.

Around the hip, assess whether there are scars, sinuses, dressings or skin changes.

Feel

Tenderness on palpation over the greater trochanter suggests trochanteric bursitis.

Tenderness over the lesser trochanter and ischial tuberosity is common in sporting injuries due to strains of the iliopsoas and hamstring muscle insertions respectively.

Move

With the patient face up on the couch, check the pelvic brim is perpendicular to the spine.

Flexion: place your left hand under the back (to detect any masking of hip movement by movement of the pelvis and lumbar spine — use Thomas's test) and check the range of flexion of each hip in turn (normal 0–120°).

Abduction and adduction: stabilize the pelvis by placing your left hand on the opposite iliac crest. With your right hand abduct the extended leg until you feel the pelvis start to tilt (normal 45°). Test adduction similarly by crossing one leg over the other and continuing to move it medially (normal 25°) (Fig. 14.44A).

Internal and external rotation: test with the leg in full extension by rolling the leg on the couch and using the foot to indicate the range of rotation. Then test with the knee (and hip) flexed at 90°. Move the foot medially to test external rotation and laterally to test internal rotation (normal 45° for each movement) (Fig. 14.44B).

Extension: ask the patient to lie face down on the couch. Place your left hand on the pelvis to detect any movement. Lift each leg in turn to assess the range of extension (normal range 0–20°) (Fig. 14.44C).

Special tests

Shortening

Shortening occurs in hip and other lower limb conditions (Box 14.26). Apparent shortening is present if the affected limb appears shortened, usually because of an adduction or flexion deformity at the hip.

■◣ Examination sequence

Measuring shortening

Ask the patient to lie supine and stretch both legs out as far as possible in equivalent positions to eliminate any soft tissue contracture/abnormal posture.

14

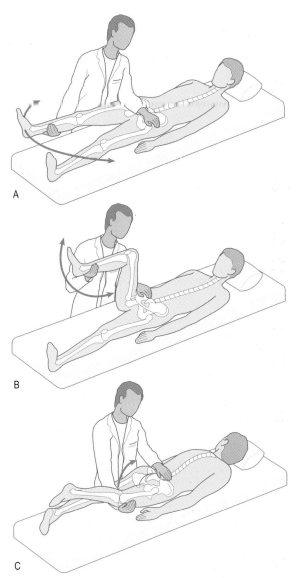

Fig. 14.44 Testing hip movement. (A) Abduction. **(B)** Flexion. **(C)** Extension.

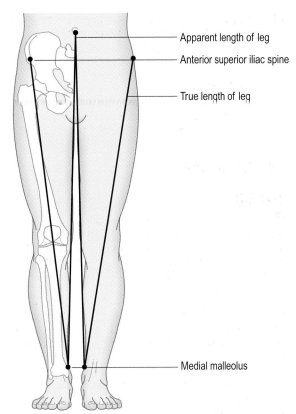

Fig. 14.45 True and apparent lengths of the lower limbs.

 Measure with a tape:
- from umbilicus to medial malleolus: the apparent length
- from anterior superior iliac spine to medial malleolus: the 'true length' (Fig. 14.45).

 Confirm any limb length discrepancy by 'block testing'. Ask the patient to stand with both feet flat on the ground.

 Raise the shorter leg using a series of blocks of graduated thickness until the pelvis is level, assessed by palpating both iliac crests.

14.26 Causes of true lower limb shortening

Hip

- Fractures, e.g. neck of femur
- Following total hip arthroplasty
- Slipped upper femoral epiphysis
- Perthes' disease (juvenile osteochondritis)
- Unreduced hip dislocation
- Septic arthritis
- Loss of articular cartilage (arthritis, joint infection)
- Congenital coxa vara
- Missed congenital dislocation of the hip

Femur and tibia

- Growth disturbance secondary to:
  Poliomyelitis
  Cerebral palsy
  Fractures
  Osteomyelitis
  Septic arthritis
  Epiphyseal injury
  Congenital causes

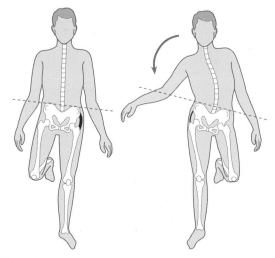

Fig. 14.46 Trendelenburg's sign. Powerful gluteal muscles maintain the position when standing on the left leg; weakness of the right gluteal muscles results in pelvic tilt when standing on the right leg.

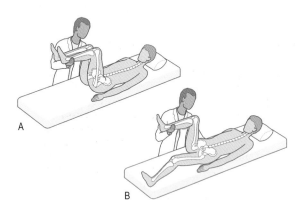

Fig. 14.47 Thomas's test: for examining the left hip.

OSCEs 14.27 Examine this patient with acute hip pain felt in the groin

1. Ask the patient to walk, and observe gait from the front and side.
2. Perform Trendelenburg's test.
3. Measure leg lengths.
4. Examine movements at the hip in all directions (abduction/adduction, internal/external rotation, flexion).
5. Perform Thomas's test for fixed flexion deformity.

Trendelenburg's test

▶ Examination sequence

Trendelenburg's test

▶ Stand in front of the patient and ask him to stand on one leg for 30 seconds.

▶ Repeat with the other leg.
▶ Watch the iliac crest on each side to see if it moves up or down.

Normally, the iliac crest on the side with the foot off the ground should rise. The test is abnormal if the hemipelvis falls below the horizontal (Fig. 14.46). It may be caused by gluteal weakness or inhibition from hip pain, e.g. osteoarthritis, or structural abnormality of the hip joint, e.g. coxa vara or developmental hip dysplasia.

Thomas's test

Do not perform the test if the patient has a hip replacement on the non-test side, as forced flexion may cause dislocation.

Thomas's test measures fixed flexion deformity (incomplete extension). This deformity may be masked by compensatory movement at the lumbar spine or pelvis and increasing lumbar lordosis.

▶ Examination sequence

Thomas's test

▶ The patient lies face up on a hard surface.
▶ Place your left hand palm upwards under the patient's lumbar spine.
▶ Passively flex both the patient's legs (hips and knees) as far as possible.
▶ Keep the non-test hip maximally flexed (you will feel that the lordotic curve of the lumbar spine remains eliminated).
▶ Now ask the patient to extend the test hip. Incomplete extension in this position indicates a fixed flexion deformity at the hip (Fig. 14.47).

Possible difficulties with Thomas's test are:

• If the contralateral hip is not flexed enough, lumbar lordosis will not be eliminated.
• Fixed flexion deformity of the ipsilateral knee will confuse the issue. In this case, perform the test with the patient lying on his or her side.

The knee

The knee is a complex hinge joint with tibiofemoral and patellofemoral components. It has a synovial capsule that extends under the quadriceps (the suprapatellar pouch), reaching about 5 cm above the superior edge of the patella. The joint is largely subcutaneous, allowing easy palpation of the patella, tibial tuberosity, patellar tendon, tibial plateau margin and femoral condyles.

For stability the knee depends on its muscular and ligamentous structures (Fig. 14.48).

Flexion is produced by the hamstring muscles. Extension requires the quadriceps muscles, quadriceps tendon, patella, patellar tendon and tibial tuberosity. Any disruption of this 'extensor apparatus' causes inability to straight leg-raise or an extensor lag (a difference between active and passive ranges of extension).

The medial collateral ligament resists valgus stress. The lateral collateral ligament resists varus stress. The anterior cruciate ligament prevents anterior subluxation of the tibia on the femur, and the posterior cruciate ligament resists posterior translation. The medial

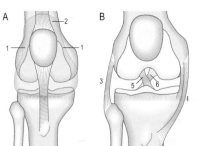
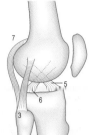
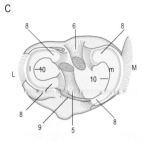
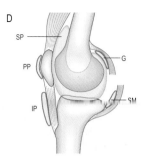

Key

L	Lateral tibiofemoral articulation	1	Extensions of synovial sheath on either side of the patella	7	Posterior ligament
M	Medial tibiofemoral articulation	2	Extension of synovial sheath at upper pole of patella	8	Horns of lateral (l) and medial (m) menisci
SP	Suprapatellar pouch (or bursa)	3	Lateral ligament	9	Connection of anterior horns
PP	Prepatellar bursa	4	Medial ligament	10	Unattached margin of meniscus
IP	Infrapatellar bursa	5	Anterior cruciate ligament		
G	Bursa under the medial head of gastrocnemius	6	Posterior cruciate ligament		
SM	Semimembranosus bursa				

Fig. 14.48 Structure of the right knee. (A) Anterior view, showing the common synovial sheath. **(B)** Anterior and lateral views, showing the ligaments. **(C)** Plan view of the menisci. **(D)** Bursae. (G, bursa under the medial head of gastrocnemius; IP, infrapatellar bursa; L, lateral tibiofemoral articulation; M, medial tibiofemoral articulation; P, patellofemoral articulation; PP, prepatellar bursa; SM, semimembranosus bursa; SP, suprapatellar pouch (or bursa).)

and lateral menisci are crescentic fibrocartilaginous structures that lie between the tibial plateaux and the femoral condyles.

There are several important bursae around the knee:

- anteriorly: the suprapatellar, prepatellar (between the patella and the overlying skin) and infrapatellar bursae (between the skin and the tibial tuberosity/patellar ligament)
- posteriorly: several bursae lie in the popliteal fossa (Fig. 14.48D).

Abnormal findings

Pain

Take a detailed history of the mechanism of injury. The direction of impact, load or deformation predicts what structures are injured. Remember that pain in the knee may be referred from the hip. Anterior knee pain, particularly after prolonged sitting or going downstairs, suggests patellofemoral joint pathology.

Swelling

An effusion indicates intra-articular pathology and may be due to synovial fluid, blood, pus or a mixture of these fluids. The normal volume of synovial fluid is 1–2 ml and is undetectable.

Bleeding into the knee (haemarthrosis) is caused by injury to a vascular structure within the joint, e.g. torn cruciate ligament or intra-articular fracture. Patients with a coagulation disorder, e.g. haemophilia, or on anticoagulant therapy are particularly prone to haemarthroses. The menisci are predominantly avascular, and unless torn at their periphery or in conjunction with some other internal derangement, do not cause a haemarthrosis.

In acute injury the speed of onset of swelling is a clue to the diagnosis.

- Rapid (<30 min), severe swelling suggests a haemarthrosis
- Swelling of a lesser degree over 24 hours is more suggestive of traumatic effusion, e.g. meniscal tear
- Septic arthritis develops over a few hours with pain, marked swelling, tenderness, redness and extreme reluctance to move the joint actively or passively. Concurrent oral steroid or non-steroidal anti-inflammatory drug (NSAID) therapy modifies these features. If you suspect that swelling is due to septic arthritis, the joint should be aspirated as an emergency and an urgent Gram stain/microscopy obtained
- Crystal-induced arthritis (gout or pseudogout) can mimic septic arthritis. Confirm the diagnosis by looking at aspirated fluid under polarized light microscopy.

Locking

This is a block to full extension. It may be longstanding or intermittent. The two predominant causes are a loose body, e.g. from osteochondritis dissecans, osteoarthritis or synovial chondromatosis, and a meniscal tear. Bucket-handle and anterior beak meniscal tears are especially associated with locking. Posterior horn tears commonly cause pain on extreme flexion and prevent the last few degrees of flexion. Meniscal tears also cause local joint-line tenderness. Congenital discoid meniscus may present with locking and clunking.

Instability ('giving way')

Any of the four main ligaments may rupture from trauma or become loose with degenerative disease. Because the normal knee has a valgus angle the patella is prone to dislocate laterally.

389

◼▶ Examination sequence

The knee
Look

◼▶ Observe the patient walking and standing, as described for gait.

◼▶ Ask the patient to lie face up on the couch. Both legs should be fully exposed. Look for:

- Scars, sinuses, redness or rashes.
- Posture and common deformities, genu valgum (knock-knee) or genu varum (bow-legs).
- Muscle wasting: quadriceps wasting is almost invariable with inflammation or chronic pain and develops within days. Measure the thigh girth in both legs 20 cm above a defined fixed bony landmark: the tibial tuberosity.
- Leg length discrepancy (Fig. 14.45).
- Flexion deformity: if the patient lies with one knee flexed, this may be caused by a hip, knee or combined problem.

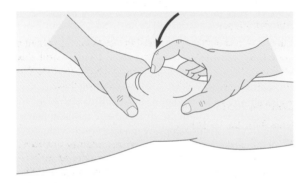

Fig. 14.49 Testing for effusion by the patellar tap.

- Swelling: an enlarged prepatellar bursa (housemaid's knee) and any effusion of the knee joint. A large effusion forms a horseshoe-shaped swelling above the knee. Swelling extending beyond the joint margins suggests infection, major injury or, rarely, tumour.
- Baker's cyst: bursa enlargement in the popliteal fossa.

Feel

◼▶ Warmth: feel the skin, comparing both sides.

◼▶ Effusion: the patellar tap: with the patient's knee extended, empty the suprapatellar pouch by sliding your left hand down the thigh until you reach the upper edge of the patella. Keep your hand there and, with the finger tips of your right hand, press down briskly and firmly over the patella (Fig. 14.49). In a moderate-sized effusion you will feel a tapping sensation as the patella strikes the femur. You may feel a fluid impulse in your left hand.

◼▶ The 'ripple test' (Fig. 14.50): with the patient's knee extended and the quadriceps muscles relaxed, empty the suprapatellar pouch, as for the patellar tap. Then, with your fingers extended, stroke the medial side of the joint. Now stroke the lateral side of the joint and watch the medial side for a bulge or ripple as fluid re-accumulates on that side.

◼▶ Synovitis: with the patient's knee extended and the quadriceps relaxed, feel for sponginess on both sides of the quadriceps tendon.

◼▶ Joint lines: feel the tibial and femoral joint lines. If there is tenderness, localize this as accurately as possible. Localized tenderness occurs over the tibial tuberosity in Osgood–Schlatter disease, a traction osteochondritis.

Move

◼▶ Active flexion and extension: with the patient supine ask him to flex the knee up to the chest and then extend the leg back down to lie on the couch (normal range 0–140°). Feel for crepitus between the patella and femoral condyles, suggesting chondromalacia patellae (especially in younger female patients) or osteoarthritis. If there is a

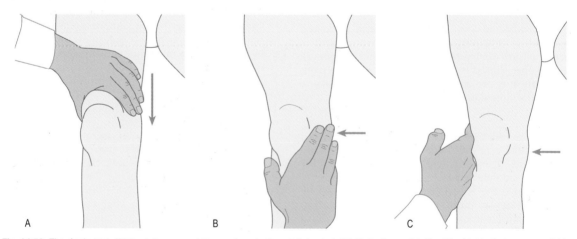

A   B   C

Fig. 14.50 The ripple test. (A) Empty the suprapatellar pouch, as for the patella tap test. **(B)** Stroke the medial side of the joint to displace excess fluid to the lateral side of the joint. **(C)** Stroke the lateral side while watching the medial side closely for a bulge or ripple as fluid re-accumulates. This test may be negative if the effusion is tense.

fixed flexion deformity of 15° and flexion is possible to 110°, record this as a range of movement of 15–110°.

- Ask the patient to lift the leg with the knee kept straight. If the knee cannot be kept fully extended an extensor lag is present, indicating quadriceps weakness or other abnormality of the extensor apparatus.

- Passive flexion and extension. Normally, the knee can extend so that the femur and tibia are in longitudinal alignment. Record full extension as 0°. A restriction to full extension occurs with meniscal tears, osteoarthritis and inflammatory arthritis. To assess hyperextension, lift both legs by the feet. Hyperextension (genu recurvatum) is present if the knee extends beyond the neutral position. Up to 10° is normal.

Ligament testing

Tests of stability

Collateral ligament stability

With the knee fully extended, there should be no abduction or adduction possible. If the ligament is lax or ruptured, movement can occur. If the ligament is strained (partially torn) but intact, pain will be produced but the joint will not open.

■▶ Examination sequence

Collateral ligament stability

- With the patient's knee fully extended, hold the ankle between your elbow and side. Use both hands to apply a valgus and then varus force to the knee.

- Use your thumbs to feel the joint line and assess the degree to which the joint space opens. Major opening of the joint indicates collateral and cruciate injury (Fig. 14.51A).

- If the knee is stable, repeat the process with the knee flexed to 30° to assess minor collateral laxity. In this position the cruciate ligaments are not taut.

■▶ Examination sequence

Cruciate ligament stability

- Flex the patient's knee to 90° and maintain this position by sitting with your thigh trapping the patient's foot.

- Check that the hamstring muscles are relaxed and look for posterior sag (posterior subluxation of the tibia on the femur). This causes a false-positive anterior drawer sign which should not be interpreted as anterior collateral ligament laxity.

The anterior drawer sign

- With your hands behind the upper tibia and both thumbs over the tibial tuberosity, pull the tibia anteriorly (Fig. 14.51B). If there is significant movement (compare with the opposite knee), the anterior cruciate ligament is lax. Movement of >1.5 cm suggests anterior cruciate ligament rupture. There is often an associated medial ligament injury.

The posterior drawer sign

- Push backwards on the tibia. Posterior movement of the tibia suggests posterior cruciate ligament laxity.

Patellar stability

Carry out the patellar apprehension test. With the patient's knee fully extended, push the patella laterally and flex the knee slowly. If the patient actively resists flexion, this suggests previous patellar dislocation or instability.

Special tests

Tests for meniscal tears

Meniscal tears in younger sporting patients are most often the result of a twisting injury to the flexed weight-bearing leg. In middle-aged patients, degenerative horizontal cleavage of the menisci is common, with no history of trauma. Associated well-localized joint-line tenderness is common. Meniscal injuries commonly have small effusions, especially on weight-bearing or after exercise. There may be localized joint-line tenderness.

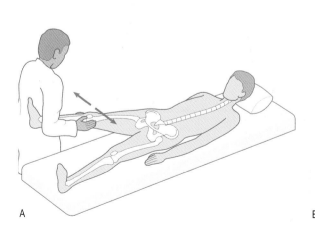
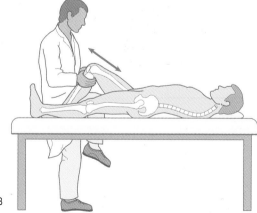

Fig. 14.51 **Testing the ligaments of the knee. (A)** Collateral ligaments. **(B)** Cruciate ligaments.

14

◼▶ Examination sequence

Meniscal provocation test

◼▶ Ask the patient to lie face up on the couch. Test the medial and lateral menisci in turn:

Medial meniscus

◼▶ Passively flex the knee to its full extent.

◼▶ Externally rotate the foot and abduct the upper leg at the hip, keeping the foot towards the midline (i.e. creating a varus stress at the knee).

◼▶ Extend the knee smoothly. In medial meniscus tears a click or clunk may be felt or heard, accompanied by discomfort.

Lateral meniscus

◼▶ Passively flex the knee to its full extent

◼▶ Internally rotate the foot and adduct the leg at the hip (i.e. creating a valgus stress at the knee).

◼▶ Extend the knee smoothly. In tears of the lateral meniscus a click or clunk may be felt or heard, accompanied by discomfort.

OSCEs 14.28 Examine this patient who complains of pain in the knee aggravated by walking

1. Ask the patient to walk, and observe gait and movement of the knee from the front and side.
2. Ask the patient to lie on the couch and expose both legs.
3. Look at the lower limbs for redness, scars, muscle wasting, deformity, swollen bursae, etc.
4. Feel both knees with the back of your hand for temperature difference — warm in septic arthritis, haemarthrosis and inflammatory arthritis.
5. Palpate for knee effusion — found in septic arthritis, trauma, haemarthrosis.
6. Feel for tenderness over joint lines and soft tissues.
7. Assess active and passive movements at both knees — note crepitus.
8. Examine collateral and cruciate ligament stability and menisci.
9. Ask the patient to squat on his heels.

◼▶ Examination sequence

Squat test

◼▶ Ask the patient to squat, keeping the feet and heels flat on the ground. If he cannot do this, it indicates incomplete knee flexion on the affected side. This may be caused by a tear of the posterior horn of the menisci.

◼▶ The extreme range of knee flexion may also be tested with the patient face down on the couch, which makes comparison with the contralateral side easy.

The ankle and foot

The ankle is a hinge joint. The talus articulates with a three-sided mortise made up of the tibial plafond and the medial and lateral malleoli. This allows dorsiflexion and plantar flexion, although some axial rotation can occur at the plantar-flexed ankle. During dorsiflexion the trochlea of the talus rocks posteriorly in the mortise and the malleoli are forced apart because the superior articular surface of the talus is wider anteriorly than posteriorly. The bony mortise is the major factor contributing to stability but the lateral, medial (deltoid) and inferior tibiofibular ligaments are also important (Fig. 14.52).

Foot movements are inversion and eversion, and principally occur at the midtarsal (talonavicular/calcaneocuboid) and subtalar (talocalcaneal) joints. Toe movements are dorsiflexion and plantar flexion.

Traumatic conditions

- A 'twisted' ankle is very common, and is usually related to a sporting injury or stepping off a kerb or stair awkwardly. Establish the exact mechanism of injury and the precise site of pain. Frequently there has been a forced inversion injury with involvement of the lateral ligament. A sprain occurs when some fibres are torn but the ligament remains structurally intact. A complete ligament tear allows

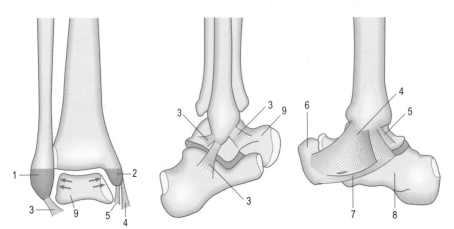

1 Lateral malleolus
2 Medial malleolus
3 Lateral (external) ligament
4 Medial ligament
5 Deep fibres of medial ligament
6 Navicular
7 Spring ligament
8 Calcaneus
9 Talus

Fig. 14.52 The ankle ligaments.

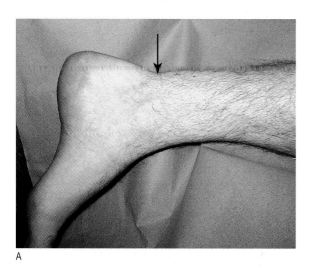

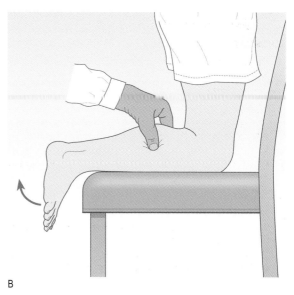

A   B

Fig. 14.53 Ruptured Achilles tendon. (A) The arrow indicates the site of a palpable defect in the Achilles tendon. **(B)** Thomson's test. Failure of the foot to plantar flex when the calf is squeezed is pathognomonic of an acute rupture of the Achilles tendon.

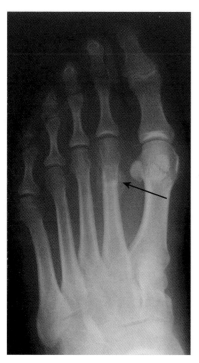

Fig. 14.54 Stress fracture of second metatarsal. Fracture site and callus are arrowed.

excessive talar movement in the ankle mortise with instability
- Achilles tendon rupture (Fig. 14.53) is associated with attempted sudden plantar flexion at the ankle. It is common in middle-aged patients doing unaccustomed activity, e.g. badminton, squash or the fathers' race at sports day and associated with some drug therapy, e.g. steroids, fluoroquinolones. Sudden pain occurs above the heel and there is often a sensation or noise of a crack. Patients may feel as if they have been kicked or even shot
- Forefoot pain, often localized to the second metatarsal, after excessive activity such as trekking, marching or dancing, suggests a stress fracture (Fig. 14.54). Symptoms are relieved by rest and aggravated by weight-bearing. X-rays in the first week may be normal.

Non-traumatic conditions
- Anterior metatarsalgia with forefoot pain is common, especially in middle-aged women. Acute joint pain with swelling suggests an inflammatory arthropathy such as rheumatoid arthritis or gout. The forefoot is commonly affected in rheumatoid arthritis. In severe cases the metatarsal heads become prominent and walking feels like 'walking on pebbles or broken glass'
- Plantar surface heel pain that is worse in the foot-strike phase of walking may be due to plantar fasciitis and tends to affect middle-aged patients
- Posterior heel pain may be caused by Achilles tendonitis, an enthesopathy which is associated with seronegative arthritides and hypercholesterolaemia
- Spontaneous lancinate pain in the forefoot radiating to contiguous sides of adjacent toes occurs with

Morton's neuroma. A common site is the interdigital cleft between the third and fourth toes. This occurs predominantly in women aged 25–45 years and is aggravated by wearing tight shoes.

Examination sequence

The ankle and foot

Ask patients to remove their socks and shoes.

Look

Examine the soles of the shoes for any abnormal patterns of wear.

Gait: observe as described previously. In particular, look for:
- Increased height of step, indicating 'foot-drop'.
- Ankle movement (dorsi-/plantar flexion).
- Position of the foot as it strikes the ground (supinated/pronated).
- Hallux rigidus — loss of movement at the MTP joints.

With the patient standing, observe:
- From behind: how the heel is aligned (valgus/varus).
- From the side: the position of the midfoot, looking particularly at the longitudinal medial arch. This may be flattened (pes planus — flat foot) or exaggerated (pes cavus). If the arch is flattened, ask the patient to stand on tiptoe, which will restore the arch in a mobile deformity, but not in one with a structural basis.

A 'splay-foot' has widening at the level of the metatarsal heads, often associated with MTP joint synovitis.

Examine the ankle and foot for scars, sinuses, swelling, bruising, callosities (an area of thickened skin at a site of repeated pressure), nail changes, oedema, deformity and position, e.g. fixed plantar flexion or foot-drop.

The toes: look for deformities of the great and other toes.
- Hallux valgus is common, has a familial pattern and may be aggravated by footwear and activities such as ballet dancing (Fig. 14.55). A bunion (a soft tissue bursal swelling) may develop over the protuberant first metatarsal head and become inflamed or infected. As the condition progresses, the hallux may rotate over the second toe.
- Gout of the first MTP joint causes marked redness and soft tissue swelling. This is followed by desquamation (peeling) of the superficial skin and pain on movement or touch.

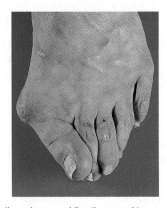

Fig. 14.55 Hallux valgus overriding the second toe.

- Swelling of the entire digit, 'sausage toe' (dactylitis), is characteristic of psoriatic arthropathy.
- Claw toes result from dorsiflexion (hyperextension) at MTP joints and plantar flexion at PIP and DIP joints.
- Hammer toes are due to dorsiflexion at MTP and DIP joints and plantar flexion at PIP joints.
- Mallet toes describe plantar flexion at DIP joints.

Feel

Feel for focal tenderness and heat. In an acute ankle injury, palpate the proximal fibula, both malleoli, the lateral ligament and base of the fifth metatarsal.

Gently compress the forefoot. Tenderness on metatarsal compression suggests Morton's neuroma or, if associated with sponginess, synovitis due to rheumatoid arthritis. If there is toe deformity, assess whether there is impingement on the other toes, e.g. overriding hallux valgus. Pain and stiffness at the first MTP joint suggest hallux rigidus.

Move

Active: assess the range of plantar flexion and dorsiflexion at the ankle and inversion/eversion of the foot by asking the patient to perform these movements.

Passive ankle dorsiflexion/plantar flexion: grip the heel with the cup of your left hand from below, with the thumb and index finger on the malleoli.

Put the foot through its arc of movement (normal range 15° dorsiflexion to 45° plantar flexion).

If dorsiflexion is restricted, assess the contribution of gastrocnemius (which functions across both knee and ankle joints) by measuring ankle dorsiflexion with the knee extended and flexed. If more dorsiflexion is possible with the knee flexed, this suggests a gastrocnemius contracture.

Passive foot inversion/eversion: examine the subtalar joint in isolation by placing the foot into dorsiflexion to stabilize the talus in the ankle mortise.

Move the heel into inversion (normal 20°) and eversion (normal 10°).

Examine the combined midtarsal joints by fixing the heel with your left hand and moving the forefoot with your right hand into dorsiflexion, plantar flexion, adduction, abduction, supination and pronation.

Special tests

Examination sequence

Achilles tendon

Ask the patient to kneel with both knees on a chair.

Palpate the gastrocnemius and Achilles tendon for focal tenderness and soft tissue swelling. Achilles tendon rupture is often palpable as a discrete gap in the tendon about 5 cm above the calcaneal insertion (Fig. 14.53).

Examination sequence

Thomson's (Simmond's) test

Squeeze the calf just distal to the level of maximum circumference. If the Achilles tendon is intact, plantar flexion of the foot will occur (Fig. 14.53B).

FRACTURES, DISLOCATIONS AND TRAUMA-RELATED PRESENTATIONS

A fracture is a breach in the structural integrity of a bone. This may arise in:

- normal bone from excessive force
- normal bone from repetitive (load-bearing) activity (stress fracture)
- bone of abnormal structure (pathological fracture) (Box 14.29) with minimal or no trauma.

The epidemiology of fractures varies geographically. In developed countries, there is an epidemic of osteoporotic fractures because of the increasing elderly population. Fractures resulting from road traffic accidents and falls are decreasing because of legislative and preventive measures, such as seat belts, air bags and improved road engineering.

Osteoporosis is systemic skeletal loss of bone mineral density with associated microarchitectural deterioration. It is the most common cause of abnormal bone structure and its incidence increases with age, particularly in postmenopausal women (Box 14.30). In the absence of complications, osteoporosis is asymptomatic. Although any osteoporotic bone can fracture, the common sites are

the distal radius (Fig. 14.56), neck of femur (Fig. 14.57), proximal humerus and the spinal vertebrae. Europeans have a lifetime risk of osteoporotic fracture of 50% in women and 20% in men.

Clinical features

A fracture may occur in the context of severe trauma. If so, examine the patient according to the system in Chapter 17.

History

Establish the mechanism of injury. For instance, a patient who has fallen from a height on to his heels may have obvious fractures of the calcaneal bones in his ankles but is also at risk of fractures of the proximal femur, pelvis and vertebral column.

Examination

Use the Look/Feel/Move approach. Observe patients closely to see if they move the affected part and are able to weight-bear.

14.29 Bone conditions associated with pathological fracture

- Osteoporosis
- Osteomalacia
- Primary or secondary tumour
- Osteogenesis imperfecta
- Renal osteodystrophy
- Parathyroid bone disease
- Paget's disease

14.30 Risk factors for osteoporosis

- Age
- Sex
  Female (female:male 3:1)
- Menstrual history
  Decreased menstrual cycling, i.e. late menarche, early menopause, amenorrhoea
- Past history
  Hypogonadism (anorexia nervosa/excessive exercise/ hyperprolactinaemia)
  Previous fragility fracture
- Drug history
  Previous or current steroid therapy
- Family history
  First-degree relative (risk increased × 2)
- Social history
  Immobilization, smoking, alcohol, low calcium/ vitamin D in diet

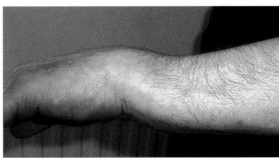

A

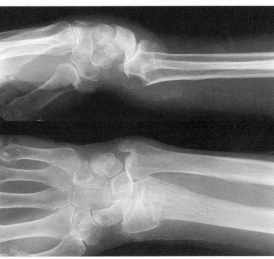

B

Fig. 14.56 Colles' fracture. (A) Clinical appearance of dinner fork deformity. **(B)** X-ray appearance.

14

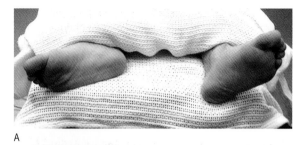

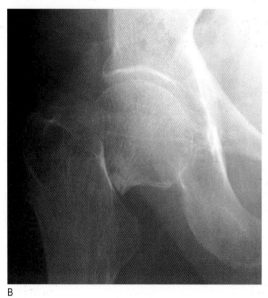

A

B

Fig. 14.57 Fracture of neck of right femur. (A) Shortening and external rotation of the leg. **(B)** X-ray showing translation and angulation.

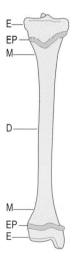

E
EP
M

D

M
EP
E

Fig. 14.58 Describing a fracture. The site of the fracture: anatomical divisions. (D, diaphysis or shaft; E, epiphysis; EP, epiphyseal plate; M, metaphysis.)

■▶ Examination sequence

Fractures, dislocations and trauma-related presentations

Look

■▶ Look to see if the skin is intact. If there is a breach in the skin and the wound communicates with the fracture, the fracture is open or compound; otherwise it is closed.

■▶ Look for associated bruising, deformity, swelling or wound infection.

Feel

■▶ Feel (gently) for local tenderness, and distal to the suspected fracture to establish if sensation and pulses are present.

Move

■▶ Try to establish whether the patient can move joints distal and proximal to the fracture.

■▶ Do not move the fracture site to see if crepitus is present; this causes additional pain and bleeding.

Investigations

For each suspected fracture, X-ray (at least) two views at perpendicular planes of the affected bone, and include the joints above and below.

Describing a fracture

- What bone(s) is/are involved?
- Is the fracture open (compound) or closed?
- Is the fracture complete or incomplete?
- Where is the bone fractured (intra-articular/ epiphysis/physis/metaphysis/diaphysis; Fig. 14.58)?

	14.31 Complications of fractures	
	Early (first 48 hours)	**Late (weeks, months, years)**
Systemic	Hypovolaemia and shock Fat embolism Acute respiratory distress syndrome	Chest infection Urinary tract infection
Bone	Osteomyelitis	Delayed or non-union Osteomyelitis Malunion Necrosis
Joint		Stiffness Osteoarthritis Instability
Soft tissues	Compartment syndrome Muscular/tendon injury Neural injury Vascular injury Adjacent structural damage	Reflex sympathetic dystrophy Peripheral and cord injury Ischaemic contracture Pneumothorax

- What is the fracture's configuration (transverse/oblique/spiral/comminuted/butterfly fragment; Fig. 14.59)?
- What components of deformity are present?
  - Translation is the shift of the distal fragment in relation to the proximal bone. The direction is defined by the movement of the distal fragment, e.g. dorsal or volar, and is measured as a percentage
  - Angulation is defined by the movement of the distal fragment, measured in degrees
  - Rotation is measured in degrees along the longitudinal axis of the bone, e.g. for spiral fracture of the tibia or phalanges.

  - Shortening: proximal migration of the distal fragment can cause shortening in an oblique fracture. Shortening may also occur if there has been impaction at the fracture site, e.g. in a Colles' fracture of the distal radius
- Is there distal nerve or vascular deficit?
- What is the state of the tissues associated with the fracture — soft tissues and joints, e.g. fracture blisters, dislocation?

Complications of fractures are summarized in Box 14.31.

INVESTIGATIONS

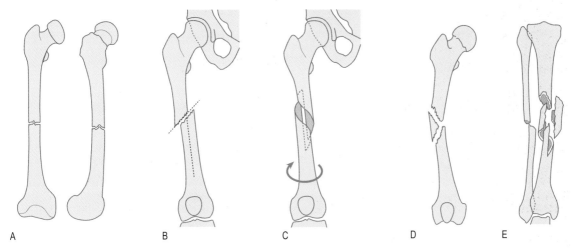

Fig. 14.59 The nature of the fracture. (A) If there is no deformity (no movement of the bone ends relative to one another), the fracture is in anatomical position. **(B)** Oblique fracture: the fracture runs at an oblique angle of 30° or more. **(C)** Spiral fracture: simple spiral fractures result from twisting forces. **(D)** Multifragmentary (comminuted) fracture: there are more than two fragments. **(E)** Multifragmentary complex fracture: there is no contact between the main fragments after reduction.

14.32 Common musculoskeletal investigations

Investigation	Indication/Comment
Bedside	
Schirmer tear test	Keratoconjunctivitis sicca (dry eyes)
Urinalysis	
Protein	Secondary amyloid in rheumatoid arthritis and other chronic arthropathies
	Drug adverse effects, e.g. myocrisin, penicillamine
Blood	Glomerular disease, e.g. SLE, vasculitis
Microscopy for red cells and casts	Glomerular disease, e.g. SLE
Haematological	
Full blood count	Anaemia in inflammatory arthritis, blood loss after trauma
	Neutrophilia in sepsis and very acute inflammation, e.g. acute gout
	Neutropenia in SLE, Felty's syndrome and adverse effects of antirheumatic drug therapy
ESR/plasma viscosity/C-reactive protein	Non-specific indicator of inflammation or sepsis
	Acute phase protein

(Continued)

14

14.32 Continued

Investigation	Indication/Comment
Biochemical	
Urea and creatinine	↑ in renal impairment, e.g. secondary amyloid in rheumatoid arthritis or adverse drug effect
Uric acid	May be ↑ in gout. Levels may be normal during an acute attack
Calcium	↓ in osteomalacia; normal in osteoporosis
Alkaline phosphatase	↑ in Paget's disease, in osteomalacia, and immediately after fractures
Angiotensin-converting enzyme	↑ in sarcoidosis
Serological	
IgM rheumatoid factor (RF)	↑ titres in 60–70% of cases of rheumatoid arthritis; occasionally low titres found in other connective diseases. Present in up to 15% of normal population
Anti-cyclic citrullinated peptides (ACPA)	Present in 60–70% of cases of rheumatoid arthritis and up to 10 years before onset of disease. Highly specific for rheumatoid arthritis. Occasionally found in Sjögren's syndrome
Antinuclear factors (ANF/ANA)	↑ titres in most cases of SLE; low titres in other connective tissue diseases and rheumatoid arthritis
Anti-Ro, Anti-La	Sjögren's syndrome
Anti-dsDNA	SLE
Anti-Sm	SLE
Anti-RNP	Mixed connective tissue disease
Antineutrophil cytoplasmic antibodies	Wegener's granulomatosis, polyarteritis nodosa, Churg–Strauss vasculitis
Imaging	
Plain radiography (X-rays)	Fractures, erosions in rheumatoid arthritis and psoriatic arthritis, osteophytes and joint space loss in osteoarthritis, bone changes in Paget's disease, pseudofractures (Looser's zones) in osteomalacia
Ultrasonography	Detection of effusion synovitis, cartilage breaks and erosions in inflammatory arthritis Detection of bursae, tendon pathology and osteophytes
Isotope bone scan	Increased uptake in Paget's disease, bone tumour
MR imaging	For joint structure and soft tissue imaging
CT scan	
Dual-energy X-ray absorptiometry (DXA)	Gold standard for determining osteoporosis. Usual scans are of lumbar spine and hip
Joint aspiration	
Polarized light microscopy	+ly birefringent rhomboidal crystals — calcium pyrophosphate −ly birefringent needle-shaped crystals — monosodium urate monohydrate
Bacteriology	Raised white cell count in infection Organism may be isolated
Biopsy and histology	Synovitis — rheumatoid arthritis and other inflammatory arthritis

14.33 Key points: the musculoskeletal system

- Establish the pattern of joint involvement.
- Use direct questioning to establish extra-articular features.
- Pain is often referred from other structures: e.g., the hip as a source of knee pain, and vice versa.
- Fever, weight loss and night pain are 'red flags' and should prompt investigation for infection, malignancy or systemic pathology.
- Steroid and NSAID therapy can mask symptoms of inflammation, infection and malignancy.
- In patients with back pain ask about sphincter disturbance and assess perianal sensation and anal tone.
- A septic joint is characteristically immobile and painful.
- Pain out of proportion to an injury suggests compartment syndrome.
- Distal pulses may be preserved in compartment syndrome.
- In aches and pains with headache or jaw pain on chewing, think of temporal arteritis.
- Joint erythema implies an acute arthritis such as crystal-induced arthritis or infection.
- Look at the hands for diagnostic extra-articular features, e.g. small muscle wasting in rheumatoid arthritis, digital infarcts in rheumatoid vasculitis, nail pitting and onycholysis in psoriatic arthritis.
- Abnormal patterns of wear on the soles of the shoes indicate underlying foot deformity.
- Inflammatory arthritis must be detected early to commence disease-modifying therapy.
- Pain 'all over' is a common feature of chronic pain syndromes.

SECTION

3

Specific situations

Ian A. Laing
Sineaid Bradshaw
James Paton

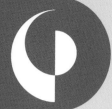

Babies and children

15

15

EXAMINATION OF NEONATES AND INFANTS

A neonate is a baby in the first few weeks of life. The term 'infant' is sometimes used instead, but this includes babies up to the age of 1 year. You need to be opportunistic when assessing neonates and infants, and should not expect to carry out an examination systematically, as in older children and adults. Defer any examination that you cannot complete and keep uncomfortable procedures to the end so that you do not disturb a contented baby. Remember the basic principles discussed in Chapter 2 and apply them to both the parents and the baby.

Assessing a newborn infant fulfills several functions (Box 15.1).

PREPARATION AND SETTING

Gather your equipment together and use a well-lit, warm, draught-free room. You need a stethoscope, an ophthalmoscope, an otoscope, a tape measure and some scales. Use a firm, comfortable surface. Do not examine the baby immediately before or after a feed.

Introductions

Introduce yourself, and find out who is going to be present during the examination and what their names are. Establish their relationships with each other and with the infant. Examine the neonate in front of both parents. This is an ideal opportunity for you to identify and address any uncertainties they have. Some parents have never handled an infant before, and some will be highly experienced. Do not be judgemental and do not be intimidated yourself.

Listening

Encourage parents to share their fears and anxieties so that you can respond to them. They may have ideas and expectations about the baby and you need to clarify what these might be. Although 9% of infants have abnormalities (mainly orthopaedic problems), many congenital disorders cannot be identified during this first examination. Inform parents of the purpose of newborn examination and emphasize that not all problems are evident at birth. Record this in writing.

Information-gathering

Establish the essential background (Box 15.2).

THE PHYSICAL EXAMINATION

Observation is the key to diagnosis, since physical signs are usually less obvious than in adults. Become familiar with what falls into the range of normal in order to be confident about what is abnormal.

Experienced paediatricians often have their own individual system of examination. With time, you may develop your own (Box 15.3). Where possible, examine the supine infant from the right side. This will allow you to be consistent in your clinical approach.

General examination

Observe the demeanour and posture of the infant before asking a parent to undress him completely and remove the nappy. A normal term infant will be flexed and symmetrical, but a preterm infant, or one who is profoundly hypotonic, may adopt a more extended position. Does the baby look well and is he

---

15.2 Essential background information

- The infant's:
  - Gender
  - Name (if already chosen)
- The previous maternal:
  - Medical history
  - Obstetric history
- History of the:
  - Current pregnancy
  - Delivery
  - Events since the infant's delivery
- Parental concerns

15.1 Functions of assessing a newborn infant

- To reassure parent and doctor that the baby:
  - Appears to be normal
  - Is feeding acceptably
  - Has passed urine and meconium
- To identify any:
  - Congenital abnormalities
  - Illnesses or infection
- To measure and record baseline data:
  - Weight
  - Head circumference
  - Length

15.3 Sequence of examination

- General inspection
- Inspection of skin and related tissues
- Head, neck, ears, nose and mouth
- Cardiovascular examination
- Respiratory examination
- Abdominal examination
- Neurological examination
- Final inspection

an appropriate size for the gestation? Look for any visible congenital abnormalities, like a rash or skin tag. Check that the respiratory rate is normal (Box 15.6) and whether the baby is resting or irritable. If the baby is crying, note whether the pitch and volume are normal.

Look at the limbs and count the digits, noting any decrease in number (oligodactyly), increase in number (polydactyly) or joined digits (syndactyly). Open the baby's fingers and look for the palmar creases in both hands. A small percentage of normal babies have single palmar creases but this may also be associated with Down's syndrome and many other chromosomal abnormalities, including trisomies 13, 16 and 18.

Measure the weight, crown–heel length and occipitofrontal circumference, and record the results on a centile chart appropriate to the infant's population.

- Ideally, weigh the baby fully undressed using electronic scales that are accurate to within 5 g
- Measure the crown–heel length using a neonatal stadiometer (Fig. 15.1). Ask a parent or assistant to hold the baby's head still, stretch out the child's legs, and ensure that he is supine and fully extended. This is the least reproducible of the three measurements

- Use a non-extendible paper tape to measure the occipitofrontal circumference round the forehead and occiput at the largest part (Fig. 15.2). Take the measurement three times and note the largest measurement to the nearest millimetre.

Skin

Look at the baby's skin characteristics (Box 15.4).

The 'stork's beak mark' (Fig. 15.3), a pink discoloration at the nape of the neck, the eyelids and the glabella, occurs in 30–50% of newborns; it is not significant. Pallor may be due to anaemia or peripheral vasoconstriction. Note any blue colour of the lips, tongue and mucous membranes of the mouth. This is central cyanosis and indicates hypoxia. By contrast, acrocyanosis is common in the early minutes and hours of life. The infant has blue peripheries but is centrally pink. Plethora describes a general red colour and occurs in vasodilatation, polycythaemia and vascular overload. Jaundice is always an abnormal finding in the first 24 hours of life and requires investigation.

The texture of the skin may be normal, dry, wrinkled or vernix-covered. Describe any blisters or bullae.

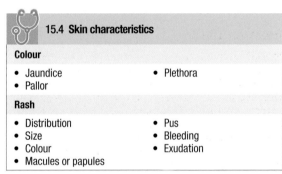

15.4 Skin characteristics

Colour

- Jaundice
- Pallor
- Plethora

Rash

- Distribution
- Size
- Colour
- Macules or papules
- Pus
- Bleeding
- Exudation

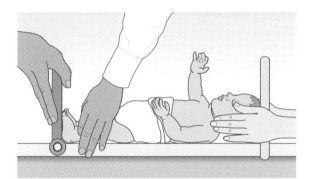

Fig. 15.1 Measuring length accurately in infants.

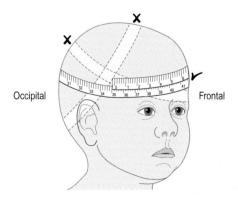

Occipital   Frontal

Fig. 15.2 Measurement of head circumference.

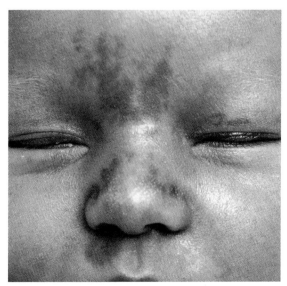

Fig. 15.3 Stork's beak mark.

A 'collodion baby' has a varnished appearance to his or her skin and may be post-mature.

Count and measure any pigmented naevi. A Mongolian blue spot (Fig. 15.4) may be found, usually over the buttocks, back and thighs. It is often large with a bluish tinge, and usually fades in the first year of life. Other common skin changes include milia due to sebaceous gland hyperplasia, acne neonatorum, erythema toxicum, nappy dermatitis and dermatitis due to *Candida* infection.

Look for evidence of trauma. Document any scalp cuts and bruises from forceps or cardiotocography leads. Subcutaneous fat necrosis occurs as hard plaques under the skin where there has been local trauma: for example, as a result of compression by forceps.

Head

Moulding of the head is common in the first 24 hours of life. Note the baby's head shape (Box 15.5) and any swellings. The anterior fontanelle is usually open (Fig. 15.5). Feel to establish whether the skin is sunken, flat or bulging. Palpate all the sutures. They may be overriding (feels like a shallow step), split apart, e.g. by raised intracranial pressure, or fused together (synostosis).

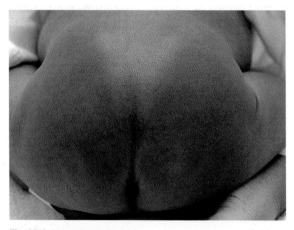

Fig. 15.4 Mongolian blue spot.

15.5 **Neonatal head shapes**	
Head shape	**Description**
Microcephalic (small-headed)	Small cranial vault
Megalencephalic (large-headed)	Large cranial vault
Hydrocephalic (water-headed)	Large cranial vault due to enlarged ventricles
Brachycephalic (short-headed)	
Dolichocephalic (long-headed)	
Plagiocephalic (oblique-headed)	Asymmetrical skull

Eyes

Look at the eyebrows, eyelashes, eyelids and lacrimal system. Note any congenital abnormality and any asymmetry. Pull the lower lid down gently and look for yellow sclerae. In pigmented races this is the best sign of neonatal jaundice. Note any discharge of pus from the eyes and any surrounding erythema.

What size are the eyes? Small eyes (microphthalmia) may suggest multiple congenital abnormalities. If the eyeball appears large, gently palpate it through the baby's closed lid, using the tip of both of your index fingers. If it is firm, this suggests glaucoma (buphthalmos).

Look at the cornea. Observe any clouding and note its colour and position. A hyphema is a red fluid level over the iris, caused by bleeding, which varies with the child's position.

Ophthalmoscopy

Keep the instrument as close as possible to your eye, shining the light into the baby's eye with your head at the same level as that of the baby. Start about 20 cm away and look through the lens to identify the baby's pupil. You should see a red or pale pink glow from the pupil — the red reflex, which is reflected light from the retina.

If you cannot see the red reflex, there may be small lens opacities (a cataract). Black spots in front of the retina may also be cataracts and you should obtain a formal ophthalmological opinion. Congenital cataract occurs in 2–3 per 10 000 births in the UK and is a cause of preventable blindness. Only 35% of congenital cataracts are identified at birth.

If the eyelids are very puffy from oedema in the first 2 days of life, you may not be able to examine the eyes. Arrange to do so later in the first week of life.

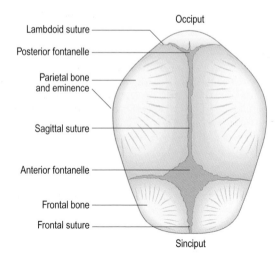

Fig. 15.5 The fetal skull from above.

Nose

Check that the nostrils are both patent. Block each one in turn with your finger and see if the infant continues to breathe through the other nostril.

Mouth

Note whether the jaw is small (hypomandibularism or micrognathia). Examining the inside of the mouth is easy in the crying infant and also in the sleeping baby, but be patient. Open the baby's mouth gently, using your finger tips to depress the lower jaw. Use the index finger and thumb of your other hand to retract the angles of the mouth. Shine a narrow-beamed torch on the palate, and feel using your little finger with the pad turned towards the palate. Do not routinely use tongue elevators and depressors, which may cause trauma.

Tongue

A large tongue protruding from the mouth is true macroglossia. In Down's syndrome the tongue is normal-sized or small, and protrudes through a small mouth (glossoptosis). Look for the lingual frenulum in the midline, joining the tongue to the floor of the mouth. True tongue tie (ankyloglossia) is an uncommon congenital condition in which the frenulum is abnormally short; the tip of the neonate's tongue cannot be protruded beyond the lower incisor teeth and, if the infant is unable to suck effectively, there may be breastfeeding difficulties.

Palate

Describe any cleft lip or palate. Is the defect midline, unilateral or bilateral, and does it involve the gum (alveolus)? Is it associated with cleft of the hard palate? Epstein's pearls are a small cluster of whitish-yellow epithelial swellings at the junction of the soft and hard palate in the midline; they are of no medical significance.

Gums

You may see eruption cysts before the neonatal teeth erupt.

Mucosa

White discoloration may be due to curdled milk from the last feed or to thrush (Candida albicans). Scrape the discoloration gently using a tongue depressor. Milk comes off easily, but thrush adheres and produces a little local bleeding when removed. A mucous cyst on the floor of the mouth is a ranula; it is related to the sublingual or submandibular salivary ducts.

Ears

Examine the size, shape and position of the ears and look for any auricular skin tags, usually anterior to the pinna. The helix may be temporarily folded due to local pressure in utero. Low-set ears occur if the helix joins the cranium below an imaginary line through the inner corners of the eye where the lids meet (the canthi).

Inspect the external auditory meatus and tympanic membrane using an otoscope. This examination may be carried out without precautions if the child is deeply asleep, but if the child is awake, seek help in restraining him (Fig. 15.24). Choose the smallest earpiece available and hold the otoscope comfortably. Gently retract the pinna posteriorly and downwards. The external auditory meatus passes up and forwards in the neonate and you need to straighten it to visualize the tympanic membrane. Insert the earpiece into the external auditory meatus to a depth of 0.5cm only, and then move the tip gently until you see the tympanic membrane.

Neck

Neck asymmetry is often due to fetal posture and usually resolves. A lump in the sternocleidomastoid muscle is often caused by a fibrosed haematoma. This may result in a wry neck (torticollis), which causes the baby to rotate the neck to gaze in the contralateral direction.

Transilluminate any swellings to see whether they are cystic (Fig. 15.9). Cystic swellings glow, as the light is transmitted through clear liquid, but solid or blood-filled swellings do not.

One-third of normal neonates have palpable lymph nodes in the cervical, inguinal and axillary areas.

CARDIOVASCULAR EXAMINATION

Cardiovascular problems often present with respiratory abnormalities. Count the respiratory rate for 15 seconds and multiply by four to give the rate per minute. This should be 20–40 breaths/min in a sleeping baby, but may be above 60 breaths/min if the baby is hungry, crying or cold.

Look for respiratory distress (p. 407). A baby with heart failure may be tachypnoeic but rarely uses the accessory muscles of respiration. Look for the apex beat, which should be visible and prominent. The apex beat of the newborn is normally in the 4th or 5th intercostal space, on or within the midclavicular line. Palpate the apex beat using the palm of your hand. Note its position relative to the midclavicular line. If it is displaced lateral to the midclavicular line, this may indicate cardiomegaly, or it may mean that the heart has been displaced to the left, e.g. by left lung atelectasis, right-sided pneumothorax or a right-sided pleural effusion. If the force of the heartbeat moves your hand

15.6 Normal ranges or values for physiological variables in the newborn

Sign	Preterm neonate	Term neonate
Heart rate (beats/min)	120–160	100–140
Respiratory rate (breath/min)	40–60	30–50

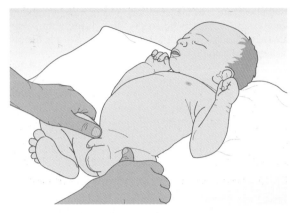

Fig. 15.6 Palpating the femoral pulses. The pulse can be difficult to feel at first; use a point halfway between the pubic tubercle and the anterior superior iliac spine as a guide.

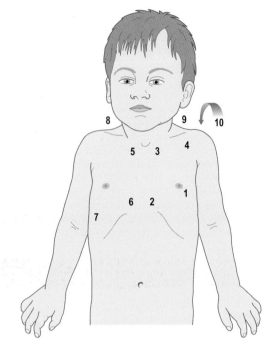

Fig. 15.7 Auscultation positions. Recommended order of auscultation: **1,** apex; **2,** left lower sternal edge; **3,** left upper sternal edge; **4,** left infraclavicular; **5,** right upper sternal edge; **6,** right lower sternal edge; **7,** right mid-axillary line; **8,** right side of neck; **9,** left side of neck; **10,** posteriorly.

up and down, this is a parasternal heave; if you can feel a vibration, it is called a thrill.

Record the heart rate by feeling the right radial or brachial pulse. Count the number of beats in 15 seconds and multiply by 4. Rates between 80 and 160/min can be normal, depending on the state of arousal of the baby.

Feel the femoral pulses by placing your thumbs gently on either femoral triangle while moderately abducting the infant's hips (Fig. 15.6). Good-volume femoral pulses indicate that there is no severe narrowing of the outflow tract from the left ventricle and no significant coarctation of the aorta detectable at the time of the examination. In neonates, you may feel the femoral pulses, even when coarctation of the aorta is present, because the ductus arteriosus is open in the early hours or days and the right ventricular outflow may contribute to arterial pulsation in the lower aorta distal to the coarctation. In older children and adults palpate the right radial and femoral pulses together in order to identify a delayed femoral pulse compared with the radial. In neonates with a heart rate of 140/min it may be impossible to detect true radiofemoral delay, and only a comparison of pulse volumes is possible. Compare the femoral pulse with the brachial pulse by palpating the infant's right femoral pulse with your right thumb and the infant's right brachial pulse with your left thumb. Refer a neonate with low-volume femoral pulses to a paediatric cardiologist to exclude coarctation of the aorta.

Auscultate the heart. Start at the apex using the bell of the stethoscope, which is best for hearing low-pitched sounds. The diaphragm is better for detecting high-pitched sounds and murmurs, and should be used in all positions (Fig. 15.7).

A murmur is heard in up to 2% of neonates, but congenital heart disease occurs in only 0.6% of live-born infants. Routine examination detects only 45% of these babies. Many murmurs are transient or benign.

The fast heart rate of the newborn makes it difficult to hear some sounds. You should still describe the rate, the quality of the first and second heart sounds, splitting of the second heart sound, additional heart sounds and the presence or absence of murmurs.

A patent ductus arteriosus may cause a murmur restricted to systole in the early days of life. This is because the pulmonary and systemic blood pressures are initially similar and left-to-right shunting of blood through the ductus is limited. The typical continuous murmur with a diastolic component is heard after a few weeks or months.

Do not measure blood pressure routinely in the newborn. It is very difficult to measure non-invasively. The baby who is well perfused and has readily palpable brachial pulses is unlikely to be hypotensive. If you do measure BP, use a cuff width of a size that is two-thirds of the distance from the baby's elbow to shoulder tip. Repeat the measurement with a different cuff if the BP is unexpectedly high.

Palpate the abdomen. Measure the size of the liver, using a tape measure in a cephalocaudal direction from the lowest rib anteriorly, in the midclavicular line.

RESPIRATORY EXAMINATION

Note any extra breathing sounds before you handle the infant.

Look for any abnormality of the shape of the chest wall and for any signs of respiratory distress. Respiratory distress in the newborn manifests as tachypnoea and suprasternal, intercostal and subcostal recession, but these signs can also be caused by cardiac problems. Stridor is a sound made in the upper respiratory tract and is predominantly inspiratory. Stridor and indrawing beginning on the second or third day of life in an otherwise well baby and getting worse may be due to laryngomalacia (softness of the larynx). Consider chest infection if there is any sign of respiratory distress.

Percussion of the newborn's chest is not helpful. It makes the baby cry, so that further respiratory examination is difficult.

Auscultate using the diaphragm symmetrically, starting anteriorly, then laterally and finally posteriorly. Compare both sides and note any crackles and wheeze.

ABDOMINAL EXAMINATION

Remove the nappy and look at the abdomen. Mild abdominal distension from gastric distension after a recent feed or swallowed air during crying is common. Because the anterior abdominal wall has poorly developed musculature in the neonate you may see the outline of the intestines. You may see clearly defined laddering of the intestines with intestinal obstruction.

Inspect the umbilicus for any lump. The cord stump should age and drop off on the fourth or fifth day.

- An umbilical hernia is common and is covered with skin and subcutaneous tissue. It usually closes spontaneously
- An omphalocoele, or exomphalos (Fig. 15.8), is an eventration through the umbilicus that contains protruding intestines covered by a thin layer of peritoneum
- Gastroschisis is a defect in the anterior abdominal wall with herniation of intestines through the defect. In contrast to exomphalos, the intestines are not covered with a membrane and the most common site of herniation is above and to the right of the umbilicus
- A granuloma appears later as a pink fleshy lump in the umbilicus when the cord remnant has separated.

A small amount of bleeding from the umbilicus is common in the neonate, but check that the infant has received vitamin K supplementation. A halo of erythema round the umbilicus suggests infection causing omphalitis, which may require urgent treatment.

Look at both groins for swellings. Hydrocoeles are the most common scrotal swelling and contain only fluid, while inguinal hernias contain bowel. These are best differentiated by palpation. Transillumination may help but can be misleading, since both a hydrocoele and a hernia of thin-walled bowel may transilluminate (Fig. 15.9). Hydrocoeles usually resolve spontaneously in the early months of life. Indirect inguinal hernias are common in the newborn, especially in boys and

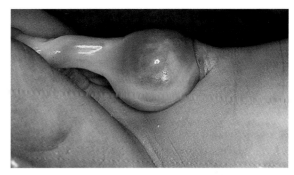

Fig. 15.8 Small exomphalos with loops of bowel in the umbilicus.

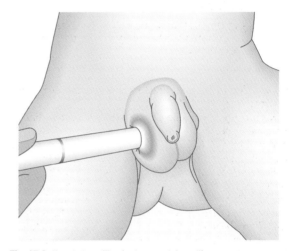

Fig. 15.9 How to transilluminate a scrotal swelling.

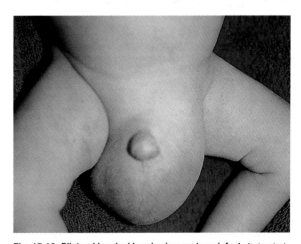

Fig. 15.10 Bilateral inguinal hernias in a preterm infant. An inguinal hernia is primarily a groin swelling; only when it is large does it extend into the scrotum.

preterm infants who develop chronic lung disease (Fig. 15.10).

Check that any hernia can be readily reduced. Gently push the hernia contents upwards from the scrotum towards the inguinal canal and abdomen. An irreducible hernia may become incarcerated and requires urgent surgical repair.

To palpate the abdomen, make sure your hands are warm and be gentle. Stand on the supine infant's right side. Use the flat of your hand rather than probing with your finger tips. Always start with superficial palpation before feeling deeper structures. In the neonate the kidneys are often palpable, especially if ballotted (Fig. 9.10, p. 229). The neonate's spleen enlarges down the left flank rather than towards the right iliac fossa. Gently palpate the suprapubic region to establish bladder fullness; the baby may respond by passing urine.

THE NEONATAL PERINEUM

Female

Lay the baby on her back, hold her thighs gently, and wait for her to relax. Gently abduct the legs and use your thumbs to separate the labia. A milky substance in the vagina is normal and not due to an infection. Later in the first week of life you may see a little vaginal bleeding (pseudomenses) as the neonatal uterus withdraws from the influence of maternal hormones. Gently retract the labia majora. You may see a mucosal tag attached to the wall of the vagina; this needs no treatment. In preterm infants the labia minora appear prominent because the labia majora are positioned laterally. This may give a masculinized appearance, which resolves spontaneously over the next few weeks.

Male

Look for any abnormality in the shape or size of the penis. Do not attempt to retract the child's foreskin, but look for the urethral meatus. This should be at the tip of the penis but may be malpositioned. In hypospadias, which occurs in 1 in 400 boys, it is on the ventral aspect of the glans, on the ventral shaft of the penis or rarely in the scrotum or further posteriorly in the perineum (Figs 15.11 and 15.12A). The meatus may occasionally be on the dorsum of the penis (epispadias). If you are in any doubt about the position of the meatus, ask the mother to watch the baby urinating.

Chordee is a tethering of the foreskin, which often causes the glans to be curved ventrally (Fig. 15.12B).

Look at the scrotum and the testes. Palpate both testes with warm hands. The right testis usually descends from the abdomen into the scrotum later than the left testis, and ends up higher in the scrotum. If the testes are larger than usual, the most common cause is a hydrocoele. Confirm this by transillumination (Fig. 15.9).

If you cannot identify the testes in the scrotum, exclude undescended or retractile testes. Using your right hand, start above the inguinal region on that side. Feel for any smooth lumps, moving your fingers down towards the scrotum, and then check the other side

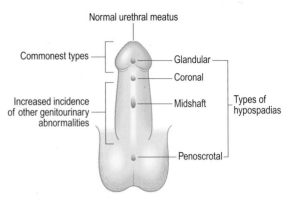

Fig. 15.11 Varieties of hypospadias.

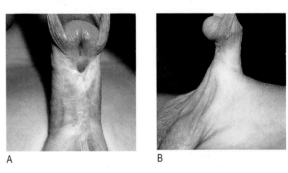

A   B

Fig. 15.12 Hypospadias and chordee. (A) Penile shaft hypospadias. **(B)** In this lateral view, the ventral curvature of the penis (chordee) can be seen.

with your left hand. The testis is smooth, soft and about 0.7×1 cm across. You may feel a retractile testis just below the inguinal canal. Try gently milking it along the line of the inguinal canal to see if you can bring it down into the scrotum. Note any cryptorchidism or maldescent of one or both testes. It may be difficult to palpate the testes if there is a large pad of suprapubic fat. If there is any doubt about the position of the testes, arrange for the infant to be examined at 6 weeks.

NEUROLOGICAL EXAMINATION

This consists principally of assessing tone, posture, movement and primitive reflexes. Sensory examination is limited.

Look at the baby and note any asymmetry in posture and movement. Erb's palsy post-delivery affects the upper brachial plexus roots (C5, C6), producing reduced movement of the arm, medial rotation of the forearm and failure to extend the wrist (Fig. 15.13). The rarer Klumpke's palsy may be seen after breech delivery and is due to damage to nerve roots C8 and T1, with weakness of the forearm and hand.

Facial nerve palsy causes reduced movement of the affected cheek muscles, and that side of the mouth does not turn down when the baby cries. Note any muscle

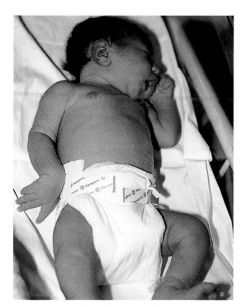

Fig. 15.13 Erb's palsy. The right arm is medially rotated and the wrist is flexed.

15.7 Hearing behaviours checklist for parents

Age	Behaviour
Shortly after birth	Startle and blink at a sudden noise, e.g. slamming of door
By 1 month	Notice sudden prolonged sounds, e.g. a vacuum cleaner, and pause and listen when they begin
By 4 months	Quieten or smile to the sound of your voice, even when they cannot see you. May also turn their head or eyes towards you if you come up from behind and speak to them from the side
By 7 months	Turn immediately to your voice across the room or to very quiet noises made on each side, as long as they are not too occupied with other things
By 9 months	Listen attentively to familiar everyday sounds and search for very quiet sounds made out of sight. Should also show pleasure in babbling loudly and tunefully
By 12 months	Show some response to their own name and to other familiar words. May respond when you say 'no' and 'bye-bye', even when they cannot see any accompanying gesture

wasting present in, for example, primary club foot (talipes equinovarus).

Check sensation by seeing whether the baby withdraws from stimuli: for example, when you are stroking the child's feet. Never inflict painful stimuli or use a pin or needle. Neonates' eyesight can be checked crudely if they are alert, by carrying them to a dark corner where they may open their eyes wide. Then take them to a brightly lit area, such as a window in daylight, and they will screw up their eyes against the bright light. If there is any doubt about vision, refer to a neonatal ophthalmologist.

Test hearing by noting the startle response to a loud sound. In the UK all neonates should undergo electronic audiological screening.

Tone is the resistance to passive movement across a joint. It is a subjective judgement and you need experience to judge it reliably. A normal infant's tone changes, so the baby may feel 'floppy' after a large feed.

- Hypotonic infants may have a frog-like posture with abducted hips and extended elbows. Causes of hypotonia include Down's syndrome and illness such as meningitis and sepsis
- Increased tone may cause back and neck arching and limb extension; the baby may feel stiff when picked up. Causes include meningitis, asphyxia or an intracranial haemorrhage
- Neonates are often tremulous, but this also occurs in subarachnoid haemorrhage or drug withdrawal if the mother has been abusing opioids in pregnancy. Infrequent jerks in light sleep are common and normal, but regular clonic or tonic jerks are abnormal.

Power is difficult to assess and depends on the infant's state of arousal. Look for strong symmetrical limb and trunk movements.

Assess the primitive reflexes in the order shown in Box 15.8.

Grasp responses

Stroke the sole of the infant's foot, and the toes will flex and curl round your examining finger. Stimulate the palm of the baby's hands by placing your finger firmly into it and observe the reflex grasping of your finger. Make sure the response is not inhibited by inadvertently stimulating the dorsal aspects of feet and hands.

Pull to sit

Hold the baby's hands and gently pull to sit (Fig. 15.14). Watch the sternocleidomastoid muscles, which should bilaterally anticipate the pull to sit; the head flexes for a moment before head lag occurs.

Ventral suspension/pelvic response to back stimulation

Turn the baby prone and look for good neck extension. Firmly stroke the skin over the vertebral column and observe the extensor response. Pelvic response to stimulation of the back and flanks should be symmetrical.

i | 15.8 **Order of assessment of the primitive reflexes**

- Grasp response of feet
- Grasp response of hands
- Pull to sit
- Ventral suspension
- Pelvic response to back stimulation
- Vestibular responses
- Place and step reflexes
- Moro reflex
- Root and suck responses
- Tonic neck reflex

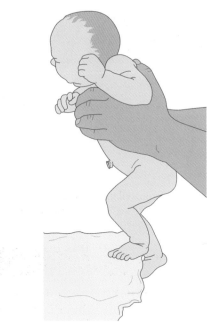

Fig. 15.15 Placing reflex.

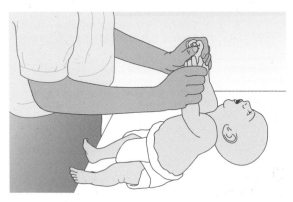

Fig. 15.14 Pulling to sit.

Vestibular responses

Hold the baby upright at your eye level, and then rotate him in an arc around your body. The baby's eyes should gaze in the direction of travel. Once the baby is a few days old, it is normal to see a horizontal jerking movement of the eyes in response to the arc rotation movement (optokinetic nystagmus).

Place and step reflexes

Hold the baby vertically and stimulate the dorsum of the foot on the edge of the examination table. The infant should flex the knee and hip, placing the sole of the foot on the table (Fig. 15.15).

Hold the baby under the arms and facing towards you, and lower him towards the surface of the table or couch. When the feet touch the surface, a walking movement occurs.

Both of these responses depend on the baby's state of arousal.

Moro reflex

Always elicit the Moro response with the infant safely on the examining couch. Support the baby's trunk and head at an angle of 70° to the couch. With your right hand supporting the baby's head, allow the head to drop 1 cm on to your right hand. The normal baby quickly throws out both arms with symmetrical abduction and spreads the fingers (Fig. 15.16). This is often followed by jerky adduction of the arms, as though the hands were reaching for an unseen source of security.

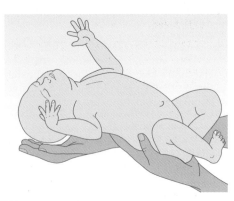

Fig. 15.16 The Moro response.

An asymmetrical Moro response may be due to a previously unsuspected fracture of the clavicle or Erb's palsy. Primitive reflexes persisting into later infancy may be the first indication of neurodevelopmental abnormality.

Root and suck responses

Efficient infant feeding depends on rooting, sucking, swallowing and defending the airway. Test the first two by gently stroking the baby's cheek. The hungry baby immediately turns to that side and opens the mouth, as though for a nipple. This is called rooting. If the baby sucks on your finger, this is often very vigorous.

Tonic neck reflex

This is the most difficult to demonstrate of all the primitive reflexes. In theory, if you turn the recumbent infant's head to the left, then the left arm and leg extend

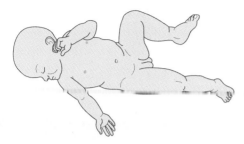

Fig. 15.17 Tonic neck reflex.

and the right arm and leg will flex. The tonic neck reflex appears at 37 weeks' gestation but is most prominent at 1 month (Fig. 15.17).

FINAL INSPECTION

The final inspection ensures that you do not omit anything and allows the parents a further opportunity to ask questions and seek clarification.

▶ Examination sequence

Neonates and infants

▶ Begin at the top of the scalp and progress down to the feet. Look at the scalp again and feel for any abnormalities. Re-inspect all aspects of the head and neck.

▶ Re-inspect the chest and abdomen. Breast engorgement is benign and resolves spontaneously.

▶ Turn the baby over and feel along the length of the vertebral column, starting at the neck. In particular, note and record the presence of the sacrum and coccyx if the mother is diabetic; sacral agenesis is associated with maternal diabetes. A hairy or pigmented patch over the lower spine may indicate spina bifida occulta. If you find a sacrococcygeal pit, visualize the bottom of it by separating the surrounding skin in good light. It is usually possible to see that the pit is lined with dry skin, which excludes pathological communication with the spinal cord.

▶ Look at the anus to confirm that it is present. Check the anal margins for a fissure, a local split in the protecting epidermis of the anal ring. The position of the anus may be abnormal: either too anterior or too posterior. Establish whether it is patent; confirm this by checking that the baby has passed meconium — the greenish-black stool passed by a neonate in the first few days of life. Meconium in the nappy does not necessarily mean that the baby has an anus; he could have a rectovaginal fistula. If the anus pouts, gently stimulate the sphincter by touching it with your finger and see that the muscle contracts.

▶ Do not routinely perform a digital rectal examination; it can cause an anal fissure. The few indications for rectal examination in a neonate include suspected rectal atresia or stenosis and delayed passage of meconium. If you do have to perform a rectal examination, put on gloves and lubricate your little finger. Gently press your finger tip against the anus until you feel the muscle resistance relax and insert your finger up to your distal interphalangeal (DIP) joint only.

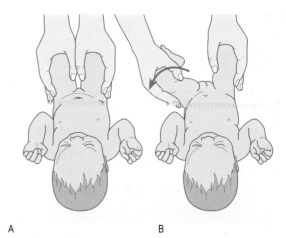

A   B

Fig. 15.18 Examination for developmental dysplasia of the hip. (A) The hip is dislocated posteriorly out of the acetabulum (Barlow manœuvre). **(B)** The dislocated hip is relocated back into the acetabulum (Ortolani manœuvre).

▶ If there is mucus or bleeding per rectum, visualize the rectal mucosa using an otoscope and a well-lubricated earpiece.

▶ Look at the baby's legs for any malformations. Hold the lower half of each leg in your hands and gently flex and extend them to gain an impression of the infant's tone. Count the toes and note whether any override each other. In talipes equinovarus the foot is plantar flexed and rotated, so that the sole is directed medially. Check that you can gently manipulate the foot and ankle into the correct position. Normal findings include forefoot adduction and tibial bowing caused by the fetal position in utero.

▶ Examine for dislocation of the hip, now called developmental dysplasia of the hip (DDH) because there is evidence that some dysplasias identified at 1 year are not evident in the first few weeks. The detection of DDH depends on the experience of the examiner, but incidence is around 1:1000 in the UK. Be particularly suspicious if there is a family history of DDH, if the delivery was by extended breech, if there is positional talipes (especially calcaneovalgus of the foot), if there is a small amount of amniotic fluid (oligohydramnios) or if the baby is a large first-born girl.

▶ Lay the baby supine on a firm but comfortable surface. Look at the thighs for symmetry of the thigh creases.

▶ Examine each hip separately. Hold the thigh with the knee flexed and your thumb on the medial aspect of the thigh. Move the proximal end of the thigh laterally and then push down towards the examining table (Barlow manœuvre) (Fig. 15.18A); a clunk implies dislocatability of the hip. Then abduct the thigh; if you feel a clunk now, this indicates that the head of the femur has been dislocated and has been returned into the acetabulum (Ortolani manœuvre) (Fig. 15.18B). Diagnose dislocated hips if the femoral head is very lax and you feel a clunk without carrying out the lateral and downward movement: that is, the Ortolani manœuvre without requiring the Barlow manœuvre.

▶ You can often feel minor clicks at the hip or knee produced by tendon movements. If you are in any doubt, refer the infant for a senior opinion, preferably that of an orthopaedic surgeon with expertise in paediatrics. An ultrasound screening programme is available in some centres (Box 15.9).

15.9 Key points: neonates and infants

- Parents appreciate it if you are enthusiastic about their new baby; remember to congratulate them.
- The neonatal clinical examination can only identify abnormalities present at the time of the examination. It does not guarantee that all congenital abnormalities are identified.
- The baby may still have congenital abnormalities, even after a normal neonatal examination.
- Always listen to the parents' concerns and address these. If a parent thinks that the baby has a problem, you must take this seriously.
- Be opportunistic and do not expect to carry out your examination systematically.
- Defer any examination that you cannot complete.
- Keep uncomfortable procedures to the end so that you do not disturb a contented baby.
- You need experience to appreciate the normal range of neonates and infants. Seek advice from a senior colleague if you are in doubt.
- If you identify any abnormalities, give parents a clear written plan of treatment and follow-up.
- Give parents information about other appropriate sources of advice that will be relevant to their infant's care in the coming days and weeks.

EXAMINATION OF CHILDREN

Children are not miniature adults; they are constantly growing and developing. Most doctors and students have an idea of the range of heights, weights and behaviours expected in adults, but because children are at various stages on a continuum leading to physical and psychological maturity, it is much more difficult to recognize deviations from normal. Parents often have similar difficulties, and when they consult the doctor they may simply want reassurance that their child is normal. In practice, even experienced paediatricians require specific tools such as growth charts to distinguish what is normal (Figs 15.19 and 15.20).

Careful observation is the key to examining children. This means much more than just formal inspection. From the time you first encounter individual children, look at them carefully, observing their interaction with people and with their environment, and taking careful note of their appearance and demeanour. This provides important clues about their growth and nutrition, their development, their relationship with their parents, and the severity of any illness. Use the general principles of family-friendly consulting and have all your equipment gathered together (Boxes 15.10 and 15.11). Often, you do not need to examine every system in detail. A combination of detailed observation and a careful history allows you to target specific systems for detailed examination.

At the start of a consultation, watch the child play while you chat to the parents. A major factor in the art

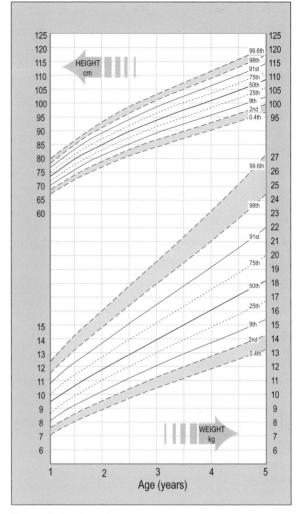

Fig. 15.19 Growth chart.

of examining children is engaging their cooperation. Capture the child's interest, by playing with a toy or talking about a television programme; this will enable you to carry out a great deal of examination without the child realizing you are doing so. Direct methods of examination, such as palpation and auscultation, are less informative than in adults because specific localized signs in children are uncommon. Always leave unpleasant examinations, such as examining the throat, to the end.

Approach your assessment using a series of logical questions. Is the child:
- ill?
- in pain?
- obviously abnormal?
- well grown and cared for?
- developing normally?

Is the child ill?

Assess illness severity in children (Fig. 15.21). Do they need resuscitation, urgent treatment or pain relief?

15.10 Equipment

- Otoscope with a bright light and selection of sizes of clean earpieces
- Disposable spatulas
- Ophthalmoscope
- Paediatric stethoscope
- Selection of sizes of blood pressure cuffs
- Stadiometer and accurate, calibrated weighing scales
- Disposable paper tape measure
- Centile charts for plotting measurements
- Developmental assessment tools
  - 8 × 2.5 cm bricks
  - Drawing equipment
  - Picture books
- Prader orchidometer

15.11 Family-friendly consulting

Environment

- Provide enough chairs for everyone (parents and siblings) and arrange them to encourage friendly interaction
- Make sure the space is safe and uncluttered
- Ensure that the space is sufficiently private
- Provide a small table and chairs with paper and crayons, and a selection of toys suitable for a range of ages

Personal

- Dressed appropriately (not overly informal)
- Wear short sleeves (bare to the elbow) to allow frequent hand-washing to minimise cross-infection
- Avoid dangling jewellery

Is the child in pain?

Parents are very sensitive to distress or pain experienced by their child. In children who cannot speak, assess the degree of pain using an appropriate pain chart (Box 15.12).

Is there any obvious abnormality?

Look for an unusual posture or gait as the child approaches you. Are there obvious dysmorphic features such as low-set ears, slanting eyes or a large tongue? Check whether the child's features are like those of their parents or siblings. You cannot remember every unusual syndrome but you should be able to describe, record and, if necessary, measure what you see.

Is the child well grown and cared for?

Healthy, well-fed and properly nurtured children grow normally. Growth therefore provides a valuable measure of overall physical and psychological well-being.

Weigh toddlers and children in their underwear, using accurately calibrated scales.

Measure height using a stadiometer, a vertical scale with a rigid armpiece (Fig. 15.23). If a child is unusually tall or short, measure the parents' heights. Calculate the child's predicted height using the following equation:

$$\text{Mid-parental height} = \frac{\text{Parental heights added} + 7\,\text{cm boy or} -7\,\text{cm girl}}{2}$$

Plot the mid-parental height on a growth chart at the furthest end of the age scale, which is usually 18 years. The range 10 cm above and below that figure is the target centile range for the child, creating a 'normal' distribution curve adjusted for this particular family spanning 2 standard deviations.

Use pubertal grading scales to evaluate a child's progress through puberty (Fig. 15.27). Every child's progress should be recorded on a growth chart

15.12 Pain assessment tool: FLACC scale

	0	1	2
Face	No particular expression or smile	Occasional grimace or frown, withdrawn, disinterested	Frequently or constantly quivering chin, clenched jaw
Legs	Normal position or relaxed	Uneasy, restless, tense	Kicking or legs drawn up
Activity	Lying quietly, normal position, moves easily	Squirming, shifting back and forth, tense	Arched, rigid or jerking
Cry	No cry (awake or asleep)	Moans or whimpers, occasional complaint	Crying steadily, screams or sobs, frequent complaints
Consolability	Content, relaxed	Reassured by occasional touching, hugging or being talked to, distractible	Difficult to console or comfort

Each category is scored on a 0–2 scale to give a total score of 0–10: 0 = no pain; 1–3 — mild pain; 4–7 = moderate pain; 8–10 = severe pain.

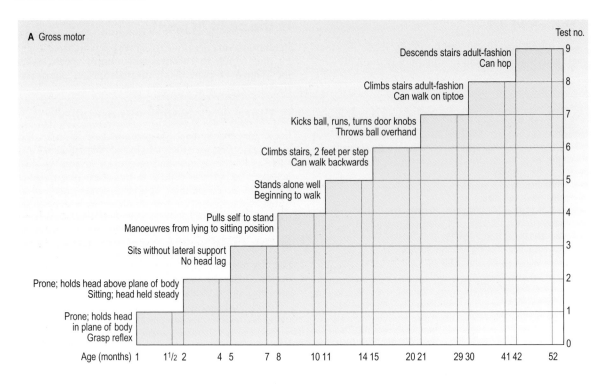

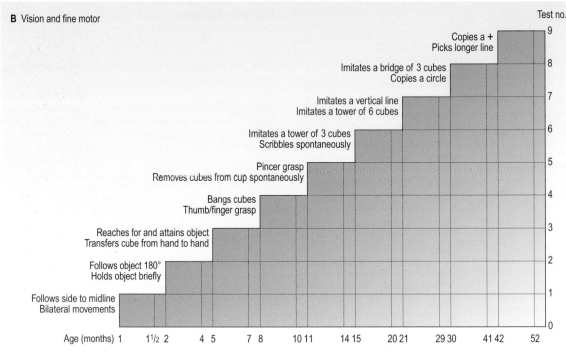

Fig. 15.20 Woodside system of developmental assessment.

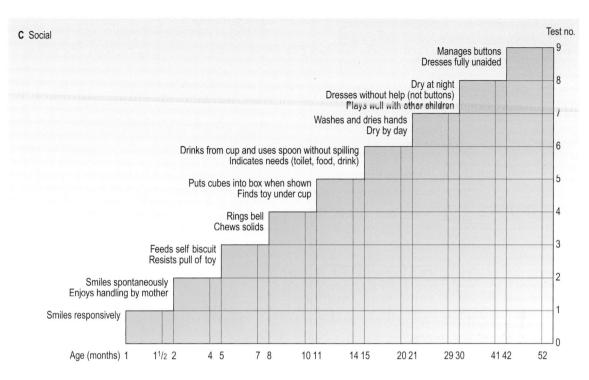

C Social

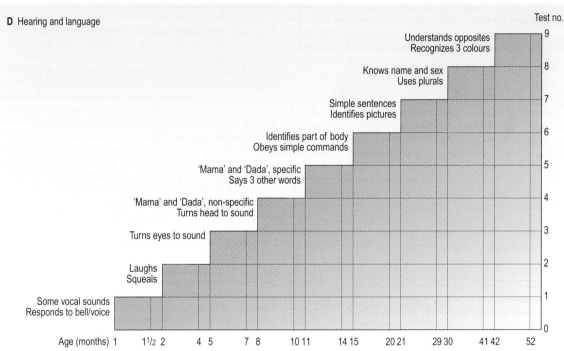

D Hearing and language

Fig. 15.20 (Continued)

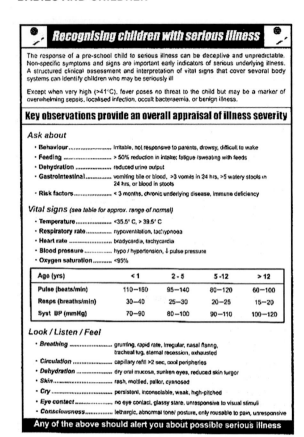

Fig. 15.21 Rapid cardiopulmonary evaluation.

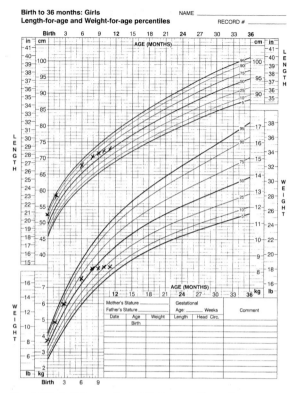

Fig. 15.22 A child's growth chart that crosses the centiles.

documenting height and weight, with head circumference in infants (Fig. 15.19). Previous measurements are often available, so serial growth over time can be plotted. Measurements crossing the centiles should raise concern (Fig. 15.22).

The child's appearance, demeanour, behaviour and interactions with carers are important indicators of well-being. Always be vigilant for signs of neglect or abuse and document any suspicious behaviours and unusual bruises or injuries. Ask how any injury occurred, decide whether the injuries are consistent with the explanation and note any delay before presentation. Child abuse may present as failure to thrive, so keeping careful growth records is important. Signs that may suggest child neglect or abuse are listed in Box 15.13.

Is the child developing normally?

Children progressively acquire movement and motor skills and develop intellectually and cognitively as the nervous system matures. Consider their development under four headings:

- movement and posture
- vision and manipulation

15.13 Signs that may suggest child neglect or abuse

Behavioural signs

- 'Frozen watchfulness'
- Passivity
- Over-friendliness
- Sexualized behaviour
- Inappropriate dress
- Hunger, stealing food

Physical signs

- Identifiable bruises, e.g. finger tips, handprints, belt buckle, bites
- Circular (cigarette) burns or submersion burns with no splash marks
- Injuries of differing ages
- Eye or mouth injuries
- Long bone fractures or bruises in non-mobile infants
- Posterior rib fracture
- Subconjunctival or retinal haemorrhage
- Dirty, smelly, unkempt child
- Bad nappy rash

- hearing and speech
- social behaviour.

Children can differ widely in the age they attain each developmental milestone (Fig. 15.20). They may be

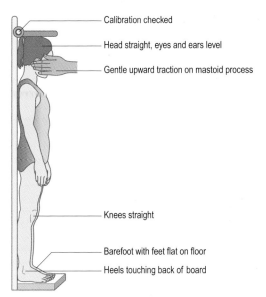

Fig. 15.23 Stadiometer for measuring height accurately in children.

slow for one milestone but advanced in another. Not achieving certain milestones at a single examination does not necessarily indicate a problem; the child may be tired or uncooperative. Carry out a more detailed developmental examination if certain warning signs are present (Box 15.14). Make allowances for prematurity, up to the age of 2 years.

Developmental delay may be global, encompassing all four categories listed above, or specific, affecting one category in particular: for example, motor delay in cerebral palsy, or social impairment and language delay in autism.

Talking with parents and listening to their concerns

Always listen carefully to the parent (or main carer) and explore his or her FIFE (p. 10). Parents and carers are the experts on their child, so explore their feelings and ideas about their child, ask whether the symptoms are affecting the child's functioning in any way, and establish what their expectations are of you and this consultation. Use the principles outlined in Chapter 2.

Clarify the relationship between historian and child, e.g. parent, childminder, grandparent, and record this in the notes. You are receiving an interpretation of events from a third party, not hearing about an experience first-hand, so clarify any ambiguous terms, e.g. fit, constipation, wheeze. Ask parents to demonstrate what they saw. Summarize your understanding to check you have understood parents correctly.

Talking to children

Talk to the child and explain what you are doing. If possible, ask him to describe the problem and tell you

15.14 Warning signs in developmental milestones

The supine infant: around 6 weeks

- Marked head lag (in cerebral palsy, excessive extensor tone can mimic advanced motor development)
- Asymmetry of limb movements
- Absence of visual fixation and following
- Excessive placidity or hyper-excitability
- Difficulty with sucking and swallowing

The sitting infant: 7–10 months

- Unable to sit unsupported
- Unable to raise head and chest when prone
- Hand preference (right or left dominance should not be present until age 2; before this, it suggests a problem with the neglected hand)
- Absence of hand transfer, unable to handle two objects
- Absence of visually directed reach
- Poor vocalization
- Unable to chew or swallow

The mobile toddler: around 2 years

- Unsteady gait
- Unable to climb stairs
- Mouthing or casting objects
- Unable to build a tower of cubes
- Lack of intelligible speech
- No meaningful three-word combinations: subject — verb — object
- Unable to name pictures

The talking child: 3–4 years

- Unable to stand on one foot
- Unable to pedal a tricycle
- Unable to copy a circle
- Unable to use sentences of at least six words
- Unable to separate from mother
- Solitary or obsessional play

about it (Box 15.15). By 12–18 months, a child normally uses single words. By 3–4 years, an average child has a vocabulary of 850–1500 words and uses three-word sentences. Children's understanding of illness changes as they get older. Pre-school children tend to attribute illness to coincidence or magic. In primary school, the idea of contagion develops and contracting disease is associated with contamination from other people or objects. Older children perceive that they fall ill through ingestion or inhalation of a 'germ'. Only in adolescence can young people fully understand psychological or pathological explanations for illness.

THE HISTORY

In children, it is often more practical to approach the history using a logical problem-based focus on the relevant facets of the history and examination, rather than the typical detailed history, full examination and differential diagnosis used for adults.

15.15 Communicating with children

- Get down to the child's eye level
- Compliment children about their clothes, hair adornments, etc.
- Refer to popular characters, e.g. Bob the Builder
- Tailor your language appropriately and talk playfully
- Play games with your equipment, e.g. listening to dolly's chest, blowing out the light of the otoscope
- Give 'I've been brave at the doctor's' stickers

15.16 Some causes of short stature in children

Intrinsic shortness

- Familial (genetic) short stature
- Turner's syndrome

Delayed growth

- Constitutional delay in growth (adult height often normal)
- Subtle undernutrition
- Physical and/or psychological abuse/child neglect
- Underlying systemic diseases of mild to moderate severity

Attenuated growth

- Chronic renal failure
- Metabolic acidosis
- Malignancy (including effects of chemotherapy and radiotherapy)
- Glucocorticoid excess
- Pulmonary disease, e.g. cystic fibrosis and severe asthma
- Congenital heart disease
- Gastrointestinal disease, e.g. coeliac disease and Crohn's disease — patients often underweight as well as short
- Hypothyroidism
- Advanced HIV infection
- Severe protein and calorie malnutrition

Presenting complaint

Confirm what name the child is known by and check his age. Knowing a child's age and sex rapidly limits the range of diagnostic possibilities. Ask the parents to describe the problem and how it developed.

Past medical history

Note significant ill health, particularly hospital referral or admission. Find out about investigations, treatment and any operations, accidents or injuries, including their outcome.

Birth history

Find out from the mother about the pregnancy, delivery and neonatal period:

- Was the pregnancy uneventful?
- Did labour start spontaneously?
- Was the baby preterm?
- How long was gestation and what was the birth weight?
- Were there any complications at delivery?
- Did the baby require resuscitation, or special or intensive care?
- Were there any other neonatal problems?
- During pregnancy, did the mother take:
    Prescribed drugs
    Non-prescribed drugs
    Alcohol?

Feeding history

This is important in children with poor appetite, faltering growth (Box 15.16), obesity, constipation, diarrhoea and vomiting, or possible food allergies, and should be explored if the parents are concerned (Box 15.17).

Vaccination history and infectious illness

Check that the child's immunizations are up to date, that BCG has been given in certain ethnic minorities and that hepatitis B immunization has been carried out if the parents have that infection or a history of intravenous drug use. If the child is not immunized, find out why not. Are there parental concerns about vaccinations? Were there previous adverse reactions? Note any contact with infectious illness or recent foreign travel.

15.17 Feeding history

- Are infant artificial feeds being prepared correctly?
- Is/was the child bottle-fed or breastfed?
    Length of exclusive breastfeeding?
    Volume and frequency of current bottle feeds (5 oz/150 ml of formula/kg/day)?
- Age at which unmodified cow's milk was introduced?
- Age at which the child was weaned?
    Which foods were given?
    Given by bottle, spoon or as finger food?
- Can the child chew, suck and swallow without difficulty?
- Associated symptoms, such as vomiting, rashes or swelling, after particular foods?

Developmental history

Record developmental progress, especially when the parents are concerned about a delay in development or if the child has epilepsy, an unusual (dysmorphic) appearance, a recognized syndrome, or an abnormal skull shape or size (Fig. 15.13). With young children, find out when they first smiled, sat, crawled, walked and talked. With school-age children, establish whether they attend an ordinary school and are making good progress. If so, significant developmental problems are unlikely.

Family history

It is important to locate the presenting illness in the context of the child's life and the family dynamics and relationships.

- Are the child's mother and father living together?
    - If not, what contact does the patient have with the absent parent?

- Who else makes up the household?
  - What are their occupations?
- How many siblings does the child have?
  - What is their age and sex?
  - Are they all healthy?
- What are the family's childcare arrangements?
- Are the family restricted because of the child's illness?

If the problem runs in the family, draw a family tree (Fig. 2.3, p. 18).

Social history

Home

- Are there any problems with housing, e.g. damp?
- Are there enough bedrooms and bathrooms?
- Are cooking facilities adequate?
- Is there room for safe play?
- How many smokers are there in the house?
- Are there any pets?

School

- How has the child's school attendance been?
- How is the child performing?
- Document the name of the school and teacher.
- Have there been bullying or behaviour problems?
- What is the impact of the symptom/s at and after school?
- Does the illness interfere with the child's day-to-day activities, e.g. play, sports, activities of daily living, and ability to keep pace with peers?

Drug history

Note the dose, route and frequency of administration of current medications, including over-the-counter and complementary remedies. Clarify any adverse reactions, particularly to antibiotics.

Psychiatric history

Emotional, behaviour or relationship problems are common, and can present with sleeping difficulties, temper tantrums, faddy eating and school refusal. Certain symptoms, such as abdominal pain or headache, may have no physical explanation, and psychiatric and emotional problems can complicate physical illness.

The aim of the psychiatric history is to elucidate the symptoms, explore their impact and look at the child's risk factors for mental health problems, along with strengths or protective factors. Children may find direct questioning about their behaviour and emotions intimidating. Usually, it is more illuminating to observe children's facial expression, body language, play, drawing and interactions sensitively as you talk with them. Once you have grasped the presenting symptoms, ask about specific symptoms of mood disorder, such as appetite and sleep disturbance, physical symptoms, attention and concentration, and separation anxiety.

Enquire about any significant events in the child's life, such as starting school, moving home, the death of a family member or parental divorce, and note how the child responds. Empathetic, open-ended questions to the child, such as 'That sounds difficult. How did it make you feel?', can be useful.

It is important to understand why a child has become a focus for concern. Sometimes problems arise because of a disturbance in the mental health and coping skills of the parents. Use the family tree to document family functioning by enquiring about relationships between parents and siblings.

15

THE PHYSICAL EXAMINATION

Examination of the skin, hair and nails

Examine the skin, hair and nails if there is any history of a rash. Make a drawing or diagram of any rash for accuracy. Arrange for photographs for medicolegal documentation of trauma due to suspected child abuse.

Inspection

Note:

- colour
- distribution
- size and nature of individual lesions
- whether lesions are separate or confluent
- itchiness
- rashes in the scalp
- nails
  fungal infection
  bitten to the quick
- hair
  alopecia.

Palpation

- Is the rash raised?
- Do the individual lesions contain clear or cloudy fluid or pus?

Examination of the lymph nodes

Parents may see or feel an enlarged lymph node, particularly in the child's neck or groin. Often, such glands are normal. 'Normal' glands are not tender, may be multiple and tend to be small ('shotty'). Parents may have unspoken anxieties about leukaemia or cancer; fortunately, malignant conditions are rare in children

15.18 Causes of lymph node enlargement

Cervical lymphadenopathy

- Tonsillitis, pharyngitis, sinusitis
- 'Glandular fever' (infectious mononucleosis/cytomegalovirus)
- Tuberculosis (uncommon in developed countries)

Generalized lymphadenopathy

- Febrile illness with a generalized rash
- 'Glandular fever'
- Systemic juvenile chronic arthritis (Still's disease)
- Acute lymphatic leukaemia
- Drug reaction
- Mucocutaneous lymph node syndrome (Kawasaki syndrome)

15.19 Respiratory rate in children (breaths/min)

Age	Normal	Tachypnoea
Neonates	30–50	>60
Infants	20–30	>50
Young children	20–30	>40
Older children	15–20	>30

(Box 15.18). Children with skin conditions such as eczema may have lymph nodes that are enlarged from draining an affected area of skin.

Inspection

- Is there a swelling?

Palpation

- Size
- Number
- Consistency
- Temperature
- Tenderness
- Mobility/attachment to skin or deeper structures.

Check all the other regional lymph node areas. If regional nodes are enlarged, make sure there are no injuries, infections or skin abnormalities within the drained area. Look for liver and spleen enlargement.

Respiratory examination

Examine the respiratory system in any child with a cough, breathing difficulties, wheezing, poor feeding or fever.

Inspection

Watch the child's breathing and count the respiratory rate over 30–60 seconds. Fast breathing (tachypnoea) is a sensitive marker for acute respiratory infection (Box 15.19).
Look for:

- Cyanosis or alteration in the child's colour. Use a pulse oximeter to measure oxygen saturation (SpO_2) to avoid missing mild desaturation. The normal level is ≥95% (p. 163)
- Respiratory rate
- Signs of more severe respiratory distress:
    Subcostal, intercostal or supraclavicular retraction
    Indrawing of the trachea in the suprasternal notch during inspiration (tracheal tug)
    Flaring of the nostrils
- Hyperinflation of the chest or asymmetry of chest wall movement. In chronic, poorly controlled asthma the chest is hyperinflated and over time the chronic diaphragmatic traction leads to fixed retraction of the lower ribs with flaring of the diaphragm (Harrison's sulcus)
- Pattern of breathing. In obstructive airway diseases such as asthma, expiration becomes more prolonged than inspiration
- A prominent cough. Does this sound moist and productive or dry? A persistent, moist cough is uncommon in children and is not a feature of asthma
- Any sputum and its colour. The colour of sputum usually correlates with the presence of infection. Neutrophils produce the enzyme myeloperoxidase, which colours the sputum green (p. 157)
- Finger clubbing. This is most common in cystic fibrosis and cyanotic congenital heart disease, but is not seen in asthma.

Palpation and percussion

Feel the position of the trachea. A shift laterally may indicate underlying mediastinal shift. Check chest expansion by watching carefully from the front.

Percussion is occasionally helpful if you suspect consolidation or an effusion from the quality of the breath sounds.

Auscultation

Respiratory noises are often audible without a stethoscope and may even be palpable.

- Note any respiratory noise, such as an expiratory grunt, inspiratory stridor or wheeze
- Establish whether the noise originates in the chest or throat, or both
- Listen to the breath sounds with your stethoscope. The respiratory sounds are usually high-pitched, so use the diaphragm. Diminished breath sounds which vary across the chest suggest underlying pathology
- Note wheezes and crackles and whether they are symmetrical or focal. Localized differences point to

| 15.20 Normal resting pulse rate in children* ||
Age	Beats/min
<1 year	110–160
2–5 years	95–140
5–12 years	80–120
>12 years	60–100

* Increased with stress, exercise, fever or arrhythmia.

15.21 Characteristics of innocent murmurs

- Soft: grades 1–3 in intensity and often mid-systolic
- Localized
- Poorly conducted
- Not usually conducted posteriorly
- Variable with position and with respiration

focal lung lesions. Generalized wheezing suggests asthma
- In children over 5 years of age, it may be useful to check peak flow rate. Normal values vary with a child's height and can be checked on reference tables.

Cardiovascular examination

Examine this in any child with shortness of breath, syncope, cyanosis, feeding difficulties or a previously noted murmur.

Inspection

Look for central cyanosis. If you are not sure about cyanosis, check the SpO_2 using a pulse oximeter. Count the respiratory rate. Look for any abnormality of the precordial area, such as a precordial bulge.

Assess:
- sweating
- finger clubbing
- peripheral oedema; check infants lying on their backs for occipital oedema.

Palpation

Feel the child's fingers and toes. Are they warm and well perfused? Record the time for capillary return (p. 444).

Feel the femoral and brachial pulses for rate, which varies with the child's age, fever, excitement, distress and exercise (Box 15.20). Normal femoral pulses are difficult to feel in small children; use your thumbs.

Assess:
- Strength and volume. Small-volume pulses are difficult to feel and distal pulses are more difficult than proximal pulses. Full-volume pulses are bounding, and peripheral pulses are easier to feel
- Whether the pulses on both sides are symmetrical
- Whether there is any brachiofemoral delay (coarctation of the aorta)
- The apex beat, which is normally found in the fourth–fifth intercostal space in the midclavicular line
- The precordium. Palpate for a heave or thrill. A thrill is a palpable murmur and always significant. Thrills from aortic stenosis may only be palpable in

the suprasternal notch, so feel in the notch with your index finger.

Auscultation

Listen to the heart at the end of the cardiovascular examination, unless children are cooperative or asleep; if that is the case, use the opportunity to listen while they are quiet.

Listen to the precordium. Identify the first and second heart sounds. Note the quality and intensity of the second sound and whether it is split. Children with an atrial septal defect can have wide splitting of the second heart sound, which does not change with respiration.

If there is a murmur, note:
- where it is loudest
- whether it is systolic or diastolic, or both
- where it is conducted.

Murmurs associated with a thrill are always pathological, but innocent murmurs are common (Box 15.21). Refer a child with a suspicious murmur to the paediatric cardiologist.

Blood pressure

Blood pressure varies with age. To take a child's BP, use a cuff that measures two-thirds of the distance from the elbow to the shoulder tip. With the child sitting or standing, keep his heart and arm and the sphygmomanometer at the same level and explain what you are going to do. Record the cuff size and whether the child was sitting or standing. Repeat a single elevated reading with a larger cuff until the cuff does not fit the arm (p. 123).

Examination of the ears, nose and throat

Examine the ears, nose and throat in children with earache, deafness or aural discharge, a runny or blocked nose, sore throat or fever.

Inspection of the ears

- Look at the shape and position of the external ears. One-third of the pinna of normal ears is above an imaginary coronal plane between the inner and outer canthi. Low-set ears have less than one-third of the pinna above this line and occur in Down's syndrome

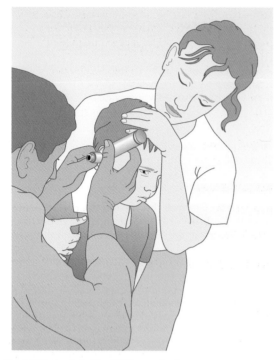

Fig. 15.24 How to hold a child to examine the ear.

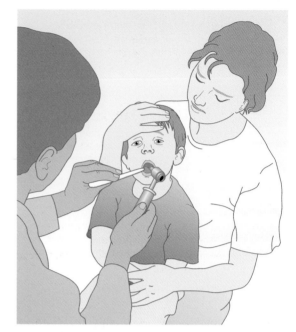

Fig. 15.25 How to hold a child to examine the mouth and throat.

- Use an otoscope to visualize the tympanic membrane. Ask parents to hold young children properly to avoid discomfort (Fig. 15.24)
- Use the largest speculum that fits in the external auditory meatus
- To straighten the auditory canal, pull the pinna down in infants, because the auditory canal is directed upwards, and back and up in older children
- Note the anatomical landmarks, bulging, retraction, perforation, redness, dullness and fluid levels (p. 337).

Inspection of the nose

- Does the nose look normal?
- Is the child breathing through the nose?
- Note any nasal discharge and whether it is clear, pussy or bloodstained. Children with allergic rhinitis may persistently rub their nose, producing a small, horizontal crease near the tip of the nose — the 'allergic salute'
- Examine the nasal mucosa. In a cooperative older child, use an otoscope with a large speculum (p. 346). Note inflammation, swelling or pus on the mucosa.

Inspection of the mouth and throat

Examine these in a child with sore throat, unexplained fever or mouth ulcer.

- Look at the tongue and jaw size. A protruding tongue is seen in a number of conditions e.g. Down's syndrome.
- Examine the throat. Leave this to the end of the examination. Use a bright light and ask the parent to hold the child firmly (Fig. 15.25). You may only have the chance for a brief look. Ask young children to do an 'alligator's yawn' or to show you what they had for breakfast by opening their mouth even wider. If they are uncooperative, slip a tongue depressor along the side of the mouth between the lips and teeth to touch the back of the throat. When the child gags you will catch a glimpse of the throat. Use this only when it is important to visualize the throat and never in a child with stridor, in case you precipitate complete obstruction.
- Look for redness, exudates or secretions in the oropharynx. Palatal petechiae are seen in glandular fever. In thrush, the white exudate is difficult to scrape away. Check for Koplik's spots (measles) on the buccal mucosa if the child has a rash.
- Check the tonsils for ulceration or exudates. Large tonsils are only significant if they produce symptoms of airway obstruction during sleep.
- Look at the palate for any cleft of the soft or hard palate. It is surprisingly easy to miss a cleft palate. If you cannot obtain a good view, use a spatula to inspect this part clearly.
- Do not examine the throat in children who have become rapidly unwell with a sore throat, or are febrile and drooling, because they may have epiglottitis and you may precipitate complete airway obstruction. Always ask whether the child has had *Haemophilus influenzae* b (Hib) immunization.

Inspection of the teeth

Check the teeth for dental caries and the gums for any abnormalities. If necessary, suggest that the child sees a dentist for full assessment.

Gastrointestinal examination

Examine the abdomen of any child with vomiting, diarrhoea, constipation, abdominal swellings, abdominal pain or urinary symptoms.

Inspection

Note jaundice or anaemia and markers of liver disease, such as spider naevi and finger clubbing.

Look for abdominal distension. The abdomen is often protuberant in normal toddlers and children because of an exaggerated lumbar lordosis. Abdominal movement with respiration is normal up to school age. Fullness in the flanks may occur if there is ascites. If a swelling is present, note its size and whether it is local or generalized. The site may suggest the cause. Fat, fluid, faeces and flatus all cause generalized swelling, while localized swellings may be due to a hernia, distended bowel loops, masses or enlarged organs. Umbilical and inguinal hernias are common. With gross ascites the umbilicus may be everted. Visible peristalsis occurs in pyloric stenosis or intestinal obstruction.

Palpation

Make sure that the child is as relaxed as possible. This takes skill and patience. Ideally, children should lie on their back. Always ask if their abdomen is sore before you start to examine them and watch their face during palpation for any sign of discomfort. Palpate:

- Methodically round the abdomen, feeling for the size and position of the abdominal organs and for any masses or fluid
- The liver, which is felt 1–2 cm below the costal margin in the midclavicular line. Start palpating in the left iliac fossa to detect a very large liver (Fig. 8.18, p. 202). Define the upper edge by percussion, then measure the distance in centimetres between the top and bottom edges in the mid-clavicular line. Record the liver breadth in centimetres and note whether the edge is soft or firm. A hyperinflated chest (as occurs in severe bronchiolitis) can flatten the diaphragm and push the liver down. Measuring the liver breadth differentiates a large liver from one of normal size that is pushed down and palpable
- The spleen, which may be felt in children who are well. Start in the right iliac fossa and work towards the left costal margin (Fig. 8.20, p. 204)
- The kidneys, keeping your left hand underneath the child and using your right hand on top for both

sides (Fig. 9.10, p. 229). The kidneys are difficult to feel in young children, except in a hypotonic neonate; if you do feel them, they are probably enlarged

- The bladder. You may feel a full bladder and sometimes see it arising from the pelvis in infants and young children
- The groins, for swellings that might indicate a hernia.

If you suspect ascites, check for shifting dullness (Fig. 8.21, p. 204).

Auscultation

Listen for bowel sounds. Bowel sounds are accentuated in intestinal obstruction and absent in peritonitis or paralytic ileus.

The anus and rectum

Look at the anus when you examine the abdomen in case the child has an imperforate anus. Do not carry out a rectal examination routinely in a child. If you have to perform one, explain clearly what you are going to do and why it is necessary. Put lubricant gel on your gloved little finger in infants and small children (index finger for older children). Feel for any masses or local tenderness, and look at your finger afterwards to check for blood or other material (p. 207).

Genitourinary examination

Genital abnormalities are common, especially in boys. If you are examining the genitalia, make sure you have a chaperone or parent with you and record their presence in the notes. If there is any suggestion of sexual abuse from the history or from your assessment of the situation, refer the child for a detailed assessment.

Inspection in boys

- Assess the size of the penis
- Check the position of the urethral opening, which should be at the penile tip
- Check that the scrotum is normal in size and rugose (wrinkled), and that both testes are visible in the scrotum. Transilluminate any swellings by placing a pen-torch against the skin over the swelling and seeing if the light is transmitted across the swelling. If so, this indicates a fluid-filled swelling, most commonly a hydrocoele (Fig. 15.9).

Palpation in boys

- Palpate the scrotum with the boy standing and confirm that both testes are in the scrotum. To help differentiate an undescended testis from a retractile one, ask the child to squat. This abolishes the

15

423

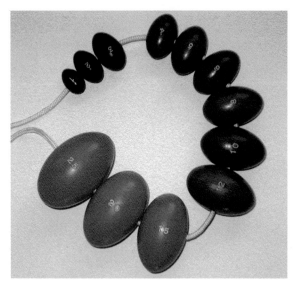

Fig. 15.26 Prader orchidometer.

cremasteric reflex and allows you to feel a retractile testis.

- Assess the testicular volume using a Prader orchidometer (Fig. 15.26).

Inspection in girls

With the child lying on her back, look for enlargement of the clitoris, labial adhesions, the position of the vagina, the presence and nature of any vaginal discharge, and any signs of trauma or scratching.

In older children, stage their progress through puberty. Pubertal staging charts make use of the extent of pubic hair growth, breast development (in girls) or penile and testicular development (in boys) to assign a pubertal stage (Figs 15.27 and 15.28).

Musculoskeletal examination

Pain in the joints, bones or limbs is common. Parents may worry about bow-legs or knock knees. Specific descriptive labels, e.g. phocomelia — a seal-like limb, talipes — club foot, are in use. Do not worry if you do not know the name, but always describe exactly what you see.

The age of the child is important in determining the likely cause of a limp (Box 15.23). In acute limp consider trauma and infection. Ask about recent vaccinations, infections and antibiotic treatment. Ask about pyrexia, early-morning stiffness and pain to help diagnose inflammatory conditions such as juvenile idiopathic arthritis.

Inspection

- Watch the child moving around. See whether infants crawl or bottom-shuffle; ask older children to hop, skip and jump and look for a waddle or a limp.

- Check for bony deformity or joint swelling or redness.
- Note any limb abnormalities. Some findings will only become obvious when a child is undressed. Make sure you do not miss extra toes or fingers.
- Look for muscle wasting or hypertrophied muscle groups.

Palpation

- Check active joint movements before attempting passive ones. Be careful to avoid causing pain or do what you can to minimize it. Ask children's permission before you touch them and watch their face during your examination.
- Feel for swelling, heat and tenderness over bones and joints.
- Note which joints are affected and whether these are proximal or distal.

Nervous system examination

Carry out a neurological examination in a child with a history of seizures, headaches, an abnormal or unsteady gait, any weakness and any increase or decrease in tone.

Full examination

Perform a detailed neurological examination in an older child as you would in an adult. In younger children, the nervous system is developing and their degree of comprehension and cooperation is lower, so the examination of development and the nervous system is intertwined.

Inspection of the head

Look at the shape and size of the head, and at the fontanelles. Is the head shape normal (Box 15.5)? Some head shapes are associated with particular syndromes.

Palpation of the head

- Measure the occipitofrontal circumference using a disposable paper tape.
- Place the tape around the head at the level of the occiput and forehead. Make sure this is at the largest circumference and then measure three times, noting the largest measurement, to the nearest millimetre (Fig. 15.2). Plot the result on a centile chart.
- Feel the fontanelles and the cranial sutures and note whether they are open or closed. The posterior fontanelle closes soon after birth, and the anterior at 15–18 months. Delay in closure suggests increased intracranial pressure, bone disease such as rickets or other abnormalities of the skull bones.

Inspection for neck stiffness

More than 80% of cases of meningitis occur in children. Neck stiffness is an important sign but is unreliable in infants and young children. It may be absent in children with severe meningitis but present in a child with tonsillitis.

15

A Female breast changes

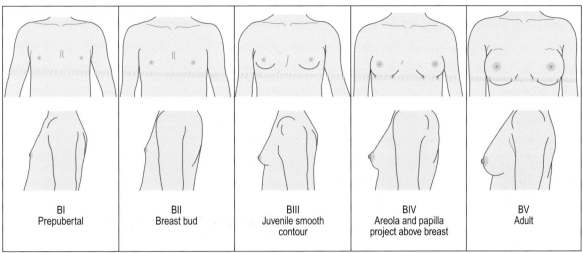

| BI
Prepubertal | BII
Breast bud | BIII
Juvenile smooth
contour | BIV
Areola and papilla
project above breast | BV
Adult |

B Pubic hair changes — female and male

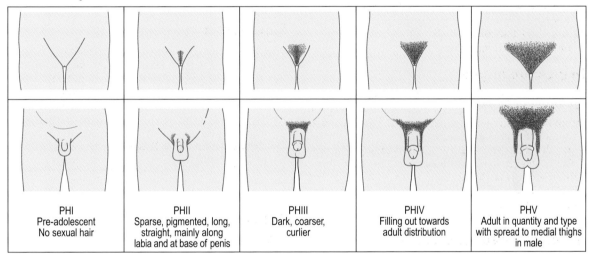

| PHI
Pre-adolescent
No sexual hair | PHII
Sparse, pigmented, long,
straight, mainly along
labia and at base of penis | PHIII
Dark, coarser,
curlier | PHIV
Filling out towards
adult distribution | PHV
Adult in quantity and type
with spread to medial thighs
in male |

C Male genital stages

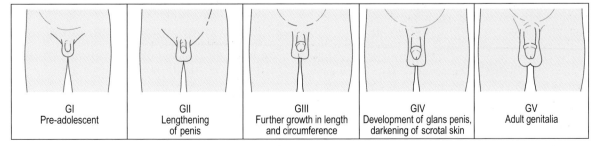

| GI
Pre-adolescent | GII
Lengthening
of penis | GIII
Further growth in length
and circumference | GIV
Development of glans penis,
darkening of scrotal skin | GV
Adult genitalia |

Fig. 15.27 Stages of puberty in males and females. Pubertal changes are shown according to the Tanner stages of puberty.

Female

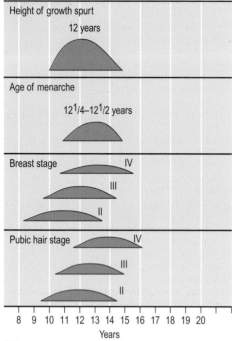

Male

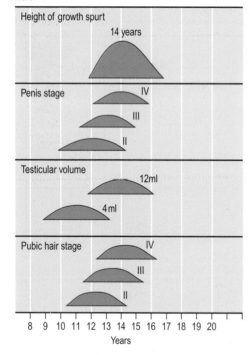

Fig. 15.28 Timing of puberty in males and females.

▪▶ Look for passive resistance. Does the child lie rigid or can he turn his head from side to side?

▪▶ Ask the child to flex the chin on to the chest. In severe meningeal irritation, he may lie with the head extended.

OSCEs 15.22 Examine this patient with enuresis at 10 years of age

1. Record height and weight on a growth chart.
2. Measure blood pressure (hypertension from renal scarring associated with chronic reflux).
3. Examine the abdomen — an indentable mass (faeces) in the left iliac fossa suggests constipation exacerbating enuresis.
4. Ballot the loins to detect enlarged kidneys.
5. Palpate the bladder and percuss to delineate a full bladder.
6. Examine the lower spine for a dimple or tuft of hair (spina bifida occulta).
7. Examine the lower limbs for muscle tone and tendon reflexes.
8. Test the urine for haematuria and proteinuria, and for diabetes.
9. Obtain a mid-stream specimen of urine (MSSU) to exclude infection.

10% of normal 5-year-olds and 5% of normal 10-year-olds wet the bed.

15.23 'The limping child': age-related conditions that cause a limp

1–3 years

- Developmental dysplasia of the hip
- Neuromuscular disease, e.g. muscular dystrophy
- Juvenile idiopathic arthritis
- Limb length discrepancy
- Child abuse
- Septic arthritis

4–10 years

- Transient synovitis — 'the irritable hip'
- Perthes' condition
- Limb length discrepancy
- Juvenile idiopathic arthritis
- Septic arthritis
- Tumour

>10 years

- Slipped upper femoral epiphysis
- Osgood–Schlatter disease
- 'Shin splints'
- Tarsal coalition
- Heel pain
- Köhler's disease

Palpation for neck stiffness

▪▶ Gently flex the child's neck by supporting the occiput with both your hands behind his head (Fig. 11.3, p. 275).

▪▶ Feel for resistance and watch the child's facial expression.

▪▶ Ask older children to kiss their knees. A child with meningism will not be able to do this without discomfort.

▪▶ Head jolt may be a more sensitive test of meningeal irritation. Standing to the right of the child and facing the child's head, place your hands on either side of the head. Turn it from side to side fairly rapidly and note any resistance.

Central nervous system

Inspection of the cranial nerves

▪▶ Watch the child making a face, smiling, crying, chewing or drinking.

▪▶ Ask the child to open his mouth and stick out the tongue.

▪▶ Does the child fix and follow with the eyes?

Does he respond to a loud sudden noise?
Can he stand on one foot and hop?

Checking the special senses

Ask the parents or carers specifically if they think the child hears and sees normally. If not, clarify exactly what they think is wrong.

Vision

- Watch to see if the child fixes and follows. Make sure there is no limitation of eye movements at the extremes of gaze. Check for nystagmus. Children follow faces, not torchlights.
- Look for a squint (Fig. 12.26, p. 322). Observe whether the light reflection is in the same position on the cornea in both eyes. By 6 weeks, both eyes should move together.
- Check the red reflex, using your ophthalmoscope (p. 325). This is absent in cataract, corneal clouding and retinal tumour.
- Test vision and manipulation together by seeing whether a child can pick up small objects such as raisins. Developmental paediatricians often use very small, coloured, edible cake decorations.
- Fundoscopy takes practice and patience in children and testing visual acuity in young children is a specialist skill.

Hearing

In the UK, universal hearing screening has been introduced in the neonatal period because detecting deafness is clinically difficult. If screening is not in place, hearing should be checked at 8 months using distraction testing. This test requires properly trained staff. Ask the parents about the child's hearing behaviour and refer if there are any concerns.

Peripheral nervous system

Inspection for motor function

- Look for abnormal postures, such as scissoring of the legs, which indicate increased tone (Fig. 15.29).
- Test for primitive reflexes. In infants, primitive reflexes, e.g. sucking and palmar grasping, are present (p. 410). They are lost before new, more advanced skills are acquired. Their persistence suggests underlying neurological abnormality.
- Watch for movements against gravity and observe sitting, crawling and walking.

Palpation for motor function

- Pick infants up and feel their tone. If they are excessively floppy, they may slip through your fingers; increased tone makes them feel stiff so they seem to move as if in one piece. Pull them to sit and look for evidence of head lag. In young children use the 180° test (Box 15.24) to assess their tone.
- Test the tendon reflexes as in an adult. Increased reflexes are easier to assess than decreased ones. If the reflexes are pathologically increased or decreased, look for evidence that the underlying tone is altered. An upgoing plantar response provides additional evidence of upper motor neurone dysfunction (Fig. 11.24, p. 291).

Sensation

A useful screening test in young children is to check whether they withdraw from tickling.

OSCEs 15.24 Examine this patient with inability to walk at 18 months

1. Movement and posture:
   Perform the 180° test: pull the supine baby by the hands to a sitting position and look for head lag.
   Does the child sit unsupported?
   Put your hands under the baby's axillae and raise him up, noting tone.
   Bring the baby's feet down to touch the table and see if the child supports his weight.
   Turn the baby quickly face down and note whether the child supports his head.
   Watch for the 'parachute reflex', whereby the baby suddenly extends the arms as if for protection as you lie him down (usually only 6–9 months).
   Does the baby push his chest up off the floor by extending the arms?
   Does he roll from front to back and from back to front?
   Note any asymmetry of movement.
2. Vision and manipulation:
   Can the baby build a tower of two blocks?
3. Hearing and speech:
   Does the baby say three words, other than mama and dada?
   Does he understand simple commands?
4. Social behaviour:
   Does the baby drink from a cup?
   Can the child feed himself with a spoon?

If all these tests are normal, the most common cause is 'bottom-shuffling' — an effective alternative to crawling occurring in 10% of children, which may delay walking until the age of 2 years. (Confirm by asking the parent how the baby moves around.)

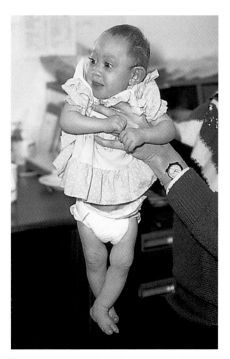

Fig. 15.29 Scissoring of the legs. A child with spastic quadriplegia showing scissoring from excessive adduction of the hips, pronated forearms and 'fisted' hands.

Coordination

Ask younger children who can stand and walk to stand on one leg or hop.

PUTTING IT ALL TOGETHER

Having looked, listened and examined, you should have a differential diagnosis. In children, this is often short. From this, plan investigation and treatment and negotiate these with the parents and child. By the end of the consultation, everyone should agree on the expected outcome and plan. In some conditions, the management plan is summarized in writing as an action plan.

Check to ensure that parents understand your discussions, and know what to look for and how to respond if things do not develop as expected. Discuss signs that suggest deterioration, along with a plan of how to respond and who to contact. This is 'safety-netting'.

Information-sharing and communication

Parents often feel that they receive insufficient information about their children's health. They want explanations and detailed advice to help them manage their sick child confidently. Address their fears, ideas

and expectations. Health professionals should educate parents and provide the information they want and need. Having parent-held records, sending copies of clinic letters to parents and involving them in case meetings all help to promote partnership between parents and clinicians (Box 15.25).

15.25 Key points: children

- Listen carefully to parents' concerns about their child. If they think there is a problem, you must take this seriously. They will usually be giving you the diagnosis.
- Observation is the key to paediatric examination; watch children closely from the first moment you see them.
- Children often do not cooperate sufficiently to allow a full formal examination. Examine what you can, when you can. Return another time if necessary.
- Always measure and chart children's growth and check on their development.
- Leave uncomfortable procedures until the end of the consultation.
- You need experience to appreciate the range of normality in children. Check with senior colleagues if you are in doubt.
- Parents want explanations and detailed advice. Address their fears, expectations and ideas. By the end of the consultation, everyone should agree on the expected outcome and plan.

Timothy Walsh

Assessment for sedation and anaesthesia

16

EXAMINATION PRIOR TO SEDATION OR ANAESTHESIA

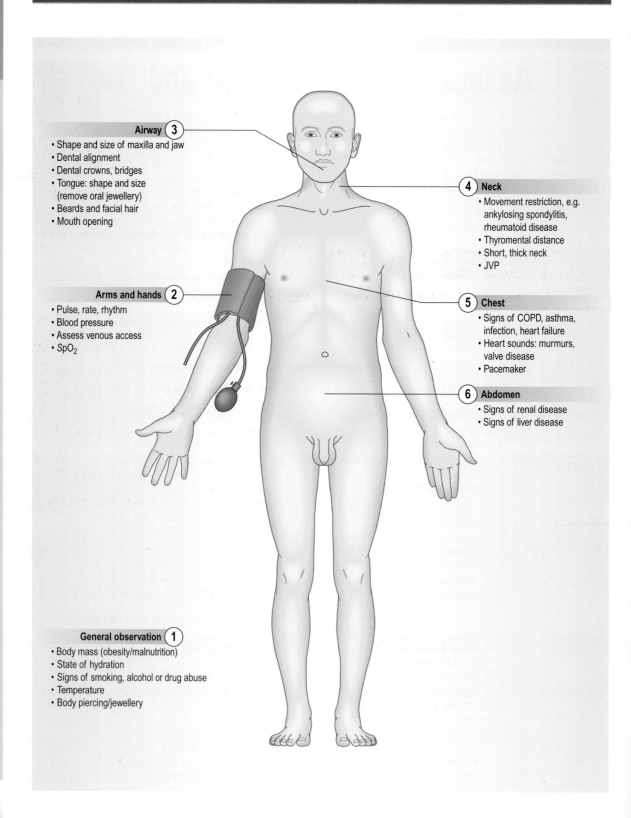

Airway (3)
- Shape and size of maxilla and jaw
- Dental alignment
- Dental crowns, bridges
- Tongue: shape and size (remove oral jewellery)
- Beards and facial hair
- Mouth opening

(4) Neck
- Movement restriction, e.g. ankylosing spondylitis, rheumatoid disease
- Thyromental distance
- Short, thick neck
- JVP

Arms and hands (2)
- Pulse, rate, rhythm
- Blood pressure
- Assess venous access
- SpO_2

(5) Chest
- Signs of COPD, asthma, infection, heart failure
- Heart sounds: murmurs, valve disease
- Pacemaker

(6) Abdomen
- Signs of renal disease
- Signs of liver disease

General observation (1)
- Body mass (obesity/malnutrition)
- State of hydration
- Signs of smoking, alcohol or drug abuse
- Temperature
- Body piercing/jewellery

Patients frequently require investigative or therapeutic procedures to be performed under sedation or anaesthesia. The clinical examination of these patients is necessary to:

- establish a rapport with the patient
- obtain relevant information about past medical, family and social history
- undertake a systematic enquiry relevant to anaesthesia
- examine relevant systems for abnormalities that could increase anaesthetic risk
- inform the patient about anaesthetic options, e.g. local versus general anaesthetic techniques, discussing patient preferences
- provide reassurance, information and advice that could decrease risk
- document consent.

THE HISTORY

Relevant elements of the systematic enquiry

A detailed cardiorespiratory system history is important to assess the status of known disease and to detect undiagnosed conditions. Ask specifically about exercise tolerance and functional limitations. Pay particular attention to symptoms suggesting recent upper or lower respiratory tract infection. These increase the risk of perioperative complications and may mean that surgery has to be delayed.

Ask about symptoms suggesting reflux (heartburn, water brash), which may need treatment with acid suppression and use of airway protection techniques to prevent aspiration.

Establish when the patient last ate or drank. In emergency cases relate this time to the onset of symptoms because pain, trauma, opioid administration and some metabolic conditions, such as diabetes mellitus and renal failure, delay gastric emptying.

During the neurological and musculoskeletal enquiry ask about any symptoms that may be relevant to regional anaesthetic techniques: for example, back problems when epidural anaesthesia is planned or pre-existing sensory abnormalities prior to peripheral nerve blockade.

Past medical history

Document previous serious illnesses and chronic conditions (Box 16.1). Cardiovascular and respiratory conditions, e.g. congenital, rheumatic or ischaemic heart

16.1 Common features of the medical history particularly relevant to anaesthesia assessment

Condition in past history	Key features relevant to anaesthesia	Reason
Angina	What is the frequency? What is the response to treatment?	Poorly controlled angina increases risk of perioperative cardiovascular complications
Myocardial infarction (MI)	How many MIs has the patient suffered? How long ago? Treatment required?	Likely to indicate degree of cardiac impairment. Risk of perioperative cardiac events greatly increased if within past 3–6 months. Effective treatment with surgery or coronary stenting reduces risk
Hypertension	How well is it controlled?	Poor control increases risk of cardiovascular and cerebrovascular events perioperatively
Heart failure/valve disease	How severe are the symptoms (exercise tolerance, breathlessness, oedema)?	Poorly controlled heart failure increases perioperative risk. Valve disease may need antibiotic prophylaxis
Cardiac arrhythmias	Is arrhythmia persistent or intermittent? How is it treated?	Anticoagulation requires management. Pacemakers may need checking and/or reprogramming and special precautions. Some anaesthetic drugs may exacerbate arrhythmias
COPD and asthma	How severe are the symptoms (exercise tolerance, breathlessness, steroid requirement, frequency of hospital admissions, lung function)?	Severe disease increases perioperative risk and influences choice of anaesthetic technique
Renal failure	Is it dialysis-dependent? What volume of urine is still passed? Are there any recent complications, e.g. hyperkalaemia, fluid overload?	Influences fluid management, choice of technique and drugs
Diabetes mellitus	Has glycaemic control been achieved? Are there any complications? If so, how severe?	Requires perioperative glycaemic control. Complications increase anaesthetic risk, e.g. cardiac disease, neuropathy, delayed gastric emptying

16

disease, pacemakers, chronic obstructive pulmonary disease (COPD) and asthma, are particularly important, but many conditions are significant and a large number of conditions are potentially relevant to anaesthesia (Box 16.2).

Previous anaesthetic history

Ask about previous anaesthetics. Document any complications or distressing side-effects. Examine available anaesthetic charts from previous procedures. Record any problems, particularly difficult intubation/airway control. If major complications have previously been noted, or there is a family history of anaesthetic reactions, consider rare genetically inherited abnormalities. The two most important are:

- Pseudocholinesterase deficiency ('scoline apnoea'): prolonged apnoea following the administration of suxamethonium chloride and some other agents. The patient may have required mechanical ventilation unexpectedly after previous surgery
- Malignant hyperpyrexia: a life-threatening condition caused by a genetic abnormality of muscle metabolism when exposed to certain anaesthetic agents. Patients with the condition or those with a family history require specialist investigation.

Drug history and allergies

Record all current drugs, including over-the-counter medications. It may be necessary to stop some drugs or modify their doses prior to surgery (Box 16.3). Patients taking oral steroid therapy may have impaired stress response and require replacement therapy perioperatively.

Document all allergies, including the nature of the reaction; some may be side-effects, such as nausea, rather than true allergy. Record any reactions to skin preparation agents, e.g. iodine, or to specific skin dressings. Food allergies, e.g. to eggs, may result in sensitivity to some anaesthetic drugs. Latex allergy requires special precautions in the operating theatre.

Take a smoking and alcohol history (Box 16.4).

16.3 Some drugs that may need to be stopped or have their dose adjusted before surgery

Drug	Reason
Aspirin Clopidogrel Warfarin	Increase bleeding risk
ACE inhibitors and other antihypertensives	Inadequate dose increases risk Some drugs may require omission in the perioperative period to decrease risk of hypotension
Diabetic treatment (especially insulin and metformin)	Glycaemic control requires specific perioperative management

16.4 Importance of the smoking and alcohol history

History	Relevance
Smoking	↑ risk of COPD ↑ risk of intra-operative bronchospasm ↑ risk of chest infection ↓ oxygen-carrying capacity of blood (COHb)
Alcohol	Risk of alcohol-related chronic disease (especially liver) ↓ sensitivity to many anaesthetic drugs Risk of alcohol withdrawal in perioperative period

16.2 Some conditions with special relevance to anaesthesia

Condition	Considerations
Rheumatoid arthritis	Neck may be unstable and mouth opening impaired; co-morbidity, e.g. respiratory and renal impairment; poor vascular access; complex drug therapy; need for careful positioning under anaesthesia
Epilepsy	Drug treatment can interact with anaesthetics; surgical stress and some anaesthetics can increase risk of seizures
Scoliosis and spinal abnormalities	Can decrease respiratory reserve; tracheal intubation can be difficult; regional anaesthesia difficult
Myasthenia gravis and other chronic neuromuscular disorders	Risk of respiratory failure; sensitivity to anaesthetic drugs; surgical and anaesthetic stress can cause acute exacerbations, e.g. multiple sclerosis
Sickle cell disease	Stress of surgery, hypoxia, hypothermia or dehydration can precipitate sickle cell crisis
Porphyria	Some anaesthetic agents e.g. barbiturates, etomidate may trigger a porphyric attack; acute porphyria may mimic a 'surgical' acute abdomen

Relevance

Inspect the patient's face, head and neck from the front and side

Note the shape of the maxilla and jaw, and alignment of teeth

Facial hair — makes mask-face seal more difficult. Difficult intubation is associated with:
- Protruding maxilla (overbite) and/or receding chin
- A short thick neck
- Obesity
- A short distance (<6.5 cm) between the prominence of thyroid cartilage and tip of the chin during head extension (thyromental distance)

Examine the range of neck movement

Assess the patient's ability to extend their head on their neck (atlanto-occipital joint function) and flex their cervical spine on the body

Airway control is more difficult in: patients who cannot achieve the "sniffing the morning air" position — with head extended and neck flexed forward on the body

Ask the patient to open their mouth fully

Document the completeness and state of the teeth, especially the position of loose teeth and those at higher risk of damage (crowns, bridges)

Assess size of mouth and degree of mouth opening possible (temporomandibular joint function)

Note size of tongue and presence of tongue or oral jewellery

Poor dentition increases risk of dental damage

More difficult to obtain a seal between mask and face in endentulous patients

Reduced mouth opening makes airway access difficult

Large tongue associated with more difficult airway. Oral jewellery should be removed

Ask patient to stick out their tongue with mouth fully open and tongue pointing at chin

Examine the view of the mouth and throat

Assess airway using Mallampati risk classification. Classes III and IV are associated with increased likelihood of difficult intubation

16

Class I   Class II   Class III   Class IV

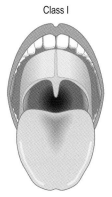 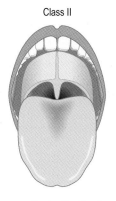 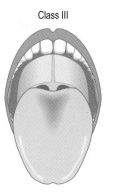 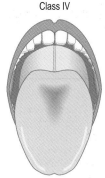

Fig. 16.1 Assessing the airway prior to anaesthesia. Classification when performing the modified Mallampati test: Class I, pharyngeal pillars, soft palate and uvula visible; Class II, only soft palate and uvula visible; Class III, only soft palate visible; Class IV, soft palate not visible.

Family and social history

Ask whether any family members have suffered problems related to anaesthesia. This may reveal important rare familial conditions or bad experiences such as nausea or pain. Patients often worry that they will experience similar problems and benefit from explanation and reassurance.

THE PHYSICAL EXAMINATION
General examination

Weigh the patient to help guide drug dosage. Calculation of body mass index (p. 59) is useful for stratifying risk. Both obesity and malnutrition significantly increase anaesthetic risk. Assess the patient's arm veins (for venous access) and other anatomy relevant to the anaesthetic technique planned, such as radial pulses (arterial catheter insertion) or thoracic/lumbar spine flexion (epidural catheter placement). Check for pyrexia, which could indicate an intercurrent infection. Note any body-piercing jewellery, which may need removal or protection to prevent it being caught, causing pressure damage or infection.

The airway

Look for and ask about loose or false teeth, dental caps and crowns, and tongue or oral jewellery. Assess potential difficulties in airway control with a face mask, laryngeal mask or tracheal intubation (Fig. 16.1).

Cardiorespiratory and other systems

Examine specifically for arrhythmias, heart murmurs and signs of heart failure. Auscultate the chest for crackles or wheezes that could indicate poorly controlled chronic disease or acute infection. Examine all systems to document known abnormalities and exclude occult disease.

SUMMARIZING RISK

Use the American Society of Anesthesiologists' (ASA) grading system to summarize the anaesthetic and peri-operative complication risk rates (Boxes 16.5 and 16.6).

PREOPERATIVE INVESTIGATIONS

Appropriate preoperative investigations depend on the type of surgery, the patient's condition and local policies. Some general guidelines are shown in Box 16.7.

16.5 The ASA risk-grading system

ASA class	Description of patient
I	Normally healthy individual
II	Patient with mild systemic disease
III	A patient with severe systemic disease that is not incapacitating
IV	A patient with incapacitating systemic disease that is a constant threat to life
V	A moribund patient who is not expected to survive 24 hours with or without an operation
E	Added as a suffix for an emergency operation (which carries greater risk)

16.6 Factors associated with significantly increased risk during anaesthesia

Type of surgery

- Emergency procedures
- Major thoracic, abdominal or cardiovascular surgery
- Perforated bowel
- Acute pancreatitis
- Palliative surgery

Patient factors

- Older age (>70 years)
- Cardiac:
    Myocardial infarction within last 6 months
    Heart failure (especially if poorly controlled)
    Aortic stenosis
- Respiratory:
    Productive cough
    Breathlessness at rest or minimal exertion
    Smoker
- Gastrointestinal:
    Jaundice
    Chronic liver disease
    Malnutrition (low weight and/or low albumin)
- Renal:
    Acute or chronic renal failure
- Haematological:
    Ongoing haemorrhage
    Anaemia (<100 g/l)
    Polycythaemia
- Neurological:
    Confusion
- Metabolic:
    Poorly controlled diabetes mellitus
    Oral steroid therapy

CONSENT AND ADVICE TO PATIENTS

Consent for anaesthesia is often linked to surgical consent. Consent is only valid if the patient:

- has capacity to give consent

16.7 Preoperative investigations

Investigation	Indication
Full blood count	Prior to major surgery Patients known to have abnormalities, e.g. anaemia or thrombocytopenia Suspected infection
Urea and electrolytes	Prior to major surgery Pre-existing disease affecting biochemistry, e.g. renal failure or liver disease Drugs that could affect electrolytes, e.g. diuretics
Coagulation	Known states that can alter coagulation, e.g. warfarin therapy, liver disease Prior to major surgery that may affect coagulation, e.g. cardiac surgery, hepatobiliary surgery
Blood cross-matching	Hospitals should have a surgical blood ordering schedule to guide requests
12-lead electrocardiograph	Known or suspected heart disease Prior to major surgery (to provide a baseline)
Chest X-ray	Selected patients with known respiratory disease
Respiratory function tests (FEV and FVC)	Prior to major thoracic surgery Selected patients with chronic respiratory disease
Echocardiography	Selected patients with heart disease (especially heart murmurs)

(FEV = forced expiratory volume; FVC = forced vital capacity.)

- has been provided with sufficient information to make a balanced decision
- can make a voluntary decision.

This requires careful explanation of procedures and their risks. More frequent or serious side-effects or complications should be discussed: for example, in relation to cannula insertion or epidural anaesthesia.

Advise smokers to stop smoking: if not permanently, then for at least 2–3 days before surgery. Provide clear advice about which medications should be stopped or continued to the day of surgery, particularly for cardiac, antihypertensive and diabetic treatments. This is particularly important for patients who will attend on the day of surgery.

Fasting

Ensure the patient knows how long to fast, referring to local policies. Most centres fast patients for solids for 4–6 hours before elective surgery, but allow clear fluids up to 2 hours before surgery.

16.8 Key points: assessment for sedation and anaesthesia

- All patients require a full history and examination before anaesthesia or sedation.
- Concentrate on the functional status of chronic diseases, especially of the cardiorespiratory systems.
- Document previous problems during anaesthesia or complications experienced by family members.
- Use the systematic enquiry and examination to elicit factors that could increase risk, e.g. gastric reflux, drug therapy, changes in chronic symptoms and signs, or new respiratory symptoms.
- Assess the airway and document anticipated problems.
- Record an overall assessment of risk using the ASA classification and additional specific features relevant to the individual patient.
- Explain clearly about the techniques planned and relevant side-effects, and document the patient's consent.
- Give clear instructions about usual medications prior to surgery.
- Ensure appropriate premedication and prophylaxis are prescribed.

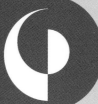

The critically ill patient

17

EXAMINATION OF THE CRITICALLY ILL PATIENT

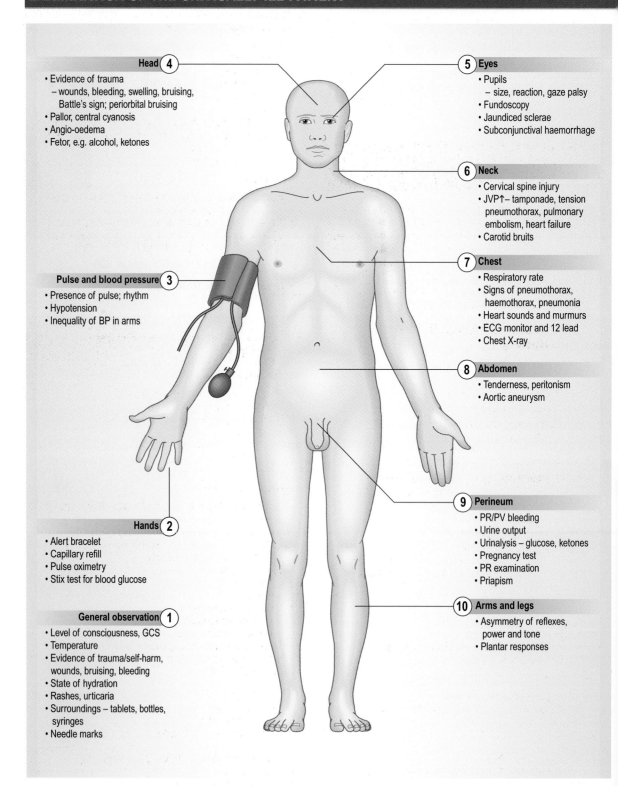

Head (4)
- Evidence of trauma
  – wounds, bleeding, swelling, bruising, Battle's sign; periorbital bruising
- Pallor, central cyanosis
- Angio-oedema
- Fetor, e.g. alcohol, ketones

(5) **Eyes**
- Pupils
  – size, reaction, gaze palsy
- Fundoscopy
- Jaundiced sclerae
- Subconjunctival haemorrhage

(6) **Neck**
- Cervical spine injury
- JVP↑– tamponade, tension pneumothorax, pulmonary embolism, heart failure
- Carotid bruits

Pulse and blood pressure (3)
- Presence of pulse; rhythm
- Hypotension
- Inequality of BP in arms

(7) **Chest**
- Respiratory rate
- Signs of pneumothorax, haemothorax, pneumonia
- Heart sounds and murmurs
- ECG monitor and 12 lead
- Chest X-ray

(8) **Abdomen**
- Tenderness, peritonism
- Aortic aneurysm

(9) **Perineum**
- PR/PV bleeding
- Urine output
- Urinalysis – glucose, ketones
- Pregnancy test
- PR examination
- Priapism

Hands (2)
- Alert bracelet
- Capillary refill
- Pulse oximetry
- Stix test for blood glucose

(10) **Arms and legs**
- Asymmetry of reflexes, power and tone
- Plantar responses

General observation (1)
- Level of consciousness, GCS
- Temperature
- Evidence of trauma/self-harm, wounds, bruising, bleeding
- State of hydration
- Rashes, urticaria
- Surroundings – tablets, bottles, syringes
- Needle marks

The systematic approach to examination is inappropriate for critically ill patients, as immediate intervention may be needed to save life, e.g. in cardiac arrest or tension pneumothorax, or to halt or stabilize processes which, untreated, would lead to death, e.g. hypovolaemic shock. Therefore, in the critically ill, examination and interventions are often performed simultaneously. This is a temporary phase, which must always be followed by a full history and clinical examination when the patient is 'stable'.

IDENTIFYING THE CRITICALLY ILL PATIENT

Critical illness, if unrecognized or untreated within the next few minutes or hours, may lead to death or serious disability. The disease process may not necessarily determine whether a patient is critically ill or not. The time course of the disease process is more relevant, and initially you may not be able to make a definitive diagnosis. Your aim is to stabilize the patient's condition to allow full diagnosis, specialist investigations and definitive therapy.

The clinical manifestations of critical illness

Clinical features of the critically ill patient are shown in Box 17.1.

Critical illness can present as:
- altered conscious state (Box 17.2)
- acute respiratory compromise (Box 17.3)
- acute cardiovascular compromise (Box 17.4).

17.1 Clinical features of the critically ill patient

Airway and breathing

- Respiratory arrest
- Obstructed or compromised airway
- Respiratory rate <8 or >35/min
- Respiratory distress: stridor, inability to speak in complete sentences, use of accessory muscles, intercostal indrawing

Circulation

- Cardiac arrest
- Pulse rate <40 or >140/min
- Systolic BP <100 mmHg
- Features of shock: altered conscious level, peripheral perfusion, urine output <0.5 ml/kg/h

Neurological

- Failure to obey commands
- Glasgow Coma Scale (GCS) <9, or fall of 2 points in GCS
- Frequent or prolonged seizures

Other

- Temperature
- Any patient you are seriously concerned about, even if they do not fulfill any of the above criteria

17.2 Common causes of altered conscious state

Non-CNS causes

- Hypoxia
- Hypovolaemia
- Hypoglycaemia
- Drugs and poisons, e.g. opioids, alcohol, carbon monoxide, benzodiazepines, tricyclic antidepressants
- Metabolic
  Type II respiratory failure ($\uparrow PaCO_2$), hepatic or renal failure
  Thyrotoxicosis/myxoedema/Addisonian crisis, non-ketotic hyperosmolar states
- Hypothermia or hyperthermia

CNS causes

- Intracranial haemorrhage, e.g. subarachnoid haemorrhage
- Ischaemia: thrombosis, embolism
- Trauma: concussion, white matter shearing (diffuse axonal injury), haemorrhage (extradural, subdural and/or intracerebral)
- Infections: meningitis, encephalitis, cerebral malaria
- Seizures
- Primary or secondary tumour
- Hypertensive encephalopathy

17.3 Common causes of acute respiratory compromise

Airway obstruction

- Altered conscious state (see Box 17.2)
- Upper airway/maxillofacial injury
- Tracheolaryngeal injury
- Foreign body
- Infections e.g. epiglottitis, quinsy
- Angio-oedema
- Tumours

Pulmonary conditions

- Pneumothorax (especially if tension is present or bilateral)
- Chest injury
  Blunt: rib fractures, flail segment, lung contusion
  Penetrating: pneumothorax, open chest wound, major vessel injury with haemothorax
- Severe acute asthma
- Pulmonary embolism
- Pneumonia
- Acute pulmonary oedema
  Cardiogenic: acute left heart failure
  Non-cardiogenic: smoke, toxic fume inhalation
- Acute respiratory distress syndrome (ARDS)
- Exacerbation of chronic obstructive pulmonary disease (COPD)
- Massive pleural effusion

Non-pulmonary conditions

- Metabolic acidosis
  Diabetic ketoacidosis
    Severe renal or hepatic failure
    Lactic acidosis
    Overdose: methanol, ethylene glycol, (late) salicylate
- Severe anaemia
- Psychogenic hyperventilation

17.4 Common causes of acute cardiovascular compromise

Cardiac

- Cardiac arrest
- Acute myocardial infarction or ischaemia
- Acute valve dysfunction, e.g. endocarditis, mechanical valve failure or obstruction
- Arrhythmia
- Pericardial tamponade
- Cardiomyopathy: viral, alcohol-related, post-partum

Vascular

- Dissection, or rupture, of abdominal or thoracic aortic aneurysm
- Mesenteric infarction

Massive pulmonary embolus

Blood loss

- Gastrointestinal
  Upper: varices, peptic ulcer, tumour, Mallory–Weiss tear, non-steroidal anti-inflammatory drugs (NSAIDs)
  Lower: diverticular disease, angiodysplasia, ischaemic bowel, Meckel's diverticulum, tumour
- Trauma
- Overt: wounds especially to scalp, face; long bone or pelvic fractures
- Concealed: chest — haemothorax; abdomen — splenic and/or hepatic injury, retroperitoneal
- Obstetric/gynaecological: placenta praevia, miscarriage, ectopic pregnancy, trauma, tumour
- Anticoagulant use or bleeding diathesis

Miscellaneous

- Anaphylaxis
- Hypothermia
- Hyperthermia
- Electric shock/lightning injury
- Envenomation (bites or stings from snakes, insects, jellyfish)

17.5 Key preliminary data

A	Allergies
M	Medication
P	Past medical history
L	Last meal
E	Events leading up to presentation and environment

THE ABCDE APPROACH

The ABCDE approach has four interlinked phases:

1. preparation before you see the patient (where possible)
2. primary survey
3. secondary survey
4. definitive care intervention.

You cannot manage a critically ill patient alone. Seek senior, experienced help immediately. If you have to work alone, only proceed to the next item once the preceding one has been adequately completed. A team can deal with the separate elements simultaneously, but the leader must ensure that all components are covered and, if a patient's condition deteriorates, must immediately review the ABCDE sequence.

Preparation

You may be unable to take a history from patients because of their condition. Use all possible sources of information for your preliminary data (Box 17.5). Include previous primary care or hospital records, relatives, friends, bystanders and emergency or ambulance personnel. Look for diabetic/steroid/anticoagulant cards and medications, and Alert bracelets and necklaces (Fig. 3.2, p. 48). If possible, contact the patient's GP — often a key source of current and background information.

Primary survey

The primary survey, investigations and interventions should take 5–10 minutes, unless a life-saving intervention such as tracheal intubation needs to be undertaken.

A: Airway

Approach patients so that they can see you, if they are conscious and able to open their eyes. This is particularly important for those who are supine and immobile because of splintage, pain or paralysis. Speak slowly and clearly. If the patient talks to you normally, the airway is clear and there is circulation of blood to the brain; if speech is lucid, cerebral function is adequate. Give the patient a high inspired concentration of oxygen by mask, and move on to B (Breathing).

In cardiac arrest, all three features are present. Some states present with a single manifestation, but if untreated, the remaining two may develop; e.g. a patient with a pneumothorax developing tension initially has respiratory symptoms. As increasing tension occurs, cardiovascular compromise develops and leads to loss of consciousness and ultimately death.

What do you do?

Initially, you may not be aware of the preceding events or time frame concerned. Concentrating on the system which appears most likely to have caused the problem may be misleading, wastes time and further compromises the patient. An ABCDE approach is simple and safe. This allows you to address and correct conditions using a logical framework.

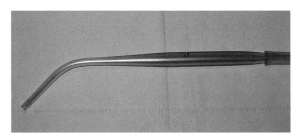

Fig. 17.1 Yankauer suction catheter.

17.6 Airway noises

No noise (the 'silent airway')

- Implies complete airway obstruction and/or absence of, or minimal, respiratory effort

Snoring

- Caused by partial upper airway obstruction from soft tissues of the mouth and oropharynx

Gurgling

- Caused by fluids (secretions, blood or vomit) in the oropharynx

Hoarseness

- Caused by partial laryngeal obstruction associated with oedema

Wheeze

- A 'musical' noise, best heard on auscultation
- When loudest in expiration, relates to obstruction in the small bronchi and bronchioles, most often in asthma and COPD

Stridor

- A harsh noise, usually loudest in inspiration, caused by partial obstruction around the larynx or main bronchi
- In febrile patients, consider epiglottitis or retropharyngeal abscess
- Otherwise, foreign bodies, laryngeal trauma, burns or tumours are possible

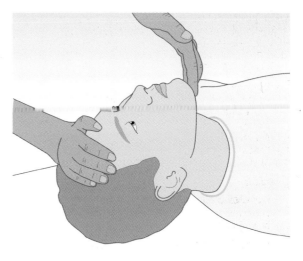

Fig. 17.2 Opening the airway by tilting the head and lifting the chin.

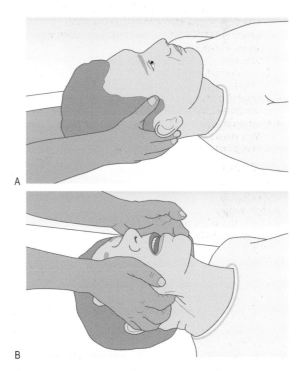

A

B

Fig. 17.3 Manœuvres in patients with suspected neck injury.
(A) Control the head and neck manually. **(B)** Open the airway using the jaw-thrust technique.

If there is no response, usually because the patient has altered consciousness, perform a more detailed assessment of the airway. Look, listen and feel. Open the mouth and remove secretions, blood, vomit or foreign material by gentle suction with a Yankauer catheter (Fig. 17.1) under direct vision. Leave well-fitting dentures or dental plates in place to maintain the normal airway anatomy. If they are loose or poorly fitting, remove them. Listen for upper airway noises (Box 17.6). Gurgling, snoring or stridor suggests partial airway obstruction. Absence of any breath sounds indicates either complete airway obstruction and/or absence of breathing.

Open the airway by tilting the patient's head and lifting the chin (Fig. 17.2). If you suspect neck injury, control the head and neck by manual in-line control and open the airway using the jaw-lift technique (Fig. 17.3). Do not move the neck. Appropriately sized airway adjuncts, such as nasopharyngeal or oropharyngeal (Guedel) airways, can maintain the airway in patients with altered consciousness (Fig. 17.4). Do not use a nasopharyngeal airway if you suspect a skull-base fracture, if epistaxis, nasal trauma or deformity is present, or if the patient is taking anticoagulants. Tracheal intubation may be needed

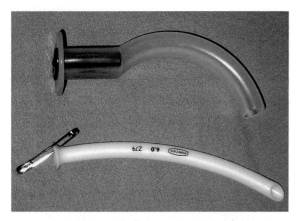

Fig. 17.4 **Airway adjuncts.** Guedel airway (top); nasopharyngeal airway (bottom).

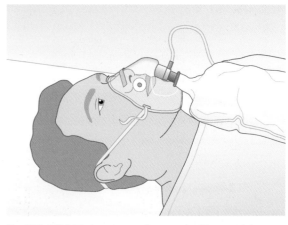

Fig. 17.5 Administering oxygen using a mask with reservoir bag.

> **i** **17.7 Principal indications for emergency advanced airway and ventilation techniques**
>
> - Apnoea
> - Airway obstruction
>   Inability to maintain airway with simple manœuvres/adjuncts
>   Facial trauma, uncontrolled vomiting/bleeding
>   GCS <9
>   Potential for subsequent clinical deterioration, e.g. facial/airway burns
> - Oxygenation and ventilation
>   Raised intracranial pressure
>   Potential environmental risk, e.g. ambulance transfer, CT/MR scan

if the patient cannot maintain a patent airway. This should only be performed by an experienced clinician (Box 17.7).

B: Breathing

Hypoxia hastens and causes death. Use an oxygen mask with reservoir bag and adjust the oxygen flow rate to maintain an SpO_2 of 94–98% (Fig. 17.5). The only exception to this initial treatment is where you know the patient has COPD with CO_2 retention (type II respiratory failure). These patients lose the hypoxic stimulus to breathe if given high concentrations of oxygen.

Recognize and treat open pneumothorax or a pneumothorax under tension. Expose the chest and abdomen, and look for wounds (usually gunshot or stab) producing an open defect in the chest wall (Fig. 17.6). Examine the back and axillae.

An open chest wound equalizes pressure between the pleural space and atmosphere, and the affected lung is unable to expand or contract normally with respiration. During inspiration and expiration, you may hear air movement and see a spray of blood at the wound. Cover the wound with a sterile occlusive dressing secured on

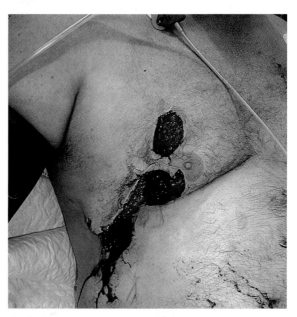

Fig. 17.6 Wound producing an open defect in the chest wall.

three sides. This allows air to escape from the pleural space during expiration and impedes air entry during inspiration. A formal tube thoracostomy with underwater seal drainage is then needed.

Tension pneumothorax occurs when lung injury produces a one-way valve effect (Fig. 17.7). On inspiration air escapes from the lung and accumulates in the pleural space. As the pleural pressure increases, the ipsilateral lung progressively collapses and the increased intrathoracic pressure reduces venous return to the heart, eventually causing cardiac arrest.

Suspect tension pneumothorax in any patient who rapidly develops severe respiratory and cardiovascular distress. It occurs most commonly in chest injury, during

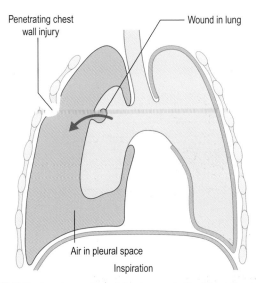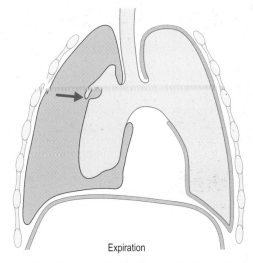

Penetrating chest wall injury — Wound in lung

Air in pleural space

Inspiration

Expiration

Fig. 17.7 Tension pneumothorax following penetrating injury. Air enters the pleural cavity via the punctured lung during inspiration. The chest wall and lung defects act as one-way valves. Air cannot escape from the pleural cavity during expiration. The right intrapleural pressure increases, collapsing the right lung, impeding venous return to the heart and occasionally shifting mediastinal structures to the contralateral side.

positive-pressure ventilation, or in those with underlying lung disease (especially when ventilated). The diagnosis is clinical. The patient appears acutely breathless and agitated, has a tachycardia and may be cyanosed. Hypotension, bradycardia and altered consciousness are preterminal features. Quickly examine for jugular venous distension, tachycardia, and absent breath sounds on the affected side. Do not delay in order to perform a chest X-ray. Immediately insert a large-bore (16 or 18 FG) intravenous cannula through the second intercostal space in the midclavicular line on the affected side. Remove the needle. A hiss of air escaping from the cannula, followed by rapid clinical improvement, confirms the diagnosis. Tube thoracostomy with underwater seal drainage is then performed.

The patient may be unable to sit up, necessitating a supine examination. If the oxygen mask is 'misting' on exhalation, the patient has (some) respiratory effort. Look for movements of the chest (including the accessory muscles) and the abdomen. Paradoxical respiration, movement of the abdomen exactly out of phase with that of the chest, indicates respiratory compromise. It is most often due to fatigue of the diaphragm and/or airway obstruction. Look for abnormal breathing patterns (Box 17.8). Seek signs of injury (bruising, pattern imprinting, wounds) and of flail segment in trauma patients. In a 'flail' segment the affected area moves paradoxically: that is, it moves outwards with respect to the rest of the chest wall during expiration and inwards during inspiration. Kneel at the patient's side and look tangentially across the chest wall. The area is often well localized and clearly seen. It is important, as it implies that at least three ribs are broken in at least two places (Fig. 17.8), and underlying lung injury is common.

17.8 Respiratory patterns: common causes

Tachypnoea

- Anxiety
- Pain
- Asthma
- Metabolic acidosis
- Chest injury
- Pneumothorax
- Pulmonary embolus
- Brainstem stroke

Bradypnoea/apnoea

- Cardiac arrest
- Opioids
- Central neurological causes (stroke, head injury)

Cheyne–Stokes respiration

- Left ventricular failure
- Central neurological causes (stroke, head injury)
- Overdose (barbiturates, γ-hydroxybutyrate, opioids)

Küssmaul respiration

- Metabolic acidosis — diabetic ketoacidosis
- Uraemia
- Hepatic failure
- Shock (lactic acidosis)
- Overdose (methanol, ethylene glycol, salicylate)

Paradoxical respiration

- Respiratory failure
- Guillain–Barré syndrome
- High spinal cord lesions

Feel in the suprasternal notch to assess the position of the trachea. In trauma patients, systematically and gently palpate the chest to identify any areas of injury. Rib and sternal fractures are associated with localized discomfort. Subcutaneous emphysema feels like 'crackling' under your fingers. Examine for consolidation, pneumothorax, pleural effusion and haemothorax.

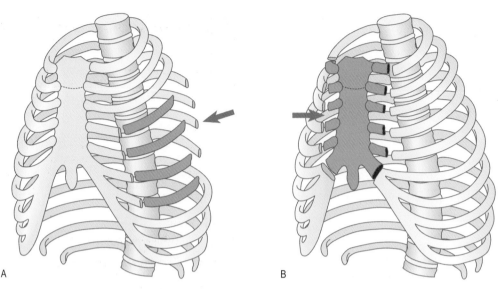

A   B

Fig. 17.8 Flail chest. (A) A direct blow (arrowed) that fractures several ribs at two points will result in a flail segment. **(B)** A severe blow to the sternum (arrowed) may cause multiple bilateral costochondral fractures, resulting in a flail chest.

17.9 Situations in which pulse oximetry may give misleading values

- Shock
- Hypotension/poor peripheral perfusion
- Hypothermia
- Excessive movement
- Nail varnish, false fingernails
- Severe anaemia
- Abnormal haemoglobins, e.g. carboxyhaemoglobin, methaemoglobin or sulphaemoglobin
- Skin pigmentation or excessively dirty fingers

Auscultate for breath sounds and added sounds. Critically ill patients may not have the signs you expect. For example, a patient with life-threatening asthma may have little or no wheeze (a silent chest) because airflow into the lungs is poor.

Central cyanosis is a late and unreliable sign of hypoxia. Even in critical hypoxia, cyanosis may be completely absent because of severe anaemia or massive blood loss.

Pulse oximetry is a simple, non-invasive method to assess peripheral oxygenation (Box 17.9). Attach a probe to a finger tip (Fig. 7.30, p. 180) or ear lobe. An SpO_2 of <94% indicates the need for oxygen therapy.

C: Circulation

If the patient is not responding, feel for a central (carotid or femoral) pulse for 10 seconds. If you cannot feel a pulse and the patient is unresponsive, treat as for cardiac arrest (Fig. 17.9). In responsive patients, feel for a peripheral (radial or brachial) pulse. If you cannot palpate a peripheral pulse, this suggests that the patient is significantly hypotensive. Note the pulse rate, rhythm, volume and character. Assess peripheral perfusion by pressing on the finger-tip pulp for a few seconds, removing your finger and estimating the capillary refill time (normal <2 s). Attach the patient to an ECG monitor and note the ventricular rate and the rhythm.

Control external blood losses from wounds or open fractures by direct firm pressure with a sterile dressing placed over the site. Minimize blood loss from long bone fractures (femur, tibia/fibula, humerus and forearm) by splintage.

Insert a large-bore (16 FG, 1.7 mm internal diameter or bigger) IV cannula and tape it securely to the skin. In trauma patients and those in whom you suspect hypovolaemia, insert and secure two large-bore cannulae. Take initial blood samples (Box 17.10) from the cannula and then attach an IV fluid-giving set. Commence volume replacement, if needed, with warmed 0.9% saline or Ringer's solution.

Examine jugular venous pressure (JVP) (Fig. 6.22, p. 125). In a sitting or semi-recumbent patient, elevation of the JVP in the presence of shock suggests a major problem with the heart's pumping ability, such as acute heart failure, cardiac tamponade, massive pulmonary embolus, tension pneumothorax or an acute valvular problem.

Check the blood pressure (p. 123).

Examine the precordium and heart, identifying the presence of added heart sounds or murmurs.

Insert a urinary catheter (unless there is evidence of urethral or prostatic injury — blood at the urethral meatus and/or a high-riding, 'boggy' prostate on rectal examination), to monitor urine output.

The term 'shock' implies that the oxygen and blood supply to an organ or tissue is inadequate for its

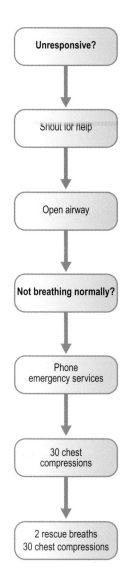

Fig. 17.9 Adult basic life-support algorithm.

17.10 Initial venous blood samples

All patients

- Stix test for blood glucose and formal blood glucose
- Blood grouping and save serum
- Full blood count
- Urea, creatinine and electrolytes

Selected patients

- Amylase
- Cross-matching
- Toxicology screen
- Coagulation screen
- Liver function tests
- Blood cultures
- Cardiac biomarkers, e.g. troponin, creatine kinase

17.11 Clinical features of shock

- Altered consciousness, confusion, irritability
- Pallor, cool skin, sweating
- Heart rate >100/min
- Hypotension (systolic BP <100 mmHg): N.B. Hypotension is a late sign
- Respiratory rate >30/min
- Oliguria (urine output <0.5–1 ml/kg/h)

17.12 Classification of shock

Hypovolaemic

- Blood loss: trauma, GI or obstetric haemorrhage, abdominal aortic aneurysm rupture
- Fluid loss: burns, GI loss (diarrhoea, vomiting), severe dehydration, diabetic ketoacidosis, 'third space' losses, e.g. sepsis, pancreatitis, ischaemic bowel

Cardiogenic

- Arrhythmia, myocardial infarction, myocarditis, acute valve failure, overdose of negatively inotropic drugs, e.g. calcium channel-blocker or β-blocker

Obstructive

- Major pulmonary embolism, tension pneumothorax, cardiac tamponade, acute valve obstruction

Neurogenic

- Major cerebral or spinal injury

Others

- Toxic causes: carbon monoxide, cyanide, hydrogen sulphide, poisons causing methaemoglobinaemia
- Anaphylaxis

metabolic requirements. Clinically, shock is recognized by a combination of features (Box 17.11). The extent to which each feature is present depends upon the cause (Box 17.12) and the time course. Signs of shock may be delayed or obscured in athletes, pregnant women, those on vasoactive drugs (β-blockers, calcium channel-blockers, angiotensin-converting enzyme (ACE) inhibitors), those with pacemakers, and the very young and old.

Tachycardia (pulse rate >100/min) and hypotension (systolic blood pressure <100 mmHg) are not required to diagnose shock. The heart rate may be normal or low in hypoxic shocked patients or those on drugs such as β-blockers. Blood pressure may be temporarily maintained by sympathetic activity and peripheral vasoconstriction. In critically ill patients non-invasive cuff blood pressure measurements are often inaccurate. Do not concentrate on absolute figures of systolic or diastolic blood pressure. Readings of 90/50 mmHg are normal in many healthy young women, while 120/70 mmHg indicates significant hypotension in a patient whose pressures are usually 195/115 mmHg.

17.13 Glasgow Coma Scale

Eye opening	
Spontaneous	4
To speech	3
To pain	2
No response	1
Verbal response	
Orientated	5
Confused: talks in sentences but disorientated	4
Verbalizes: words not sentences	3
Vocalizes: sounds (groans or grunts) not words	2
No vocalization	1
Motor response	
Obeys commands	6
Localizes to pain, e.g. brings hand up beyond chin to supra-orbital pain	5
Flexion withdrawal to pain: no localization to supra-orbital pain but flexes elbow to nail bed pressure	4
Abnormal flexion to pain	3
Extension to pain: extends elbow to nail bed pressure	2
No response	1

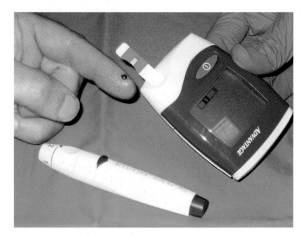

Fig. 17.10 Monitoring blood glucose with a testing strip and meter.

Trends in pulse and BP give far more information than initial or isolated readings. If a patient thought to have hypovolaemia has a rising pulse rate, with a falling blood pressure and reduced urine output, this strongly implies continuing volume loss and inadequate replacement.

In a trauma patient the most likely cause of shock is blood loss. External blood loss from wounds and compound fractures is usually apparent, but haemorrhage into the abdomen and chest, or from closed long bone or pelvic fractures, will be less obvious.

D: Disability

Assess the patient's Glasgow Coma Score (GCS). Record the three components: eye opening, verbal response and motor response (Box 17.13). Examine the limbs for localizing signs or paraplegia. Check the pupils for size, reactivity and equal reaction to light. In structural causes of coma (intracranial haemorrhage, infarction) the light reflex is usually absent; in metabolic causes (poisoning, hypoglycaemia, sepsis) it is usually present. A difference in pupillary diameters >1 mm suggests a structural cause.

Hypoglycaemia

Check the blood glucose using a Stix test (Fig. 17.10). Hypoglycaemia usually causes a global neurological deficit with reduced consciousness, but may present with irritability, erratic or violent behaviour (sometimes mistaken for alcohol or drug intoxication), seizures or focal neurological deficits, e.g. hemiplegia.

If the Stix test reading is <3 mmol/l, take a venous sample for formal blood glucose measurement, but do not wait for this result before giving treatment. Give 25–50 ml of 50% dextrose IV. If you cannot obtain venous access rapidly, give 1 mg glucagon by subcutaneous or intramuscular injection. If hypoglycaemia is the cause of the altered mental state, the patient's conscious level should start to improve in 10–20 minutes. Repeat the Stix test to confirm correction of hypoglycaemia. Persistent altered consciousness where hypoglycaemia has been adequately corrected implies co-existent pathology, e.g. stroke, or cerebral oedema from prolonged neuroglycopenia. In patients with hypoglycaemia where you suspect chronic alcohol use or withdrawal, or malnutrition, give 100 mg IV thiamine to prevent and treat Wernicke's encephalopathy (confusion, ataxia and eyes signs — nystagmus and conjugate gaze palsies).

Overdose

If you cannot clearly identify a cause for the patient's altered conscious state, consider drug overdose. The most common drugs to threaten life acutely are opioids, which cause altered consciousness, respiratory depression (reduced respiratory rate and volume) and small pupils. Give 0.8–2 mg IV naloxone (a specific opioid antagonist) as a diagnostic aid and definitive treatment to any patient with no clear cause for altered consciousness. In opioid intoxication, a response is seen within 30–60 seconds of IV administration. If IV access is difficult, give naloxone subcutaneously or intramuscularly. If the patient responds, further doses will be needed, as naloxone has a short duration (minutes), while the half-life of most opioids and their active metabolites is hours/days.

Seizures (fits)

Give immediate treatment to stop active focal or generalized seizures. First-line therapy is IV lorazepam (0.5–1 mg/min up to 4 mg) or diazepam (1–2 mg/min

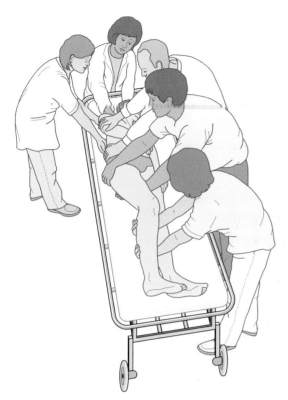

Fig. 17.11 Deployment of personnel and hand positions used when 'log-rolling' a patient from the supine to the lateral position.

17.14 The primary survey: investigations and interventions

ABCDE

A Administer high-flow oxygen

B Measure respiratory rate and SpO_2

C Monitor the ECG continuously and measure BP every 5 min
Insert and secure large-bore IV cannula(e) and take blood samples
'Stix' test for blood glucose

D Record GCS
Record pupil size and reactivity

E Measure core (rectal or tympanic membrane) temperature

Others

- Arterial blood gas measurement
- 12-lead ECG
- Chest X-ray (+ pelvic and cervical spine views in multiply injured)
- Urinary catheter[1] (and measure urine output hourly)
- Urinalysis (Stix test) for blood, protein, glucose, ketones, nitrite, bilirubin and urobilinogen
- Urine pregnancy test in females
- Nasogastric tube[2]

[1]Contraindicated if urethral injury suspected.
[2]Contraindicated if skull-base fracture suspected.

up to 10–20 mg). If seizures continue despite this, other agents may be required, e.g. phenytoin.

Manage seizures in pregnancy using the ABCDE approach but consider the fetus as well. Seek senior obstetric and neonatal support immediately. In women >20 weeks' gestation, position the patient in the left lateral position (most easily achieved by placing one or two pillows under the right hip). This prevents the gravid uterus from obstructing venous return to the heart with consequent hypotension. Eclamptic seizures in pregnant and post-partum patients are associated with hypertension (diastolic BP >100 mmHg), oedema (usually generalized and often affecting hands and face) and proteinuria. IV magnesium sulphate is a first-line treatment.

E: Exposure and environment

If patients are not fully undressed, remove remaining clothing. Cover them with a gown and warm blankets to prevent hypothermia and maintain dignity. Critically ill patients lose heat rapidly and cannot maintain normal body temperature. Trauma patients may arrive on a rigid spinal board with neck immobilization. Remove them from the board to reduce the chance of pressure sores and facilitate radiological examination. If patients are conscious, tell them what you are going to do before

they are 'log-rolled' and lifted (Fig. 17.11). The process needs five people. One holds the head/neck and directs the procedure; one removes the spinal board and other debris, and examines the back and spine; the remaining three roll and hold the patient. While the patient is rolled, perform a rectal examination, assess anal tone and perianal sensation, and check the core temperature.

Examine the patient's skin surface rapidly but comprehensively. Look for bruises and wounds. In particular, examine the scalp, perineum and axillae. Note open fractures and rashes, e.g. the non-blanching purpuric rash of meningococcal septicaemia (Fig. 17.13), and hyperpigmentation (hypoadrenalism).

Investigations and interventions of the primary survey are summarized in Box 17.14.

Secondary survey

The secondary survey reassesses the patient after examination and emergency interventions of the primary survey are complete. This is a systematic and detailed top-to-toe examination that fully documents additional signs and identifies injuries in the trauma patient. Only start the secondary survey once you are confident that there is no immediate need for resuscitation and if the patient does not require immediate transfer for definitive care, e.g. to theatre for a patient with a ruptured abdominal aortic aneurysm.

Adequate analgesia is needed for all patients in pain. There is no 'standard' dose. Slowly titrate an opioid drug, e.g. morphine, IV in 1–2 mg aliquots to achieve pain relief. The amount needed varies according to the patient's response and adverse effects, e.g. respiratory depression, hypotension. An antiemetic, e.g. cyclizine, may be required.

Examine the entire body surface, including the scalp, eyes, ears, mouth and face. Carry out a detailed examination of all relevant systems. Organize further investigations and treatment to confirm the cause of the patient's condition. Continually re-evaluate to assess the response to treatment. If they deteriorate or you are unsure about clinical status, return to the primary survey.

Start by examining the head. In the trauma patient palpate the scalp for swelling, and look for wounds which may be hidden in thick or tangled hair. Look for signs of skull-base fracture. These include periorbital bruising ('raccoon' or 'panda' eyes) (Fig. 17.12A), subconjunctival haemorrhage (usually without a posterior margin) (Fig 17.12B), otorrhoea or rhinorrhoea, and bleeding from the ear or behind the tympanic membrane (haemotympanum). Battle's sign (bruising over the mastoid process) (Fig. 17.12C) may take 1–3 days to develop. Examine the eyes for foreign bodies, including retained contact lenses (remove them at this stage), and signs of chronic disease, such as jaundice or anaemia. If corneal abrasions are suspected, stain the eye with fluorescein to identify them. Assess the pupils for size, shape, reactivity to light and accommodation. Examine the eye movements, visual acuity and optic fundi. Refer any patient with penetrating injury, disruption of the globe or loss of vision urgently to a specialist ophthalmologist.

Look in the mouth for injury to the palate, tongue and teeth. Check the ears and throat for potential sources of infection. Smell the patient's breath. The sweet odour of ketones in diabetic ketoacidosis is unmistakable, but not everyone can detect it. Severe uraemia causes a 'fishy' smell, and hepatic failure a 'mousy' smell (fetor hepaticus) due to methyl mercaptan. Note whether a patient smells of alcohol, but never attribute altered conscious level to alcohol alone.

Assume that the spine and/or spinal cord is injured in all trauma patients, especially those with altered consciousness. Conscious patients may complain of localized neck or back pain, but may be distracted by pain from other injuries. Maintain spinal immobilization until you can exclude underlying injury. This is rarely possible in the initial assessment period, and many cases will need imaging to exclude cord or bony injury.

If there is no history of trauma, ask patients to flex the neck to touch their chin on their chest. If this causes discomfort, gently flex the neck passively. Meningeal irritation causes spasm of the paraspinal neck muscles with neck stiffness. Meningitis and subarachnoid haemorrhage are common causes and may be

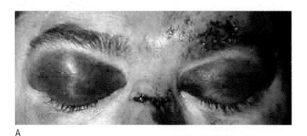

A

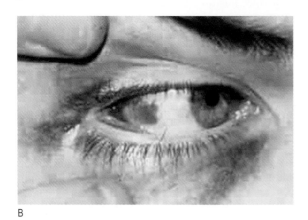

B

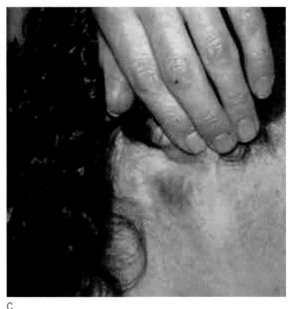

C

Fig. 17.12 **Signs of skull-base fracture.** **(A)** Periorbital bruising ('raccoon' or 'panda' eyes). **(B)** Subconjunctival haemorrhage. **(C)** Battle's sign.

associated with photophobia and a positive Kernig's sign (Fig. 11.3, p. 275). Neck stiffness may be absent in early presentations of these conditions or if the patient has altered consciousness.

Re-examine the chest and precordium in detail, as outlined in Chapters 6 and 7. Examine the back of the chest during the log-roll process. A 12-lead ECG and chest X-ray are needed in all patients.

Examine the abdomen with the pelvis and perineum. Perform a rectal and vaginal examination if necessary. A rectal examination, to help identify gastrointestinal bleeding, is mandatory in patients presenting with signs of hypovolaemia. In trauma patients examine the perineum, rectum and urethral orifice before inserting a urinary catheter.

Check perianal sensation and rectal sphincter tone to assess potential spinal cord injury. Perform a urinary pregnancy test in all women of child-bearing age and consider toxic shock syndrome due to a retained tampon in all menstruating females. Clinical assessment of the pelvis is often misleading. A pelvic X-ray is required in patients with significant injury, as major blood loss can occur from the pelvis. Do not 'spring' the pelvis to assess stability, as this may precipitate further bleeding.

Examine each limb in turn. Look for wounds, swelling and bruising; palpate all bones and joints for tenderness and crepitus, and assess passive and active joint movements. Always examine the neurovascular integrity of the limb distal to any injury.

Perform a full neurological examination. This is particularly important in patients with altered conscious level or possible spinal injury. Do not omit examination of the genital area and perineum.

Certain skin colours may give clues to the underlying diagnosis, including pallor (blood loss or anaemia), jaundice (hepatic failure), vitiligo or pigmentation in sun-exposed areas, recent scars and skin creases (Addison's disease). Look for rashes (in particular, the non-blanching purpuric rash of meningococcal disease) (Fig. 17.13), foci of infection (cellulitis, abscesses, erysipelas), bruising and wounds. Examine joints for swelling suggesting septic or reactive arthritis.

Ensure tetanus prophylaxis for all trauma patients who are non-immune. Give IV antibiotic therapy to patients with presumed meningococcal disease, septic shock and open fractures.

Accurately document all investigations, therapy and response to treatment. Stop the assessment process if you identify the need for immediate definitive care or investigation. Let the receiving team know exactly which stage of the assessment process you have reached when you hand over care of the patient.

Definitive treatment

Once stable, the patient will be moved to a critical care area, theatre, scanning room or another hospital. This is a high-risk process and you need to ensure you are sufficiently trained to accompany the patient. The critically ill patient needs to be adequately monitored and as 'stable' as possible. All relevant documentation and investigation results should go with the patient, with clear lines of communication between clinicians.

If you discover that the patient is terminally ill and that this crisis is not unexpected, it may not be appropriate for the patient to be given aggressive or 'heroic' treatment. Recognizing and preparing for a patient's death is difficult but essential. Communicate with the family, the GP and the senior clinician previously involved in the patient's care. The patient must be cared for in a dignified manner, with the emphasis on analgesia, relief of distressing symptoms and the highest quality of nursing care.

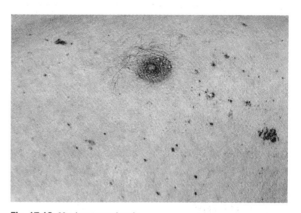

Fig. 17.13 Meningococcal rash.

17.15 Key points: the critically ill patient

- Get senior experienced help now.
- Simple things save lives; follow the ABCDE approach.
- 'Classical' signs of shock are unreliable and late.
- A patient in pain needs appropriate, adequate analgesia.
- Trends in parameters (heart rate, blood pressure, respiratory rate, SpO_2) are more important than isolated values.
- If the patient deteriorates, re-evaluate from the beginning of the ABCDE sequence.

Jamie Douglas
Graham Douglas

Confirming death

18

EXAMINATION TO CONFIRM DEATH

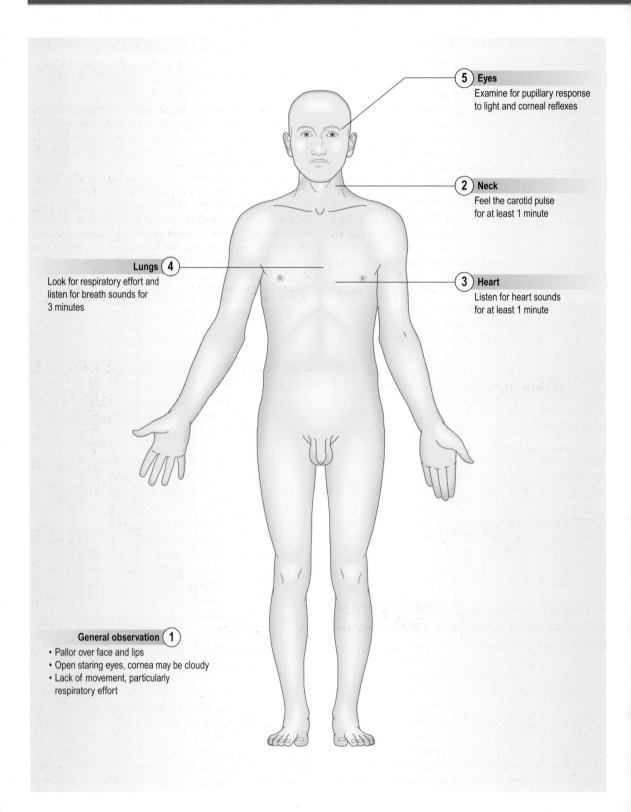

5 **Eyes**
Examine for pupillary response
to light and corneal reflexes

2 **Neck**
Feel the carotid pulse
for at least 1 minute

Lungs **4**
Look for respiratory effort and
listen for breath sounds for
3 minutes

3 **Heart**
Listen for heart sounds
for at least 1 minute

General observation **1**
• Pallor over face and lips
• Open staring eyes, cornea may be cloudy
• Lack of movement, particularly
  respiratory effort

In the UK there is no legal definition of death and it is the clinician's responsibility to declare when a patient has died. Death is defined medically by the UK Academy of Medical Royal Colleges as: 'the irreversible loss of the capacity for consciousness, combined with irreversible loss of the capacity to breathe'.

Death used to be synonymous with the sudden and unexpected loss of spontaneous cardiac activity and respiration (cardiac arrest); however, appropriate and prompt cardiopulmonary resuscitation (CPR) can successfully resuscitate some of the people in this category. The exact timing of death is rarely predictable, but is sometimes anticipated and accepted: for example, in a patient with advanced metastatic cancer. Start CPR (Fig. 17.9, p. 445) provided resuscitation is appropriate and he has not signed a Do Not Attempt Resuscitation (DNAR) directive.

Death is not always easy to diagnose when vital functions and general metabolism are greatly reduced (Box 18.1).

Although it may appear obvious that a patient has died, the body should be carefully and systematically examined. Confirmation of death has significant medicolegal implications and is extremely important for relatives. Your approach and manner must always be professional.

While you are doing this, watch the chest wall for any movement.
Listen to the chest for breath sounds for 3 minutes.
Watch for any spontaneous movement during your examination.
Check there is no motor response to supra-orbital pressure.
Simultaneously retract both eyelids, shine a bright light into each eye in turn and check that both pupils are fixed and unreactive.
Check the corneal reflexes, which should be absent (Fig. 11.9, p. 281).

In certain situations, additional investigations may be available and confirmatory: for example, an ECG monitor trace showing asystole, absence of pulsatile flow from an intra-arterial line, or absence of contractile motion on echocardiography.

Other clinical features associated with death include unnatural pallor, particularly of the face and lips, relaxation of the facial muscles with drooping of the lower jaw and open staring eyes. Eye changes after death include cloudiness of the cornea, reduced eyeball tension and, on fundoscopy, segmentation of blood within the retinal veins. This is known as 'cattle-trucking', 'railroading' or 'boxcars' (Fig. 18.1). None of these changes should be used in isolation as a marker of death. Other post-mortem changes gradually develop (Box 18.2).

18

18.1 Situations that can 'mimic' death

- Hypothermia
- Drug overdose
  - Opioids
  - Tricyclic antidepressants
  - Barbiturates
  - Alcohol
  - Anaesthetic agents
- Near drowning, cold water immersion
- Severe hypoglycaemia
- Severe hepatic encephalopathy
- Myxoedema coma
- Severe catatonic state

PROTOCOL FOR CONFIRMING DEATH

Death has occurred if there is no spontaneous cardiac function, no spontaneous respiratory effort and no central nervous system activity, including no pupillary response to light.

Examination sequence
Confirming death

Feel for a major (carotid or femoral) pulse for at least 1 minute.
Listen for heart sounds over the cardiac apex for at least 1 minute.

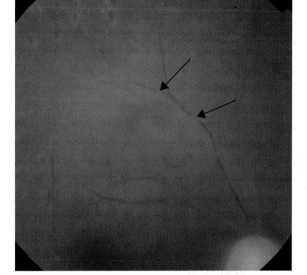

Fig. 18.1 Optic fundus after death: showing segmentation of blood within retinal vessels (arrowed).

Brainstem death

Modern resuscitative devices and techniques can maintain the function of the heart, lungs and visceral organs, even when the centres of brainstem function

18.2 Post-mortem changes

Body cooling

Varies according to:
- Temperature before death: fever, hypothermia
- Clothing/coverings
- Environmental temperature and air movement
- Body surface area

Post-mortem lividity

- Dark red/purple skin discoloration in gravity-dependent parts of the body develops within 20–30 minutes of death and becomes 'fixed' after about 12 hours

Rigor mortis

- Generalized muscular stiffening of voluntary and involuntary muscles of variable onset (up to 12 hours) and duration

Putrefaction

- Soft-tissue breakdown caused by commensal bacteria and enzymes
- Rate of putrefaction depends upon the body type, disease processes before death and environmental conditions, including temperature and humidity
- In conditions of dehydration and dry heat, mummification can occur

Fig. 18.2 Example of a medical death certificate.

have stopped. Patients receiving mechanical ventilation require additional tests to confirm brainstem death, which should be carried out by two experienced doctors on two occasions 24 hours apart:

- There is no motor response to painful stimuli, e.g. supra-orbital pressure or ear lobe pinching
- There is no response to corneal stimulation by cotton wool
- There is no response to the presence of the tracheal tube, nor any cough response or gag reflex to suction applied to the trachea
- No eye movements (oculovestibular reflexes/nystagmus) occur when 20 ml of ice-cold water are injected into the external auditory meati
- No respiratory effort occurs when ventilation is stopped long enough to allow PCO_2 to rise to >6.7 kPa. Continue 100% oxygenation, given by a cannula in the endotracheal tube. Failure of respiratory effort indicates medullary brainstem failure.

Prior to such testing establish that:

- the patient has irreversible brain injury of known cause producing deep coma and apnoea requiring artificial ventilation
- potentially reversible causes have been excluded, e.g. hypothermia, depressant drugs, and circulatory, metabolic and endocrine causes (Box 18.1).

WHAT TO DO AFTER YOU HAVE CONFIRMED DEATH

Record the death in the patient's medical notes, along with the date and time at which you pronounced life extinct, and sign the notes legibly, including your designation. If possible, state what you believe to be the cause of death.

It is essential to inform the close family or next of kin about the death. Wherever possible, do this in person rather than by telephone. 'Breaking bad news' is one of the most difficult situations you will face. Always speak to the bereaved in a quiet and private environment, avoid interruption (ask someone to take your telephone and pager) and, wherever possible, involve a nurse or counsellor. Relatives need time to understand and accept the situation. Use great care and sensitivity to try to support them (p. 13). Inform the family doctor as soon as is reasonable. Remember that the followers of some faiths have procedures and rituals that should

18.3 Deaths that may require further enquiry

These include:

- Death caused by an accident arising from use of a vehicle, e.g. aircraft, ship, train or car
- Death of a person while at work
- Death due to an industrial disease, e.g. mesothelioma
- Death due to poisoning
- Death where the circumstances suggest suicide
- Death following abortion or attempted abortion
- Death thought to be due to sudden infant death syndrome
- Death of a child in the care of a local authority or on an 'at risk' register
- Death in legal custody
- Death by drowning
- Death due to a disease, infectious disease or syndrome which poses a serious public health risk, e.g. hepatitis A, B, C or E, food poisoning, legionnaire's disease, any hospital acquired infection
- Death by burning or scalding or as a result of fire or explosion
- Any drug-related death
- Any death occurring in a GP's surgery or health centre
- Death which might have arisen from medical mishap
- Any death where a complaint has been received at the health board about the medical treatment given to the deceased
- Any other death with a violent, suspicious or unexplained cause

be followed after a death and which require the involvement of an appropriate religious leader.

Preferably before the patient dies, ask senior colleagues if they think a post-mortem is necessary, so that you can be prepared to ask the relatives when the time comes. You cannot force next of kin to agree to a post-mortem but many will agree if the reasons are made clear.

DEATH CERTIFICATION

Where the circumstances of death are unexpected or where death has occurred in suspicious or prescribed circumstances, the legal authorities must be informed and death certification must await inquiry and possibly forensic procedures: for example, laboratory results in suspected overdose, or post-mortem examination (Box 18.3).

If the cause of death is clear, complete a medical certificate showing the cause of death — the 'death certificate'. Certification of death is the responsibility of the medical practitioner who pronounces death and should be carried out as soon as possible after confirmation of death (Fig. 18.2). The death certificate has two functions; it is a legal document and a public health record, so if you are not sure about the cause of death, always ask a senior colleague involved in the case.

The format for certifying the cause of death has been defined by the World Health Organization and is followed in most countries. The certifier should state in Part I of the form, 'to the best of his/her knowledge and belief', the conditions that led directly to death: for example, myocardial infarction, community-acquired pneumonia or colon cancer; other conditions that have contributed to death, such as diabetes mellitus, hypertension or chronic obstructive pulmonary disease, should be listed in Part II of the certificate. Certifying the mode of death as 'cardiac arrest' or 'coma' is inappropriate, as is certifying death due to 'natural causes'. Undertakers and relatives find it very helpful if you explain the causes of death that you are putting on the certificate. This avoids misunderstandings and enhances communication.

18.4 Key points: confirming death

- When faced with an unconscious patient with absence of cardiac activity and respiration, start CPR immediately.
- Remember there are several potentially reversible situations that can 'mimic death'.
- Confirmation of death has medico-legal implications and is important to relatives — always be professional.
- Use a standard protocol when examining to confirm death.
- Patients receiving mechanical ventilation require additional tests to confirm brainstem death.
- Record the date and time at which life was pronounced extinct in the patient's notes.
- Always use great care and sensitivity when speaking to bereaved relatives.
- Certification of death is the responsibility of the doctor who pronounces death.
- When death is unexpected or has occurred in suspicious or prescribed circumstances, the legal authorities must be informed.

18

Index

NB: Page numbers in **bold** refer to boxes, figures and tables

B